Musculoskeletal Diseases 2017-2020

Juerg Hodler • Rahel A. Kubik-Huch
Gustav K. von Schulthess
Editors

Musculoskeletal Diseases 2017-2020

Diagnostic Imaging

49th International Diagnostic Course in Davos (IDKD)
Davos, March 26–30, 2017

including the
Nuclear Medicine Satellite Course "Diamond"
Davos, March 25–26, 2017

Pediatric Radiology Satellite Course "Kangaroo"
Davos, March 25, 2017

Breast Imaging Satellite Course "Pearl"
Davos, March 25, 2017

and additional IDKD Courses 2017–2020

Presented by the Foundation for the
Advancement of Education in Medical Radiology, Zurich

Springer

Editors
Juerg Hodler
Department of Radiology
University Hospital of Zurich
Zürich, Switzerland

Gustav K. von Schulthess
Medical Radiology
University Hospital of Zurich
Zürich, Switzerland

Rahel A. Kubik-Huch
Department of Radiology
Cantonal Hospital of Baden
Baden, Switzerland

ISBN 978-3-319-54017-7 ISBN 978-3-319-54018-4 (eBook)
DOI 10.1007/978-3-319-54018-4

Library of Congress Control Number: 2017936691

Printed on acid-free paper

This Springer imprint is published by Springer Nature
The registered company is Springer International Publishing AG
The registered company address is: Gewerbestrasse 11, 6330 Cham, Switzerland

Preface

The International Diagnostic Course in Davos (IDKD) is a unique learning experience for imaging specialists and clinicians. The course is useful for experienced radiologists and nuclear physicians, imaging specialists in training, and clinicians wishing to be updated on the current state of the art in all relevant fields of musculoskeletal imaging.

This IDKD syllabus includes imaging of joints, bones, soft tissue, and the spine. In addition, there will be satellite courses covering pediatric radiology and nuclear medicine in more depth. These courses are also represented in the current Syllabus, as well as our traditional breast imaging satellite course.

During the last few years there have been considerable advances in the field of musculoskeletal imaging driven by clinical as well as technological developments. These will be highlighted in the workshops given by internationally known experts in their field. The presentations encompass all relevant imaging modalities including CT, MRI, hybrid imaging, sonography, and standard radiography.

This Syllabus contains condensed versions of the more than two dozen topics discussed in the IDKD workshops. As a result, this book offers a comprehensive review of the state-of-the-art musculoskeletal imaging.

The IDKD Syllabus was initially designed to summarize the relevant information for the course participants and to allow them to fully concentrate on the lectures and participate in the workshop discussions without the need of taking notes. However, the Syllabus has developed into a complete update in musculoskeletal imaging for radiologists, radiology residents, nuclear physicians, and clinicians interested in imaging.

Additional information on IDKD courses can be found on the IDKD website: www.idkd.org

Zürich, Switzerland — Juerg Hodler
Baden, Switzerland — Rahel A. Kubik-Huch
Zürich, Switzerland — Gustav K. von Schulthess

Contents

Part I

Workshops

Adult Bone and Soft Tissue Tumors: Fundamental Concepts

Mark J. Kransdorf and Mark D. Murphey

Introduction

Although the choices available for imaging evaluation of musculoskeletal masses have changed dramatically, the basic objective of this assessment has remained constant: diagnosis and staging. The fundamental principles of evaluating musculoskeletal masses and achieving these objectives also have not changed. This review addresses application of the current imaging methods in assessment of adult bone and soft tissue musculoskeletal masses, emphasizing fundamental concepts. We do not intend to provide a comprehensive review of imaging techniques or diagnoses, but rather to provide a useful review of the fundamental concepts needed to select and protocol the appropriate studies to optimize diagnostic information and allow local staging.

Clinical History

The clinical history is an important factor in establishing an accurate diagnosis and should not be overlooked. In many circumstances it provides key information that suggests or allows a specific diagnosis when imaging is nonspecific and begins with how and why the patient came to medical attention. Additional information includes a history of previous lesions or underlying malignancy, surgery, radiation, significant trauma, or anticoagulation. The differential diagnostic considerations are markedly reduced if multiple lesions are present (Table 1). As a generalization, an incidental finding on an examination for an unrelated cause is more likely (although not invariably) benign. Similarly, lesions that have remained stable in size over time are also more likely benign, while a history of continued growth is always suspicious for malignancy.

Table 1 Differential diagnoses: multiple musculoskeletal lesions

Bone tumors	Soft tissue tumors
Metastases	Neurofibromatosis
Myeloma	Schwannomatosis
Lymphoma	Myxomas (Mazabraud syndrome)
Enchondromatosis (including variants)	Angiomatosis
Multiple hereditary exostoses	Lipomas (including hereditary lipomatosis)
Langerhans cell histiocytosis	Desmoid tumors
Multifocal osteomyelitis	
Hyperparathyroidism with brown tumors	

Initial Imaging Evaluation

Initial assessment of a suspected musculoskeletal bone or soft-tissue mass begins almost invariably with radiographic evaluation, a fundamental concept that is emphasized by the American College of Radiology Appropriateness Committee [1, 2]. The radiograph accurately predicts the biologic activity of a bone lesion, which is reflected in the appearance of the lesion's margin and the type and extent of accompanying periosteal reaction. In addition, the pattern of associated matrix mineralization (osteoid or chondroid) may be a key to the underlying histology [3–5]. Although other imaging modalities (MR and CT) are superior to radiographs in staging, the radiograph remains the single best modality for establishing a diagnosis, for formulating a differential, and for accurately assessing the biologic activity.

M.J. Kransdorf (✉)
Department of Radiology, Mayo Clinic,
5777 E Mayo Blvd, Phoenix, AZ 85054, USA
e-mail: kransdorf.mark@mayo.edu

M.D. Murphey
American Institute for Radiologic Pathology,
1100 Wayne Ave, Suite 1020, Silver Spring, MD 20910, USA

Department of Radiology and Nuclear Medicine,
Uniformed Services University of the Health Sciences,
Bethesda, MD 20814, USA
e-mail: mmurphey@acr.org

J. Hodler et al. (eds.), *Musculoskeletal Diseases 2017-2020*, DOI 10.1007/978-3-319-54018-4_1

Radiographs are typically considered unrewarding in the assessment of soft tissue masses; however, a recent study 281 patients showed calcification in 27%, bone involvement in 22% and fat in 11% of cases [6]. Such features may be essential in establishing an imaging diagnosis or differential. Radiographs may also be diagnostic of a palpable lesion caused by an underlying skeletal deformity (such as exuberant callus related to prior trauma) or exostosis, which may masquerade as a soft tissue mass. The soft tissue calcifications and/or ossification identified on radiographs can be suggestive, and at times highly characteristic, of a specific diagnosis, such as phleboliths within a hemangioma, the multiple intraarticular osteocartilaginous masses of synovial chondromatosis, or the peripherally more mature ossification of myositis ossificans.

Advanced Imaging Techniques

MRI has become the technique of choice for detecting and characterizing musculoskeletal masses. Its improved soft tissue contrast and multiple-image-plane capabilities have provided significant advantages for lesion conspicuity, characterization, and local staging.

MR Imaging

The protocoling of the MR imaging examination has become far more complex. The old "one size fits all" approach should be avoided as it often leads to less than optimal results. Appropriate protocoling should be based on the initial review of clinical history, physical evaluation, and initial (pre-MR) imaging, in conjunction with the patient age and lesion location, which allows a suspected diagnosis or at least a reasonable differential diagnosis. Equally important, an initial review will allow selection of the appropriate field of view (FOV), imaging planes, MR imaging sequences, and necessity for contrast material. These parameters are truly fundamental in achieving the most diagnostic imaging and deserve special emphasis.

Field of View

One of the most important parameters in tumor imaging is FOV. Although it is applicable to all cross-sectional imaging, it has received relatively little attention until recently [7]. Referring providers often order an MR study by anatomic area. MR imaging for a small mass around the hip may be ordered as a pelvis study or a lesion in the intertrochanteric region as a femur; examinations which are typically performed with a large (36–40-cm) FOV. Imaging the hip, for example, would typically be evaluated with a 20-cm FOV, allowing increased spatial resolution by as much as a factor of four, allowing markedly improved anatomic delineation of adjacent vessels, nerves, fascial planes, and other anatomic structures.

As a general guide, FOV is dictated by the size and location of the mass being studied and must be large enough to evaluate the entire lesion and allow appropriate local staging. Cases which require evaluation of an entire long bone, such as with suspected osteosarcoma, small FOV images can be supplement with limited large FOV images. Similarly, for example, when no discrete lesion is identified at initial imaging and a superficial unencapsulated lipoma is suspected, limited large FOV imaging of both sides is useful for comparison to allow confident identification of asymmetry and a definitive diagnosis.

Imaging Planes

MR imaging is invariably performed using a multiplanar technique. In the vast majority of locations neurovascular structures and muscles can be optimally identified and followed in the axial plane. Consequently, we generally use this as the primary imaging plane. This is augmented with long-axis images giving the best assessment of the entire lesion in "profile," assisting in its characterization as well as its relationship to the important surrounding anatomic structures; information required for diagnosis and surgical planning. Lesions such as those of the chest wall may be problematic due to its curved nature, and images in the standard coronal or sagittal plane may be less useful than imaging perpendicular to the chest wall. To avoid confusion during image acquisition, unusual oblique planes must be clearly defined to the imaging technologist.

MR Imaging Sequences

Most musculoskeletal masses are well evaluated with T1-weighted and fat-suppressed fluid-sensitive images. We generally prefer fat-suppressed proton-density–weighted FSE images to fat-suppressed T2-weighted FSE images due to the increased signal-to-noise ratio of the former. It is important to remember that the main purpose of fat suppression in fluid-sensitive imaging is enhancement of lesion conspicuity. In reality, conspicuity is typically not an issue in tumor imaging, and non-fat-suppressed T2-weighted images may be a useful adjunct for comparison of signal intensity to that of internal controls of muscle (low), fat (intermediate), and fluid (high). This is often helpful in better assessing the nature of the mass; for example, myxoid lesions generally follow fluid signal intensity, whereas collagenous/fibrous lesions generally have low to intermediate signal intensity. As FSE imaging tends to blur the signal intensity difference between fat and water, strongly T2-weighted parameters are required in such cases for non-fat-suppressed T2-weighted sequences (TR > 4000/TE100–110).

Gradient-echo (GRE) imaging has less fluid conspicuity but is particularly useful in identifying evidence of prior intralesional hemorrhage, revealing hemosiderin deposition as a result of its greater magnetic susceptibility [8]. In addition to hemosiderin, gradient-echo imaging is useful in identifying increased susceptibility artifacts from metal and air [8].

We find short τ inversion-recovery (STIR) images especially useful in areas where fat suppression is heterogeneous. Heterogeneous fat suppression can be particularly problematic in evaluation of off-center extremity musculoskeletal masses, as well as in areas where air pockets form adjacent to curves in the extremity or torso, such as adjacent to the perineum. STIR imaging is more susceptible to degradation from patient or respiratory motion and has lower signal-to-noise ratio than spin-echo imaging; however, it can increase lesion conspicuity and is a useful adjunct [9–11].

Contrast Material

The use of contrast material for evaluation of musculoskeletal tumors is well established, and its efficacy in improving diagnostic accuracy is well documented [10, 12, 13]. Contrast material is also useful in assessment of the vascular anatomy as well as lesion vascularity [12, 14]. We find contrast material useful not only in giving greater confidence in diagnosis, but also in identifying the most suitable location of the vascularized solid elements that will provide diagnostic tissue from subsequent biopsy if required.

Contrast-enhanced imaging is especially useful in assessment of hematomas and in distinguishing the hemorrhagic component of a neoplasm from the solid elements that may not be easily distinguished on conventional imaging. Subtraction imaging is a relatively recent innovation that has received little attention in the literature [15–17]; however, we find it invaluable in such cases, since this technique eliminates the possibility of misinterpreting the T1 shortening associated with hemorrhagic change as vascular enhancement.

Patient Motion

The above MR imaging techniques are applicable for the vast majority of cases; however, the relatively long imaging acquisition times of these standard sequences limit their use in anatomic areas that are susceptible to respiratory motion [10]. Recent advances in software and imaging applications now allow a variety of techniques that can capture a complete set of images in a single breath hold [18]; techniques that not only allow rapid image acquisition but are extremely fluid sensitive. Many musculoskeletal radiologists are not familiar with these techniques, although they are routinely used by our abdominal and thoracic imaging colleagues.

We generally prefer the gradient version of single-shot imaging (true FISP [true fast imaging with steady-state precession], FIESTA [fast imaging employing steady-state acquisition], balanced FFE [fast field echo]), which provides high-signal-intensity flowing blood and increased signal-to-noise ratio. When used without fat-suppression, its mixed T1/T2 weighting can be confusing due to the increased signal intensity from fat, water, and flowing blood; however, its quick acquisition time makes it a valuable adjunct.

Rapid fluid-sensitive images can also be acquired using a spin-echo single-shot technique (HASTE [half-Fourier acquisition single-shot turbo spin-echo], turbo spin-echo, single-shot FSE). These sequences are motion insensitive, ideal for breath-hold imaging, and exquisitely fluid sensitive [19–21]. The most significant limitation of HASTE and similar sequences is the decreased signal-to-noise ratio, typically requiring thicker section thickness and larger-FOV imaging.

Quantitative MR Imaging Evaluation

In MR imaging, the term *quantitative technique* is usually applied to an imaging method in which there is a measureable outcome. Those that are most applicable to clinical practice are chemical shift and diffusion-weighted imaging, both of which allow qualitative (visual) assessment as well as a quantitative (measurable) result. Most recently, MR spectroscopy has been added to this list of available quantitative techniques; however, the inherent technical challenges have limited its widespread adoption.

Chemical Shift Imaging

Chemical shift imaging is a well-established technique based on the observation that at gradient-echo imaging, the signals from similar quantities of fat and water in a single voxel will reinforce each other when in phase and cancel each other when out of phase cancel each other out [22, 23]. This allows qualitative and quantitative (measured as percentage change in signal intensity on opposed-phase relative to in-phase images) assessment of the amount of microscopic fat in any lesion. Initially used in separating adrenal adenoma from other adrenal masses [24], this technique has proved itself useful in assessment of musculoskeletal osseous masses [25]. In a retrospective study of 50 osseous pelvic lesions Kohl et al. [25] found chemical shift imaging to be highly sensitive in identifying malignant disease and, despite its lower specificity, found its use could have eliminated the need for biopsy in more than 60% of patients with benign disease. Its application for soft tissue is more limited, but it is useful in distinguishing reactive marrow changes from tumor and microscopic fat in higher-grade liposarcoma [26].

Diffusion-weighted Imaging

Diffusion-weighted imaging has been well documented to be a useful technique in MR imaging of the brain and has more recently received greater acceptance in the musculoskeletal community [27, 28]. Diffusion-weighted imaging allows qualitative and quantitative assessment of the movement of water molecules through tissue. This technique can identify when that normal random motion is restricted, such as by an abnormally increased number and/or size of cells. This restricted motion of water is detected by application of diffusion-probing gradients of different strength (expressed as the *b* value) and can be visually assessed as signal intensity, with restricted diffusion showing increased signal intensity and measured as the apparent diffusion coefficient (ADC), with restricted diffusion demonstrating decreased signal on ADC maps [22].

Although qualitative assessment of diffusion-weighted imaging readily recognizes restricted diffusion and ADC values are reproducible [29], the quantitative distinction between benign and malignant based on ADC value is not yet well-defined, with variable results reported [30–33]. There is no universally applicable "one size fits all" ADC value. Razek et al. [34] recently suggested a value of 1.34×10^{-3} mm^2/s as a threshold for distinguishing between benign and malignant masses. Using this value, they obtained a sensitivity, specificity, and accuracy of 94%, 88%, and 91%, respectively. A more recent study by Surov et al. [35] documented the variability of ADC value with tumor type, noting that if a value of 1.34×10^{-3} mm^2/s were used in their assessment, 35.1% of their malignancies would have been incorrectly categorized. Such results underscore the influence of tumor morphology (cellularity and matrix composition) in diffusion-weighted imaging, as has been previously noted [32, 36]. Although the value of diffusion-weighted imaging in distinguishing benign from malignant lesions is as yet somewhat unsettled, it can identify restricted diffusion, which is also quite useful in identifying small pelvic lymph nodes [18].

Spectroscopy

Another quantitative method for assessment of soft-tissue tumors is proton MR spectroscopy. Unlike the previous quantitative techniques, there is no real qualitative component. In musculoskeletal spectroscopy, choline, a marker for cell membrane turnover, is measured and is recognized to be elevated in malignancies. Although spectroscopy can provide useful information, it is a technically demanding and time-consuming technique. Accordingly, it is not usually used in routine practice.

CT Imaging

While MR imaging is generally the preferred imaging method for diagnosis and staging of musculoskeletal masses; CT remains an important adjunct. It is readily available, fast, and much more patient-friendly than MR imaging.

Mineralization Characterization

As previously noted, CT is particularly useful in assessment and characterization of mineralization, especially in areas where the osseous anatomy is complex. It allows distinction of ossification from calcification and identification of characteristic patterns of mineralization. CT is also superior to radiography in detecting the zonal pattern of mineralization, essential to radiologic diagnosis of early myositis ossificans, a pattern that can be identified at CT, while radiographs remain nonspecific [37].

Dual-energy CT

This is a relatively new technology that has proved itself as a useful adjunct in evaluation of musculoskeletal masses. Using the differences in energy attenuation of soft tissue at 80 and 140 kVp, dual-energy CT allows distinction of urate crystal deposits from other soft-tissue calcifications [38]. Although it may seem that the diagnosis of chronic tophaceous gout should be obvious, such is not invariably the case. The diagnosis can be challenging, especially in those without a history of gout or hyperuricemia, and cases of gout referred to tertiary-care centers as a suspected soft-tissue sarcoma are not rare [39]. Dual-energy CT has also proved to be a useful method to evaluate metal implants by generating images acquired by monoenergetic high energy quanta, reducing metal artifact [40]. Utilization of this technique can significantly reduce metal artifact in the assessment of metal implants, improving the diagnostic value of imaging [40]. Most recently, it has shown application in the assessment of marrow edema [41, 42] and has been investigated in the distinction of marrow edema from intramedullary tumor invasion [43].

The rapid image acquisition capability of modern scanners also allows accurate assessment of lesion vascularity. In a comparison with MR angiography by Mori et al. [44], CT angiogaphy with three-dimensional reconstruction was found equivalent to MR angiography in its ability to demonstrate neurovascular involvement. CT was also superior to MR in its ability to identify cortical/ marrow involvement. Finally, CT may be the most appropriate modality for very large patients and patients with pacemakers when MRI is not feasible or contraindicated.

Diagnosis of Bone Tumors

As previously noted, the radiograph remains the most diagnostic imaging study. While more advanced imaging provides the information needed for accurate staging, diagnosis (or differential diagnosis) begins with the radiograph and is based on the morphology of the lesion, the lesion's location and the patient's age.

Morphology characterizes the presence and character of the lesion's margin and periosteal reaction; features which are a function of the interaction between the lesion and the host, and are a key to biologic behavior. Morphology also includes an analysis of matrix mineralization and may be a key to the lesion histology.

The location of a lesion is a major consideration in establishing a diagnosis and structuring a differential diagnosis. There are two components to the location of an osseous lesion: the anatomic location (which bone) and the longitudinal location within the bone (epiphysis, metaphysis, metadiaphysis or diaphysis). The latter is critical in assessment of long bone lesions and is an essential principle of diagnosis pictorially presented in Fig. 1. Age is also an important consideration, with specific lesions tending to occur in specific age groups (Tables 2 and 3). For example, Langerhans cell histiocytosis localized to bone typically occurs in children and adolescents, while osseous lymphoma is most often encountered in mature adults, usually in the sixth and seventh decades. The final diagnosis, or differential, is based on the integration of the all of the above factors, taken in consideration of the prevalence of tumors within the population.

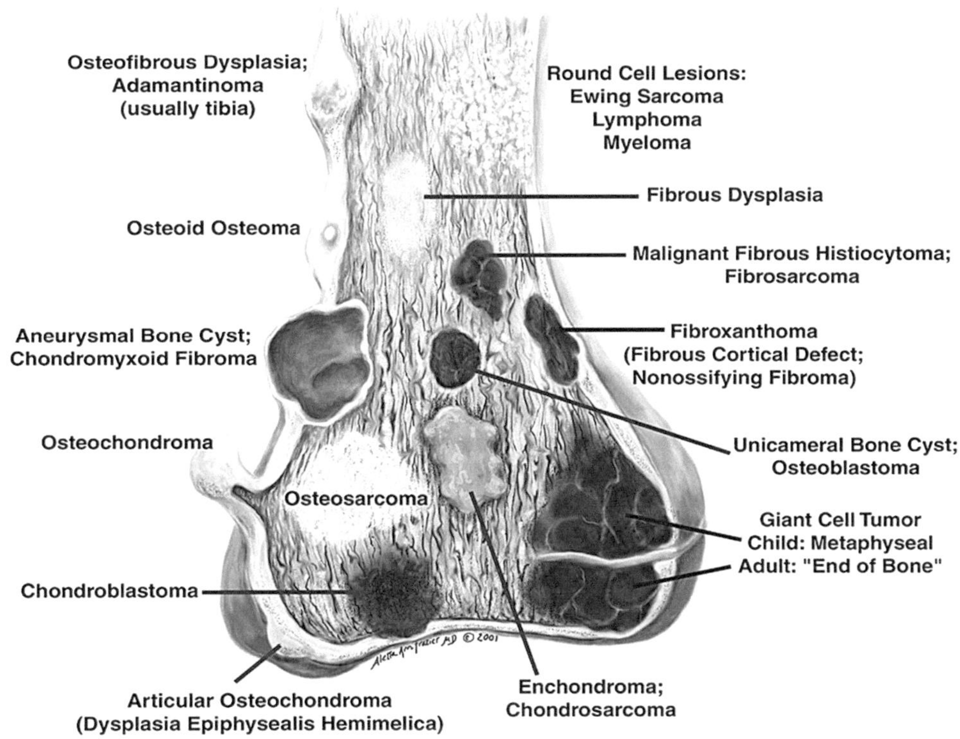

Fig. 1 Schematic diagram of the end of a long bone showing the typical sites for common primary bone tumors

Table 2 Age distribution of malignant osseous tumors[a]

Tumor type	Overall incidence (%)	Incidence by decade (%) 1	2	3	4	5	6	7	8	9+
Osteosarcoma	29.2	4.6	46.0	17.2	8.8	7.6	6.5	6.7	2.4	0.3
Chondrosarcoma	15.8	0.6	4.8	12.3	21.4	20.3	20.1	14.0	5.6	0.8
Myeloma	14.4		0.1	1.2	5.2	15.7	29.2	29.2	15.8	3.4
Lymphoma	12.3	2.7	8.9	10.8	10.2	14.7	20.3	17.5	12.0	2.7
Ewing Sarcoma	9.5	16.2	59.6	16.8	4.7	2.0	0.8			
Chordoma	6.3	1.1	4.2	6.2	13.5	18.5	24.4	20.5	9.3	2.2
Fibrosarcoma	4.5	3.1	11.4	13.3	19.2	14.5	16.7	12.9	6.3	2.4
Chondrosarcoma, dedifferentiated	2.1		1.7	2.5	6.7	18.3	32.5	17.5	16.7	4.2
Malignant fibrous histiocytoma	1.5	1.2	15.7	10.8	13.3	19.3	9.6	21.7	6.0	2.4
Osteosarcoma, parosteal	1.2		17.4	39.1	27.5	10.1	5.8			
Chondrosarcoma, mesenchymal	0.6		17.6	32.4	29.4	11.8	2.9		2.9	
Adamantinoma	0.6	2.9	29.4	44.1	5.9	5.9	5.9		5.9	

[a]Adapted from Reference 51, based on an analysis of 5656 malignancies, including 814 cases of myeloma diagnosed on the basis of surgical biopsy. Not included in Table 4 are 2935 cases of myeloma diagnosed on the basis of bone marrow aspirate, for a total of 8591 malignancies and an overall incidence of myeloma of 43.6%

Table 3 Age distribution of benign osseous tumors[a]

Tumor type	Overall incidence (%)	Incidence by decade (%)								
		1	2	3	4	5	6	7	8	9+
Osteochondroma	34.9	11.8	47.8	18.5	10.6	5.4	3.6	1.4	0.9	
Giant cell tumor	22.8	0.5	15.1	37.0	24.6	13.3	6.2	2.5	0.9	
Chondroma (enchondroma)	13.4	10.7	21.8	17.0	17.0	17.3	8.1	6.6	1.2	0.3
Osteoid osteoma	13.3	13.6	51.4	21.8	9.1	1.5	0.9	1.2	0.6	
Chondroblastoma	4.8	2.5	58.8	14.3	10.9	4.2	8.4	0.8		
Hemangioma	4.3	3.7	9.3	13.9	15.7	25.9	16.7	11.1	3.7	
Osteoblastoma	3.5	6.9	41.4	32.2	10.3	3.4	3.4	1.1	1.1	
Chondromyxoid fibroma	1.8	11.1	24.4	31.1	13.3	8.9	8.9		2.2	

[a]Adapted from Ref. [45], based on an analysis of 2496 benign tumors

Diagnosis of Soft Tissue Tumors

Despite the superiority of MR imaging in delineating soft-tissue tumors, it remains limited in its ability for precise diagnosis. There are instances, however, in which a specific diagnosis may be made or strongly suspected on the basis of MR features alone (Table 4). This is usually done on the basis of lesion signal intensity, pattern of growth, location and associated "signs" and findings. The MR imaging appearance of these lesions has been well reported, and is not reviewed here.

DeSchepper et al. [46] performed a multivariate statistical analysis of ten imaging parameters, individually and in combination. These researchers found that malignancy was predicted with the highest sensitivity when lesions had a high signal intensity on T2-weighted images, were larger than 33 mm in diameter, and had heterogeneous signal intensity on T1-weighted images. Signs that had the greatest specificity for malignancy included tumor necrosis, bone or neurovascular involvement, and mean diameter of more than 66 mm. In a recent study of 548 patients by Gielen and colleagues [47] in which imaging and clinical data were available, an accuracy of 85% was reported in differentiating between benign and malignant lesions.

When a specific diagnosis is not possible, MR is often useful to formulate a suitably ordered differential diagnosis on the basis of imaging features, suspected biological potential and a knowledge of tumor prevalence based on the patient age and lesion anatomic location. This can be further refined by considering clinical history and radiologic features, such as pattern of growth, signal intensity and localization (subcutaneous, intramuscular, intermuscular, etc.). The most common malignant and benign lesions, by tumor location and patient age, are shown in Tables 5 and 6.

Table 4 Specific diagnoses which may be made or suspected on the basis of MR imaging

Vascular lesions:	*Tumor-like lesions:*
Aneurysm and pseudoaneurysm	Abscess
Arteriovenous hemangioma (avm)	Calcific myonecrosis
Glomus tumor	Cystic adventitial disease
Hemangioma	Epidermal inclusion cyst
Hemangiomatosis (angiomatosis)	Fat necrosis
Lymphangioma	Ganglion
Lymphangiomatosis	Granuloma annulare
	Hematoma
Bone and cartilage forming lesions:	Hydroxyapatite crystal disease
Extraskeletal chondroma	Intramuscular myxoma
Myositis ossificans	Myonecrosis
Panniculitis ossificans	Popliteal (synovial) cyst
Synovial chondromatosis	Tophus
	Tumoral calcinosis
Fibrous lesions:	
Elastofibroma	*Peripheral nerve lesions:*
Fibroma of tendon sheath	Morton neuroma
Fibromatosis colli	Neurofibroma
Musculoaponeurotic fibromatosis	Schwannoma
Superficial fibromatosis	Traumatic neuroma
Lipomatous lesions:	*Synovial lesions:*
Lipoma	Giant cell tumor of tendon sheath
Lipoma arborescens	Nodular synovitis
Lipoma of tendon sheath	Pigmented villonodular synovitis
Lipomatosis	Synovial chondromatosis
Lipomatosis of nerve	Synovial sarcoma
Lipoblastoma	
Lipoblastomatosis	
Liposarcoma	
Periosteal lipoma	
Synovial lipoma	

Table 5 Distribution of common benign soft tissue tumors by anatomic location and age

Ages	Hand and wrist	No (%)	Upper extremity	No (%)	Axilla and shoulder	No (%)	Foot and ankle	No (%)	Lower extremity	No (%)
0–5	Hemangioma	15(15)[a]	Fibrous hamartoma infancy	15(16)	Fibrous hamartoma infancy	23(29)	Granuloma annulare	23(30)	Granuloma annulare	42(23)
	Granuloma annulare	14(14)	Granuloma annulare	15(16)	Hemangioma	12(15)	Infantile fibromatosis	11(14)	Hemangioma	26(14)
	Infantile fibromatosis	13(13)	Hemangioma	14(15)	Lipoblastoma	11(14)	Hemangioma	8(11)	Myofibromatosis	16(9)
	Infantile digital fibroma	8(8)	Infantile fibromatosis	12(13)	Fibrous hamartoma	7(9)	Fibromatosis	8(11)	Fibrous histiocytoma	15(8)
	Fibromatosis	8(8)	Fibrous histiocytoma	6(6)	Myofibromatosis	6(8)	Infantile digital fibroma	7(9)	Lipoblastoma	13(7)
	Aponeurotic fibroma	7(7)	Juvenile xanthogranuloma	6(6)	Lymphangioma	5(6)	Lipoblastoma	6(8)	Lymphangioma	10(6)
	Fibrous histiocytoma	5(5)	Myofibromatosis	6(6)	Nodular fasciitis	4(5)	Lipoma	4(5)	Juvenile xanthogranuloma	10(6)
	Other	27(28)	Other	20(21)	Other	12(15)	Other	9(12)	Other	48(27)
6-15	Fibrous histiocytoma	32(14)	Fibrous histiocytoma	41(23)	Fibrous histiocytoma	25(34)	Fibromatosis	35(22)	Hemangioma	47(22)
	Hemangioma	31(13)	Nodular fasciitis	39(21)	Nodular fasciitis	18(25)	Granuloma annulare	21(13)	Fibrous histiocytoma	34(16)
	Aponeurotic fibroma	25(11)	Hemangioma	24(13)	Hemangioma	7(10)	Hemangioma	21(13)	Nodular fasciitis	22(10)
	Fibroma tendon sheath	22(9)	Granuloma annulare	12(7)	Granular cell tumor	4(5)	Fibrous histiocytoma	14(9)	Granuloma annulare	20(9)
	GCT tendon sheath[b]	17(7)	Fibromatosis	11(6)	Neurofibroma	3(4)	GCT tendon sheath	13(8)	Fibromatosis	14(6)
	Fibromatosis	13(6)	Neurofibroma	7(4)	Lymphangioma	2(3)	Chondroma	11(7)	Lipoma	13(6)
	Lipoma	9(4)	Neurothekeoma	6(3)	Myofibromatosis	2(3)	Lipoma	9(6)	Neurofibroma	8(4)
	Other	86(37)	Other	42(23)	Other	12(16)	Other	37(23)	Other	58(27)
16–25	GCT tendon sheath	84(20)	Nodular fasciitis	130(35)	Fibrous histiocytoma	62(36)	Fibromatosis	46(22)	Fibrous histiocytoma	118(24)
	Fibrous histiocytoma	57(14)	Fibrous histiocytoma	87(23)	Nodular fasciitis	35(20)	GCT tendon sheath	29(14)	Nodular fasciitis	61(13)
	Hemangioma	40(10)	Hemangioma	36(10)	Fibromatosis	16(9)	Granuloma annulare	25(12)	Hemangioma	55(11)
	Fibroma tendon sheath	40(10)	Neurofibroma	24(6)	Lipoma	14(8)	Fibrous histiocytoma	24(12)	Neurofibroma	48(10)
	Nodular fasciitis	26(6)	Granuloma annulare	20(5)	Neurofibroma	12(7)	Hemangioma	13(6)	Fibromatosis	38(8)
	Granuloma annulare	21(5)	Granular cell tumor	17(5)	Hemangioma	4(2)	PVNS[c]	12(6)	Lipoma	22(5)
	Ganglion	20(5)	Schwannoma	11(3)	Schwannoma	4(2)	Neurofibroma	11(5)	Schwannoma	20(4)
	Other	132(31)	Other	51(14)	Other	25(15)	Other	45(22)	Other	122(25)
26–45	Fibrous histiocytoma	167(18)	Nodular fasciitis	309(38)	Lipoma	105(28)92(24)	Fibromatosis	99(21)	Fibrous histiocytoma	245(25)
	GCT tendon sheath	148(16)	Fibrous histiocytoma	145(18)	Fibrous histiocytoma	55(14)	Fibrous histiocytoma	74(16)	Nodular fasciitis	229(23)
	Fibroma tendon sheath	106(11)	Angiolipoma	48(6)	Nodular fasciitis	29(8)	GCT tendon sheath	41(9)	Lipoma	101(10)
	Hemangioma	86(10)	Hemangioma	43(5)	Fibromatosis	17(4)	Hemangioma	36(8)	Neurofibroma	71(7)
	Nodular fasciitis	79(8)	Schwannoma	43(5)	Hemangioma	13(3)	Schwannoma	30(6)	Schwannoma	59(6)
	Fibromatosis	46(5)	Neurofibroma	37(5)	Neurofibroma	12(3)	Neurofibroma	24(5)	Myxoma	53(5)
	Chondroma	42(4)	Lipoma	32(4)	Schwannoma	57(15)	Chondroma	23(5)	Hemangioma	52(5)
	Other	269(29)	Other	153(19)	Other		Other	135(29)	Other	185(19)

(continued)

Table 5 (continued)

Ages	Hand and wrist	No (%)	Upper extremity	No (%)	Axilla and shoulder	No (%)	Foot and ankle	No (%)	Lower extremity	No (%)
46–65	GCT tendon sheath	143(23)	Nodular fasciitis	86(20)	Lipoma	189(58)	Fibromatosis	83(25)	Lipoma	157(23)
	Fibrous histiocytoma	63(10)	Lipoma	80(19)	Fibrous histiocytoma	28(9)	Fibrous histiocytoma	43(13)	Myxoma	109(16)
	Hemangioma	61(10)	Fibrous histiocytoma	44(10)	Myxoma	16(5)	Lipoma	35(11)	Fibrous histiocytoma	93(14)
	Lipoma	59(9)	Schwannoma	30(7)	Fibromatosis	14(4)	Schwannoma	25(8)	Nodular fasciitis	40(6)
	Chondroma	52(8)	Neurofibroma	24(6)	Nodular fasciitis	13(4)	GCT tendon sheath	21(6)	Schwannoma	39(6)
	Fibromatosis	43(7)	Myxoma	24(6)	Schwannoma	12(4)	Chondroma	21(6)	Neurofibroma	31(5)
	Fibroma tendon sheath	37(6)	Hemangioma	19(4)	Granular cell tumor	12(4)	Hemangioma	16(5)	Proliferative fasciitis	28(4)
	Other	172(27)	Other	125(29)	Other	44(13)	Other	89(27)	Other	186(27)
66 & up	GCT tendon sheath	51(21)	Lipoma	39(22)	Lipoma	83(58)	Fibromatosis	16(14)	Lipoma	68(26)
	Hemangioma	24(10)	Myxoma	19(11)	Myxoma	14(10)	Schwannoma	15(13)	Myxoma	44(17)
	Schwannoma	24(10)	Nodular fasciitis	18(10)	Schwannoma	6(4)	Fibrous histiocytoma	13(11)	Fibrous histiocytoma	33(13)
	Chondroma	24(10)	Schwannoma	17(9)	Fibromatosis	5(3)	Chondroma	11(9)	Schwannoma	31(12)
	Neurofibroma	21(9)	Glomus tumor	12(7)	Fibrous histiocytoma	5(3)	Lipoma	10(8)	Hemangiopericytoma	10(4)
	Fibromatosis	14(6)	Neurofibroma	10(6)	Proliferative fasciitis	5(3)	Granuloma annulare	8(7)	Neurofibroma	9(4)
	Lipoma	13(5)	Angiolipoma	10(6)	Hemangioma	4(3)	GCT tendon sheath	6(5)	Hemangioma	8(3)
	Other	71(29)	Other	55(31)	Other	22(15)	Other	39(33)	Other	56(22)

Ages	Hip, groin & buttocks	No (%)	Head and neck	No (%)	Trunk	No (%)	Retroperitoneum	No (%)
0–5	Fibrous hamartoma infancy	14(20)	Nodular fasciitis	47(20)	Hemangioma	36(18)	Lipoblastoma	7(37)
	Lipoblastoma	14(20)	Hemangioma	43(18)	Juvenile xanthogranuloma	24(12)	Lymphangioma	5(26)
	Myofibromatosis	8(11)	Myofibromatosis	27(11)	Myofibromatosis	24(12)	Hemangioma	4(21)
	Lymphangioma	7(10)	Fibromatosis	17(7)	Nodular fasciitis	17(8)	Ganglioneuroma	2(11)
	Fibrous histiocytoma	5(7)	Granuloma annulare	14(6)	Lipoblastoma	17(8)	Fibrous hamartoma infancy	1(5)
	Nodular fasciitis	4(6)	Fibrous histiocytoma	13(5)	Infantile fibromatosis	15(7)		
	Infantile fibromatosis	4(6)	Infantile fibromatosis	13(5)	Fibrous hamartoma infancy	15(7)		
	Other	14(20)	Other	63(27)	Other	55(27)		
6-15	Nodular fasciitis	15(27)	Nodular fasciitis	75(33)	Nodular fasciitis	54(28)	Lymphangioma	7(37)
	Fibroma	7(13)	Fibrous histiocytoma	34(15)	Fibrous histiocytoma	43(22)	Ganglioneuroma	4(21)
	Fibrous histiocytoma	6(11)	Neurofibroma	23(10)	Hemangioma	25(13)	Schwannoma	2(11)
	Fibromatosis	5(9)	Hemangioma	21(9)	Lipoma	9(5)	Fibromatosis	2(11)
	Lipoma	5(9)	Myofibromatosis	14(6)	Neurofibroma	7(4)	Paraganglioma	1(5)
	Lipoblastoma	3(5)	Fibromatosis	12(5)	Fibromatosis	6(3)	Hemangioma	1(5)
	Neurofibroma	3(5)	Lipoma	6(3)	Granular cell tumor	6(3)	Inflammatory pseudotumor	1(5)
	Other	11(20)	Other	43(19)	Other	45(23)	Other	1(5)

16–25	Neurofibroma	20(16)	Nodular fasciitis	61(21)	Nodular fasciitis	112(24)	Fibromatosis	14(20)
	Fibromatosis	18(15)	Hemangioma	48(17)	Fibromatosis	72(16)	Schwannoma	10(14)
	Fibrous histiocytoma	18(15)	Fibrous histiocytoma	45(16)	Fibrous histiocytoma	71(15)	Neurofibroma	9(13)
	Nodular fasciitis	12(10)	Neurofibroma	37(13)	Hemangioma	52(11)	Hemangiopericytoma	8(11)
	Hemangioma	9(7)	Schwannoma	19(7)	Neurofibroma	38(8)	Lymphangioma	8(11)
	Lipoma	8(7)	Fibromatosis	11(4)	Lipoma	21(5)	Ganglioneuroma	6(8)
	Hemangiopericytoma	8(7)	Lipoma	10(4)	Schwannoma	17(4)	Hemangioma	4(6)
	Other	29(24)	Other	56(19)	Other	79(17)	Other	12(17)
26–45	Lipoma	57(17)	Lipoma	168(22)	Lipoma	178(19)	Schwannoma	38(23)
	Neurofibroma	38(12)	Nodular fasciitis	145(19)	Nodular fasciitis	150(16)	Fibromatosis	30(18)
	Fibrous histiocytoma	37(11)	Fibrous histiocytoma	137(18)	Fibromatosis	148(16)	Hemangiopericytoma	25(15)
	Fibromatosis	36(11)	Hemangioma	97(13)	Fibrous histiocytoma	98(10)	Neurofibroma	13(8)
	Nodular fasciitis	31(9)	Neurofibroma	57(8)	Hemangioma	78(8)	Angiomyolipoma	10(6)
	Hemangiopericytoma	24(7)	Hemangiopericytoma	37(5)	Neurofibroma	65(7)	Hemangioma	9(5)
	Myxoma	22(7)	Schwannoma	27(4)	Schwannoma	51(5)	Sclerosing retroperitonitis	7(4)
	Other	83(25)	Other	91(12)	Other	180(19)	Other	34(20)
46–65	Lipoma	76(35)	Lipoma	306(46)	Lipoma	290(44)	Schwannoma Fibromatosis	33(19)
	Myxoma	36(17)	Nodular fasciitis	66(10)	Fibromatosis	63(9)	Sclerosing retroperitonitis	25(14)
	Fibrous histiocytoma	17(8)	Hemangioma	55(8)	Nodular fasciitis	44(7)	Hemangiopericytoma	25(14)
	Schwannoma	17(8)	Fibrous histiocytoma	42(6)	Hemangioma	31(5)	Angiomyolipoma Lipoma	21(12)
	Nodular fasciitis	11(5)	Neurofibroma	30(4)	Fibrous histiocytoma	29(4)	Paraganglioma	12(7)
	Hemangiopericytoma	11(5)	Schwannoma	25(4)	Neurofibroma	28(4)	Other	10(6)
	Hemangioma	9(4)	Myxoma	23(3)	Schwannoma	28(4)		9(5)
	Other	40(18)	Other	120(18)	Other	151(23)		40(23)
66 & up	Lipoma	22(21)	Lipoma	158(50)	Lipoma	124(42)	Schwannoma	19(26)
	Myxoma	16(15)	Hemangioma	22(7)	Fibromatosis	26(9)	Hemangiopericytoma	14(19)
	Neurofibroma	13(12)	Schwannoma	18(6)	Neurofibroma	20(7)	Lipoma	6(8)
	Schwannoma	10(9)	Fibrous histiocytoma	17(5)	Schwannoma	18(6)	Mesothelioma	6(8)
	Hemangiopericytoma	10(9)	Neurofibroma	16(5)	Elastofibroma	17(6)	Sclerosing retroperitonitis	5(7)
	Hemangioma	8(8)	Nodular fasciitis	13(4)	Myxoma	16(5)	Fibromatosis	4(6)
	Nodular fasciitis	4(4)	Myxoma	12(4)	Hemangioma	14(5)	Paraganglioma	4(6)
	Other	23(22)	Other	58(18)	Other	61(21)	Other	14(19)

Based on an analysis of 18,677 cases seen in consultation by the department of soft tissue pathology, AFIP, over 10 years. (Modified from AJR 1995;164:395–402)

[a]15(15) indicates there were 15 hemangioma in the hand and wrist of patients 0–5 years, and this represents 15% of all benign tumors in this location and age group

[b]Giant cell tumor of tendon sheath

[c]Pigmented villonodular synovitis

Table 6 Distribution of common malignant soft tissue tumors by anatomic location and age

Ages	Hand and wrist	No (%)	Upper extremity	No (%)	Axilla and shoulder	No (%)	Foot and ankle	No (%)	Lower extremity	No (%)
0–5	Fibrosarcoma	5(45)[a]	Fibrosarcoma	9(29)	Fibrosarcoma	9(56)	Fibrosarcoma	5(45)	Fibrosarcoma	24(45)
	Angiosarcoma	1(9)	Rhabdomyosarcoma	7(23)	Rhabdomyosarcoma	4(25)	DFSP	2(18)	Rhabdomyosarcoma	8(15)
	Epithelioid sarcoma	1(9)	Angiomatoid MFH	3(10)	Angiomatoid MFH	1(6)	MPNST	2(18)	Giant cell fibroblastoma	5(9)
	Malig GCT tendon sheath[b]	1(9)	DFSP	2(6)	Chondrosarcoma	1(6)	Rhabdomyosarcoma	2(18)	MPNST	5(9)
	DFSP[c]	1(9)	Giant cell fibroblastoma	2(6)	MPNST	1(6)			Angiomatoid MFH	3(6)
	MPNST[d]	1(9)	MPNST	2(6)					DFSP	3(6)
	Rhabdomyosarcoma	1(9)	MFH	2(6)					Angiosarcoma	2(4)
			Other	4(13)					Other	3(6)
6–15	Epithelioid sarcoma	9(21)	Angiomatoid MFH	30(33)	Angiomatoid MFH	8(21)	Synovial sarcoma	11(21)	Synovial sarcoma	28(22)
	Angiomatoid MFH	7(16)	Synovial sarcoma	14(15)	MFH	5(13)	DFSP	9(17)	Angiomatoid MFH	22(17)
	Synovial sarcoma	5(12)	Fibrosarcoma	8(9)	Ewing sarcoma	4(10)	Rhabdomyosarcoma	5(9)	MFH	13(10)
	MFH	4(9)	MPNST	7(8)	MPNST	4(10)	Angiosarcoma	4(8)	Liposarcoma	11(9)
	Angiosarcoma	3(7)	MFH	7(8)	Rhabdomyosarcoma	4(10)	Clear cell sarcoma	4(8)	MPNST	9(7)
	Rhabdomyosarcoma	3(7)	Rhabdomyosarcoma	7(8)	Fibrosarcoma	3(8)	Fibrosarcoma	4(8)	DFSP	8(6)
	Clear cell sarcoma	2(5)	Epithelioid sarcoma	4(4)	Synovial sarcoma	3(8)	Chondrosarcoma	3(6)	Rhabdomyosarcoma	6(5)
	Other	10(23)	Other	15(16)	Other	8(21)	Other	13(25)	Other	31(24)
16–25	Epithelioid sarcoma	25(29)	Synovial sarcoma	32(23)	Synovial sarcoma	13(18)	Synovial sarcoma	27(30)	Synovial sarcoma	76(22)
	MFH	11(13)	MFH	19(14)	DFSP	12(16)	Clear cell sarcoma	10(11)	Liposarcoma	45(13)
	DFSP	7(8)	MPNST	16(12)	MPNST	11(15)	Fibrosarcoma	7(8)	MPNST	44(13)
	Synovial sarcoma	7(8)	Fibrosarcoma	12(9)	Fibrosarcoma	8(11)	DFSP	7(8)	MFH	36(11)
	Rhabdomyosarcoma	7(8)	Angiomatoid MFH	10(7)	MFH	8(11)	MFH	6(7)	Fibrosarcoma	24(7)
	Angiomatoid MFH	5(6)	Epithelioid sarcoma	9(7)	Rhabdomyosarcoma	4(5)	Hemangioendothelioma	6(7)	DFSP	18(5)
	Hemangioendothelioma	5(6)	Hemangioendothelioma	6(4)	Angiomatoid MFH	3(4)	MPNST	5(6)	Angiomatoid MFH	15(4)
	Other	19(22)	Other	34(25)	Other	15(20)	Other	22(24)	Other	80(24)
26–45	MFH	26(18)	MFH	65(28)	DFSP	55(33)	Synovial sarcoma	50(26)	Liposarcoma	196(28)
	Epitheliod sarcoma	24(16)	MPNST	29(12)	MFH	30(18)	Clear cell sarcoma	25(13)	MFH	151(21)
	Synovial sarcoma	21(14)	Fibrosarcoma	25(11)	Liposarcoma	22(13)	MFH	25(13)	Synovial sarcoma	78(11)
	Fibrosarcoma	17(12)	Synovial sarcoma	23(10)	MPNST	21(12)	Hemangioendothelioma	14(7)	MPNST	70(10)
	Clear cell sarcoma	9(6)	Liposarcoma	20(8)	Fibrosarcoma	10(6)	DFSP	13(7)	DFSP	47(7)
	Liposarcoma	9(6)	DFSP	18(8)	Synovial sarcoma	7(4)	Liposarcoma	13(7)	Leiomyosarcoma	35(5)
	MPNST	7(5)	Epithelioid sarcoma	13(6)	Chondrosarcoma	6(4)	MPNST	11(6)	Fibrosarcoma	33(5)
	Other	33(23)	Other	43(18)	Other	18(11)	Other	38(20)	Other	98(14)
46–65	MFH	16(19)	MFH	133(46)	MFH	66(35)	MFH	39(25)	MFH	399(43)
	Synovial sarcoma	12(14)	Liposarcoma	34(12)	Liposarcoma	39(21)	Synovial sarcoma	27(17)	Liposarcoma	232(25)
	Fibrosarcoma	8(10)	Leiomyosarcoma	22(8)	DFSP	22(12)	Leiomyosarcoma	19(12)	Leiomyosarcoma	63(7)
	Epithelioid sarcoma	7(8)	Fibrosarcoma	18(6)	MPNST	20(11)	Kaposi sarcoma	14(9)	Synovial sarcoma	40(4)
	Liposarcoma	7(8)	MPNST	17(6)	Leiomyosarcoma	14(7)	Liposarcoma	9(6)	MPNST	38(4)
	Chondrosarcoma	7(8)	Synovial sarcoma	16(5)	Fibrosarcoma	8(4)	Fibrosarcoma	8(5)	Chondrosarcoma	37(4)
	Clear cell sarcoma	5(6)	Hemangioendothelioma	9(3)	Synovial sarcoma	4(2)	Clear cell sarcoma	7(5)	Fibrosarcoma	24(3)
	Other	22(26)	Other	43(15)	Other	15(8)	Other	32(21)	Other	87(9)

66 & up	MFH	28(35)	MFH	183(60)	MFH	67(50)	Kaposi sarcoma	49(37)	MFH	455(55)
	Leiomyosarcoma	8(10)	Liposarcoma	25(8)	Liposarcoma	30(23)	MFH	26(19)	Liposarcoma	178(22)
	Synovial sarcoma	6(8)	Leiomyosarcoma	23(8)	MPNST	12(9)	Leiomyosarcoma	20(15)	Leiomyosarcoma	86(10)
	Kaposi sarcoma	5(6)	MPNST	20(7)	DFSP	6(5)	Fibrosarcoma	9(7)	Fibrosarcoma	22(3)
	DFSP	4(5)	Kaposi sarcoma	10(3)	Fibrosarcoma	4(3)	Chondrosarcoma	6(4)	Chrondrosarcoma	16(2)
	MPNST	4(5)	Fibrosarcoma	8(3)	Leiomyosarcoma	3((2)	MPNST	5(4)	MPNST	15(2)
	Clear cell sarcoma	3(4)	Angiosarcoma	6(2)	Chondrosarcoma	2(2)	Liposarcoma	3(2)	Synovial sarcoma	11(1)
	Other	21(27)	Other	29(10)	Other	9(7)	Other	16(12)	Other	43(5)

Ages	Hip, groin & buttocks	No (%)	Head and neck	No (%)	Trunk	No (%)	Retroperitoneum	No (%)
0–5	Fibrosarcoma	7(32)	Fibrosarcoma	22(37)	Fibrosarcoma	13(26)	Fibrosarcoma	4(20)
	Giant cell fibroblastoma	3(14)	Rhabdomyosarcoma	20(33)	Giant cell fibroblastoma	8(16)	Neuroblastoma	4(20)
	Rhabdomyosarcoma	3(14)	Malig hemangiopericytoma	3(5)	Rhabdomyosarcoma	8(16)	Rhabdomyosarcoma	4(20)
	DFSP	2(9)	Alveolar soft part sarcoma	2(3)	Angiomatoid MFH	6(12)	Ganglioneuroblastoma	3(15)
	MFH	2(9)	DFSP	2(3)	DFSP	4(8)	Angiosarcoma	2(10)
	Leiomyosarcoma	1(5)	MPNST	2(3)	Ewing sarcoma	3(6)	Leiomyosarcoma	2(10)
	Synovial sarcoma	1(5)	Giant cell fibroblastoma	2(3)	Neuroblastoma	3(6)	Alveolar soft part sarcoma	1(5)
	Other	3(14)	Other	7(12)	Other	5(10)		
6–15	Angiomatoid MFH	8(21)	Rhabdomyosarcoma	17(26)	Angiomatoid MFH	14(15)	Rhabdomyosarcoma	9(31)
	Synovial sarcoma	7(19)	Fibrosarcoma	13(20)	Fibrosarcoma	13(14)	MPNST	5(17)
	Rhabdomyosarcoma	6(16)	Synovial sarcoma	7(11)	Ewing sarcoma	12(13)	Neuroblastoma	4(14)
	MFH	4(11)	MPNST	6(9)	DFSP	12(13)	Ewing sarcoma	2(7)
	Epithelioid sarcoma	2(5)	MFH	6(9)	MPNST	9(10)	Fibrosarcoma	2(7)
	Fibrosarcoma	2(5)	Angiomatoid MFH	4(6)	Rhabdomyosarcoma	8(9)	MFH	2(7)
	MPNST	2(5)	DFSP	2(3)	MFH	3(3)	Malig hemangiopericytoma	2(7)
	Other	7(18)	Other	10(15)	Other	20(22)	Other	3(10)
16–25	Synovial sarcoma	15(18)	Fibrosarcoma	15(17)	DFSP	37(23)	MPNST	9(20)
	MPNST	13(16)	DFSP	14(16)	MFH	21(13)	Ewing sarcoma	8(18)
	Liposarcoma	8(10)	MPNST	8(9)	MPNST	19(12)	Leiomyosarcoma	6(14)
	DFSP	6(7)	Synovial sarcoma	8(9)	Fibrosarcoma	15(9)	Ganglioneuroblastoma	4(9)
	MFH	6(7)	Rhabdomyosarcoma	8(9)	Synovial sarcoma	13(8)	Neuroblastoma	4(9)
	Rhabdomyosarcoma	5(6)	MFH	7(8)	Ewing sarcoma	12(7)	Rhabdomyosarcoma	3(7)
	Leiomyosarcoma	4(5)	Angiomatoid MFH	6(7)	Angiomatoid MFH	6(4)	Malig hemangiopericytoma	2(5)
	Other	26(31)	Other	23(26)	Other	38(24)	Other	8(18)
26–45	Liposarcoma	45(18)	DFSP	59(30)	DFSP	129(30)	Leiomyosarcoma	57(32)
	DFSP	42(17)	MPNST	27(14)	MFH	77(18)	Liposarcoma	52(29)
	MFH	38(16)	Liposarcoma	18(9)	MPNST	45(10)	MFH	22(12)
	Leiomyosarcoma	26(11)	MFH	15(8)	Liposarcoma	41(9)	MPNST	11(6)
	MPNST	15(6)	Fibrosarcoma	14(7)	Fibrosarcoma	36(8)	Fibrosarcoma	7(4)
	Synovial sarcoma	13(5)	Synovial sarcoma	10(5)	Synovial sarcoma	20(5)	Malig hemangiopericytoma	7(4)
	Fibrosarcoma	12(5)	Angiosarcoma	9(4)	Angiosarcoma	15(3)	Ewing sarcoma	3(2)
	Other	53(22)	Other	42(22)	Other	70(16)	Other	20(11)

(continued)

Table 6 (continued)

Ages	Hip, groin & buttocks	No (%)	Head and neck	No (%)	Trunk	No (%)	Retroperitoneum	No (%)
46–66	Liposarcoma	67(24)	MFH	54(28)	MFH	131(31)	Liposarcoma	170(33)
	MFH	66(23)	DFSP	28(15)	Liposarcoma	80(19)	Leiomyosarcoma	154(30)
	Leiomyosarcoma	40(14)	MPNST	23(12)	DFSP	60(14)	MFH	111(22)
	DFSP	20(7)	Liposarcoma	22(12)	MPNST	35(8)	MPNST	23(5)
	Fibrosarcoma	16(6)	Angiosarcoma	16(8)	Leiomyosarcoma	27(6)	Malignant mesenchymoma	10(2)
	Synovial sarcoma	14(5)	Atypical fibroxanthoma	12(6)	Fibrosarcoma	24(6)	Fibrosarcoma	9(2)
	Chondrosarcoma	14(5)	Leiomyosarcoma	11(6)	Angiosarcoma	15(4)	Malign hemangiopericytoma	7(1)
	Other	46(16)	Other	24(13)	Other	50(12)	Other	27(5)
66 & up	MFH	111(46)	MFH	82(34)	MFH	137(44)	Liposarcoma	164(39)
	Liposarcoma	49(20)	Atypical fibroxanthoma	41(17)	Liposarcoma	56(18)	Leiomyosarcoma	118(28)
	Leiomyosarcoma	24(10)	Angiosarcoma	27(11)	Leiomyosarcoma	23(7)	MFH	93(22)
	Angiosarcoma	11(5)	Liposarcoma	20(8)	MPNST	20(6)	MPNST	13(3)
	MPNST	11(5)	MPNST	16(7)	DFSP	17(5)	Fibrosarcoma	8(2)
	Fibrosarcoma	10(4)	Leiomyosarcoma	13(5)	Fibrosarcoma	12(4)	Osteosarcoma	6(1)
	Chondrosarcoma	7(3)	Fibrosarcoma	10(4)	Chondrosarcoma	11(4)	Malignant mesenchymoma	5(1)
	Other	20(8)	Other	31(13)	Other	35(11)	Other	9(2)

Based on an analysis of 12,370 cases seen in consultation by the department of soft tissue pathology, AFIP, over 10 years. (Modified from AJR 1995;164:129–134)

[a]5(45) indicates there were five fibrosarcomas in the hand and wrist of patients 0–5 years, and this represents 45% of all malignant tumors in this location and age group

[b]Malignant giant cell tumor of tendon sheath

[c]Dermatofibrosarcoma protuberans

[d]Malignant peripheral nerve sheath tumor

Summary

In this brief review we have summarized the fundamental principles needed for the accurate assessment of musculoskeletal masses. Despite the wide variety of imaging modalities available today, adherence to these principles will provide the user with the optimal images for diagnosis and staging.

References

1. Morrison WB, Weissman BN, Kransdorf MJ et al (2013) ACR Appropriateness Criteria® Primary Bone Tumors. Available at https://acsearch.acr.org/docs/69421/Narrative/. American College of Radiology. Accessed December 30, 2016
2. Zoga AC, Weissman BN, Kransdorf MJ et al (2012) ACR Appropriateness Criteria® Soft-Tissue Masses. Available at https://acsearch.acr.org/docs/69434/Narrative/. American College of Radiology. Accessed December 30, 2016
3. Madewell JE, Ragsdale BD, Sweet DE (1981) Radiologic and pathologic analysis of solitary bone lesions. Part I: internal margins. Radiol Clin N Am 19(4):715–748
4. Ragsdale BD, Madewell JE, Sweet DE (1981) Radiologic and pathologic analysis of solitary bone lesions. Part II: periosteal reactions. Radiol Clin N Am 19(4):749–783
5. Sweet DE, Madewell JE, Ragsdale BD (1981) Radiologic and pathologic analysis of solitary bone lesions. Part III: matrix patterns. Radiol Clin N Am 19(4):785–814
6. Gartner L, Pearce CJ, Saifuddin A (2008) The role of the plain radiograph in the characterisation of soft tissue tumours. Skelet Radiol 38(6):549–558
7. Manaster BJ (2013) Soft-tissue masses: optimal imaging protocol and reporting. AJR Am J Roentgenol 201(3):505–514
8. Fujimoto H, Murakami K, Ichikawa T, Matsubara T, Tsumurai Y, Masuda S et al (1993) MRI of soft-tissue lesions: opposed-phase T2*-weighted gradient-echo images. J Comput Assist Tomogr 17(3):418–424
9. Dwyer AJ, Frank JA, Sank VJ, Reinig JW, Hickey AM, Doppman JL (1988) Short-Ti inversion-recovery pulse sequence: analysis and initial experience in cancer imaging. Radiology 168(3):827–836
10. Rubin DA, Kneeland JB (1994) MR imaging of the musculoskeletal system: technical considerations for enhancing image quality and diagnostic yield. AJR Am J Roentgenol 163(5):1155–1163
11. Shuman WP, Baron RL, Peters MJ, Tazioli PK (1989) Comparison of STIR and spin-echo MR imaging at 1.5 T in 90 lesions of the chest, liver, and pelvis. AJR Am J Roentgenol 152(4):853–859
12. Beltran J, Chandnani V, McGhee RA Jr, Kursunoglu-Brahme S (1991) Gadopentetate dimeglumine-enhanced MR imaging of the musculoskeletal system. AJR Am J Roentgenol 156(3):457–466
13. van Rijswijk CS, Geirnaerdt MJ, Hogendoorn PC, Taminiau AH, van Coevorden F, Zwinderman AH et al (2004) Soft-tissue tumors: value of static and dynamic gadopentetate dimeglumine-enhanced MR imaging in prediction of malignancy. Radiology 233(2): 493–502
14. Verstraete KL, De Deene Y, Roels H, Dierick A, Uyttendaele D, Kunnen M (1994) Benign and malignant musculoskeletal lesions: dynamic contrast-enhanced MR imaging-parametric "first-pass" images depict tissue vascularization and perfusion. Radiology 192(3):835–843
15. Park MY, Jee WH, Kim SK, Lee SY, Jung JY (2013) Preliminary experience using dynamic MRI at 3.0 Tesla for evaluation of soft tissue tumors. Korean J Radiol 14(1):102–109
16. Vanel D, Shapeero LG, Tardivon A, Western A, Guinebretiere JM (1998) Dynamic contrast-enhanced MRI with subtraction of aggressive soft tissue tumors after resection. Skelet Radiol 27(9):505–510
17. Watson TA, Olsen OE (2015) Fusion and subtraction post-processing in body MRI. Pediatr Radiol 45(2):273–282
18. Kransdorf MJ, Bridges MD (2013) Current developments and recent advances in musculoskeletal tumor imaging. Semin Musculoskelet Radiol 17(2):145–155
19. Outwater EK (1999) Ultrafast MR imaging of the pelvis. Eur J Radiol 29(3):233–244
20. Rumboldt Z, Marotti M (2003) Magnetization transfer, HASTE, and FLAIR imaging. Magn Reson Imaging Clin N Am 11(3): 471–492
21. Van Epps K, Regan F (1999) MR cholangiopancreatography using HASTE sequences. Clin Radiol 54(9):588–594
22. Bitar R, Leung G, Perng R, Tadros S, Moody AR, Sarrazin J et al (2006) MR pulse sequences: what every radiologist wants to know but is afraid to ask. Radiographics 26(2):513–537
23. Shah LM, Hanrahan CJ (2011) MRI of spinal bone marrow: part I, techniques and normal age-related appearances. AJR Am J Roentgenol 197(6):1298–1308
24. Bilbey JH, McLoughlin RF, Kurkjian PS, Wilkins GE, Chan NH, Schmidt N et al (1995) MR imaging of adrenal masses: value of chemical-shift imaging for distinguishing adenomas from other tumors. AJR Am J Roentgenol 164(3):637–642
25. Kohl CA, Chivers FS, Lorans R, Roberts CC, Kransdorf MJ (2014) Accuracy of chemical shift MR imaging in diagnosing indeterminate bone marrow lesions in the pelvis: review of a single institution's experience. Skelet Radiol 43(8):1079–1084
26. Kransdorf MJ, Murphey MD (2016) Imaging of soft-tissue musculoskeletal masses: fundamental concepts. Radiographics 36(6): 1931–1948
27. Koh DM, Collins DJ (2007) Diffusion-weighted MRI in the body: applications and challenges in oncology. AJR Am J Roentgenol 188(6):1622–1635
28. Koh DM, Collins DJ, Orton MR (2011) Intravoxel incoherent motion in body diffusion-weighted MRI: reality and challenges. AJR Am J Roentgenol 196(6):1351–1361
29. El Kady RM, Choudhary AK, Tappouni R (2011) Accuracy of apparent diffusion coefficient value measurement on PACS workstation: a comparative analysis. AJR Am J Roentgenol 196(3): W280–W284
30. Dalinka MK, Zlatkin MB, Chao P, Kricun ME, Kressel HY (1990) The use of magnetic resonance imaging in the evaluation of bone and soft-tissue tumors. Radiol Clin N Am 28(2):461–470
31. Einarsdottir H, Karlsson M, Wejde J, Bauer HC (2004) Diffusion-weighted MRI of soft tissue tumours. Eur Radiol 14(6): 959–963
32. Subhawong TK, Jacobs MA, Fayad LM (2014) Diffusion-weighted MR imaging for characterizing musculoskeletal lesions. Radiographics 34(5):1163–1177
33. van Rijswijk CS, Kunz P, Hogendoorn PC, Taminiau AH, Doornbos J, Bloem JL (2002) Diffusion-weighted MRI in the characterization of soft-tissue tumors. J Magn Reson Imaging 15(3):302–307
34. Razek A, Nada N, Ghaniem M, Elkhamary S (2012) Assessment of soft tissue tumours of the extremities with diffusion echoplanar MR imaging. Radiol Med 117(1):96–101
35. Surov A, Nagata S, Razek AA, Tirumani SH, Wienke A, Kahn T (2015) Comparison of ADC values in different malignancies of the skeletal musculature: a multicentric analysis. Skelet Radiol 44(7):995–1000
36. Maeda M, Matsumine A, Kato H, Kusuzaki K, Maier SE, Uchida A et al (2007) Soft-tissue tumors evaluated by line-scan diffusion-weighted imaging: influence of myxoid matrix on the apparent diffusion coefficient. J Magn Reson Imaging 25(6):1199–1204

37. Kransdorf MJ, Murphey MD (2000) Radiologic evaluation of soft-tissue masses: a current perspective. AJR Am J Roentgenol 175(3):575–587
38. Bongartz T, Glazebrook KN, Kavros SJ, Murthy NS, Merry SP, Franz WB 3rd et al (2015) Dual-energy CT for the diagnosis of gout: an accuracy and diagnostic yield study. Ann Rheum Dis 74(6):1072–1077
39. Upadhyay N, Saifuddin A (2015) The radiographic and MRI features of gout referred as suspected soft tissue sarcoma: a review of the literature and findings from 27 cases. Skelet Radiol 44(4):467–476
40. Bamberg F, Dierks A, Nikolaou K, Reiser MF, Becker CR, Johnson TR (2011) Metal artifact reduction by dual energy computed tomography using monoenergetic extrapolation. Eur Radiol 21(7):1424–1429
41. Peltola EK, Koskinen SK (2015) Dual-energy computed tomography of cruciate ligament injuries in acute knee trauma. Skelet Radiol 44(9):1295–1301
42. Reagan AC, Mallinson PI, O'Connell T, McLaughlin PD, Krauss B, Munk PL et al (2014) Dual-energy computed tomographic virtual noncalcium algorithm for detection of bone marrow edema in acute fractures: early experiences. J Comput Assist Tomogr 38(5):802–805
43. Chen H, Jia M, Xu W (2015) Malignant bone tumor intramedullary invasion: evaluation with dual-energy computed tomography in a rabbit model. J Comput Assist Tomogr 39(1):70–74
44. Mori T, Fujii M, Akisue T, Yamamoto T, Kurosaka M, Sugimura K (2005) Three-dimensional images of contrast-enhanced MDCT for preoperative assessment of musculoskeletal masses: comparison with MRI and plain radiographs. Radiat Med 23(6):398–406
45. Unni KK (1996) Introduction and scope of study. Dahlin's bone tumors general aspects and data on 11,087 cases, 5th edn. Lippincott-Raven Publishers, Philadelphia, pp 1–9
46. De Schepper AM, Ramon FA, Degryse HR (1992) Statistical analysis of MRI parameters predicting malignancy in 141 soft tissue masses. Rofo 156(6):587–591
47. Gielen JL, De Schepper AM, Vanhoenacker F, Parizel PM, Wang XL, Sciot R et al (2004) Accuracy of MRI in characterization of soft tissue tumors and tumor-like lesions. A prospective study in 548 patients. Eur Radiol 14(12):2320–2330

Imaging the Foot

Andrew J. Grainger

Introduction

The foot is a complex structure with multiple bones and joints, supported by ligaments and tendons. The bone and articular structures are challenging to image with conventional radiographs due to the multi-angular nature of the tarsal bones and differing planes the joints lie in. While a standard radiographic set of images for the foot should include DP, DP-oblique and lateral views, with standing radiographs obtained unless contraindicated; cross-sectional imaging with CT has a particularly useful role when imaging the foot, particularly for bone trauma. The complex ligamentous, nerve and tendon anatomy of the foot readily lends itself to assessment with ultrasound due to the superficial nature of these structures. However, MRI has an important role to play when assessing the foot given its ability to visualise the internal structure of joints, assess the bones/bone marrow and visualise the soft tissue components of the foot. Scintigraphy techniques continue to have a role, particularly when dealing with infection and also occasionally for the assessment of subtle bone pathology, including trauma and the arthritides.

The foot contains many joints and enthesis sites and is therefore an important structure when dealing with arthritis. It is also a common site for soft tissue, joint and bone infection. The foot is also a site where bone and soft tissue tumours and pseudotumours may be seen. However, bone and soft tissue oncology, musculoskeletal infection and peripheral arthritis form the subjects of other modules and will not be further addressed in this chapter.

A.J. Grainger
MSK Radiology, Chapel Allerton Orthopaedic Centre, Leeds Teaching Hospitals and The University of Leeds, Leeds, West Yorkshire LS7 4SA, UK
e-mail: andrewgrainger@nhs.net

Bone Anatomy and Variants

The complex bone anatomy and supporting soft tissue structures are integral to the form and function of the foot. However, in addition to the anatomy of the principal bones, the radiologist needs to be aware of the multiple normal variants to the bone anatomy and in particular an understanding of the large number of accessory and sesamoid bones seen in the foot many of which may simulate abnormality, although as will be seen these structures can also give rise to symptoms.

Sesamoid Bones

These lie within tendons and the most consistently seen are the medial (tibial) and lateral (fibular) hallux sesamoid bones seen at the first metatarsal phalangeal (MTP) joint on the plantar aspect of the metatarsal head. Bipartite and even multipartite hallux sesamoids are a frequent finding, with the medial sesamoid being more commonly bipartite than the lateral. Other sesamoid bones are seen in the foot and radiologists should familiarise themselves with common locations and appearances, referring to an atlas of normal variants if in doubt [1].

Accessory Ossicles

Anatomically the os peroneum is also a sesamoid bone, embedded in the peroneus longus tendon as it passes around the cuboid bone. Apart from the os peroneum other accessory and bipartite ossicles which are important to consider include the os trigonum and the accessory navicular. The accessory navicular may be symptomatic and three types are described, type 2 being most frequently symptomatic.

J. Hodler et al. (eds.), *Musculoskeletal Diseases 2017-2020*, DOI 10.1007/978-3-319-54018-4_2

- Type 1: Lies in the distal tibialis posterior tendon close to the navicular insertion.
- Type 2: The most common (also called an os naviculare) is a navicular unfused secondary ossification centre fused to the navicular through a synchondrosis.
- Type 3: A prominent medial tuberosity arising from the medial navicular and representing a fused type 2 ossicle.

Other accessory ossicles are not infrequently encountered and may occasionally give rise to symptoms, but the principle difficulty encountered by the radiologist is often distinguishing these variants from fractures [1].

Tarsal Coalitions

Tarsal coalition refers to the congenital fusion of two or more tarsal bones which may be complete, or partial and may involve a bony, fibrous or cartilaginous union. In childhood these are often asymptomatic but may become symptomatic in early adulthood, typically with a painful flat foot deformity. Altered biomechanics within the foot may lead to secondary osteoarthritis. Calcaneonavicular coalition is the most frequent followed by talonavicular coalition, together making up 90% of coalitions in total. Coalition can be difficult to diagnose on conventional radiographs due to the complex 3D anatomy involved but features described include:

- Calcaneonavicular coalition: A prominent prolongation of the anterior process of the calcaneus (the anteater nose sign), best observed on the DP oblique view.
- Talocalcaneal coalition: This usually involves the middle facet and may be seen as sclerosis of the middle facet. The C-sign is also described, where a complete posterior "C-shaped" ring is seen around the talus and sustentaculum tali. Restricted movement at the subtalar joint may lead to premature degeneration at the talonavicular joint and a talar beak (osteophyte) (Fig. 1a).

CT and MRI are both effective modalities for demonstrating coalitions. CT will directly show an osseous coalition (Fig. 1b). Fibrous coalitions can be more challenging to demonstrate using CT, although narrowing of the space between the bones and reactive bone change are important features. MRI is better suited for demonstrating all types of coalition and has the advantage of also being able to demonstrate stress reaction (in the form of bone oedema across the coalition) and soft tissue inflammatory changes, pointing to the coalition being a cause of pain. MRI may struggle to distinguish synovitis at an articulation between two bones from a fibrous coalition [2, 3].

Appearance of Bone Marrow on MRI

It is important for the radiologist to recognise the normal MRI appearances of bone marrow in the paediatric foot. Bone marrow in the foot and ankle undergoes progressive

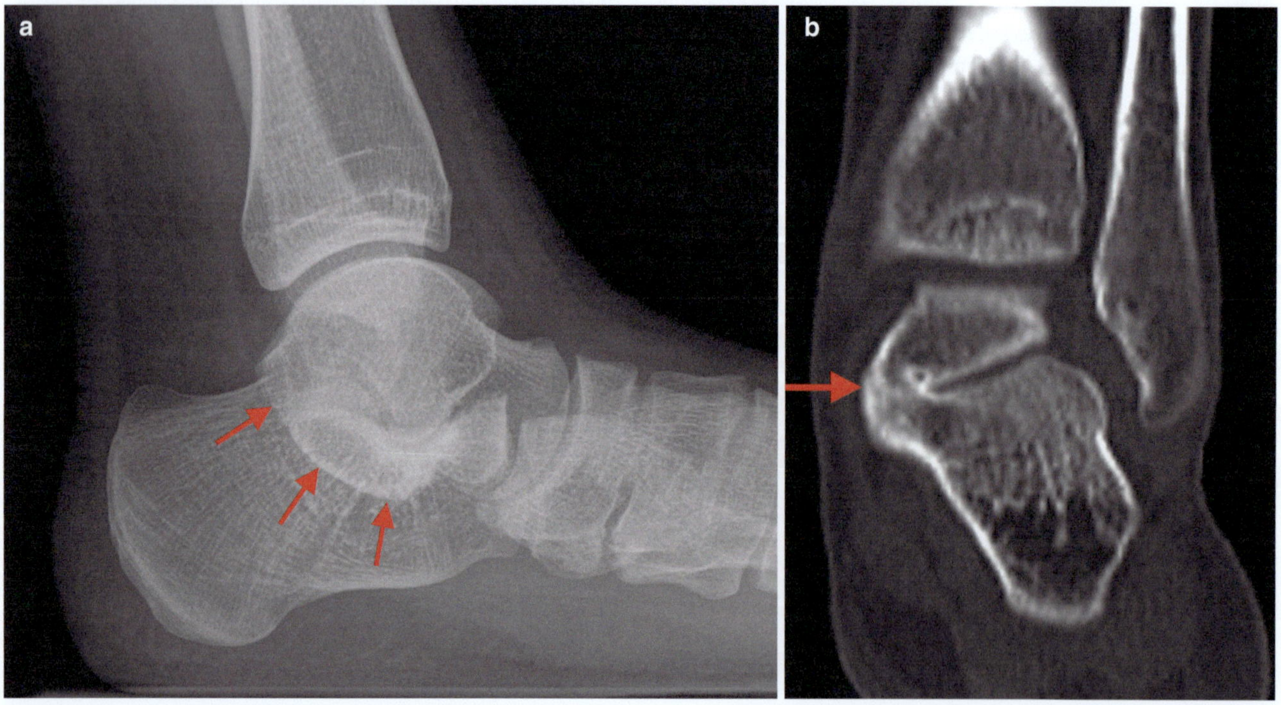

Fig. 1 Talocalcaneal coalition. (**a**) Lateral radiograph demonstrates the "C" sign (*arrows*) due to coalition across the middle subtalar joint between talus and the sustentaculum tali of the calcaneus. (**b**) CT scan in the coronal plane demonstrates the bony coalition directly (*arrow*)

conversion from red to fatty marrow during childhood [4–6]. While conversion of marrow is nearly complete by the age of 5 years isolated foci of red marrow can persist in the tarsal bones until the age of 15. These appear as multiple foci (or more confluent areas) of high signal intensity on water sensitive imaging (sometimes termed spotty bone marrow) and risk being interpreted as pathology (Fig. 2). Useful for making this distinction is review of T1 weighted imaging where these foci appear of intermediate signal compared to the surrounding high signal yellow marrow. However, they are still iso or hyperintense compared to muscle, whereas pathological marrow infiltration will usually give rise to T1 signal which is hypointense to marrow. Persistent foci of red marrow will also usually be symmetrical and should resolve by the time the patient reaches 15 years old [5].

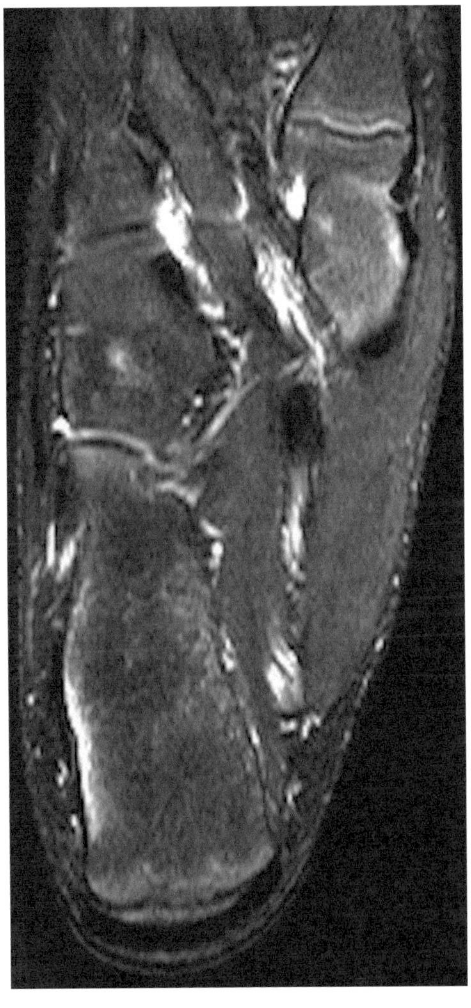

Fig. 2 Normal heterogeneity of adolescent bone marrow in the foot. Long axis STIR imaging of the foot in a 13 year old male. Note the normal "spotty" pattern of bone marrow with multiple foci of high signal

Bone Trauma

Fractures in the foot are a frequent occurrence and careful review of radiographic images is required when a fracture is suspected, assessing bone integrity and joint alignment.

Some fracture patterns are particularly common.

Fractures of the 5th Metatarsal Base

The peroneus brevis tendon inserts onto the 5th metatarsal base and the insertion site is at risk of avulsion fracture, associated with pulling off of the tendon. This is frequently seen in association with inversion injury at the ankle where the peroneus brevis contracts forcefully in a reflex attempt to stabilize the ankle as it inverts. It is sometimes termed a dancer's fracture. The 5th metatarsal base should be included on the lateral ankle radiograph and carefully reviewed in cases of ankle inversion, with additional views of the foot obtained if necessary.

A second pattern of 5th metatarsal base fracture is seen occurring distal to the articulation between the 5th and 4th metatarsals as a result of an inversion injury to the foot and is susceptible to non-union.

Both these fractures tend to have a transverse configuration, a useful feature to distinguish them from an unfused proximal 5th metatarsal apophysis which has a longitudinal configuration. They can normally be diagnosed using conventional radiographs alone.

Lisfranc Fracture Dislocation

The Lisfranc joint is the tarsometatarsal articulation between the metatarsal bases and the tarsal bones (cuneiforms and cuboid). The joint is susceptible to trauma which can occur with minimal energy but lead to lifelong disability. The tarsometatarsal joints are stabilized by a series of tarsometarsal and intermetatarsal ligaments [7]. Importantly there is no intermetatarsal ligament between the 1st and 2nd metatarsal bases, the main stabilizer here being the Lisfranc ligament running from the medial cuneiform to the second metatarsal base. Disruption of this ligament complex is frequently associated with avulsion fractures which can be extremely subtle requiring CT for accurate diagnosis. If a bone avulsion is seen at any of the medial four TMT joints a dislocation should be suspected. Pure ligamentous injury does occur and is best detected with MRI although may be evident on the conventional radiograph in the form of joint subluxation or dislocation [7]. This may only be apparent on weight-bearing radiographs. In the normal situation on a DP radiograph the medial border of the 2nd metatarsal base should line up with the medial border of the intermediate cuneiform and, on a

DP oblique radiograph, the same is true of the medial border of the 3rd metatarsal and the medial aspect of the lateral cuneiform.

Different patterns of Lisfranc dislocation may be seen depending on the injury mechanism.

Stress and Insufficiency Fractures

Stress fractures are common in the foot. Calcaneal stress fractures may be confused with a diagnosis of plantar fasciitis and should always be considered in the differential diagnosis for heel pain. Typically they occur in the posterior calcaneus and have a vertical orientation appearing as a linear zone of sclerosis on the lateral radiograph.

Navicular stress fractures are a particularly challenging injury because of the difficulty of identifying them on conventional radiographs and the significant consequences to the patient if missed. They typically occur in the sagittal plane in an athletic population and will often require MRI and/or CT to make the diagnosis.

Stress and insufficiency fractures may be seen in the other tarsal bones and may only be evident on cross sectional imaging. However, the most common stress and insufficiency fractures in the foot occur in the metatarsals. These occur with prolonged repetitive activities such as running, walking and dancing; but may also result from altered biomechanics in the foot as a result of surgery or foot deformity. These fractures may involve any metatarsal and may be multiple. The fracture itself is rarely evident on conventional radiographs, the diagnosis usually being made by the detection of new bone formation at the fracture site. However, MRI may detect the stress reaction in the metatarsal as edema signal in the bone marrow and/or periosteum, before the fracture itself has occurred.

Sesamoid Fractures

One or both hallux sesamoid bones may be fractured, the medial more commonly than the lateral. Since the normal hallux sesamoids may be bi- or even multi-partite distinction needs to be made between this normal variant and a fracture. Generally this can be done on the conventional radiograph where a bipartite sesamoid will have smooth corticated margins at the synchondrosis as opposed to the jagged, irregular fracture margins. A bipartite sesamoid will generally be larger than its neighboring non-bipartite sesamoid whereas the two components of a fractured sesamoid will make up a normal sized sesamoid. If diagnosis is difficult MRI or bone scintigraphy may be required [1].

Acute and Chronic Soft Tissue Injury

The soft tissues of the foot are subject to both acute and chronic injury. Both MRI and ultrasound are readily able to demonstrate the majority of these structures and their pathology.

The Plantar Fascia

The plantar fascia arises from the plantar surface of the calcaneus and comprises medial, central band and lateral bands. The central band itself is functionally the most important and covers flexor digitorum brevis. It divides into bands which pass towards each of the metatarsal heads. The lateral band covers abductor digiti minimi and has an insertion onto the 5th metatarsal base.

Plantar fasciitis is a common cause of heel pain and is more commonly seen in runners and dancers, but there is an association with obesity. On ultrasound plantar fasciitis is seen as thickening (>4 mm) of the plantar fascia in association with low reflective change (Fig. 3), while MRI demonstrates thickening with increased T1 and T2 signal. There may be associated adjacent soft tissue edema or bone edema in the calcaneus. In advanced disease partial or even full thickness tears may occur. The plantar fascia enthesis is also a common site of involvement in seronegative arthropathy and this should be considered in the differential diagnosis, especially if there is bone edema or erosion present.

Plantar fasciitis can occasionally involve the lateral band; in which case it is a cause of symptoms on the lateral aspect of the foot. The insertion to the fifth metatarsal is close to that of the peroneus brevis and symptoms can be confused clinically with peroneus brevis pathology.

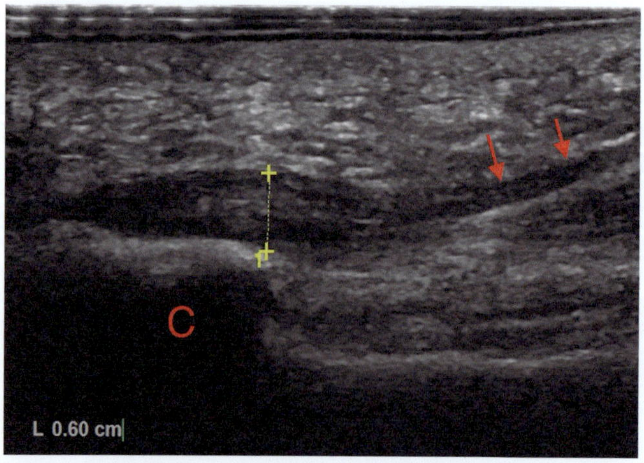

Fig. 3 Plantar fasciitis. Long axis ultrasound shows a thickened low reflective plantar fascia at its calcaneal origin (between callipers). More distally the plantar fascia shows normal thickness (*arrows*). C = Calcaneus

Plantar fibromatosis refers to nodular thickenings which develop on the plantar fascia. The condition has a genetic predisposition and is closely related to other fibromatoses including Dupuytren's disease in the hands. The nodular thickenings are readily evident on MRI and ultrasound.

Tendons

The long tendons of the foot more commonly give symptoms at and around the ankle but can give rise to symptoms in the foot. The flexor hallucis longus and flexor digitorum longus pass in the tissue plane superficial to quadratus plantae, crossing each other on the medial/plantar aspect of the foot at the knot of Henry where occasionally tenosynovitis may be seen. It should be noted that fluid in the flexor hallucis tendon sheath is a normal finding (as it communicates with the ankle joint itself) and this can pass from the ankle into the sole of the foot.

On the lateral aspect of the foot the peroneus longus passes around the cuboid into the sole of the foot. Symptoms may relate to the os peroneum which is subject to both acute and chronic injuries giving rise to the painful os peroneum syndrome (POPS). Acute fracture is rare, but chronic injury includes friction syndromes and avascular necrosis. Tendinopathy and tears may be seen and may occur in association with acute or chronic os peroneum injury. Rupture of the peroneus longus not uncommonly occurs close to the os peroneum which may result in the os retracting with the torn tendon. Distal peroneus brevis disease can also give rise to lateral foot pain and is readily demonstrated on MRI and ultrasound. The peroneus tertius is variably present anteriorly, passing laterally to insert on the dorsum of the base of 5th metatarsal. Tendinopathy of peroneus tertius is a rare cause of dorsolateral foot pain.

Dorsally tendinopathy and tears of the tibialis anterior, extensor hallucis longus and extensor digitorum may cause symptoms. Tibialis anterior has a complex insertion onto the medial cuneiform and/or 1st metatarsal and does not have a tendon sheath being surrounded by a paratenon. Tendinopathy and rupture is most commonly seen in overweight patients, athletes and in association with inflammatory arthritis. The normal tibialis anterior should be less than 5 mm thick within 3 cm of its insertion and tendon thickening (assessed on MRI or ultrasound) is a feature of tendinopathy on ultrasound and MRI. MRI may also demonstrate bone edema at the insertion and both modalities may show peritendinous inflammation including hypervascularity on ultrasound.

Tendinopathy and tenosynovitis of the extensor hallucis longus and extensor digitorum longus are both causes of pain and or swelling on the dorsum of the foot.

Tibialis posterior inserts at and around the medial navicular. As noted above an accessory navicular may be seen at the insertion and give rise to symptoms, but tendinopathy in the tendon itself may be seen close to the insertion in isolation or associated with a symptomatic accessory navicular. Longstanding tendinopathy may progress to rupture of the tendon and is a precipitating cause of a collapsed medial arch and flat foot deformity. MRI reliably demonstrates the distal tendon and has the advantage of demonstrating associated pathology relating to an accessory navicular. Ultrasound can also show the distal tendon, although care is needed as the broad and often complex tendon insertion can give rise to anisotropic artefact mimicking tendinopathy.

The Spring Ligament

The spring (plantar calcaneonavicular) ligament plays an important role in stabilizing the medial arch of the foot supporting the talar head and talocalcaneonavicular joint. The ligament complex has three components passing from the calcaneus to the navicular:

- Superomedial
- Medioplantar oblique
- Inferoplantar

While the superomedial and inferoplantar ligaments are well demonstrated on MRI, the medioplantar oblique ligament is less reliably shown [8, 9]. Only the superomedial ligament is reliably on ultrasound, but this is clinically the most important component. Using both ultrasound and MRI it is identified deep to the tibialis posterior tendon, passing from the sustentaculum to the navicular.

Isolated acute injuries to the spring ligament are rare and assessment mainly relates to the evaluation of patients with acquired flat foot deformity where both the tibialis posterior and spring ligament may be implicated. Careful assessment of these structures is important when determining further management. Patients with spring ligament insufficiency will show thickening of the ligament proximally, thinning distally or disruption of the ligament; while the changes seen in the tibialis posterior range from tenosynovitis to full thickness disruption [8, 9]. In the more advanced stages of flat foot deformity changes in the sinus tarsi and deltoid ligament complex may become evident.

Sinus Tarsi Syndrome

The sinus tarsi lies between the calcaneus and talus. Its contents include fat, blood vessels nerve endings, roots of the inferior extensor retinaculum and the cervical and interosseous talocalcaneal ligaments. Sinus tarsi syndrome is a cause of lateral foot pain thought to be due to haemorrhage, fibrosis or inflammatory change in the sinus tarsi, frequently related to talocalcaneal ligament injury. There is strong association with lateral collateral ligament injuries to the ankle. MRI characteristically demonstrates oedematous change/inflammatory tissue within the sinus tarsi, with loss of normal fat signal. Associated ligamentous disruption may be evident. In the long term osteoarthritis may develop in the subtalar joint with consequent cartilage damage and typical subchondral bone changes.

Turf Toe and Plantar Plate Disruption

The first metatarsal phalangeal joint has a complex anatomy with a capsuloligamentous complex which includes the medial and lateral sesamoid bones and a fibrocartilaginous plantar plate. The sesamoids are connected to the 1st metatarsal and proximal phalanx by the metatarso-sesamoid and sesamoid-phalangeal ligaments, while the intersesamoid ligament and plantar plate lie between the two sesamoids. Injury to this plantar capsular complex has been termed Turf Toe and results from forced hyperextension of the joint. Conventional radiographs will demonstrate fractures of the sesamoid bones. Ultrasound allows a dynamic assessment of the complex and will demonstrate disruption of the plantar plate, but MRI will often be used in the acute situation allowing assessment of bone and soft tissue components (Fig. 4) [10].

All the toes have plantar plates reinforcing the plantar aspect of the joint capsule. Rupture of the plantar plate of the minor toes rarely occurs acutely, usually developing over time as a chronic process leading to toe deformities such as clawing. The second toe is most commonly affected and both ultrasound and MRI can be used to assess the plantar plate with some authors also advocating the use of MR arthrography [11, 12]. Ultrasound has an advantage by allowing dynamic assessment which can be helpful when distinguishing partial from full thickness tears. Plantar plate disruption is also seen as a feature of inflammatory arthritis [13].

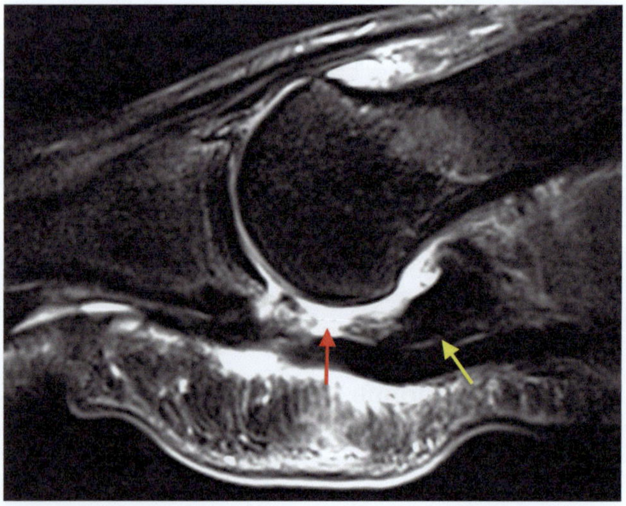

Fig. 4 Turf Toe. Sagittal T2(fs) MRI of the 1st MTP joint shows disruption of the plantar mechanism (*red arrow*) with retraction of the plantar plate (*yellow arrow*)

Nerve Entrapment

The foot has a complex cutaneous innervation and nerve entrapments may give rise to paresthesia and pain in specific distributions (Fig. 5) [14, 15]. Motor symptoms are rare in the foot. Ultrasound and MRI allow direct visualization of the nerves and associated pathology. Ultrasound offers particular advantages with its ability to easily follow a nerve in high resolution over a long length. Both modalities may demonstrate causes of nerve compression and changes within the nerve itself.

The most common nerve lesion seen in the foot is the intermetatarsal (Morton's) neuroma, most frequently seen in the intermetatarsal space between the 2nd and 3rd or 3rd and 4th metatarsal heads. The neuroma is often associated with an adjacent bursa. Both can be appreciated on MRI and Ultrasound, although ultrasound also provides a means to guide therapeutic injection.

Entrapment neuropathy most frequently involves the posterior tibial nerve in the fibro-osseous tarsal tunnel posterior to the medial malleolus. The posterior tibial nerve divides into its terminal branches within the tunnel which include the lateral and medial plantar nerves which may also be entrapped independently. Entrapment can be due to a variety of causes including ganglia and accessory muscles

The first branch of the lateral plantar nerve is the inferior calcaneal nerve which supplies sensation to the heel and the motor supply to abductor digiti minimi. Runners are particularly susceptible to entrapment of this nerve (known as Baxter's neuropathy) and experience heel pain (often indistinguishable from plantar fasciitis). MRI may reveal isolated atrophy of the abductor digiti minimi (Fig. 6).

Less frequently neuropathy may be found involving the sural and superficial peroneal nerves. Entrapment of these nerves generally occurs above the ankle and may relate to certain types of footwear, although neuropathy can also follow inversion injuries or, in the case of the sural nerve, be a complication of Achilles tendon surgery.

The deep peroneal nerve passes over the dorsum of the foot and may be subject to neuropathy as a result of footwear or impingement, for instance from osteophyte.

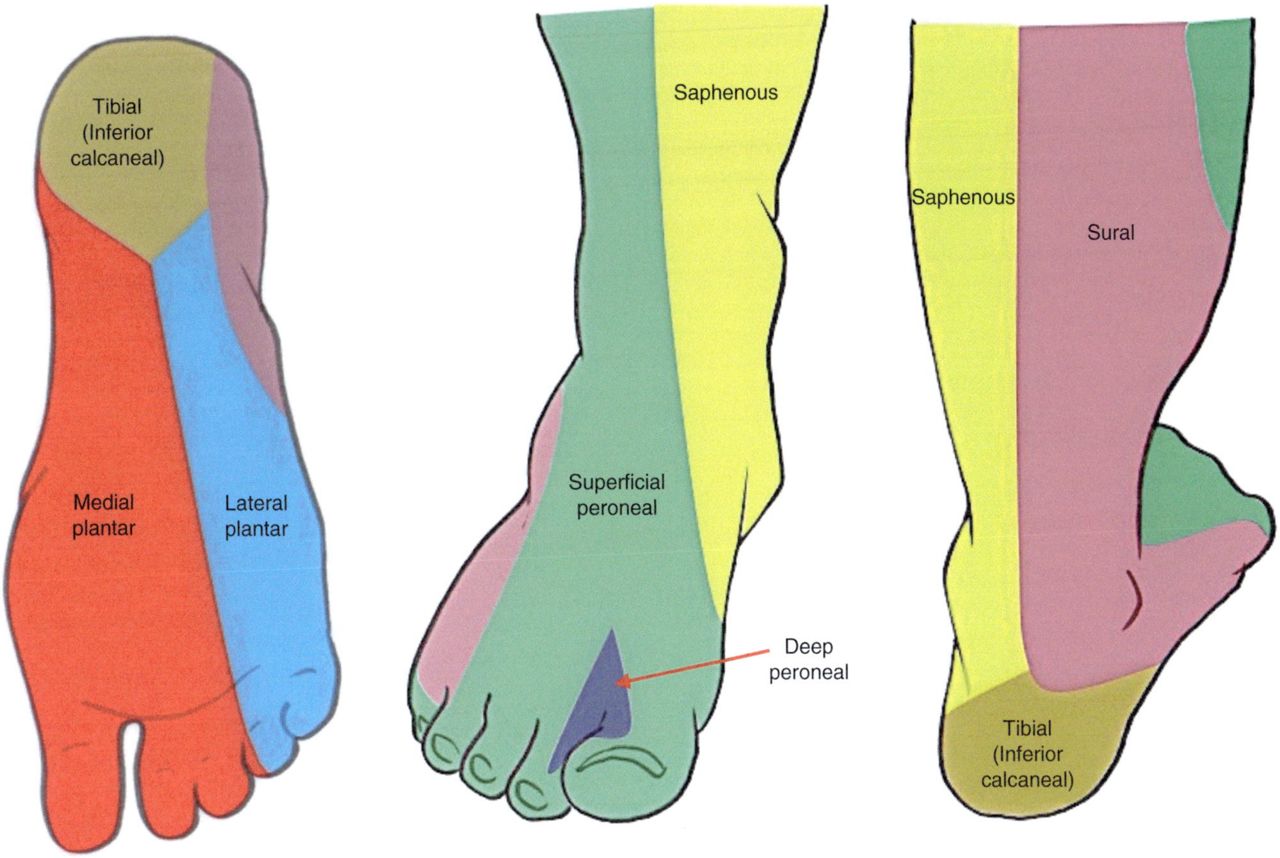

Fig. 5 Distribution of nerves providing sensation to the foot and ankle

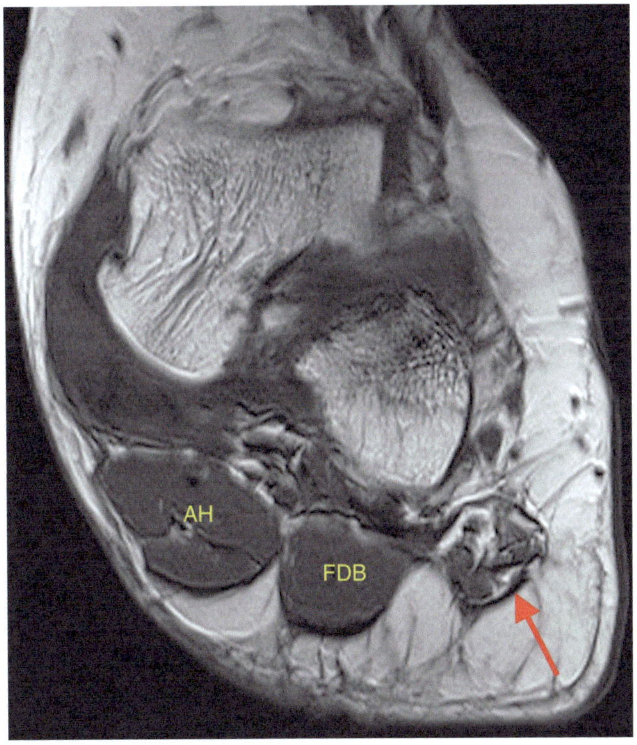

Fig. 6 Baxter's neuropathy. Short axis T1w image shows fat infiltration and atrophy of the abductor digiti minimi muscle (*arrow*). Contrast with the normal appearances of Abductor hallucis (AH) and Flexor digitorum brevis (FDB)

Summary

This chapter has reviewed common pathologies affecting the foot. As stated in the introduction tumors, infection and arthritis, also seen in the foot, are reviewed in other modules of the course. While conventional radiographs will continue to play an important role in the investigation of foot pathology, cross-sectional imaging modalities are particularly useful given the complex bone structure of the foot with multiple small bones and joints. Ultrasound and MRI are particularly valuable modalities for the investigation of soft tissue pathology.

References

1. Nwawka OK, Hayashi D, Diaz LE et al (2013) Sesamoids and accessory ossicles of the foot: anatomical variability and related pathology. Insights Imaging 4:581–593
2. Newman JS, Newberg AH (2000) Congenital tarsal coalition: multimodality evaluation with emphasis on CT and MR imaging. Radiographics 20:321–332
3. Wechsler RJ, Schweitzer ME, Deely DM et al (1994) Tarsal coalition: depiction and characterization with CT and MR imaging. Radiology 193:447–452
4. Laor T, Jaramillo D (2009) MR imaging insights into skeletal maturation: what is normal? Radiology 250:28–38
5. Shabshin N, Schweitzer ME, Morrison WB et al (2006) High-signal T2 changes of the bone marrow of the foot and ankle in

children: red marrow or traumatic changes? Pediatr Radiol 36: 670–676
6. Weishaupt D, Schweitzer ME (2002) MR imaging of the foot and ankle: patterns of bone marrow signal abnormalities. Eur Radiol 12:416–426
7. Castro M, Melão L, Canella C et al (2010) Lisfranc joint ligamentous complex: MRI with anatomic correlation in cadavers. Am J Roentgenol 195:W447–W455
8. Mengiardi B, Pinto C, Zanetti M (2016) Spring ligament complex and posterior tibial tendon: MR Anatomy and Findings in Acquired Adult flat foot deformity. Semin Musculoskelet Radiol 20:104–115
9. Williams G, Widnall J, Evans P et al (2013) MRI features most often associated with surgically proven tears of the spring ligament complex. Skelet Radiol 42:969–973
10. Crain JM, Phancao J-P, Stidham K (2008) MR imaging of turf toe. Magn Reson Imaging Clin N Am 16:93–103
11. Umans H, Elsinger E (2001) The plantar plate of the lesser metatarsophalangeal joints: potential for injury and role of MR imaging. Magn Reson Imaging Clin N Am 9: 659–69, xii
12. Mohana-Borges AV, Theumann NH, Pfirrmann CW et al (2003) Lesser metatarsophalangeal joints: standard MR imaging, MR arthrography, and MR Bursography—initial results in 48 cadaveric joints. Radiology 227:175–182
13. Siddle HJ, Hodgson RJ, Redmond AC et al (2012) MRI identifies plantar plate pathology in the forefoot of patients with rheumatoid arthritis. Clin Rheumatol 31:621–629
14. Beltran LS, Bencardino J, Ghazikhanian V et al (2010) Entrapment neuropathies III: lower limb. Semin Musculoskelet Radiol 14: 501–511
15. Martinoli C, Bianchi S, Gandolfo N et al (2000) US of nerve entrapments in osteofibrous tunnels of the upper and lower limbs. Radiographics 20:S199–S217

Ankle

Mario Maas

Ankle Anatomy

The **osteology** of the ankle joint comprises three bones and three articulations. The tibia and the fibula both articulate at their distal ends with the talus, making the true ankle articulation. On the proximal part, there is a tiny surface connection between fibula and tibia, the so called **syndesmosis** that is extending from the articular surface of the distal fibula (i.e., lateral malleolus), including a small synovial recess. This explains why synovial joint fluid might extend into a completely normal syndesmosis. Lateral malleolus extents 1 cm more distal than the medial malleolus, the distal part of the tibia. This medial malleolus consists of two colliculi separated by a groove. The ventral colliculus extends 0.5 cm farther then the posterior colliculus. The third malleolus is the prominence of the distal tibia, known as posterior malleolus or malleolus tertius. The tibia and fibula are tightly bound, constituting a fork: medial malleolus, tibial plafond and lateral malleolus cover the talus on three sides. This is known as the "mortise" configuration. So the talus is intercalated, no tendons attach. Talus is cylindrical with more convexity in the a-p direction. Trochlea of talus is more wide anterior than posterior. This morphology leads to movements of talus in the mortise of 20 degree dorsiflexion and 50 degree of plantar flexion.

This intercalated talar bone firmly is attached to tibia, fibula and calcaneus by **ligamentous** network. On the medial side there is the important *deltoid* ligament, consisting of a deep layer connecting tibia with posteromedial talus. More superficial the deltoid comprises of less strong components making connection with navicular, spring ligament and calcaneus. On the lateral side tibia and fibula connect anterior to posterior with anterior tibiofibular ligament (ATiFL), interosseous membrane and the posterior tibiofibular ligament (PTiFL): together the *syndesmotic* complex. Posterior tibiofibular ligament is considered a posterior labrum, with two separate components superior band and deep transverse band. Final ligaments on the lateral side attach the fibula to the talus, with anterior (ATFL) and posterior (PTFL) talofibular ligament and to the calcaneus with the calcaneofibular ligament (CFL).

The **cartilage** of the tibiotalar joint comprises of three separate compartments, the tibiotalar compartment, the medial compartment and the lateral compartment. In analyzing pathology each compartment needs a separate check.

Extra articular structures that are of interest to us as radiologists are muscles and more specifically accompanying **tendons** (Fig. 1). Following the anatomy anteriorly we find from medial to lateral the tendons **Ti**bialis anterior, the Extensor **H**allucis and the Extensor **D**igitorum (**T**om **H**ates **D**ick) tendon. Originating posterior and extending into the medial aspect of the ankle we encounter from anterior to posterior the tendons of the **T**ibialis Posterior, Flexor **D**igitorum, Flexor **H**allucis Longus (**T**om **D**ick and **H**arry). It is important to recognize that these tendon originate posteriorly, implying that posterior ankle pain can easily be caused by them. Posterior we encounter the Achilles tendon, a tendon that lies far back from the ankle joint, yet cause of severe posterior ankle pain. The Achilles tendon is anatomically different from the other tendon around the ankle for the absence of a tendon sheet, instead it is enveloped within a tiny highly permeable peritendinium. The lateral compartment comprises the peroneal tendons, peroneal Longus on the outside and the peroneal brevis on the inside. From an anatomical point of view this side of the ankle hosts anatomical variations quite often with additional peroneal muscles and tendons.

M. Maas
Professor of Radiology, University of Amsterdam,
Academic Medical Center, Meibergdreef, 1105 AZ, Amsterdam,
The Netherlands

Department of Radiology, Division of Musculoskeletal Radiology
Amsterdam Movement Sciences, Academic Center for Evidence
Based Sports Medicine, Meibergdreef 9, 1105 AZ, Amsterdam,
The Netherlands

J. Hodler et al. (eds.), *Musculoskeletal Diseases 2017-2020*, DOI 10.1007/978-3-319-54018-4_3

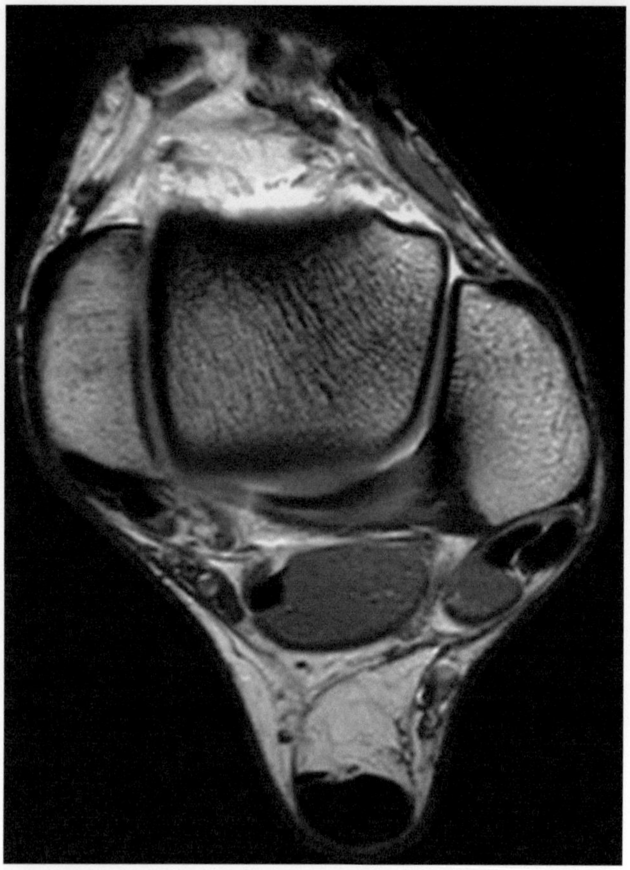

Fig. 1 Axial PD weighted 3 T image showing the normal appearance of the tendons medial, anterior lateral and the Achilles tendon posterior

Ankle Pathology

From a patients perspective the above mentioned anatomical separation is quite irrelevant. The patient almost always presents itself with a specific location of the ankle problem. This may be extremely obvious, such as inversion injury with immediate lateral ankle pain, or less obvious, such as an inversion injury with late posteromedial ankle pain or deep ankle pain. After a careful anamnesis and clinical assessment the referring medical specialist might know the anatomical structure that is suspected of pathology, yet quite often the request for MR lists a suggested Differential Diagnosis. We, as reading radiologists might feel the need to clear all mentioned anatomical structures. In my opinion the knowledge of the several pathological entities, distributed by their anatomical location, is more helpful in arriving at the right diagnosis.

I choose to focus the pathology section on some pathological entities that are frequently seen in our tertiary referral center for ankle and sports pathology.

Impingement Syndromes

Ankle impingement (AI) is an important cause of chronic ankle pain. AI is a painful mechanical limitation of full-ankle movement, secondary to osseous and/or soft-tissue pathology. Radiologists are frequently encountered with requests for MRI of the ankle, an investigation that needs to answer important preoperative questions. The presence of multiple ligaments, tendons and joint extensions make interpretation of MRI challenging. Anatomy of this small joint is considered difficult, yet crucial knowledge to interpret these MRI's adequately. Using anatomical landmarks, AI is divided as (1) anterior impingement, with a subdivision in anteromedial and anterolateral impingement and (2) posterior impingement, also divided in posterior and posteromedial impingement.

Anterior impingement can be caused both by osseous as well as soft tissue pathology. In our experience the osseous pathology often occurs medial and soft tissue impingement anterolateral. Both axial and sagittal planes are needed. Be aware: soft tissue impingement can be of a low signal intensity due to fibrotic changes. So the chosen protocol in the axial plane needs not only fat suppressed images.

Posteromedial impingement is very frequently overlooked. Because of a traumatized deep deltoid ligament fibers secondary fibrosis. This fibrotic tissue is more form, will not easily adapt to the various movement and will cause pain and blockage. Secondary reaction of the deep flexors can occur, leading to the diagnosis of tenosynovitis, and with the help of the *Satisfaction of search mechanism* we might fail to detect the ligamentous abnormality.

Although plain film is mainstay in daily practice AI is not easily detected. Guidelines on improving use of plain film are provided. Also value of easy to perform additional plain films with low costs are explained, of which the posterior impingement view in 25 degrees of exorotation is one of (Fig. 2). Since MR is thought essential in workup of chronic ankle pain, guidelines for standardized interpretation and reporting are provided. Together with demonstrating the typical imaging features, the reading radiologist is comfortable to be able to provide the surgeon with the necessary answers. In our daily practice, MRI holds several orthopedic limitations, which are discussed. MDCT of both ankles, in neutral and maximal plantar flexion are thought of important additional value. Typical MDCT features of various AI subtypes are displayed. When radiologists are able to closely interact with the clinical colleagues, optimal care in chronic ankle pain can be provided.

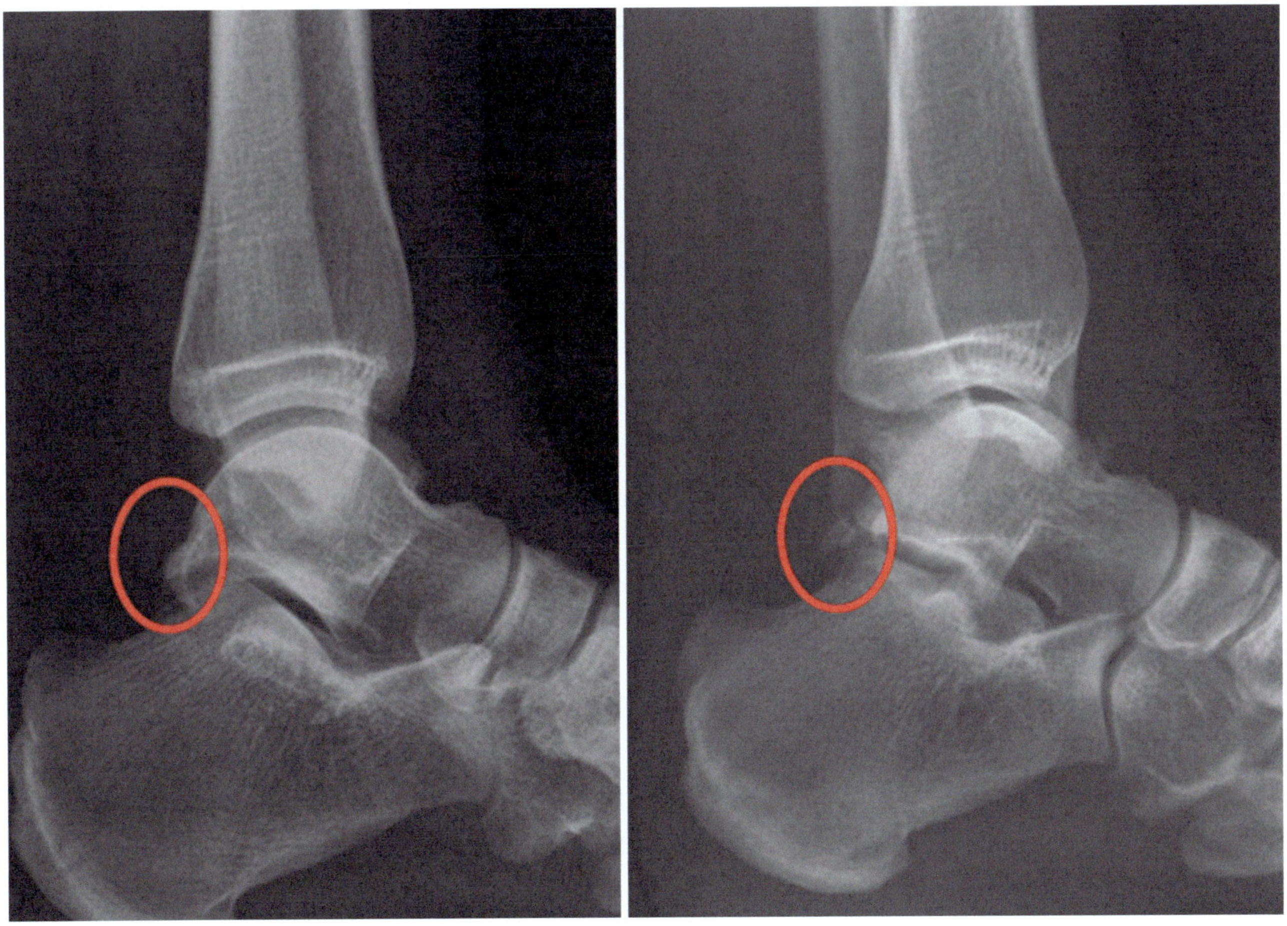

Fig. 2 New lateral film, posterior Impingement view, with 25 degrees of exorotation. So called PIM, posterior impingement view

Osteochondral Defects

An osteochondral defect (OCD) is a lesion of the joint involving the cartilage and the subchondral bone plate. Already in 1743 it was stated: "if we consult the standard chirurgical writers from Hippocrates down to the present age we shall find that an ulcerated cartilage is universally allowed to be a very troublesome disease; that is admits of a cure with more difficulty than a carious bone and that when destroyed will never recover". So it is considered an ongoing quest. An ankle trauma is widely accepted as the most important etiological factor of OCD of the talus. Berndt and Harty clearly described in cadaveric ankles the occurrence of lateral defects by strong inversion of sa dorsiflexed ankle.leading to compression of the lateral border against the fibula. A medial lesion was reproduced by plantarflexion of the ankle in combination with a slight anterior displacement of the talus on the tibia.

The patients present themselves with a persisting deep ankle pain during or after activity. Reactive swelling caused by synovitis often is present. With maximal plantar flexion the talar surface can be palpated and is painful.

In Using MR Imaging fat suppressed sagittal sequences clearly detect the zone of bone marrow edema. T1 or PD weighted sequences will better define the clear area of the defect, that might be overcalled by the fat suppressed images (Fig. 3). In our experience preoperative CT scanning, performed in maximal dorsiflexion and in maximal plantar flexion is crucial for surgical planning (Figs. 4 and 5).

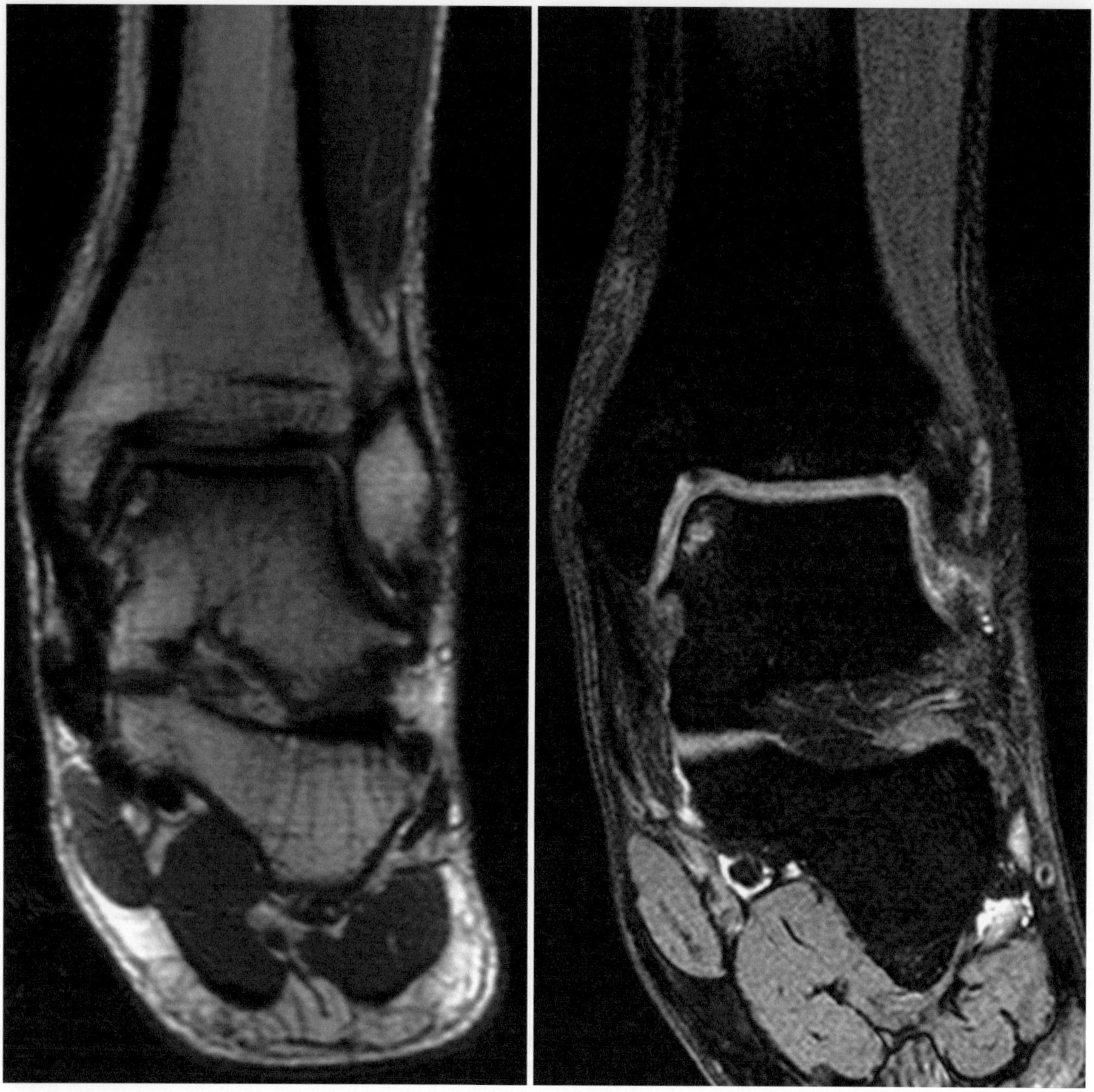

Fig. 3 Osteochondral defect of medial talar dome on coronal PD and T2 weighted sequences. PD weighing clearly delineates the lesion

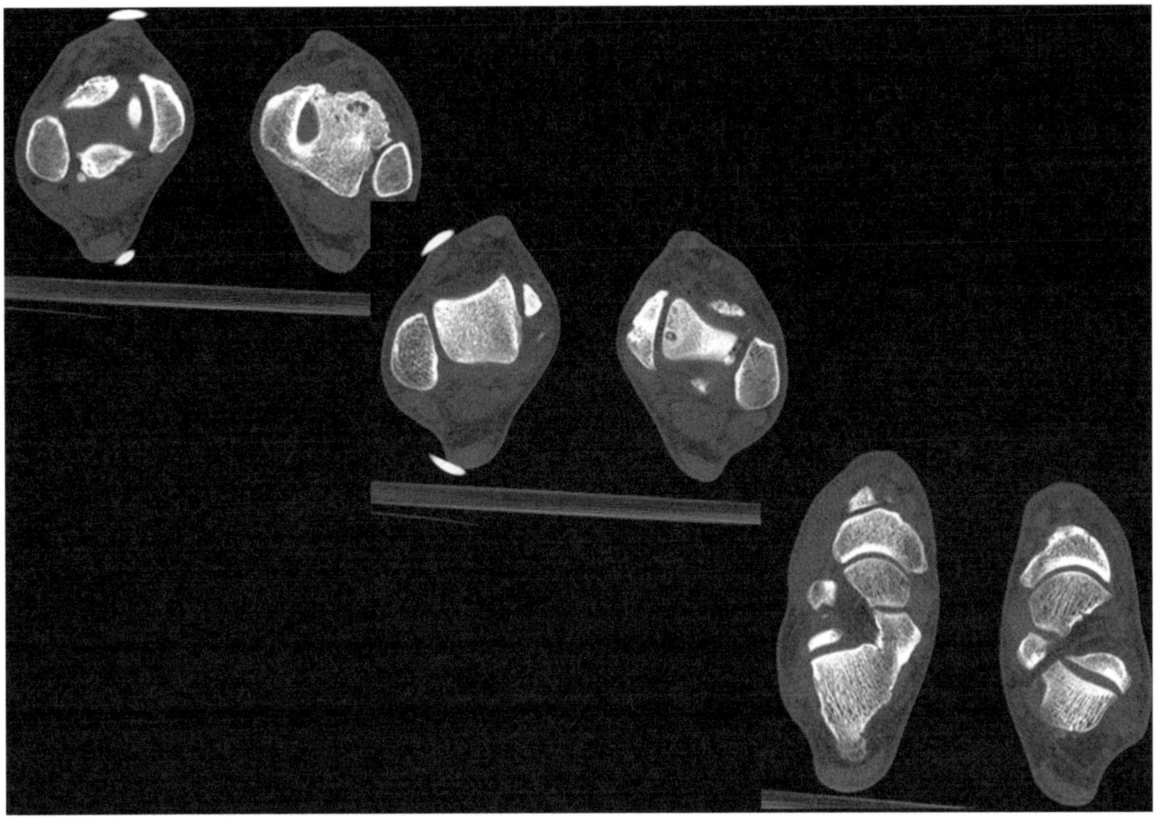

Fig. 4 Axial HRCT 0.5 mm of two ankles, mark up of the right one showing OCD in the left talar bone

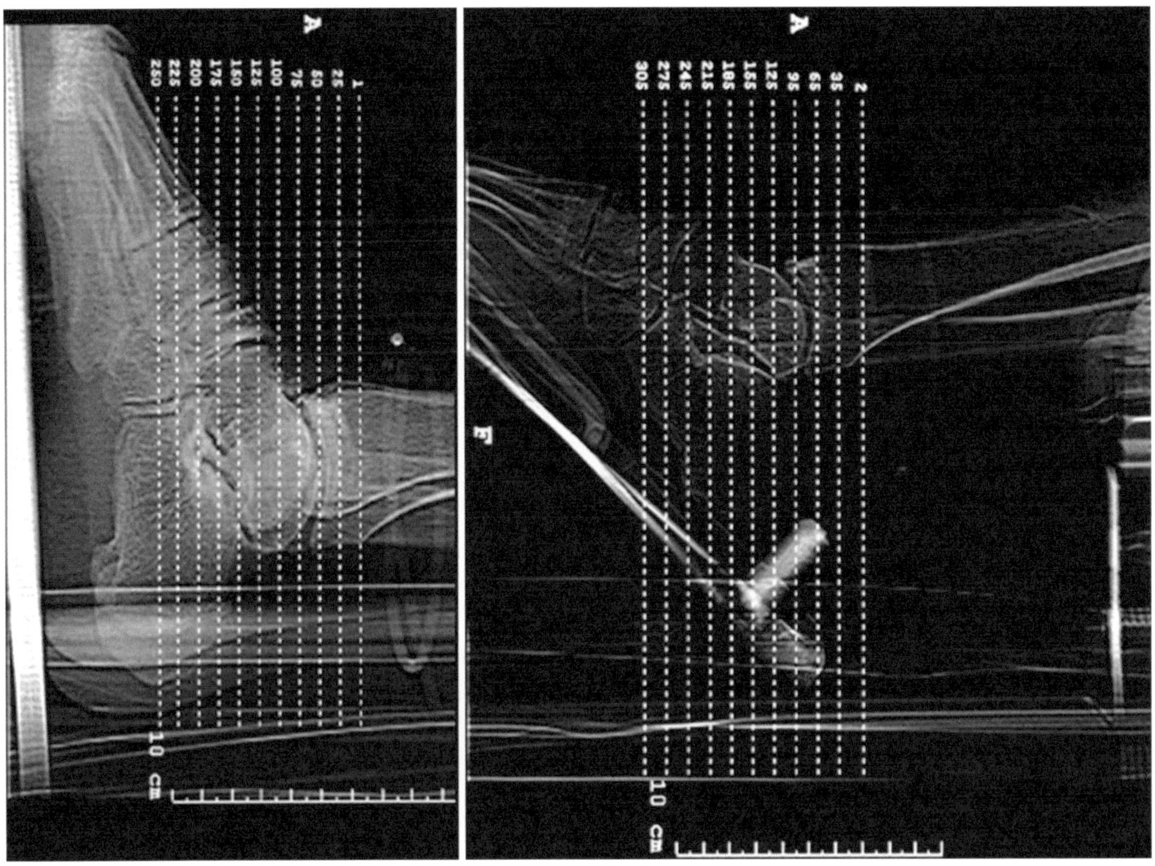

Fig. 5 Scout views of the general CT in dorsiflexion and the CT in maximal plantar flexion

Sports Injury

The ankle is prone for various sports related and sports specific injuries. Obviously the acute inversion injury in which following the trauma mechanism the classification of Lauge Hansen is helpful in detecting and ruling out both less visible bone and soft tissue lesions. Plain film is mainstay, yet the increasing use of CT scanning in early trauma of small joints allows assessment of both osseous, subchondral bone plate as well as soft tissues. This however needs CT scanning of the ankle using both bone and soft tissue Kernel reconstruction filters. Scanning two sides in our experience is quite helpful. Early detection of OCD is feasible.

Another important sportsspecific (mailnly soccer) lesions is the bony and soft tissue impingement anteriorly. The bony impingement often is anteromedial, yet 2 cm more lateral than the medial malleolus. Also mark the osteophyte at the talar surface distally. Soft btissue impingement almost exclusively occurs anterolateral. Treatment during season by US guided injection therapy shows good results.

The stress fracture of the medial aspect of the distal tibia should be known to us when reading sports imaging. We might mistake it for a simple bone bruise (however in my opinion hardly existing!) when we are not aware of this entity. The second common stress fracture is the navicular boen stress fracture.

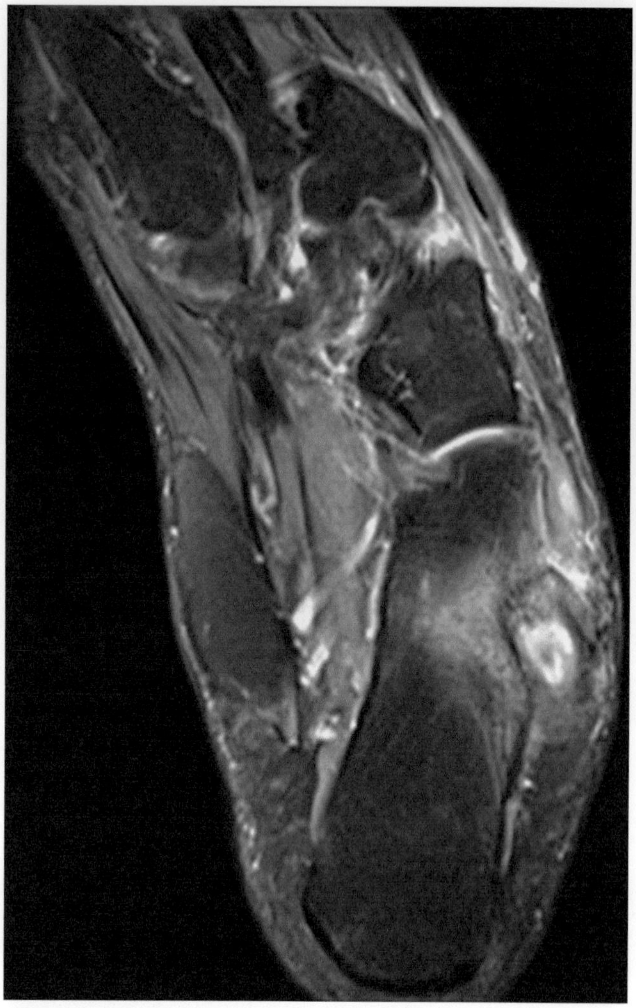

Fig. 6 Peroneal tendon pathology with accompanying edema in the calcaneal bone

Peroneal Tendons

Tendon pathology around the ankle can be thought of as a predominantly chronic process, as a response to repetitive loading in combination with ageing of tendons and occurs more frequently occur in females. That might also go for the peroneal tendons pathology, in which the peroneal split tear is frequently seen and easily overlooked. Since signal intensity change not always is seen, we need to focus on morphology of the tendons. So be sure that the rond on all sequences low signal intensity is present. The longitudinal split of most often the peroneus brevis tendon often is related to chronic instability of this tendon. Unique for the peroneal tendon is the (sub) luxation due to shallow groove as anatomical factor together with biomechanical items. Peroneal tendon pathology is more frequently associated with ankle instability trauma. Also when dealing with calcaneal fractures, please assess the position of the peroneals, since they can get caught within the fracture. More focal pathology most often occurs at the calcaneocuboid joint (Fig. 6).

Suggested Readings

1. Stufkens SAS (2014) Posttraumatic ankle osteoarthritis. PhD thesis, University of Amsterdam
2. Sarrafian SK (2014) Anatomy of the foot and ankle: descriptive, topographic functional. Lippincott Williams & Wilkins, Philadelphia
3. Reilingh M (2016) The role of bone in osteochondral talar defects. PhD thesis, University of Amsterdam
4. Reilingh ML, van Bergen CJ, Blankevoort L, Gerards RM, van Eekeren IC, Kerkhoffs GM, van Dijk CN (2016) Computed tomography analysis of osteochondral defects of the talus after arthroscopic debridement and microfracture. Knee Surg Sports Traumatol Arthrosc 24(4):1286–1292. PubMed PMID: 26713327
5. Kerkhoffs GM, Reilingh ML, Gerards RM, de Leeuw PA (2016) Lift, drill, fill and fix (LDFF): a new arthroscopic treatment for talar osteochondral defects. Knee Surg Sports Traumatol Arthrosc 24(4):1265–1271

6. Reilingh ML, Blankevoort L, van Eekeren IC, van Dijk CN (2013) Morphological analysis of subchondral talar cysts on microCT. Knee Surg Sports Traumatol Arthrosc 21(6):1409–1417
7. van Dijk CN, Reilingh ML, Zengerink M, van Bergen CJ (2010) The natural history of osteochondral lesions in the ankle. Instr Course Lect 59:375–386
8. van Dijk CN, Reilingh ML, Zengerink M, van Bergen CJ (2010) Osteochondral defects in the ankle: why painful? Knee Surg Sports Traumatol Arthrosc 18(5):570–580
9. Reilingh ML, Beimers L, Tuijthof GJ, Stufkens SA, Maas M, van Dijk CN (2010) Measuring hindfoot alignment radiographically: the long axial view is more reliable than the hindfoot alignment view. Skelet Radiol 39(11):1103–1108
10. Hopper MA, Robinson P (2008) Ankle impingement syndromes. Radiol Clin N Am 46(6):957–971
11. Robinson P (2007) Impingement syndromes of the ankle. Eur Radiol 17(12): 3056–3065. Review.
12. Messiou C, Robinson P, O'Connor PJ, Grainger A (2006) Subacute posteromedial impingement of the ankle in athletes: MR imaging evaluation and ultrasound guided therapy. Skelet Radiol 35(2):88–94
13. Robinson P, White LM (2005) The biomechanics and imaging of soccer injuries. Semin Musculoskelet Radiol 9(4):397–420. Review
14. Robinson P, White LM (2002) Soft-tissue and osseous impingement syndromes of the ankle: role of imaging in diagnosis and management. Radiographics 22(6):1457–1469; discussion 1470–1. Review
15. Stone AV, Little KJ, Glos DL, Stringer KF, Wall EJ (2016) Repetitive stresses generate osteochondral lesions in skeletally immature rabbits. Am J Sports Med 44(11):2957–2966
16. Wong GN, Tan TJ (2016) MR imaging as a problem solving tool in posterior ankle pain: a review. Eur J Radiol 85(12):2238–2256
17. LiMarzi GM, Scherer KF, Richardson ML, Warden DR 4th, Wasyliw CW, Porrino JA, Pettis CR, Lewis G, Mason CC, Bancroft LW (2016) CT and MR imaging of the postoperative ankle and foot. Radiographics 36(6):1828–1848
18. Yammine K (2015) The accessory peroneal (fibular) muscles: peroneus quartus and peroneus digiti quinti. A systematic review and meta-analysis. Surg Radiol Anat 37(6):617–627
19. Galli MM, Protzman NM, Mandelker EM, Malhotra AD, Schwartz E, Brigido SA (2015) An examination of anatomic variants and incidental peroneal tendon pathologic features: a comprehensive MRI review of asymptomatic lateral ankles. J Foot Ankle Surg 54(2):164–172
20. Galli MM, Protzman NM, Mandelker EM, Malhotra AD, Wobst GM, Schwartz E, Brigido SA (2014) Examining the relationship between pathologies of the peroneal, Achilles, and posterior tibial tendons: an MRI review in an asymptomatic lateral ankle population. Foot Ankle Spec 7(4):277–285
21. Lee SJ, Jacobson JA, Kim SM, Fessell D, Jiang Y, Dong Q, Morag Y, Choo HJ, Lee SM (2013) Ultrasound and MRI of the peroneal tendons and associated pathology. Skelet Radiol 42(9):1191–1200. doi:10.1007/s00256-013-1631-6
22. Galli MM, Protzman NM, Mandelker EM, Malhotra AD, Schwartz E, Brigido SA (2014) Examining the relation of osteochondral lesions of the talus to ligamentous and lateral ankle tendinous pathologic features: a comprehensive MRI review in an asymptomatic lateral ankle population. J Foot Ankle Surg 53(4): 429–433
23. Mansour R, Jibri Z, Kamath S, Mukherjee K, Ostlere S (2011) Persistent ankle pain following a sprain: a review of imaging. Emerg Radiol 18(3):211–225
24. van Dijk PA, Gianakos AL, Kerkhoffs GM, Kennedy JG (2016) Return to sports and clinical outcomes in patients treated for peroneal tendon dislocation: a systematic review. Knee Surg Sports Traumatol Arthrosc 24(4):1155–1164
25. van Dijk PA, Madirolas FX, Carrera A, Kerkhoffs GM, Reina F (2016) Peroneal tendons well vascularized: results from a cadaveric study. Knee Surg Sports Traumatol Arthrosc 24(4):1140–1147
26. http://www.radiologyassistant.nl/en/p420a20ca7196b/ankle-fracture-weber-and-lauge-hansen-classification.html
27. Nosewicz TL, Beerekamp MS, De Muinck Keizer RJ, Schepers T, Maas M, Niek van Dijk C, Goslings JC (2016) Prospective computed tomographic analysis of osteochondral lesions of the ankle joint associated with ankle fractures. Foot Ankle Int 37(8): 829–834

Arthritis

Charles S. Resnik and Klaus Bohndorf

Introduction

The World Health Organization (WHO) lists rheumatoid arthritis and osteoarthritis as the top two chronic rheumatic conditions with the greatest impact on society. A large number of disorders are subsumed under the terms "arthritis" or "rheumatism" but present quite different manifestations and pose different diagnostic and therapeutic challenges.

Correctly diagnosing arthritis involves consideration of numerous factors, including clinical features (age and sex of the patient, duration of symptoms, clinical appearance of involved joint or joints, presence or absence of associated diseases such as skin disease, uveitis, urethritis), laboratory values (e.g., markers for inflammation, serum rheumatoid factor, serum uric acid level), and imaging features.

Radiographs represent the mainstay for diagnosis and follow up of joint damage. However, in the last two decades, magnetic resonance imaging (MRI) and sonography have emerged as powerful evaluation tools for early diagnosis and staging of rheumatic diseases. They also may give information about the prognosis of rheumatic diseases and may help in differential diagnosis. To establish a correct diagnosis of rheumatic disease, many imaging features have to be systematically addressed:

1. The distribution of joint involvement (mono-, oligo-, or polyarticular, symmetrical or asymmetrical, proximal or distal, associated axial involvement, associated involvement of ligaments, tendons, tendon attachments, and muscles).
2. Soft tissue swelling (periarticular, fusiform, nodular, around tendons and tendon attachments).
3. Joint space narrowing (uniform, non-uniform).
4. Bone erosion (marginal, central, periarticular, well-defined, symmetrical, asymmetrical).
5. Bone proliferation (subchondral sclerosis, osteophytes, syndesmophytes, enthesophytes, periosteal new bone).
6. Joint deformity, destruction, ankylosis.
7. Subchondral osteolytic lesions (cysts).
8. Calcification (periarticular, intraarticular).
9. Vacuum phenomenon.
10. Periarticular and overall osteoporosis (including loss of subchondral bone plate).

Rheumatoid Arthritis (RA)

Rheumatoid arthritis (RA) is a systemic auto-immune disease which originates primarily in the synovial membrane of affected joints and may progress to joint destruction. Extra-articular manifestations involving lungs, heart, pericardium, and nerves may occur. The auto-immune reaction may possibly be related to a prior infection, and many patients are found to be carriers of certain HLA-DBRI genes. Activated T-lymphocytes stimulate B-lymphocytes to produce immunoglobulins (rheumatoid factor and anti-cyclic citrullinated peptides [anti-CCP]) and macrophages to form cytokines (interleukin-1, interleukin-6, and tumor necrosis factor α). This results in the proliferation of mesenchymal tissue elements (fibroblasts) and the influx of inflammatory cells from the blood into the synovial membrane, so that aggressive granulation tissue (pannus) develops. Synovitis develops at certain sites of predilection in joints and tendon sheaths, which probably depends on the number of synovial B-cells present and tissue perfusion. This may result in destruction of adjacent cartilage with joint space narrowing. At areas with absent or thinned hyaline cartilage covering adjacent bone (bare areas), early osseous erosion (marginal erosions) may develop, related to inflammation that stimulates

C.S. Resnik (✉)
Department of Diagnostic Radiology, University of Maryland School of Medicine, 22 S. Greene St, Baltimore, MD 21201, USA
e-mail: cresnik@umm.edu

K. Bohndorf
MR High Field Center, Department of Biomedical Imaging and Image-guided Therapy, Medical University of Vienna, Lazarettgasse 14, 1090 Wien, Austria
e-mail: klaus.bohndorf@meduniwien.ac.at

J. Hodler et al. (eds.), *Musculoskeletal Diseases 2017-2020*, DOI 10.1007/978-3-319-54018-4_4

osteoclasts via another cytokine, the RANK ligand. Furthermore, osteoclastic activity may result in juxta-articular osteoporosis or a more generalized arthritis-related osteoporosis of the entire skeleton. Furthermore, collagen-splitting enzymes may damage the ligaments, resulting in subluxation or dislocation, especially in the hands, feet, and atlantodental joint. Early secondary osteoarthritis may develop as a result of joint deformity and destruction. Less commonly ankylosis occurs following complete erosion of articular surfaces.

The initial radiographic manifestations of RA are soft tissue swelling and periarticular osteoporosis. These features represent indirect evidence of synovial inflammation, and their assessment is quite subjective. During the first 3 months of disease onset (referred to as early arthritis), timely initiation of treatment can favorably affect prognosis. However, standard radiographs will usually appear normal, since the disease is still predominantly confined to the synovial membrane. This can be confirmed by ultrasound or MRI.

RA typically begins in the peripheral joints, usually the metacarpophalangeal (MCP) and proximal interphalangeal (PIP) joints, the wrists, and the metatarsophalangeal (MTP) joints, with a predominantly symmetrical left/right distribution. As the disease progresses, it affects more proximal joints. Early marginal erosions of bone may occur at the radial aspect of the second and third metacarpal heads, at the ulnar styloid process, and at the metatarsal heads, especially at the lateral aspect of the fifth metatarsal head. This is followed by diffuse narrowing of PIP, MCP, MTP, and wrist joints. Characteristically, the distal interphalangeal (DIP) joints are spared. There is no osseous proliferation and no involvement of entheses.

The development of new, powerful but expensive therapeutic agents for RA, such as the anti–tumor necrosis factor (TNF) agents, has created new demands on radiologists to identify patients with aggressive rheumatoid arthritis at an early stage. Sonography is often used to detect synovitis and tenosynovitis at specific joints, whereas MRI is a more global way to evaluate the small synovial joints of the appendicular skeleton and is more sensitive than radiography in detecting synovitis, bone marrow edema, and bone erosions. MRI is also an excellent means to assess spinal complications of RA, in particular subluxation at the atlantoaxial joint. Both MRI and sonography may be used to demonstrate the soft tissue changes of RA, such as tenosynovitis and rheumatoid nodules.

Spondyloarthritis

The spondyloarthritides are a group of rheumatic diseases, each with characteristic clinical findings and a common genetic predisposition, especially for the antigen HLA-B27. The terms seronegative spondyloarthritis or seronegative spondyloarthopathy may also be used, with seronegative referring to the serum rheumatoid factor not being elevated.

Forms of spondyloarthritis include ankylosing spondylitis (Bechterew's disease), (infectious) reactive arthritis, psoriatic arthritis, the enteropathic arthropathies, SAPHO (synovitis, acne, pustulosis, hyperostosis, osteitis) syndrome, Type 2 juvenile oligoarthritis, and undifferentiated spondyloarthritis. Chronic, non-bacterial osteomyelitis (chronic recurrent multifocal osteomyelitis, or CRMO) should also be mentioned, even though it is not included in the official classifications. These diseases frequently cause symptoms in the axial skeleton, but the appendicular skeleton may also be affected, in isolation or in combination. Radiographically, these diseases differ from rheumatoid arthritis by the absence or mild nature of periarticular osteoporosis, the involvement of entheses with erosions and with new bone formation, and the asymmetrical involvement of the peripheral skeleton.

The cause of spondyloarthritis remains hypothetical, possibly taking origin from a bacterial infection. Overloading of the endoplasmic reticulum with misfolded HLA-B27 proteins is believed to result in a proinflammatory response. Whereas with rheumatoid arthritis the center of the inflammation is located in the synovial membrane and the clinical course, if left untreated, is progressive and destructive, with spondyloarthritides, the disease is predominantly located in and around the insertions of ligaments and tendons and has an intermittent course with juxtaposed bone destruction and proliferation.

Axial spondyloarthritis is characterized by inflammatory back pain along with other features such as uveitis, dactylitis, or psoriasis. In addition to characteristic radiographic features, "positive" or "highly probable" MRI findings of bone marrow edema or osteitis help make a definitive diagnosis.

Ankylosing Spondylitis

Ankylosing spondylitis (synonym: Bechterew's disease) is the prototype of spondyloarthritis, with target areas primarily involving the axial skeleton (especially the sacroiliac joints), the entheses (tendon-bone junction), and the peripheral joints.

Radiography may demonstrate arthritis and enthesitis with erosive changes and osseous proliferation. MRI is well suited for demonstrating the early spinal and sacroiliac changes of ankylosing spondylitis. High T2 signal (edema) at the corners of vertebral bodies and in the subchondral bone of the sacroiliac joints is a typical feature. Later, osseous erosion at the sacroiliac joints and ultimately fusion of the sacroiliac joints and spine may be seen. Sites of previous inflammation may be evident as fatty change within the bone marrow, typically seen at the corners of vertebral bodies.

At an early stage of the disease, sonography and MRI may be useful in showing peripheral inflammatory changes at entheses, including extra-articular sites such as the calcaneal attachments of the Achilles tendon and plantar fascia. While sonography will show synovitis and erosive change along with enthesophytes, MRI will additionally demonstrate edema within the bone marrow. Costovertebral disease is a common finding on MRI.

Psoriatic Arthritis

The extent of psoriatic arthritis often does not correlate with the degree of psoriatic skin disease, and in some cases, skin manifestations may occur several years after arthritis is evident or may never develop. Psoriatic arthritis tends to involve the small joints of the hands and feet, and the process is characteristically asymmetrical. Involvement of the DIP joints of the fingers and toes, usually in association with psoriatic changes of the nails, is characteristic. Involvement of one entire digit (MCP + PIP + DIP, "sausage digit") is very suggestive of psoriatic arthritis. This arthritis is not necessarily associated with periarticular osteoporosis, and erosions are often small. In contrast, extensive osseous proliferation at entheses and periostitis are common.

At an early stage, sonography and MRI may show synovitis, tenosynovitis, and bursitis that are similar to those seen in rheumatoid arthritis. In addition, MRI may demonstrate extensive signal abnormality in the bone marrow and soft tissues far beyond the joint capsule, related to enthesitis. These features may be useful in patients with inflammatory polyarthralgia of the hands for differentiating rheumatoid arthritis from psoriatic arthritis. Sacroiliitis is common and resembles that seen in ankylosing spondylitis, except that it is more often asymmetrical. Spinal involvement is less common, and the paravertebral ossification that occurs in psoriatic spondylitis is typically broad, coarse, and asymmetrical in contrast to the symmetrical syndesmophytes of ankylosing spondylitis.

Reactive Arthritis

Reactive arthritis (synonym: Reiter's syndrome; the term formerly used for the triad "urethritis, arthritis, and conjunctivitis") is a form of spondyloarthritis secondary to a bacterial infection usually with a self-limiting course covering 3–12 months. If no connection can be established with a bacterial infection, then it is referred to as an undifferentiated arthritis or simply spondyloarthritis. In general, the radiographic manifestations are identical to those of psoriatic arthritis, except that the axial skeleton is not as commonly affected, and changes in the upper extremities are exceptional. The most prominent involvement is in the lower extremities, particularly the feet.

Enteropathic Arthritis

Enteropathic arthritis is associated with chronic inflammatory bowel diseases, usually Crohn's disease, less commonly ulcerative colitis, and infrequently other intestinal disorders, such as celiac disease, collagenous colitis, or primary biliary cirrhosis. The most common manifestation is sacroiliitis, which is identical to but not as extensive as that in ankylosing spondylitis, with bilateral symmetrical involvement. Patients are rarely symptomatic, and the radiographic findings of sacroiliitis are often noted incidentally on abdominal radiographs obtained as part of a small bowel or colon examination. Peripheral arthritis is uncommon.

Undifferentiated Spondyloarthritis

Together with ankylosing spondylitis, undifferentiated spondyloarthritis is the most common form of spondyloarthritis. The clinical, laboratory, and imaging findings of undifferentiated spondyloarthritis, reactive arthritis, and ankylosing spondylitis overlap.

The diagnosis "undifferentiated spondyloarthritis" is made when the clinical criteria suggest spondyloarthritis but more specific criteria for ankylosing spondylitis, psoriasis, or enteropathic spondyloarthritis are absent, and a bacterial trigger is not evident. There are no pathognomonic clinical or laboratory findings. Some patients with the diagnosis "undifferentiated spondyloarthritis" eventually develop more specific signs of ankylosing spondylitis and are then reclassified.

Osteoarthritis (OA)

The term "osteoarthritis" refers to various degenerative joint diseases which are characterized by progressive articular dysfunction. Although osteoarthritis has so far been classified as a non-inflammatory arthropathy, many authors are now asserting that intermittent episodes of inflammation strongly affect the disease course and clinical presentation.

For purposes of clinical classification, idiopathic and secondary types of OA should be distinguished. From a pathophysiological view, however, this concept must be called into question. Today it is assumed that a trigger causes early changes to the joint and subsequently initiates catabolic as well as reparative mechanisms. Such triggers may include direct or indirect injury to the joint, joint inflammation, chronic overuse, and other systemic factors (e.g., obesity, age and gender, genetic predisposition, nutrition). The concept of OA as a purely primary cartilage disease has been abandoned, given that multiple structures within a joint are involved in the disease process. In particular, a close link between articular cartilage and subchondral bone has been recognized. Nevertheless, OA is phenotypically characterized by a progressive loss of cartilage.

The diagnosis of OA is based on both radiographic and clinical features. Radiography remains the diagnostic standard, both to establish the diagnosis and to assess the progression of disease. OA mainly affects the interphalangeal joints of the fingers (characteristically sparing the MCP joints) and the weight-bearing joints (hips and knees). Standing (weight-bearing) views of the joints of the lower limbs should be obtained. This is particularly important to assess for associated limb malalignment.

The general radiographic features of OA are non-uniform joint space narrowing, subchondral sclerosis of bone, marginal osteophytes, and subchondral cysts. Narrowing of the joint space in OA is almost invariably uneven and more pronounced in that portion of the joint where weight-bearing stresses are greatest. In general, the greater the degree of narrowing, the more severe the associated findings of subchondral sclerosis and osteophytosis. Calcified or ossified fragments (loose bodies) may be identified within the joint and are particularly common in the knee. Other features include soft-tissue swelling, joint effusion, and joint deformity or attrition (increased concavity or flattening of the joint surfaces).

Atlases with illustrative examples can be of great assistance for reporting purposes (e.g., the atlas by Altman and coworkers from 1995 or the revised version from 2007).

The Kellgren-Lawrence classification uses the anteroposterior radiograph of the knee to grade the severity of OA:

Grade 0: no osteophytes, no joint space narrowing
Grade 1: possible small, marginal osteophyte
Grade 2: definite osteophyte formation
Grade 3: joint space narrowing
Grade 4: complete loss of joint space (bone-to-bone contact)

Clinical and radiographic features are usually straightforward, and MRI is not used for primary diagnosis. There is currently no universally accepted MRI-based definition and classification of OA. It should be recognized that some MRI features may be misleading, including extensive edema of subchondral bone marrow, signal changes of subchondral bone located on only one side of a joint, enhancement of subchondral cysts after intravenous gadolinium administration, and heterogeneous signal intensity of joint fluid.

Erosive osteoarthritis is an inflammatory form of OA that occurs primarily in postmenopausal women, usually limited to the interphalangeal joints of the hand. Clinically, the joints are acutely inflamed. Erosions of the central portion of articular surfaces, often more pronounced at the PIP joints, are prominent and are superimposed on the standard radiographic features of OA. Involved joints may eventually undergo osseous ankylosis, which does not occur in noninflammatory osteoarthritis.

Metabolic Joint Disease

Gout

The symptoms of gout are triggered by localized deposits of monosodium urate crystals. Uric acid is the end product of purine metabolism. Reduced renal excretion of uric acid or, more rarely, its increased production results in hyperuricemia. Genetic alterations of urate transport proteins are regarded as triggers for the impaired renal excretion. The effect of nutrition (protein- and purine-rich nutrition, alcohol consumption) has been confirmed. Over-saturation with uric acid results in precipitation of sodium urate crystals, which induces a local acute inflammation-like reaction. Characteristic sites of precipitation include the synovial membrane, joint fluid, tendon sheaths, bursae, subcutaneous tissues, and kidneys. Asymptomatic crystal deposits can precede an acute crystal-induced synovitis.

The first MTP joint is the joint most often affected (greater than 70%). Involvement of the tarsometatarsal and carpometacarpal joints frequently occurs. Over time, chronic tophaceous gout develops with typical asymmetrical joint involvement. Tophaceous deposits occur in periarticular soft tissues and sometimes in synovium and subchondral bone. These can produce hard masses that may cause ulceration of the overlying skin and extrusion of chalky material.

Radiographic features include eccentric nodular soft tissue swelling. Soft tissue masses are especially suggestive of tophi when they have high density on radiographs due to microcalcifications often related to chronic renal disease. Soft tissue tophi may produce erosion of subjacent bone, including characteristic deposition in the olecranon bursa that may be associated with erosion of the olecranon.

Erosions are suggestive of gout if they are located at a distance from any joint. In many cases, though, they may be intra-articular and may be marginal in location, mimicking rheumatoid arthritis. However, other features are helpful for the diagnosis of gout: erosions are often large in size (greater than 5 mm), they are frequently oriented along the long axis of the bone, they are characteristically surrounded by a sclerotic border due to the long duration of disease, and there may be an "overhanging edge" of new bone partially surrounding them. Also, there is commonly relative preservation of joint space due to focal rather than diffuse loss of articular cartilage, and there is not extensive osteoporosis.

Sonography may demonstrate soft tissue tophi before they are radiographically evident. They appear as hyperechoic or heterogeneous masses, sometimes with acoustic shadowing due to calcifications, which may demonstrate hyperemia on power Doppler evaluation. The double contour sign, which is a hyperechoic irregular band over the superficial margin of cartilage and the presence of hypo- to hyperechoic, inhomogeneous material surrounded by a small anechoic rim, may also be suggestive of gout. Sonography may also be used to guide aspiration of a joint.

Computed tomography (CT) may be helpful to confirm the high density of a soft tissue tophus (often about 160 Hounsfield units), which is less than the density of hydroxyapatite deposits in calcific tendinitis. Dual-energy CT is a newer technology that is more specific in identifying urate deposits. MRI features may be misleading, as there may be hypointense masses within the synovium on T2-weighted images, mimicking pigmented villonodular synovitis.

Calcium Pyrophosphate Dihydrate (CPPD) Crystal Deposition Disease

CPPD crystal deposition disease is generally observed in middle-aged and elderly patients. The disease probably begins within the hyaline cartilage, where cartilaginous matrix is replaced by chondromucoid material, followed by crystal deposition. The crystals are then released into the joint. It is still not clear what actually triggers this process, but there does appear to be a correlation with aging. Many affected persons are asymptomatic, but in others, intermittent acute attacks of arthritis resemble gout (pseudogout). The correct diagnosis is established by the identification of typical CPPD crystals in synovial fluid. Sonography may also be helpful by demonstrating multiple sparkling hyperechoic dots without acoustic shadows in the joint fluid that are very suggestive of CPPD crystals.

CPPD deposition may be associated with two types of radiographic features, which are frequently combined: articular/periarticular calcification and arthropathy. Chondrocalcinosis is the presence of intra-articular calcium-containing salts, most commonly CPPD, within hyaline cartilage and/or fibrocartilage. Radiographically, calcium within the fibrocartilage is characteristically somewhat irregular, as seen in the menisci of the knee or the triangular fibrocartilage of the wrist. Calcification of hyaline cartilage along an articular surface appears as a fine, linear radiodensity closely paralleling the subjacent cortical margin. Capsular, synovial, ligament, and tendon calcifications are less frequent.

The joints most commonly involved with pyrophosphate arthropathy are the knee, the radiocarpal and midcarpal joints of the wrist, the MCP joints of the hand, the shoulder, and the hip. The joint changes that occur in this disorder resemble osteoarthritis, with joint space narrowing, bone sclerosis, and subchondral cyst formation. The unusual distribution of these findings, the small size of the osteophytes contrasting with the severity of the arthropathy, and the presence of chondrocalcinosis allow a specific diagnosis to be made. Involvement of the MCP joints, particularly the second and third, is characteristic of this disorder. Hemochromatosis also affects the MCP joints in a similar fashion, but all MCP joints are characteristically affected, and there may be large "hook-like" osteophytes along the radial aspect of the metacarpal heads.

Suggested Readings

1. Aletaha D, Neogi T, Silman AJ et al (2010) Rheumatoid arthritis classification criteria: an American College of Rheumatology/ European league against rheumatism collaborative initiative. Arthritis Rheum 62(9):2569–2581
2. Altman RD, Gold GE (2007) Atlas of individual radiographic features in osteoarthritis, revised. Osteoarthr Cartil 15(Suppl. A):A1–A56
3. Bohndorf K, Anderson A, Davies M, Imhof H, Woertler K (eds) (2016) Imaging of bones and joints. Thieme, NY, Stuttgart, pp 418–484
4. Buchmann RF (2004) Imaging of articular disorders in children. Radiol Clin N Am 42(1):151–168
5. Greenspan A (2003) Erosive osteoarthritis. Semin Musculoskelet Radiol 7(2):155–159
6. Gupta KB (2004) Radiographic evaluation of osteoarthritis. Radiol Clin N Am 42(1):11–41
7. Guermazi A, Hayashi D, Eckstein F et al (2013) Imaging osteoarthritis. Rheum Dis Clin N Am 39(1):67–105
8. Klecker RJ, Weissman BN (2003) Imaging features of psoriatic arthritis and Reiter's syndrome. Semin Musculoskelet Radiol 7(2):115–126
9. Klippel JR, Stone JH, Crofford LJ et al (2008) Primer on the rheumatic diseases, 13th edn. Springer, New York
10. Monu JU (2004) Gout: a clinical and radiologic review. Radiol Clin N Am 42(1):169–184
11. Rowbotham EL, Grainger AJ (2011) Rheumatoid arthritis: ultrasound versus MRI. AJR 197(3):541–546
12. Rudwaleit M, Landewé R, van der Heijde D et al (2009) The development of assessment of SpondyloArthritis international society classification criteria for axial spondyloarthritis (part I): classification of paper patients by expert opinion including uncertainty appraisal. Ann Rheum Dis 68(6):770–776
13. Rudwaleit M, van der Heijde D, Landewé R et al (2009) The development of assessment of SpondyloArthritis international society classification criteria for axial spondyloarthritis (part II): validation and final selection. Ann Rheum Dis 68(6):777–783
14. Rudwaleit M, van der Heijde D, Landewé R et al (2011) The assessment of SpondyloArthritis international society classification criteria for peripheral spondyloarthritis and for spondyloarthritis in general. Ann Rheum Dis 70(1):25–31
15. Sieper J, Rudwaleit M, Baraliakos X et al (2009) The assessment of SpondyloArthritis international society (ASAS) handbook: a guide to assess spondyloarthritis. Ann Rheum Dis 68(Suppl. 2):ii1–ii44

Multimodality Elbow Imaging with Emphasis on Magnetic Resonance Imaging

Michael J. Tuite and Laura W. Bancroft

Introduction

The elbow is a complex joint that may be affected by overuse, acute trauma, arthritis, inflammation and infection. When imaging is warranted for evaluation of pathology, radiographs are essential in the initial workup and cross-sectional imaging may be helpful for further evaluation depending on the suspected pathology. Sonography is particularly useful in assessing ligament and tendon injuries, identifying effusions or synovitis, and guiding percutaneous therapeutic injections. Computed tomography (CT) may be indicated in evaluating complex osseous injury after initial radiographs, and CT arthrography is an alternative to MRI in assessing tendons and ligaments when contraindications exist. For the purpose of this discussion, the normal and pathologic imaging characteristics of osseous and soft tissue elbow disorders will be focused on trauma, with an emphasis on magnetic resonance imaging (MRI) and MR arthrography.

Bones and Cartilage

Normal Anatomy

The elbow is composed of three individual joints, all within a single synovial-lined joint capsule [1–4]. The largest of these is the ulnotrochlear joint, where the trochlea (or medial condyle of the humerus) articulates with the sigmoid notch of the proximal ulna. The sigmoid notch forms a 190° arc when viewed from the side, and its distal margin is the coronoid process and its proximal margin the olecranon process. The trochlea is covered with articular cartilage throughout its 330° arc when viewed from the side. Above the trochlea anteriorly is the coronoid fossa, into which the coronoid process sits in full flexion. Above the trochlea posteriorly is the olecranon fossa into which the olecranon process sits in full extension.

Some of the stability of the elbow joint results from the shape of the trochlear and sigmoid notch articular surfaces. The sigmoid notch has medial and lateral surfaces that both slope upward to meet in the middle to form a longitudinally-oriented ridge (Fig. 1). The trochlea has corresponding medial and lateral surfaces that slope downward to form a longitudinally-oriented trough. This trough-like shape of the trochlea has been described as being like the groove in a pulley, and it provides medial-lateral stability to the elbow joint.

The second largest articulation in the elbow joint is the radiocapitellar joint. This joint does not contribute as much to the stability of the elbow because the radial head has a shallow articular surface, but the joint surfaces allow for forearm pronation-supination. The capitellum (or lateral condyle of the humerus) is covered by articular cartilage along its anterior and distal surfaces, but not posteriorly because the relatively small radial head does not contact the posterior capitellum even in full extension. This can be a source of confusion on coronal MR images because the posterior capitellum can appear irregular like an osteochondritis dissecans (OCD) lesion, when in fact this is the "bare area" where there is no articular cartilage (Fig. 2).

The third and smallest articulation in the elbow is the proximal radioulnar joint. This joint is between the peripheral margin of the radial head, and a small concavity in the lateral coronoid process termed the semilunar (or lesser sigmoid) notch. The semilunar notch is lined with articular cartilage, as is a variable portion of the medial radial head. This allows the joint surfaces to slide on each other during pronation and supination [1, 4].

M.J. Tuite (✉)
Department of Radiology, University of Wisconsin, 600 Highland Ave, Madison, WI 53792, USA
e-mail: mjtuite@wisc.edu

L.W. Bancroft
Department of Radiology, Florida Hospital, 601 E. Rollins, Orlando, FL 32803, USA
e-mail: Laura.bancroft.md@flhosp.org

J. Hodler et al. (eds.), *Musculoskeletal Diseases 2017-2020*, DOI 10.1007/978-3-319-54018-4_5

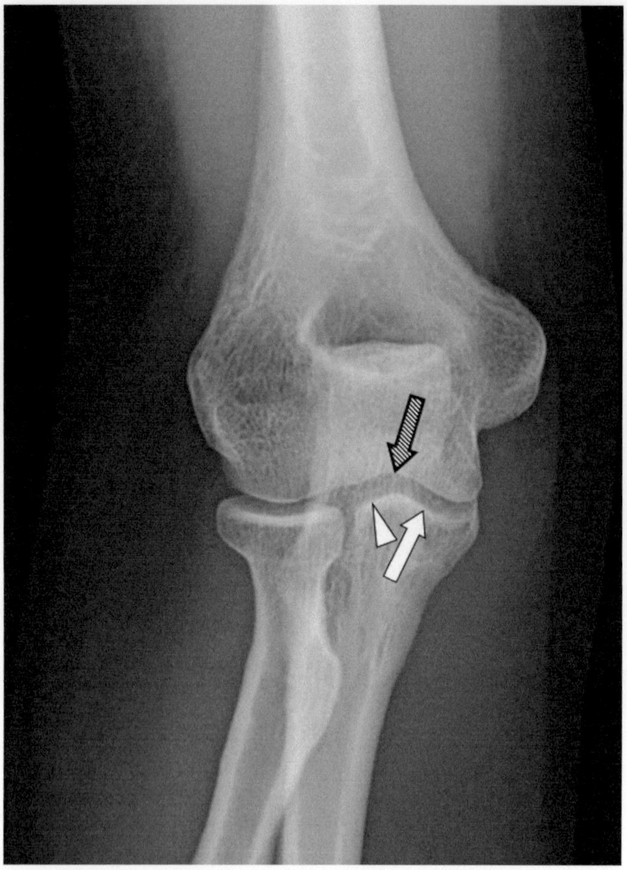

Fig. 1 Normal elbow. AP radiograph shows the medial (*white arrow*) and lateral (*arrowhead*) articular surfaces in the sigmoid notch that angle up to form a longitudinally-oriented ridge. The trochlea has corresponding sloped articular surfaces that angle down to meet in a longitudinally-oriented trough (*striped arrow*), that has been likened to the groove in a pulley

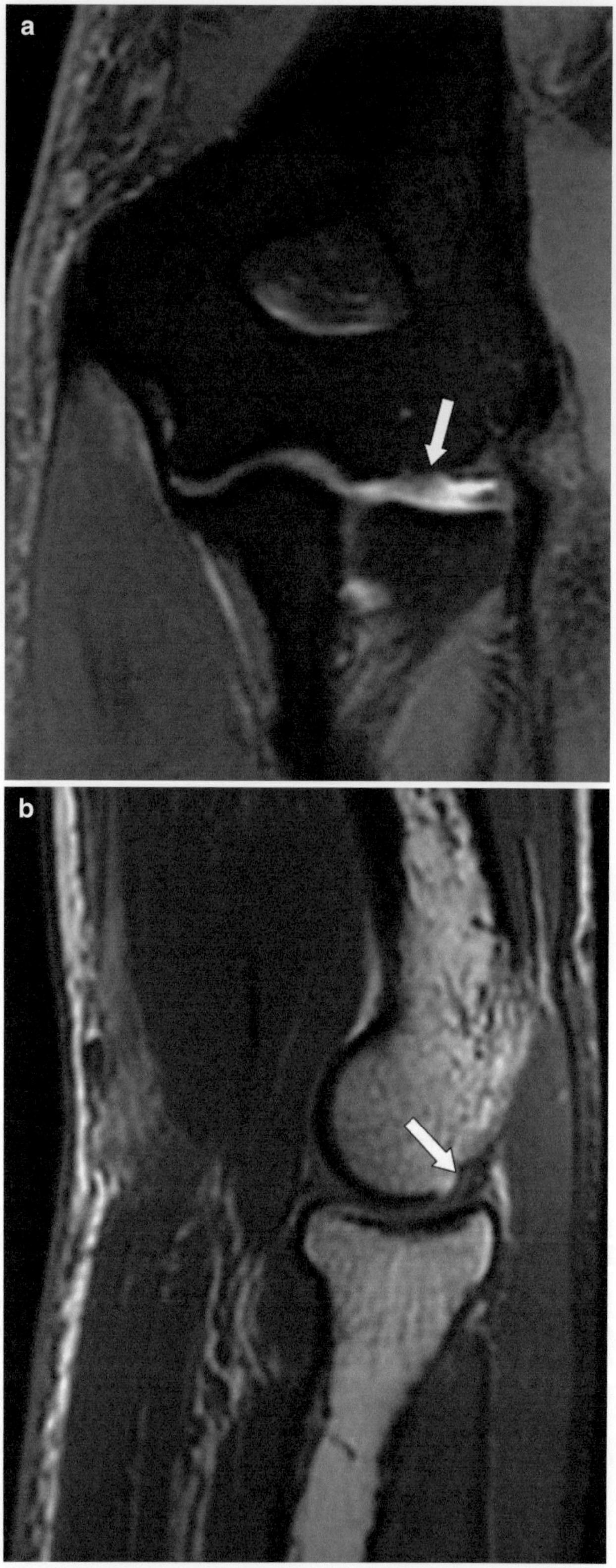

Fig. 2 (**a–b**) Pseudo-OCD of the capitellum. (**a**) Coronal fat-suppressed (FS) intermediate-weighted image shows apparent irregularity of the articular surface, or "pseudo-OCD" (*arrow*) of the capitellum. (**b**) Sagittal proton density image shows the normal bare area of the posteroinferior capitellum (*arrow*). The radial head articulates anterior to the bare area even when the elbow is fully extended

Above the elbow joint on the medial and lateral surfaces of the humerus sit the larger medial, and smaller lateral epicondyles. The medial epicondyle is the origin of the common flexor/pronator tendons, and the anterior and posterior bundles of the ulnar collateral ligament. The lateral epicondyle is the origin of the common extensor/supinator tendons, the radial collateral ligament, and the lateral ulnar collateral ligament (LUCL).

Bones and Cartilage: Normal Variants

There are several normal osseous variants of the elbow [3, 4]. Some individuals can have a ridge that runs transversely across the middle of the sigmoid notch dividing it into proximal and distal halves (Fig. 3). This ridge is variable in size and can be absent. The thickness of the articular cartilage on the ridge can be very thin, knowing this helps avoid confusing the ridge with a central osteophyte. At the medial and/or lateral margins of this ridge, there can be a small groove, which should not be confused with an osteochondral lesion (Fig. 4). Another osseous normal variant is when there is no osseous separation between the olecranon and coronoid fossae, called an olecranon foramen.

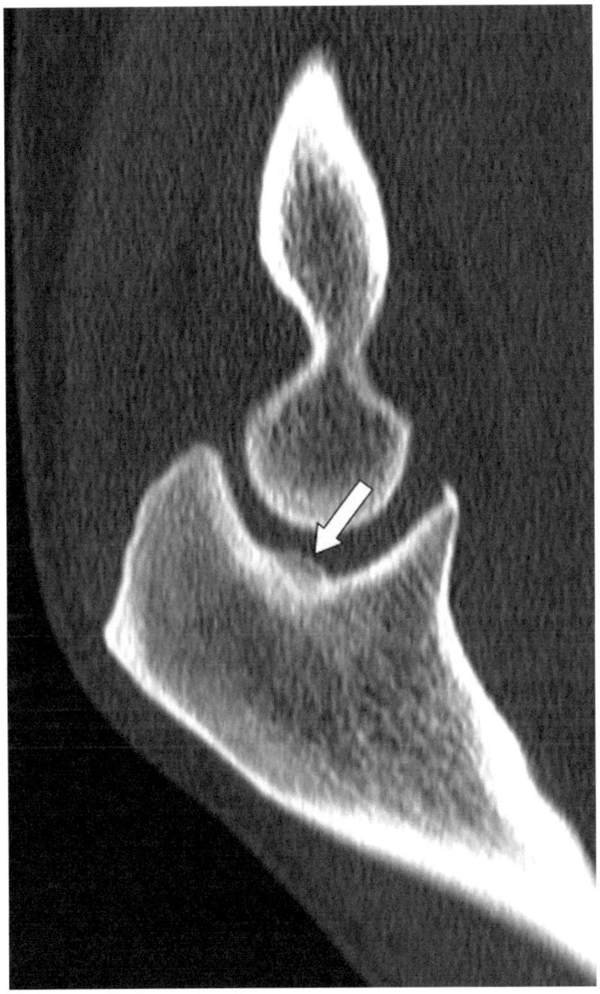

Fig. 3 Normal transverse sigmoid ridge. Sagittal reformatted CT image shows a normal variant transverse sigmoid ridge (*arrow*). This can be covered with imperceptibly-thin articular cartilage, and should not be confused with a pathologic central osteophyte

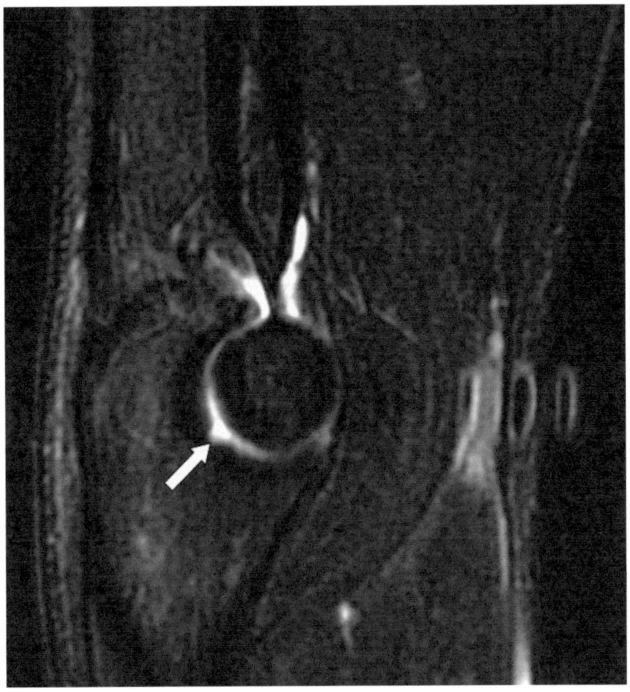

Fig. 4 Normal sigmoid groove. Sagittal T2-weighted FS image shows a normal variant sigmoid groove. These occur at the site of the fused olecranon physis, and should not be confused with a pathologic osteochondral defect

Bones and Cartilage: Pediatric Throwing Injuries

Because the ligaments and tendons in children are relatively strong relative to bone, pediatric throwers tend to get more osseous overuse elbow injuries compared to adult throwing athletes. The two main injuries in young throwers are therefore capitellar osteochondritis dissecans (OCD), and Little Leaguer's Elbow. The OCD in pediatric throwers typically involves the anterolateral aspect of the capitellum [5–8]. Although it usually occurs in the dominant throwing arm of 12–17 year old boys who are baseball pitchers, it can also be seen in young gymnasts and in other overhead sports such as tennis (Fig. 5). The OCD in gymnasts is often bilateral, and is felt to be due to similar repetitive shear forces to the elbow during hand springs or walking on their hands.

Most authors stress the difference between OCD and Panner disease. Panner disease is typically found in younger boys under 10 years old, and there is rarefaction and fragmentation of the entire capitellum rather than only the anterolateral portion. The condition is treated conservatively with rest, and is usually self-limited with reconstitution of

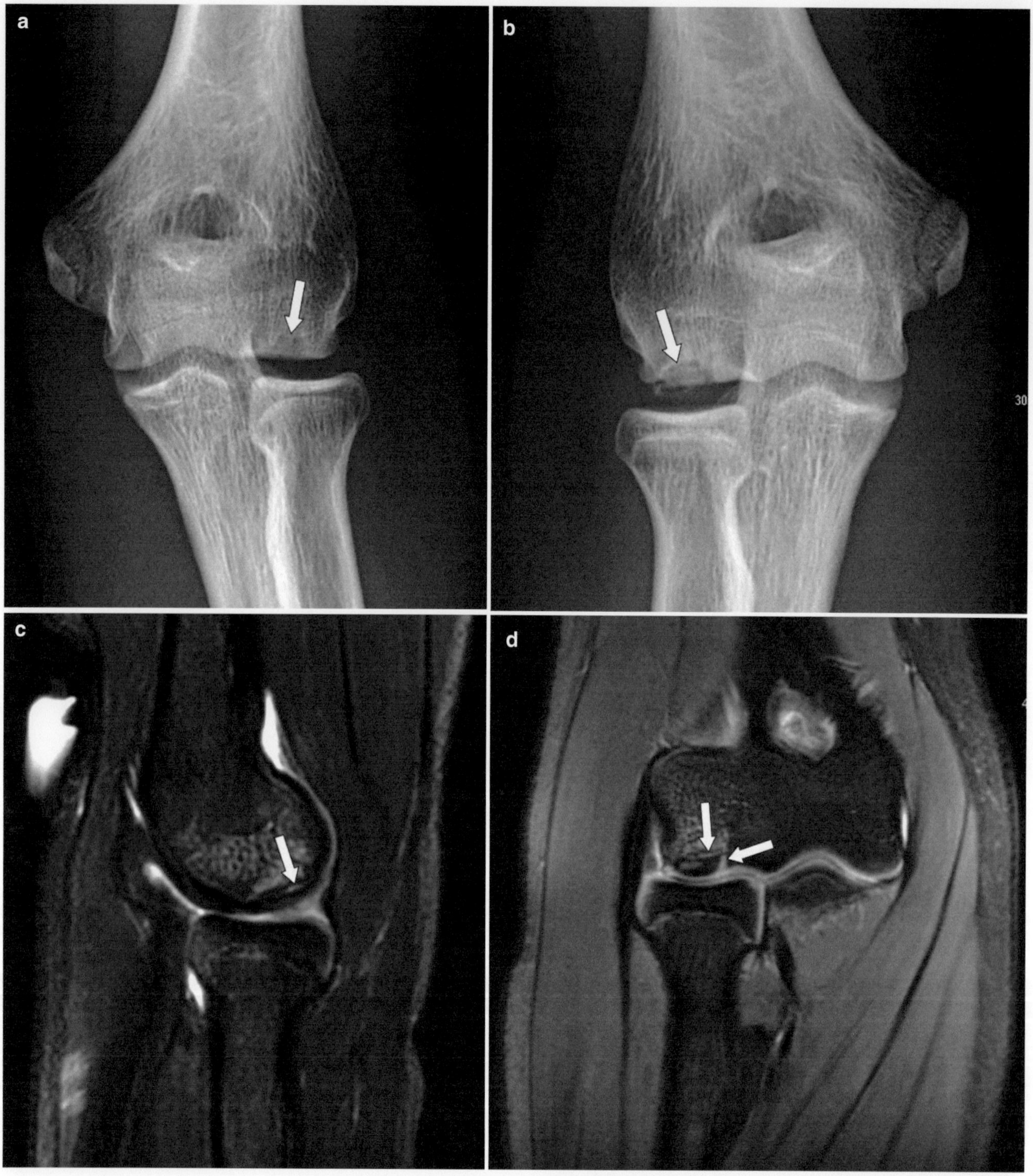

Fig. 5 (**a**–**d**) Bilateral osteochondritis dissecans in 12-year-old female gymnast. AP radiographs of the *left* (**a**) and *right* (**b**) elbow show bilateral osteochondritis dissecans (OCD) lesions (*arrows*) of the capitellum. On the *right elbow*, sagittal T2-weighted FS (**c**) and coronal intermediate-weighted FS (**d**) images show high signal at the interface (*arrows*) of the OCD fragment with the adjacent epiphysis. Because the capitellar physis is fused, this high signal indicates that the OCD is unstable

the capitellum and no long term sequelae. Although some authors report no history of trauma, others believe Panner disease is probably a similar manifestation of repetitive valgus load onto the capitellum, but in younger boys with an open capitellar physis [9].

Capitellar OCD can appear on radiographs as either a subtle area of osteopenia in the capitellum, flattening of the subchondral bone plate, or fragmentation. The subtle focal osteopenia of early OCDs can be difficult to see on radiographs, with some authors reporting that only about 1/2–2/3 are seen prospectively [7]. There are several radiographic, MR and arthroscopic grading systems for capitellar OCD that are used to separate early lesions from more advanced disease. The most important imaging determinant for the surgeon, however, is whether the OCD is stable or unstable. This is best determined with MR, and can often be done on routine T2-weighted images without intravenous or intraarticular contrast [1, 5, 8, 10]. Unstable capitellar OCD lesions will have linear increased T2 signal along most of the interface between the OCD fragment and the underlying epiphysis, or have cysts at this interface [6, 8]. If the increased signal involves only a portion of the interface in a child with an open capitellar physis, it may be stable [1, 8]. A full thickness articular cartilage fissure around the circumference of the OCD fragment is sometimes considered an additional sign of an unstable OCD.

Most capitellar OCD lesions do not heal with conservative management. Several authors have found that conservative treatment should only be pursued on patients who meet all three of the following criteria: (1) stable OCD on MR, (2) open capitellar physis, and (3) near-normal elbow motion [10, 11]. Because the majority of capitellar OCD lesions do not meet all three criteria, most either need surgery or will have a poor long term prognosis. About half of patients with a capitellar OCD will go on to have pain, reduced range of motion, or elbow degenerative change [11, 12].

Another injury in skeletally immature baseball pitchers is medial epicondyle apophysitis, also known as Little Leaguer's elbow [13, 14]. This is felt to be a chronic stress injury to the medial epicondylar physis from repetitive traction on the apophysis by the common flexor tendons and UCL from the valgus stress during throwing. The radiographic finding is abnormal widening of the physis, usually greater than 3 mm. The size of the apophysis is also often larger than that in the contralateral non-throwing elbow, probably from chronic hyperemia. On MRI in patients with Little Leaguer's elbow, the physis is wide and higher signal than normal, and there is typically adjacent bone marrow edema (Fig. 6).

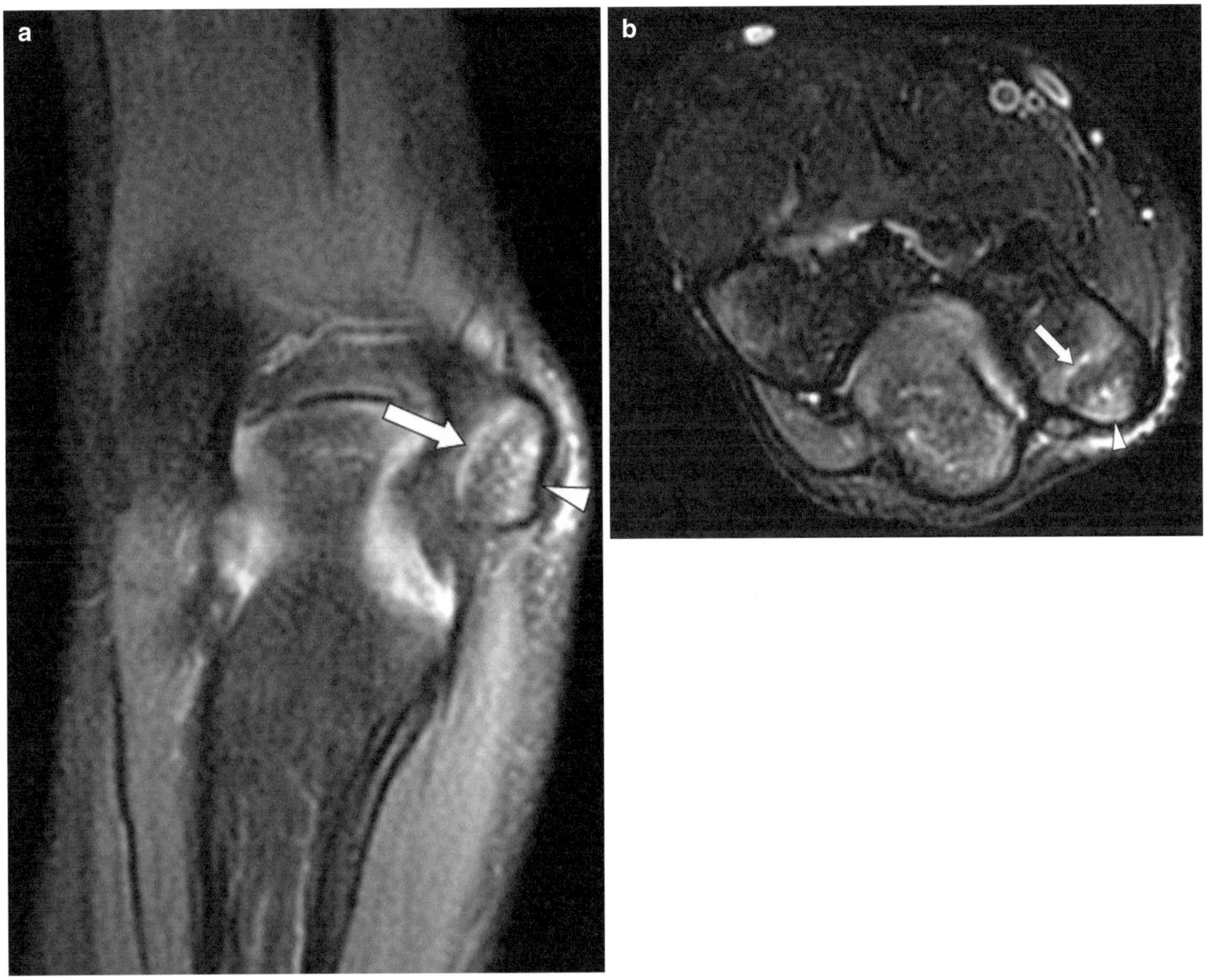

Fig. 6 (**a**, **b**) Little Leaguer's elbow in 13-year-old right-handed baseball pitcher with medial epicondyle pain. Coronal intermediate-weighted FS (**a**) and axial T2-weighted FS (**b**) images show increased high signal at the physis (*arrows*) and apophyseal marrow edema (*arrowhead*) consistent with little leaguer's elbow or medial apophysitis

Bones and Cartilage: Other Osseous and Chondral Abnormalities

The most common sites for fractures around the elbow after acute trauma are the radial head/neck and the olecranon process in adults, and supracondylar fractures in children [1]. MR can be helpful in imaging some patients with acute elbow trauma, particularly if a fracture is suspected clinically but the radiographs only show an effusion (Fig. 7). Radiographically, occult fractures will appear as linear low signal on T1-weighted images, with a variable signal-intensity fracture line on T2-weighted images with surrounding marrow edema.

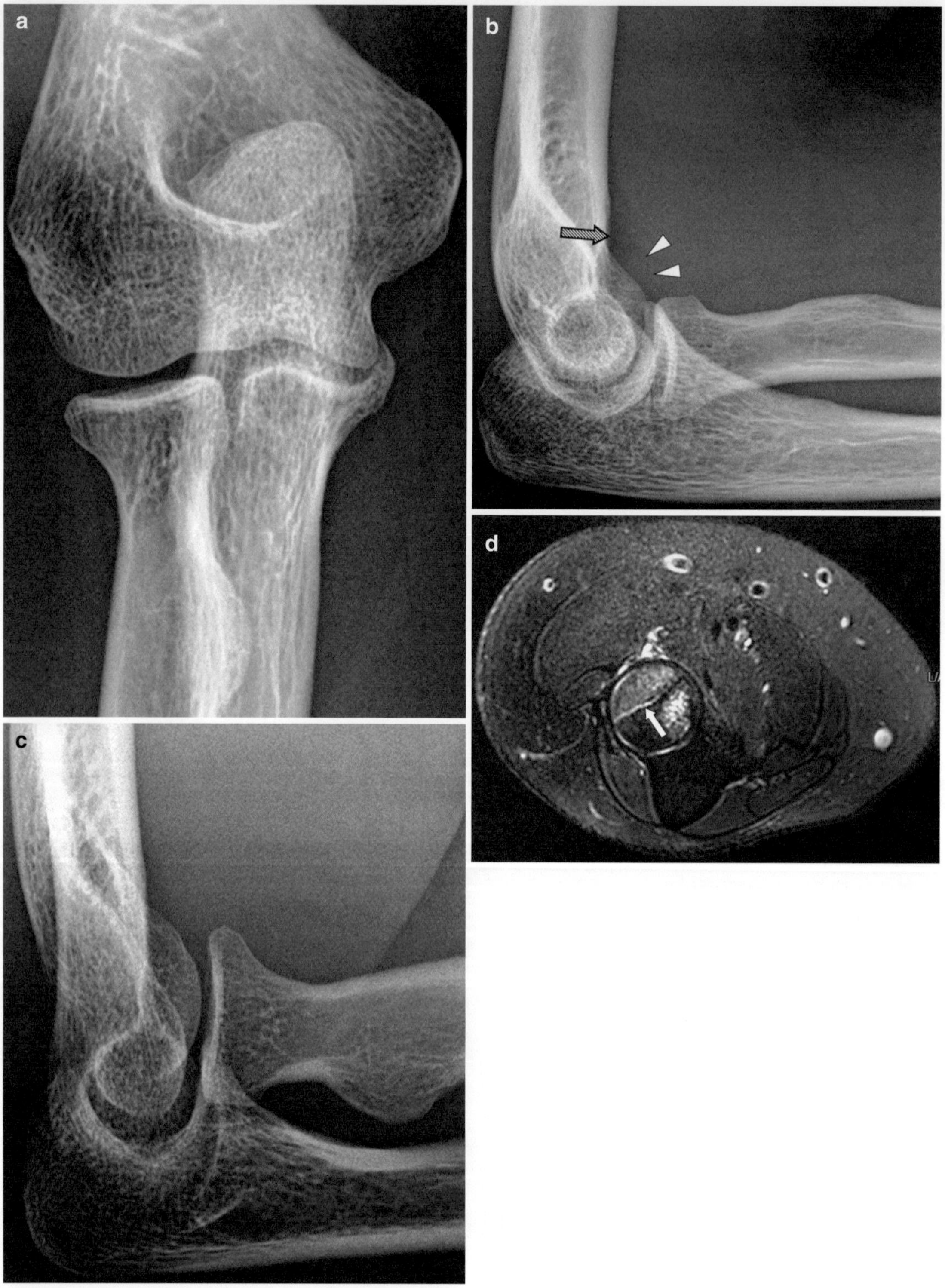

Fig. 7 (**a–d**) Radial head fracture in 33-year-old woman with elbow pain after fall. (A) Anteroposterior (**a**), lateral (**b**), and radial head (**c**) radiographic views show the anterior fat pad (*striped arrow*) becomes obscured distally (*arrowheads*) by an effusion. No fracture was seen. (**d**) Axial T2-weighted FS image 1 month later shows a subacute minimally-displaced radial head fracture (*arrow*)

Elbow dislocations can also result in fractures, often involving the coronoid process. Isolated coronoid process fractures can be small yet the patients can have significant ligamentous injuries [15]. Although patients with a small isolated coronoid process fracture after elbow dislocation may do well with casting and conservative management, those that demonstrate a "drop sign" on lateral radiographs often require surgery [16]. The injury of a coronoid process fracture, radial head fracture, and posterior dislocation is called the elbow "terrible triad," and these patients are at high risk for chronic instability [15]. Another osteochondral injury that can be seen after elbow dislocation is the Osborne-Cotterill lesion, an osteochondral fracture of the posterolateral capitellum with or without an impaction defect of the radial head. These patients often do not heal their LUCL and thus have posterolateral rotary instability.

MR can also be helpful in patients with degenerative change who have pain and restricted range of motion. MR is more sensitive for detecting loose bodies within the elbow, which can be removed arthroscopically to give patients improved range of motion.

Muscles and Tendons

Normal Anatomy

The muscles and tendons around the elbow can be divided into four main groups [2]. Medially, many of the wrist and hand flexors and pronators make up the common flexor-pronator tendon which arises from the medial epicondyle [17]. The flexor carpi ulnaris, and to a lesser extent the flexor digitorum superficialis, overlie the anterior bundle of the ulnar collateral ligament and provide secondary dynamic stabilization against varus stress.

The lateral tendon origins are more complex. The extensor carpi radialis brevis, extensor carpi ulnaris, and extensor digitorum superficialis arise from the lateral epicondyle as the common extensor/supinator tendon. The extensor carpi radialis longus and the brachioradialis arise from the anterolateral aspect of the distal humerus, anterior to the lateral epicondyle proper. The supinator muscle also has part of its origin from the lateral epicondyle, although portions also arise more distally including from the lateral proximal crest of the ulna. The supinator muscle wraps around, and then inserts broadly onto the ulna.

The main anterior muscles/tendons are the biceps and the brachialis. The deeper brachialis inserts onto the proximal ulna including at the base of the coronoid process. The more superficial biceps tendon dives lateral to the brachialis to insert onto the bicipital tuberosity located along the posteromedial aspect of the radius distal to the radial head. The two heads of the biceps sometimes have well defined continuations distally. In these cases, the tendinous continuation of the long head inserts more proximally onto the bicipital tuberosity and has a broad attachment. The short head of the biceps inserts more distal and posteriorly, so has greater mechanical advantage as a supinator of the forearm. The bicipitoradialis bursa separates the distal tendon from the anteromedial radius. The lacertus fibrosis (or bicipital aponeurosis) is a thickening of the anteromedial fascia of the biceps muscle that then courses superficial to the brachial artery and median nerve to insert onto the deep fascia of the anterior forearm.

The main posterior muscles/tendons are the triceps and the anconeus. The triceps is comprised of the long, medial, and lateral heads, and has a broad insertion onto the olecranon process. The long head originates from the infraglenoid tubercle of the scapula, while the medial and lateral heads originate from the humerus. The long head has the longest tendon distally before inserting onto the olecranon process, while the medial and lateral heads remain as muscles fairly distally with short tendons forming just proximal to their insertions. The anconeus is a small muscle that arises posterior to the lateral epicondyle and inserts onto the lateral aspect of the olecranon process. The anconeus muscle is superficial to the annular ligament and therefore may help stabilize the radial head.

Muscles and Tendons: Normal Variant

A muscle normal variant is an absent palmaris longus tendon. This variant can be important to note on MR images because the palmaris longus tendon is often used in surgical reconstructions of the wrist and hand.

Muscles and Tendons: Muscle Injuries

Muscle injuries about the elbow are uncommon, but range from delayed-onset muscle soreness (DOMS), strain, and ultimately rupture at the extreme end of the spectrum [18]. Patients with delayed-onset muscle soreness typically present with muscle pain hours to days after eccentric muscle contractions, with maximal symptoms 2 days after imaging. Consideration for imaging after overuse does not usually occur unless there is a diagnosis of rhabdomylosis or other complicating features. Abnormalities will be evident as enlarged, edematous muscles on MRI of the affected muscle groups, usually in the anterior compartment (Fig. 8).

Muscle strain is most common along the myotendinous junction, but can also occur peripherally within the muscle belly. Of note, peripheral strains typically result in extended time until return to play. Frank muscle rupture about the elbow is very rare, and is often secondary to traumatic elbow dislocation (Fig. 9) or crush injury. MRI is useful in delineating the extent of involvement, providing quantitative measurement of muscle tearing for treatment decisions, and assessing healing on subsequent followup.

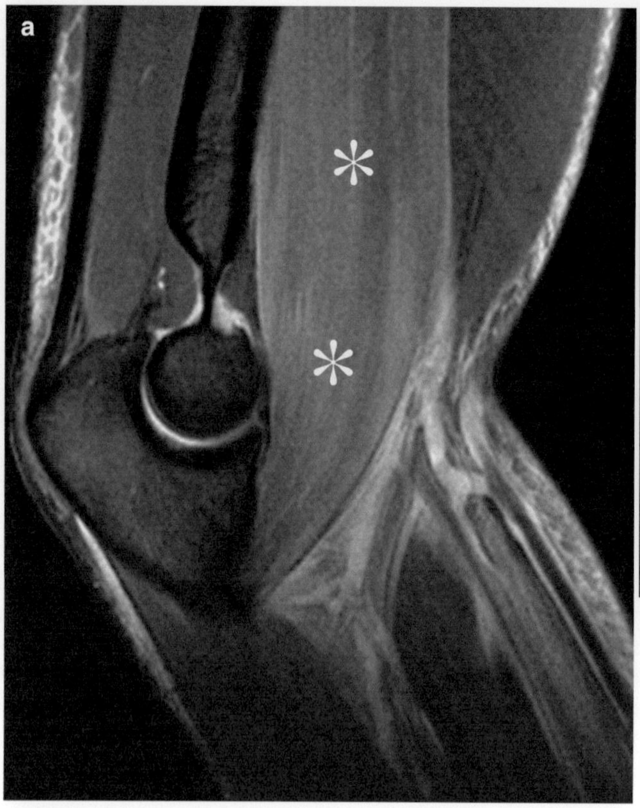

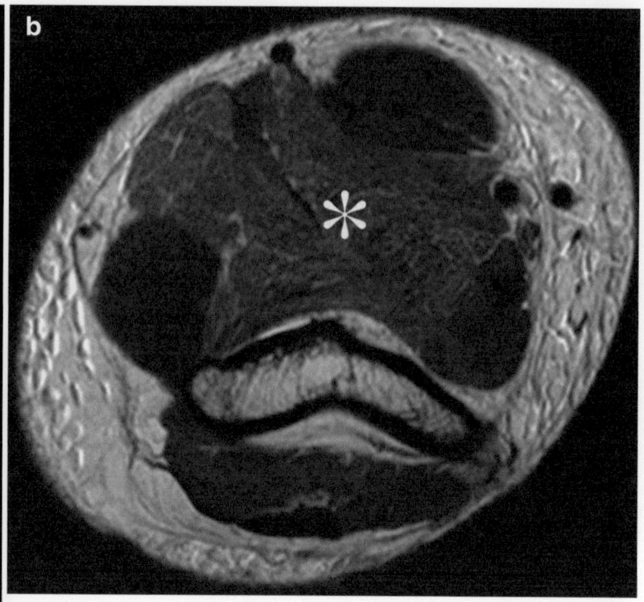

Fig. 8 (**a**–**b**) Brachialis rhabdomyolysis in 25-year-old man with arm pain and swelling 2 days after crossfit workout. Sagittal (**a**) and axial. (**b**) PD images demonstrate increased signal intensity within the enlarged brachialis muscle (*asterisks*) and subcutaneous edema-like signal changes. Patient had an elevated creatine kinase level of 33,840 units/l

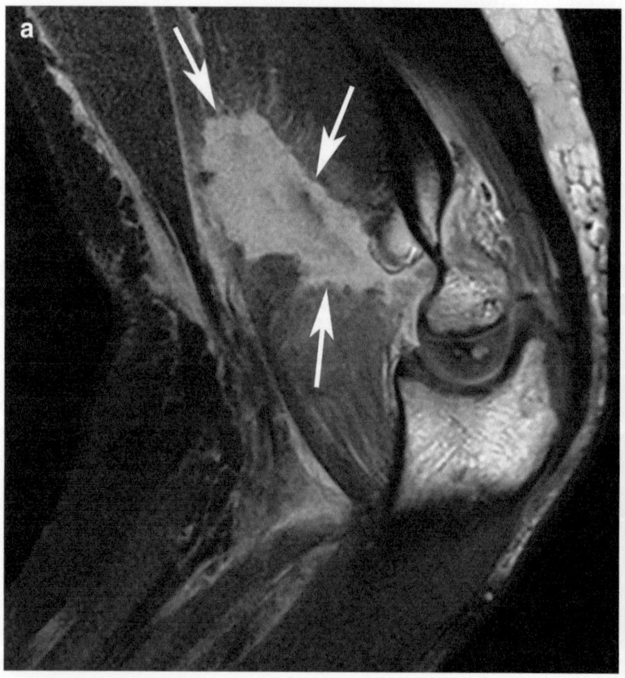

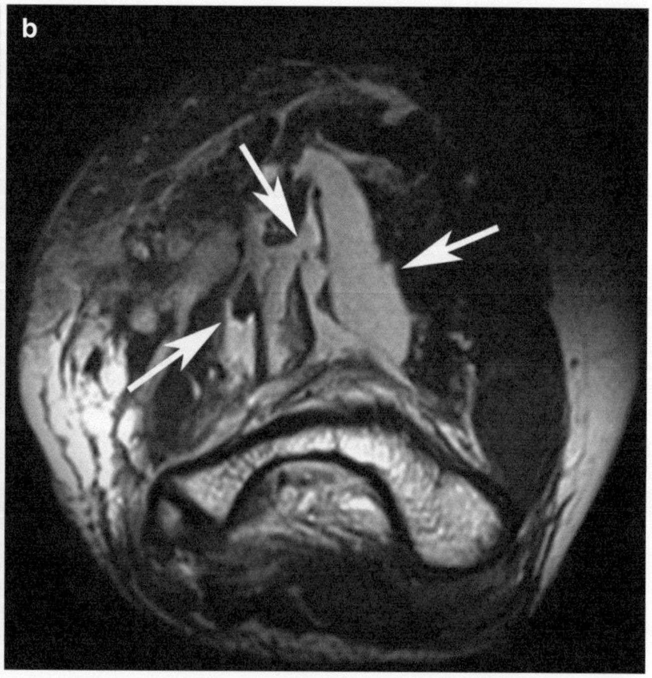

Fig. 9 (**a**–**d**) Brachialis muscle tear and brachial artery occlusion in 13-year-old boy after elbow dislocation. Sagittal (**a**) and axial (**b**) PD images show rupture of nearly the entire distal brachialis muscle (*arrows*). (**c**) Coronal 2D reconstruction from computed tomographic arteriogram (CTA) shows occlusion of the brachial artery (*arrowhead*) and adjacent hemorrhage (*asterisk*) in the brachialis defect. (**d**) 3D maximum intensity projection (MIP) from CTA shows occlusion of the brachial artery (*arrowhead*), with distal reconstitution (*arrow*)

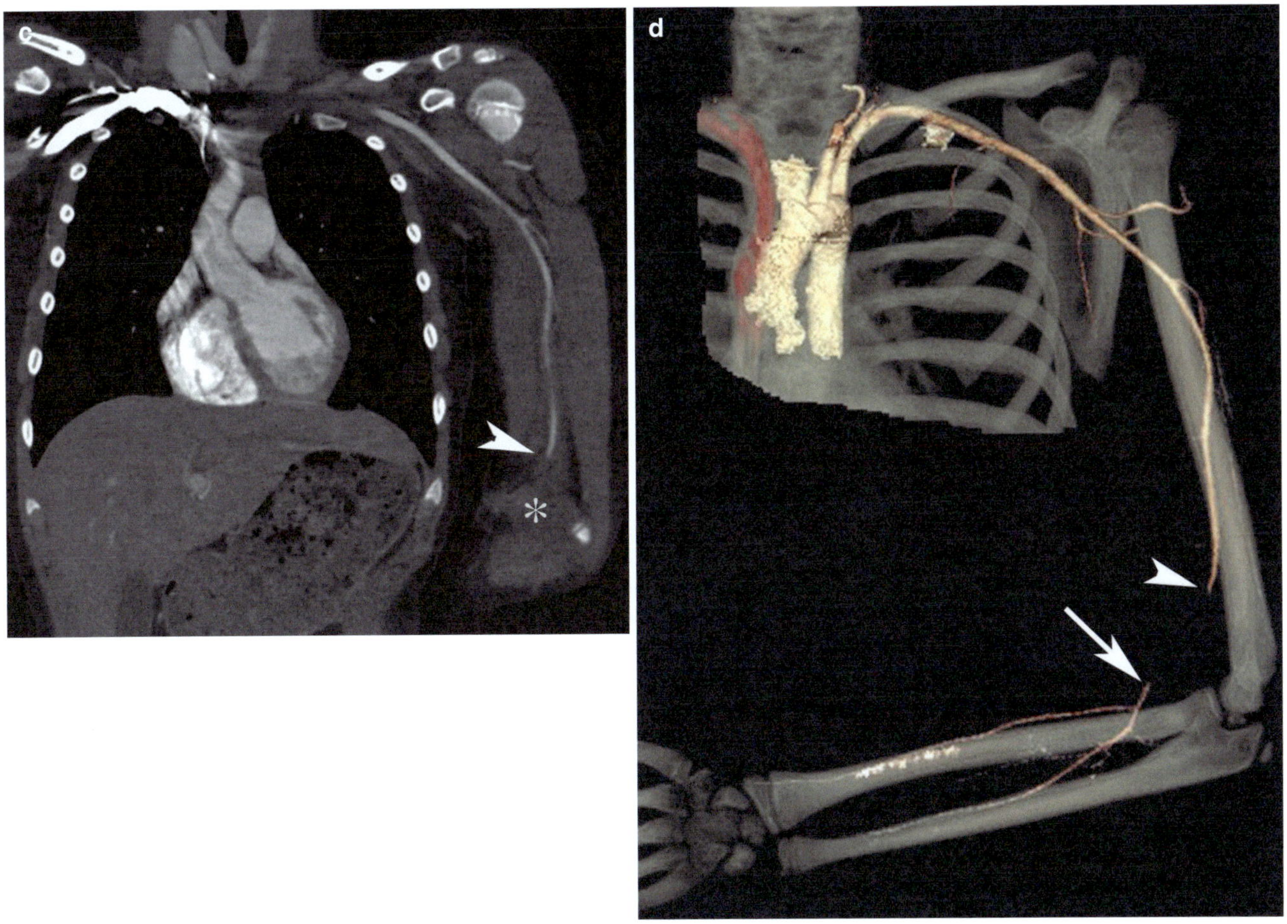

Fig. 9 (continued)

Muscles and Tendons: Tendon Injuries

Common Extensor Tendon Origin

The most common cause of elbow pain is "tennis elbow," otherwise known as "lateral epicondylitis." Common extensor tendon origin pathology classically presents in patients in the 4th or 5th decades with pain and point tenderness overlying the lateral epicondyle and pain with resisted wrist extension [19–22]. This degenerative process caused by repetitive microtrauma and is typically diagnosed clinically. If imaging is performed in equivocal or recalcitrant cases, findings include thinning, partial-thickness tearing or rupture of the common extensor tendon origin. Tendinosis will be evident as either tendon thickening or thinning, and intermediate T1- and T2-weighted signal intensity on MRI.

Partial- or full-thickness tears will demonstrate fluid signal within the discontinuous portion of the tendon [19–22]. Of importance, MRI or sonography may be helpful to exclude concomitant lateral ulnar collateral ligament complex tears, which can result in persistent instability and pain.

Common Flexor-Pronator Tendon Origin

Common flexor-pronator tendon origin pathology is also called "golfer's elbow." Repetitive overuse and microtearing of the flexor-pronator tendons in middle-aged and older individuals can result in progressive degeneration [17, 20]. Medial sided tendon injury is far less common than lateral sided pathology, and can occur in golfers, bowlers, swimmers, tennis players, and throwing athletes. Clinically, patients present with gradual onset of medial elbow pain and weakened grip. MRI or sonography may be warranted in patients with refractory medial elbow pain, and can exclude other etiologies.

Biceps Tendon

Biceps tendon injuries can be caused by caused by overuse from repetitive throwing, overhead activities or forced elbow flexion. Football players, weight-lifters and bodybuilders have the highest reported distal biceps tendon injuries, and risk further increases in men who smoke or use anabolic steroids [17, 23]. Injuries of the distal biceps are much less common than those involving the proximal biceps, and usually occur near the insertion onto the radial tuberosity. Partial-thickness tears are more common than full-thickness rupture, and tears can involve either the long or short head of the biceps. MRI and sonography are useful in presurgical planning of full-thickness tears, and imaging reports should include the degree of proximal retraction and the quality of the tendinous remnant (Fig. 10).

Triceps Tendon

Injuries of the triceps tendon are very rare, are often caused by a fall on an outstretched hand and usually occur near the olecranon insertion. Triceps tendon rupture can be partial or complete, can range from millimeters to centimeters in width, and almost always involve the lateral head insertion. Triceps tendon rupture will have adjacent soft tissue swelling, and may have olecranon bursal fluid and/or an associated small olecranon tip avulsion fracture, (Fig. 11). MRI is useful in excluding concomitant radial head fracture, capitellar fracture and ulnar collateral ligament rupture that can be associated with triceps tendon injuries [17, 20].

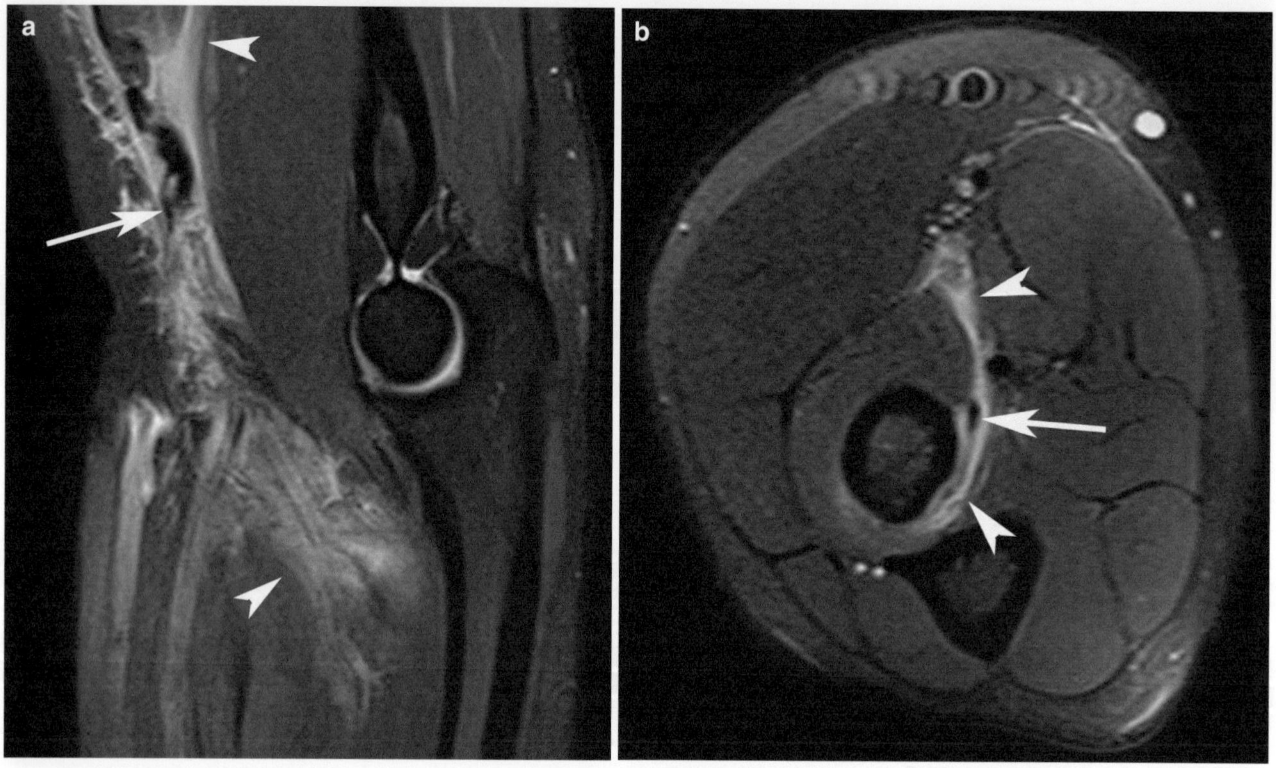

Fig. 10 (**a**, **b**) Distal biceps rupture in 44-year-old man after lifting heavy couch. (**a**) Sagittal PD FS image shows proximal retraction of both heads of the ruptured biceps tendon (*arrow*) and hyperintense hemorrhage (*arrowheads*) throughout the anterior arm and elbow soft tissues. (**b**) Axial PD FS image shows the distal biceps remnant (*arrowhead*) near its attachment onto the bicipital tuberosity and surrounding hemorrhage (*arrowheads*)

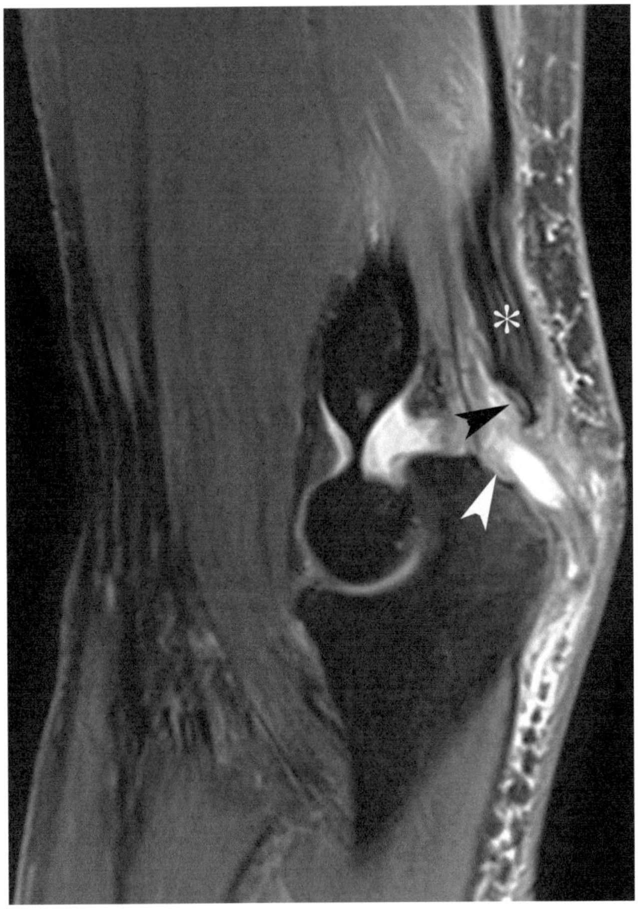

Fig. 11 Triceps tendon rupture and avulsion fracture in 54-year-old woman after fall. Sagittal PD FS image demonstrates small olecranon avulsion fracture (*arrowheads*) at the attachment of the triceps (*asterisk*)

Ligaments

Normal Anatomy

On the medial side of the elbow joint, the ulnar collateral ligament is comprised of three bundles—the anterior, posterior and transverse bundles. The anterior bundle originates from the undersurface of the medial epicondyle and inserts onto the sublime tubercle of the ulna. The anterior bundle can be separated into two bands which are taut during different portions of flexion/extension. The anterior band of the anterior bundle is the main static stabilizer of the elbow against valgus and internal rotation stress. The posterior bundle originates from the posterior aspect of the medial epicondyle and inserts on the medial aspect of the olecranon process, and forms the floor of the cubital tunnel. The transverse bundle originates from the medial tip of the olecranon process and inserts along the medial aspect of the coronoid process. Because the transverse bundle connects two points on the ulna and does not cross the elbow joint, it plays a minor role in stabilizing the elbow.

On the lateral side of the elbow joint, the lateral collateral ligament complex is made up of the radial collateral, the LUCL, and the annular ligaments [24]. The radial collateral ligament arises from the lateral epicondyle and inserts on the anterolateral aspect of the annular ligament. The annular ligament originates from the anterior margin of the semilunar notch, encircles the periphery of the radial head, and inserts onto the supinator crest of the ulna. The LUCL originates with, and is indistinguishable from, the lateral epicondylar origin of the radial collateral ligament, and inserts with the annular ligament onto the supinator crest of the ulna (Fig. 12). Although these three components of the lateral collateral ligament complex are described separately, studies show that they function as a continuous sheet to resist excessive varus and external rotational stress [24].

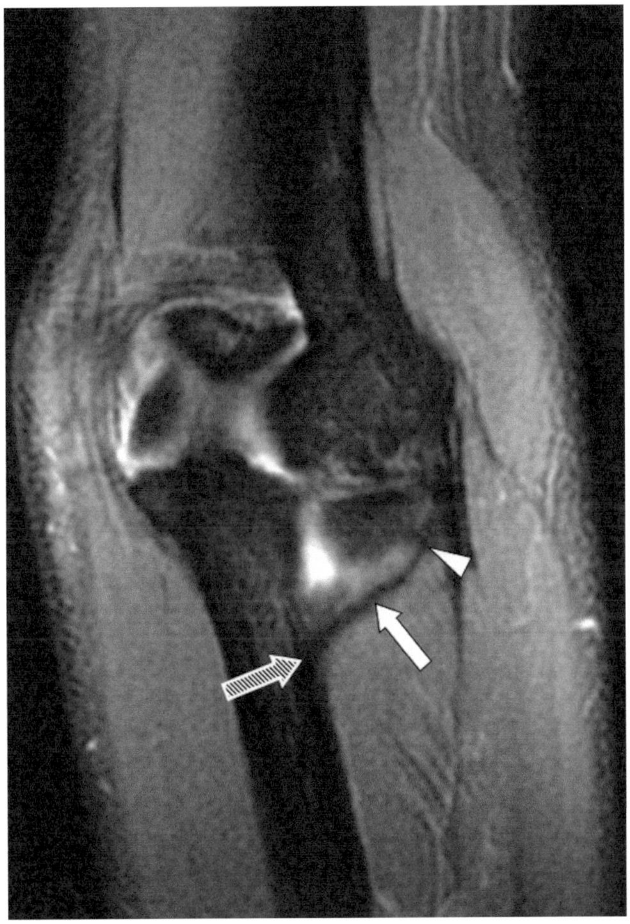

Fig. 12 Normal lateral ulnar collateral ligament. Coronal intermediate-weighted FS image shows the distal portion of the lateral ulnar collateral ligament (LUCL) (*arrow*) as it wraps around the posterior aspect of the radial neck (*arrowhead*) and inserts onto the supinator crest of the ulna (*striped arrow*)

Ligaments: Normal Variants

There are several ligament normal variants around the elbow [25]. Twenty-three percent of people have an accessory ulnar collateral ligament which originates on the posterior joint capsule and inserts onto the transverse bundle. Laterally in the elbow, one third of individuals have an accessory lateral collateral ligament which runs from the annular ligament to the supinator crest of the ulna. Also, some people may lack a LUCL. In addition, there is often a synovial fold (also called a plica or synovial fringe) in the posterolateral portion of the joint [4]. This is thickened in some people, and a subset of patients can have posterolateral elbow pain.

Ligament Injuries

Radial Collateral Ligament

Injuries to the radial collateral ligament complex can occur in conjunction with advanced cases of tennis elbow or trauma leading to posterolateral rotary subluxation. Tears can involve one or more of the three bundles (Fig. 13), but the lateral ulnar collateral ligament (LUCL) is the most important in terms of stability [14]. LUCL tears usually involve the humeral origin, and failure to recognize radial collateral ligament tears (particularly the LUCL) prior to surgical treatment of tennis elbow will lead to persistent postoperative symptoms (Fig. 14).

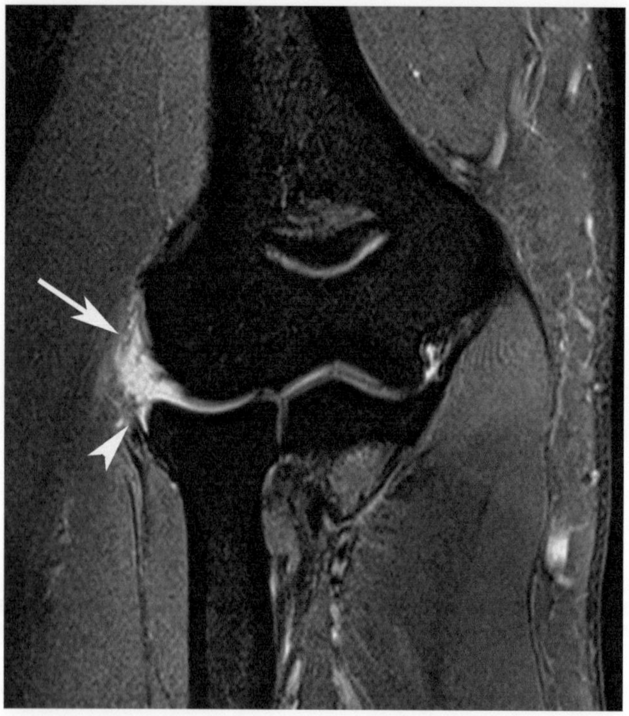

Fig. 13 Radial collateral ligament (RCL) and common extensor tendon rupture in 41-year-old man. Coronal PD FS image shows avulsion of the common extensor tendon origin (*arrow*) and the distal remnant of the ruptured RCL proper (*arrowhead*)

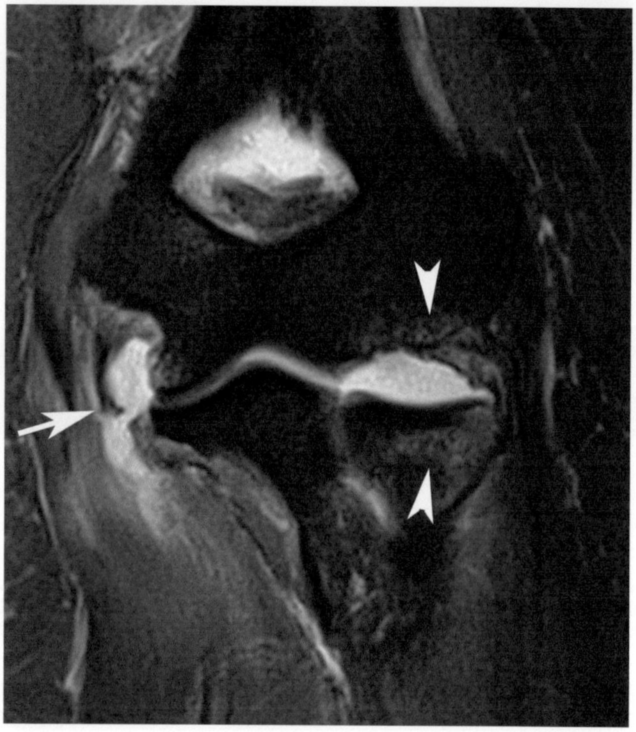

Fig. 14 Ulnar collateral ligament (UCL) rupture in 48-year-old woman with severe elbow pain and decreased range of motion. Coronal PD FS image shows distal avulsion of the anterior band of the UCL (*arrow*) and contusions (*arrowheads*) of the capitellum and radial head

Ulnar Collateral Ligament

Overhead throwing sports can result in medial elbow tension overload, lateral compression and extension overload. Medial elbow pain caused by excessive valgus forces and high pitching velocities can occur in overhead throwing athletes of all ages, and have been reported with baseball, football, javelin throwing, volleyball, golf and polo [14]. Injury to the ulnar (medial) collateral ligament is a common cause of medial elbow pain and valgus instability in athletes. Sonography may demonstrate hypoechoic and thickened ligaments with tendinosis, as well as classic findings for partial or complete ligamentous disruption. MRI may demonstrate increased T2-weighted signal within the ligament, most commonly the anterior band. Articular sided tears may occur anywhere along the tendon, and stripping of the distal ligamentous attachment may result in a "T sign" with contrast extension between the sublime tubercle and UCL [14, 20]. Complete rupture will show discontinuity of the ligament and extravasation of joint fluid or contrast through the ligamentous defect (Fig. 12).

Ligaments: Postoperative

Ligaments that have been either primarily repaired with sutures, reattached with bioabsorable or metallic suture anchors, or reconstructed with cadaveric or autologous grafts will not have the normal imaging appearance as native ligaments. It is important to recognize that intact postoperative ulnar and lateral collateral ligaments may be thicker and more heterogeneous in signal intensity than native ligaments, but tears can be detected by the same criteria of partial or complete ligamentous discontinuity (Fig. 15). High-level athletes with ulnar collateral ligament insufficiency may undergo "Tommy Johns" surgery or UCL reconstruction (Fig. 16). In a study of 51 patients who underwent MRI after UCL reconstruction, Wear and colleagues found that the normal intact UCL graft was thickened (because of double-bundle grafts and suturing of the graft to the native ligament) and variable in signal, but almost three fourths of the graft were homogeneously low signal on both T1- and T2-weighted images [26]. Intact grafts should be taut, and wavy grafts may be torn or insufficient. The Birmingham group

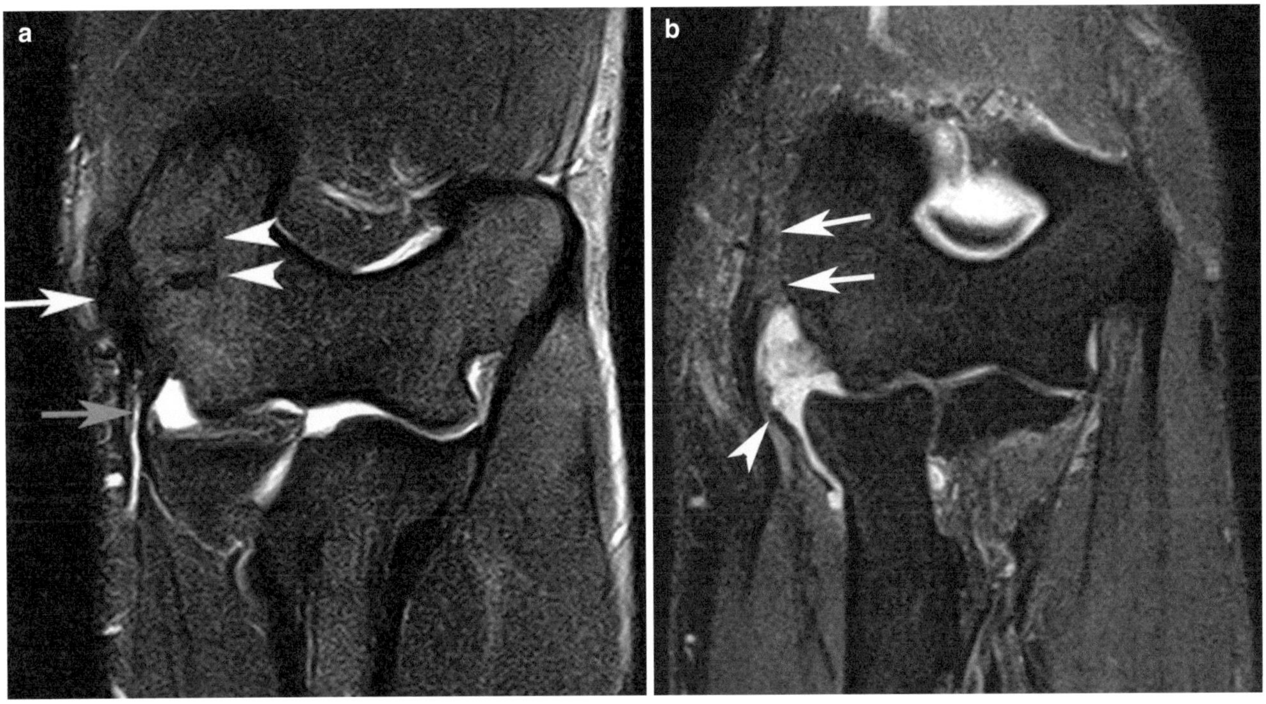

Fig. 15 (**a**, **b**) Intact common extensor tendon repair in two patients. (**a**) Coronal PD FS shows mild thickening of the intact, reattached common extensor tendon origin (*white arrow*) and underlying bioabsorbable suture anchors (*arrowheads*). Note the intact radial collateral ligament proper (*gray arrow*). (**b**) Coronal PD FS image in a 60-year-old man shows an intermediate signal but intact common extensor tendon (*arrows*) and torn underlying RCL complex (*white arrowhead*). Patient had recurrent pain and instability after undergoing fasciotomy, debridement and repair of the common extensor tendon 10 months previously

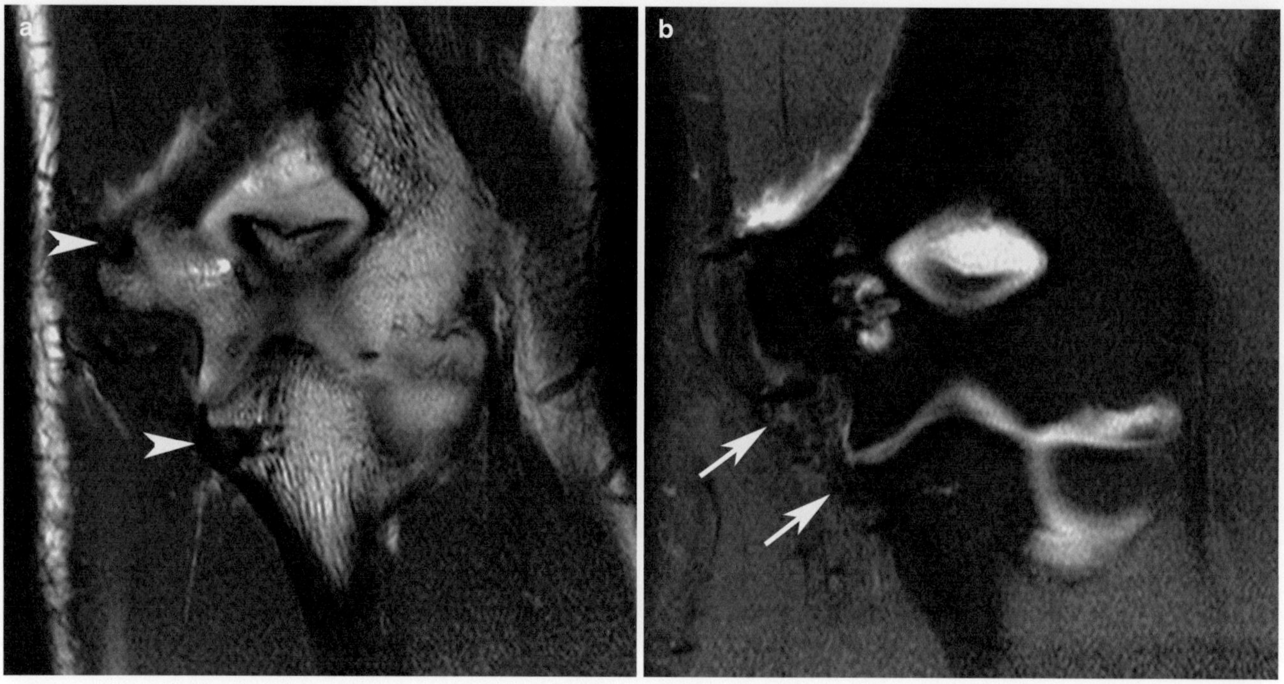

Fig. 16 Intact UCL reconstruction in 27-year-old professional baseball pitcher. (**a**, **b**). Coronal T1-weighted arthrographic images without (**a**) and with fat suppression (**b**) show the osseous tunnels (*arrowheads*) and intact UCL ligament graft (*arrows*). Grafts are thicker and typically more heterogeneous than native ligaments, and are anchored slightly distal to the sublime tubercle

prefers MR arthrographic evaluation of grafts since it can detect extension of contrast through discontinuous grafts. Of note, contrast may extend between the distal reconstructed UCL and the sublime tubercle due to distal attachment of the graft compared with the native ligament, and should not be interpreted as partial thickness tearing [26].

Nerves

Normal Anatomy

The three major nerves that course near the elbow are the ulnar, radial and median nerves. The ulnar nerve passes by the elbow joint within the cubital tunnel, which is posterior to the medial epicondyle. The floor of the cubital tunnel is made up of the posterior cortex of the medial epicondyle and the posterior bundle of the UCL. Most people have a retinaculum that covers the cubital tunnel and the ulnar nerve, and extends between the tip of the medial epicondyle and the medial aspect of the olecranon process.

The radial nerve at the level of the elbow runs within the radial tunnel, which is a space bounded mainly between the brachioradialis and brachialis muscles. Within the radial tunnel it passes by the fascial edge of the brachioradialis muscle, the tendinous edge of the extensor carpi radialis brevis muscle, and recurrent radial artery branches (the Leash of Henry). Just distal to the elbow the nerve divides into two branches, a motor branch which then dives deep to the superficial head of the supinator muscle which is called the posterior interosseous nerve (PIN), and a sensory branch called the superficial radial nerve. Proximal to the supinator muscle, motor branches arise to innervate the brachioradialis and supinator muscles, and sometimes the extensor carpi radialis longus and brevis muscles [27]. After passing the superficial head of the supinator muscle, the PIN typically innervates the extensor digitorum, extensor carpi ulnaris, anconeus, extensor pollicis longus and brevis, extensor indicis, and abductor pollicis longus muscles. The superficial radial nerve provides sensation to the dorsal forearm distal to the lateral epicondyle, as well as the back of the hand.

The median nerve runs deep to the lacertus fibrosis and medial to the brachial artery and biceps brachii muscles in the antecubital fossa. The nerve gives off motor branches to multiple muscles at the level of the elbow before it gives off the anterior interosseous nerve (AIN), a motor branch like the PIN. The AIN innervates the flexor pollicis longus muscle and the lateral portion of the flexor digitorum profundus muscle.

Nerves: Normal Variants

A small percentage of patients do not have a cubital tunnel retinaculum. Not having a retinaculum can allow the ulnar nerve to sublux out of the cubital tunnel, although this is typically asymptomatic [28]. The accessory anconeus (or anconeus epitrochlearis) muscle is a normal variant that is present in 3–28% of people. It replaces the cubital tunnel retinaculum, and originates from the posterior aspect of the medial epicondyle of the humerus and inserts onto the medial aspect of the olecranon process.

In addition to asymptomatic subluxation of the ulnar nerve, another normal variant for nerves around the elbow is where the median nerve distal to the elbow courses posterior to the brachial (ulnar) artery instead of running alongside it, although still between the pronator teres and brachialis muscles [4].

Non-Throwing Nerve Abnormalities

Ulnar Nerve

Cubital tunnel syndrome is the second most common neuropathy in the upper extremity, after carpal tunnel syndrome. In cubital tunnel syndrome, the patient has pain with or without muscle weakness due to irritation or compression of the ulnar nerve within the cubital tunnel. The irritation can be from overuse as is seen in overhead throwers and certain occupations, or entrapment due to structures that decrease the cross sectional area of the cubital tunnel. Entrapment can be from medial osteophytes, which is not only seen in overhead throwers with posteromedial impingement but also in people with osteoarthritis. Entrapment can also result from ganglia, inflamed synovium, or from an accessory anconeus muscle. An accessory anconeus muscle can be diagnosed if there is a thick, muscle signal intensity mass replacing the normal medial flexor retinaculum. In patients with a normal retinaculum there should be at least one axial image through the cubital tunnel below the triceps muscle and proximal to the medial flexor muscles where there is no muscle overlying the ulnar nerve. This axial section with no muscle in the cubital tunnel is lost in patients with an accessory anconeus muscle.

Ulnar neuropathy can also result from direct trauma. The ulnar nerve is particularly exposed to trauma at the cubital tunnel because the nerve is not protected by overlying muscles. Ulnar neuropathy is diagnosed on MR imaging by either size and signal-intensity changes of the nerve, or evidence of denervation edema of the innervated muscles. It is important to recognize that the ulnar nerve can normally be higher signal intensity on T2-weighted images within the cubital tunnel compared to that of the nerve just proximal or distal to the tunnel. Several authors have found that ulnar neuropathy should be considered only if the T2 signal intensity is twice that of the nerve outside the tunnel. Ulnar neuropathy should also be considered if the cross sectional area of the nerve is greater than 8 mm^2. Because the ulnar nerve has motor branches in the forearm to the flexor carpi ulnaris and flexor digitorum profundus muscles, edema within these muscles may also be seen on elbow MR images in patients with ulnar neuropathy (Fig. 17). If chronic, there may be atrophy and fat replacement of these two muscles.

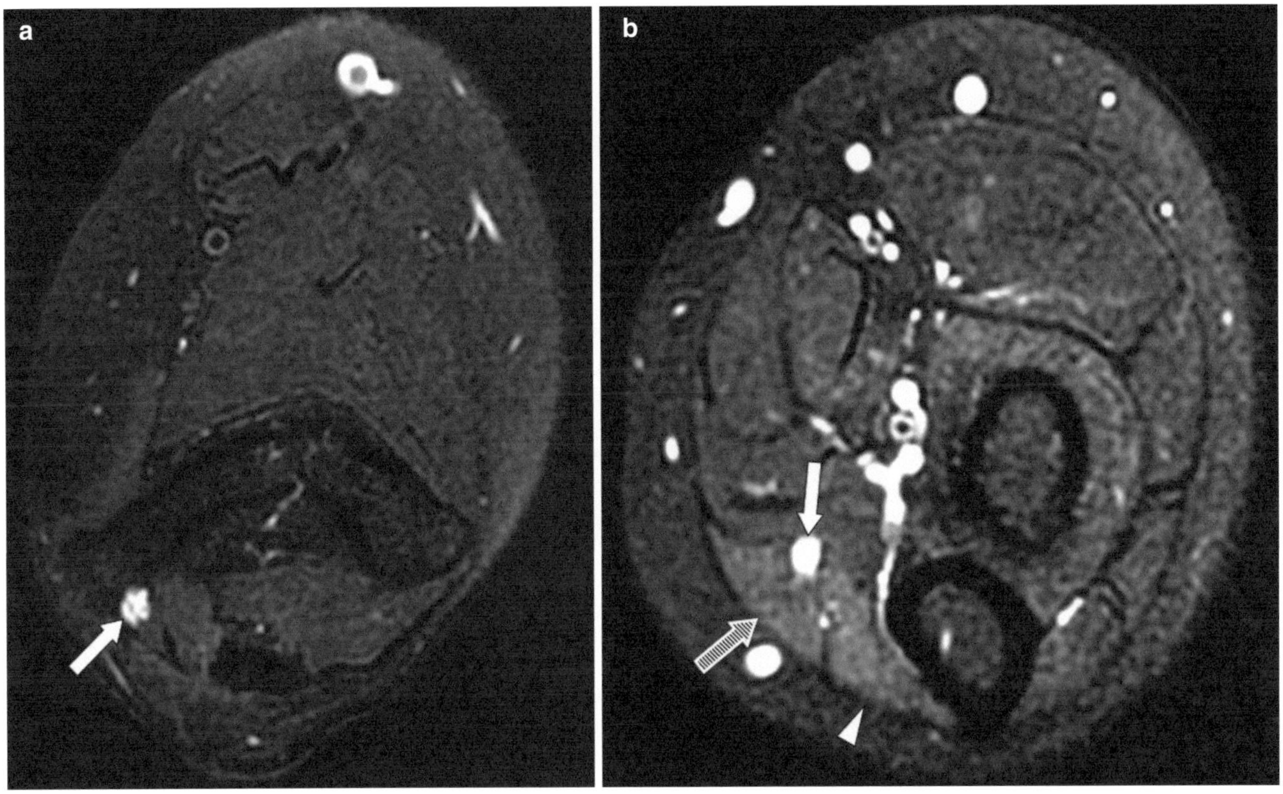

Fig. 17 (**a, b**) Ulnar neuritis in 16-year-old woman with numbness of the 5th and ulnar-aspect of the 4th fingers and hand weakness. Patient is active in martial arts and was lifting heavy boxes the prior day. Axial T2-weighted FS images through the elbow (**a**) and the proximal forearm (**b**) show a large and abnormally high signal ulnar nerve (*arrow*) and mild edema of the flexor digitorum profundus (*arrowhead*) and flexor carpi ulnaris (*striped arrow*) muscles. The symptoms resolved with physical therapy

Subluxation and dislocation of the ulnar nerve can be seen in up to 15% of individuals, and are usually asymptomatic. Dislocation out of the cubital tunnel usually occurs in individuals with an absent retinaculum and is worse in flexion. In patients with symptomatic ulnar nerve dislocation, there are typically signs of ulnar neuropathy with an enlarged and T2 high signal ulnar nerve.

Radial Nerve

There are two main entrapment neuropathies of the radial nerve at the elbow—*radial tunnel syndrome* and *posterior interosseous nerve* (PIN) syndrome [14]. Radial tunnel syndrome can be due to entrapment of the nerve at any point within the radial tunnel, and is typically due to repetitive rotatory movement of the forearm in individuals working in certain occupations. The symptoms are usually pain without much muscle weakness, as the sensory fibers tend to be effected worse than the motor fibers. The pain is in the dorsolateral aspect of the proximal forearm, several centimeters distal to the lateral epicondyle which helps distinguish it from lateral epicondylitis. The MR appearance of the radial nerve in the tunnel is often normal in these patients. It should be noted that the normal radial nerve is more difficult to see on MR images than the ulnar nerve because the radial nerve is not surrounded by fat.

The proximal edge of the superficial head of the supinator muscle is called the "Arcade of Frohse," particularly when it is fibrous and somewhat rigid as occurs in 30% of individuals [29]. The posterior interosseous branch of the radial nerve (PIN) passes adjacent to this proximal edge when it dives deep to the superficial head of the supinator muscle, and can be a site of nerve entrapment. Posterior interosseous nerve syndrome typically presents with weakness of the extensor muscles of the wrist and fingers. The posterior interosseous nerve is a purely motor nerve, so pain is less common. The most common cause of PIN syndrome is compression of the PIN as it dives deep past the proximal edge of the superficial head of the supinator muscle. PIN syndrome is more common in individuals with an Arcade of Frohse fibrous proximal edge of the superficial head of the supinator muscle [29]. Just proximal to the supinator muscle, the motor nerve branch to the supinator muscle can also be compressed, and this is sometimes also considered part of PIN syndrome. PIN syndrome can not only cause muscle weakness, but can cause denervation changes on MR images. This is seen as either edema within the supinator muscle, or within the extensor muscles such as the extensor digitorum, the extensor carpi ulnaris, the extensor pollicis longus and brevis, and the extensor indicis muscles (Fig. 18). For the supinator muscle, it is important not to overcall the slight increased signal seen normally in some individuals [30].

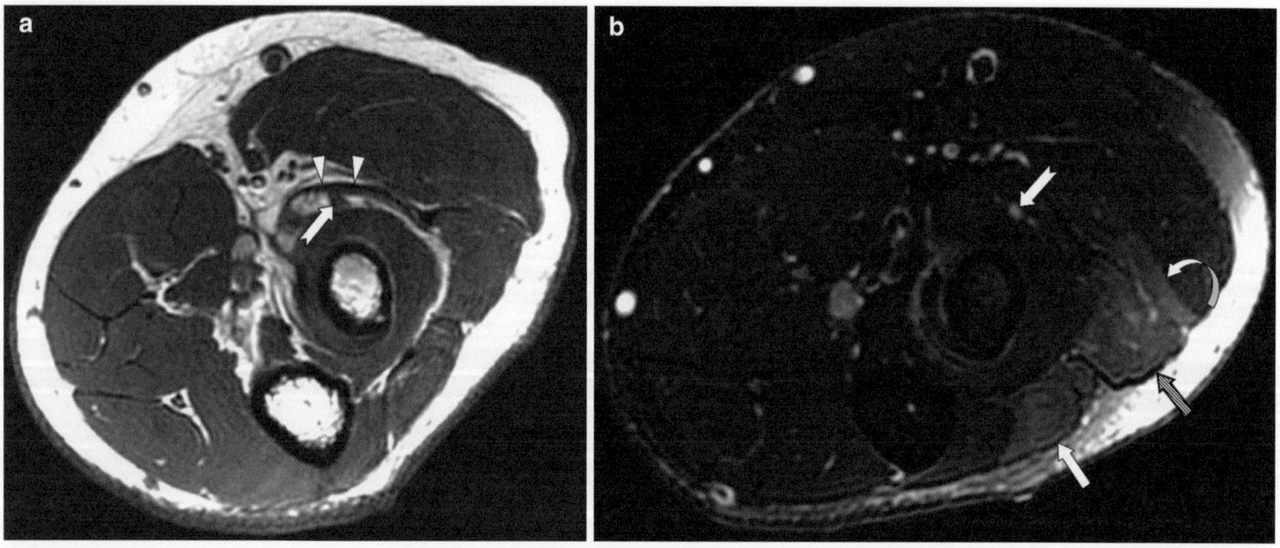

Fig. 18 (**a**, **b**) 46-year-old woman with "wrist drop" on exam and posterior interosseous nerve (PIN) abnormality on nerve conduction study. (**a**) Axial T1-weighed image shows the "Arcade of Frohse" fibrous proximal edge of the superficial head of the supinator muscle (*arrowhead*), and the PIN (*notched arrow*). (**b**) Axial T2-weighted FS image slightly more distal shows edema within the extensor carpi ulnaris (*white arrow*), extensor digitorum (*striped arrow*), and extensor carpi radialis brevis (*curved arrow*) muscles consistent with PIN syndrome. The PIN (*notched arrow*) is again seen between the superficial and deep heads of the supinator muscle

Median Nerve

There are two main entrapments that can affect the median nerve—*pronator syndrome* and *anterior interosseous nerve* (AIN) syndrome. Pronator syndrome refers to compression of the median nerve either where it crosses between the superficial and deep heads of the pronator teres muscle, or caused by a fibrous arch at the proximal margin of the flexor digitorum superficialis muscle. Like radial tunnel syndrome, this is seen usually in certain occupations with repetitive pronation/supination. People with pronator syndrome usually complain of pain in the volar aspect of the forearm, with motor weakness less common.

Anterior interosseous nerve syndrome is uncommon, and results from compression of the AIN typically by fibrous bands deep to the ulnar head of the pronator teres muscle or at the origin of the flexor digitorum superficialis muscle. The AIN is a purely motor nerve, so patients with AIN syndrome will have weakness of the flexor pollicis longus, the flexor digitorum profundus, and pronator quadratus muscles. On MR imaging, there will be denervation edema of these muscles, or atrophy and fatty replacement of the muscles.

References

1. Kijowski R, Tuite M, Sanford M (2004) Magnetic resonance imaging of the elbow. Part I: normal anatomy, imaging technique, and osseous abnormalities. Skelet Radiol 33(12):685–697
2. Morrey B (1993) Anatomy of the elbow joint. In: Morrey B (ed) The elbow and its disorders. Saunders, Philadelphia, pp 16–52
3. Sampaio ML, Schweitzer ME (2010) Elbow magnetic resonance imaging variants and pitfalls. Magn Reson Imaging Clin N Am 18(4):633–642
4. Stein JM, Cook TS, Simonson S et al (2011) Normal and variant anatomy of the elbow on magnetic resonance imaging. Magn Reson Imaging Clin N Am 19(3):609–619
5. Bancroft LW, Pettis C, Wasyliw C et al (2013) Osteochondral lesions of the elbow. Semin Musculoskelet Radiol 17(5):446–454
6. Bowen RE, Otsuka NY, Yoon ST et al (2001) Osteochondral lesions of the capitellum in pediatric patients: role of magnetic resonance imaging. J Pediatr Orthop 21(3):298–301
7. Kijowski R, De Smet AA (2005) Radiography of the elbow for evaluation of patients with osteochondritis dissecans of the capitellum. Skelet Radiol 34:266–271
8. Kijowski R, De Smet AA (2005) MRI findings of osteochondritis dissecans of the capitellum with surgical correlation. AJR Am J Roentgenol 185(6):1453–1459
9. Singer KM, Roy SP (1984) Osteochondrosis of the humeral capitellum. Am J Sports Med 12:351–360
10. Jans LB, Ditchefield M, Anna G et al (2012) MR imaging findings and MR criteria for instability in osteochondritis dissecans of the elbow in children. Eur J Radiol 81(6):1306–1310
11. Baker CL 3rd, Romeo AA, Baker CL Jr (2010) Osteochondritis dissecans of the capitellum. Am J Sports Med 38(9):1917–1928
12. Takahara M, Ogino T, Fukushima S et al (1999) Nonoperative treatment of osteochondritis dissecans of the humeral capitellum. Am J Sports Med 27:728–732
13. Hang DW, Chao CM, Hang YS (2004) A clinical and roentgenographic study of little league elbow. Am J Sports Med 21:79–84
14. Kijowski RM, Tuited M, Sanford M (2005) Magnetic resonance imaging of the elbow. Part II: abnormalities of the ligaments, tendons, and nerves. Skelet Radiol 34(1):1–18
15. Pierce JL, McCrum EC, ROzas AK et al (2015) Tip-of-the-iceberg fractures: small fractures that mean big trouble. AJR Am J Roentgenol 205(3):24–32
16. Sheehan SE, Dyer GS, Sodickson AD et al (2013) Traumatic elbow injuries: what the orthopedic surgeon wants to know. Radiographics 33(3):869–888
17. Chung CB, Chew FS, Steinbach L (2004) MR imaging of tendon abnormalities of the elbow. Magn Reson Imaging Clin N Am 12(2):233–245
18. Evans GF, Haller RG, Wyricks PS et al (1998) Submaximal delayed-onset muscle sorenesss: correlations between MR imaging findings and clinical measures. Radiology 208:815–820
19. Kotnis NA, Chiavaras MM, Harish S (2012) Lateral epicondylitis and beyond: imaging of lateral elbow pain with clinical-radiologic correlation. Skelet Radiol 41(4):369–386
20. Anderson MW, Alford BA (2010) Overhead throwing injuries of the shoulder and elbow. Radiol Clin N Am 48(6):1137–1154
21. Hayter CL, Adler RS (2012) Injuries of the elbow and the current treatment of tendon disease. AJR Am J Roentgenol 199(3):546–557
22. Frick MA, Murthy NS (2010) Imaging of the elbow: muscle and tendon injuries. Semin Musculoskelet Radiol 14(4):430–437
23. Brigido MK, De Maeseneer M, Morag Y (2013) Distal biceps brachii. Semin Musculoskelet Radiol 17(1):20–27
24. Seki A, Olsen BS, Jensen SL et al (2002) Functional anatomy of the lateral collateral ligament complex of the elbow: configuration of Y and its role. J Shoulder Elb Surg 11(1):53–59
25. Beckett KS, McConnell P, Lagopoulos M et al (2000) Variations in the normal anatomy of the collateral ligaments of the human elbow joint. J Anat 197(Pt 3):507–511
26. Wear SA, Thornton DD, Schwartz ML et al (2011) MRI of the reconstructed ulnar collateral ligament. AJR Am J Roentgenol 197(5):1198–1204
27. Andreisek G, Crook DW, Burg D et al (2006) Peripheral neuropathies of the median, radial, and ulnar nerves: MR imaging features. Radiographics 26(5):1267–1287
28. O'Driscoll SW, Horli E, Carmichael SW et al (1991) The cubital tunnel and ulnar neuropathy. J Bone Joint Surg Br 73(4):613–617
29. Posner MA (1990) Compressive neuropathies of the median and radial nerves at the elbow. Clin Sports Med 9(2):343–363
30. Gyftopoulos S, Rosenberg ZS, Petchprapa C (2010) Increased MR signal intensity in the pronator quadratus muscle: does it always indicate anterior interosseous neuropathy? AJR Am J Roentgenol 194(2):490–493

Hip

Mini N. Pathria and Klaus Woertler

Avascular Necrosis

Avascular necrosis (AVN) of the femoral head is a common disorder with an incidence of approximately 0.01%. It represents a progressive disease which is the cause for 5–10% of all hip replacement procedures. Males are affected four times more often than females. Most patients are between 30 and 50 years of age with bilateral hip involvement in 50% of cases. Pain with loading is the most common initial symptom. Later, pain at rest and by night, decreased mobility, muscle atrophy and contracture might be evident. Progressive disease and collapse of the femoral head are observed within 2 years after diagnosis in 85% and 50% of cases, respectively [1–3].

Traumatic AVN is caused by direct interruption of arterial blood supply and is most commonly seen unilaterally following femoral neck fracture and hip dislocation. Various conditions have been associated with the development of atraumatic AVN. The most common among these are corticosteroid medication and alcoholism. Other causes include metabolic and hematologic disorders, renal disease, pancreatitis, marrow storage disorders, chemotherapy, radiation, and Caisson disease. The exact pathomechanisms leading to AVN in all these different conditions remain unclear. It appears likely that there is more than one pathogenetic factor and that the underlying circulatory disturbance of the femoral head can occur at different vascular sites (arterioles, marrow sinus, veins) [1].

Histopathologic examinations show a subchondral segment of necrosis which becomes more and more demarcated from normal bone by a reactive interface. At later stages of the disease the linear interface consist of two parallel zones: an inner zone of hypervascular fibrous tissue and an outer zone of sclerosis. Progressive collapse of the femoral head is initiated by a fracture within the necrotic segment which is oriented parallel to the bone surface [1–3].

AVN of the femoral head can be staged on the basis of imaging findings. The most widely used staging system is the ARCO (Association Research Circulation Osseous) classification, which incorporates radiographic features (as described in the older classification by Ficat and Arlet) as well MR imaging, CT and scintigraphic findings (Table 1).

Imaging findings reflect the histopathologic features of AVN described above and have a great impact on treatment decisions. Radiographs are negative in ARCO stage 1, but might show the sclerotic zone of the reactive interface in stage 2, a subchondral fracture ("crescent sign") and collapse in stage 3 (Fig. 1), and secondary osteoarthritis (OA) of the hip joint in stage 4. Similar findings can be seen on CT with a higher sensitivity for the detection of subchondral fractures. As soon as fracture has occurred, preservation of the femoral head is usually futile and arthroplasty has to be performed in the majority of cases [1, 3].

M.N. Pathria
Department of Radiology, University of California San Diego,
200 West Arbor Drive, San Diego, CA 92103-8756, USA
e-mail: mpathria@ucsd.edu

K. Woertler (✉)
Department of Diagnostic and Interventional Radiology,
Technische Universität München,
Ismaninger Strasse 22, Munich D-81675, Germany
e-mail: klaus.woertler@tum.de

J. Hodler et al. (eds.), *Musculoskeletal Diseases 2017-2020*, DOI 10.1007/978-3-319-54018-4_6

Table 1 ARCO classification (modified) [4, 5]

Stage	ARCO 1	ARCO 2	ARCO 3	ARCO 4
Radiograph	Normal	Sclerosis and osteolysis in necrotic segment, sclerotic margin	Fracture (crescent sign), flattening of femoral dome	Osteoarthritis
MRI	Demarcated necrotic segment	Necrosis with reactive margin, double-line sign	Fracture	Osteoarthritis
CT	Normal	Sclerosis and osteolysis in necrotic segment, sclerotic margin	Fracture, deterioration of spherical head shape	Osteoarthritis
Scintigraphy	Diffuse or cold spot	Cold in hot pattern	Hot in hot pattern	Hot spot

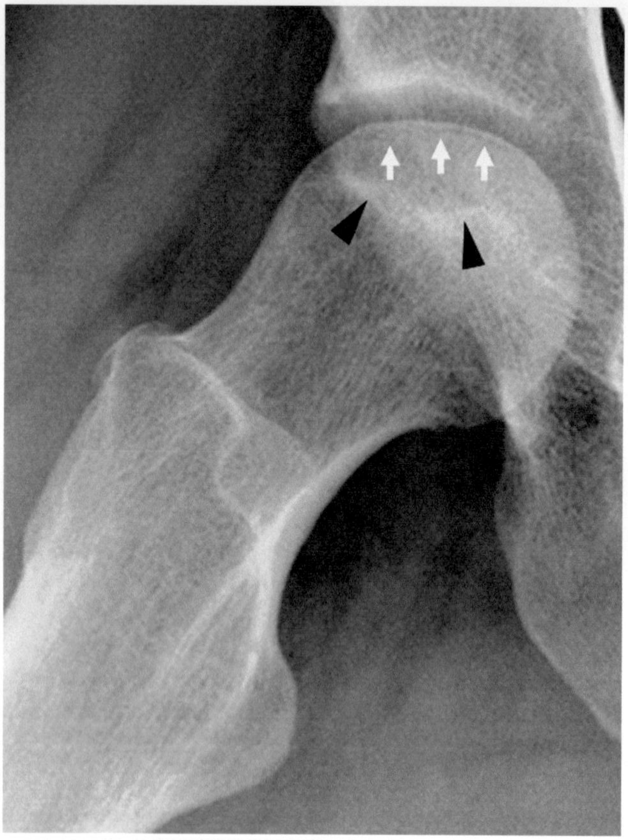

Fig. 1 AVN of the femoral head (ARCO stage 3). Frog-leg lateral view shows sclerotic line (*black arrowheads*) of reactive interface between necrotic segment and normal bone. The curved subchondral radiolucent line (*white arrows*) indicates fracture of the femoral head ("crescent sign")

On MR imaging (Fig. 2), ARCO stage 1 is characterized by the presence of a subchondral area of signal loss ("band lesion"), which in stage 2 is separated from normal bone marrow by an interface consisting of two parallel lines ("double-line sign"). This sign can be seen on images with T2 contrast and on gadolinium-enhanced T1-weighted images and describes the presence of an inner hyperintense line (fibrovascular tissue) and an outer hypointense line (osteosclerosis) bordering the avascular bone segment. In stage 3, a fracture line might become visible within the area of necrosis which typically runs parallel to the surface of the femoral head. Similar to radiographs and CT, femoral head collapse and OA are features indicative of stages 3 and 4 [1, 3, 6, 7]. Bone marrow edema can be associated with AVN of the femoral head but does not occur before the demarcation of necrosis and thus, does not represent an early sign of ischemia as previously believed [2, 3, 7]. In patients with AVN, bone marrow edema has been shown to be associated with pain, femoral head collapse and a poor prognosis [8–10]. A recent study demonstrated that bone marrow edema adjacent to the demarcated necrotic fragment represents a secondary sign of subchondral fracture and therefore indicates ARCO stage 3, even if the fracture line is not visible on MR imaging [3].

The most important tasks of imaging in patient with suspected AVN of the femoral head are the verification of the diagnosis and the differentiation of AVN from other causes of hip pain, such as transient bone marrow edema syndrome (TBMES) and subchondral insufficiency fracture (SIF), and, if AVN is diagnosed, the distinction between ARCO stage 2 and 3.

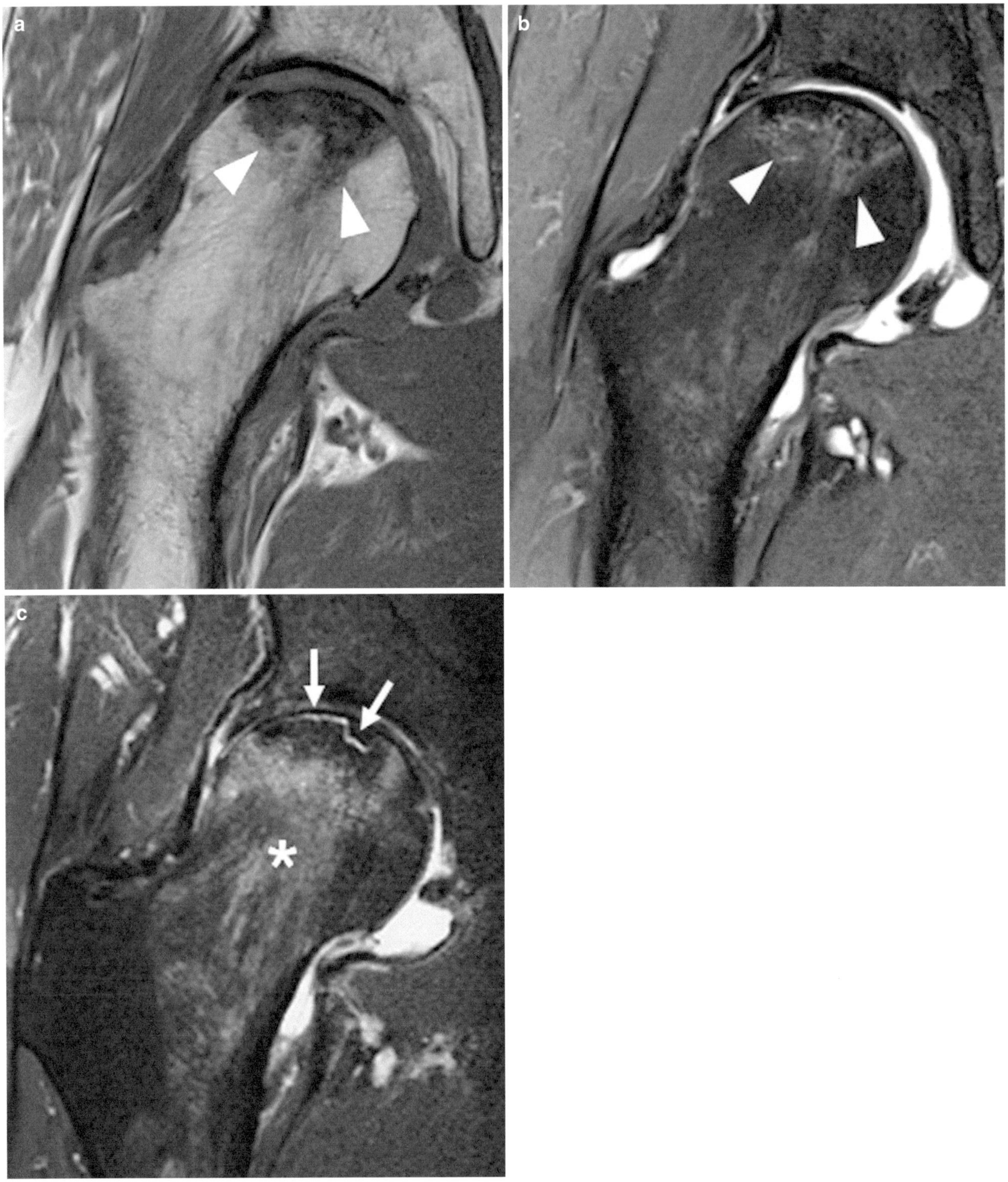

Fig. 2 (**a**–**c**) AVN of the femoral head: progression from ARCO stage 2 to stage 3. (**a**) Coronal T1-weighted TSE image and (**b**) corresponding intermediate weighted TSE image with fat suppression show hypointense subchondral segment of osteonecrosis demarcated by a reactive interface (*arrowheads*). Note absence of femoral head collapse and bone marrow edema (ARCO stage 2). (**c**) Coronal intermediate weighted TSE image with fat suppression obtained five months later demonstrates hyperintense subchondral fracture line (*arrows*) within necrotic segment as well as bone marrow edema (*asterisk*) extending to the femoral neck and intertrochanteric area (ARCO stage 3)

Transient Bone Marrow Edema Syndrome

Transient bone marrow edema syndrome of the hip is a self-limited condition, which before the advent of MR imaging was referred to as transient osteoporosis (TO). It is almost exclusively observed in healthy middle-aged men and women in the third trimester of pregnancy or immediately postpartum. Unilateral, bilateral and migratory forms have been reported. The disease is characterized by the acute onset of hip pain and limited range of motion without previous trauma. Complete restitution can be expected after a period of 6–8 months. TBMES is nowadays regarded as a distinct clinical entity separate from avascular necrosis (AVN). Although different etiological mechanisms have been discussed, there is some evidence that the basic pathomechanism is venous congestion with an increase of intraosseous pressure. Histologic examinations have shown increased vascularity, interstitial edema, and signs of an abnormal bone turnover [1, 11, 12].

Radiographs are usually normal at the initial onset of symptoms and show reversible osteopenia over the ensuing few months. Bone scintigraphy reveals increased perfusion as well as abnormal tracer uptake in the femoral head and neck [1]. On MR imaging (Fig. 3), bone marrow edema is seen extending from the femoral head and neck to the intertrochanteric region in the absence of segmental or linear subchondral changes. Edema might spare the subchondral bone marrow particularly at the medial aspect of the femoral head. Accompanying joint effusion and synovitis are the rule [1, 6, 11, 12]. Perfusion studies typically show an increased contrast accumulation with a prolonged plateau phase in the femoral head supporting the theory of venous congestion [7]. As a sequel of demineralization, insufficiency fractures can occur during the course of the disease, in particular if unloading is inadequate or terminated following core decompression with relief of symptoms. On MR images, fractures are typically seen as linear areas of low signal intensity within the subchondral bone marrow [6, 11, 12]. On the basis of imaging findings, it is virtually impossible to distinguish TBMES with secondary insufficiency fracture from primary SIF. Patient age, sex and clinical history help to differentiate between the two entities.

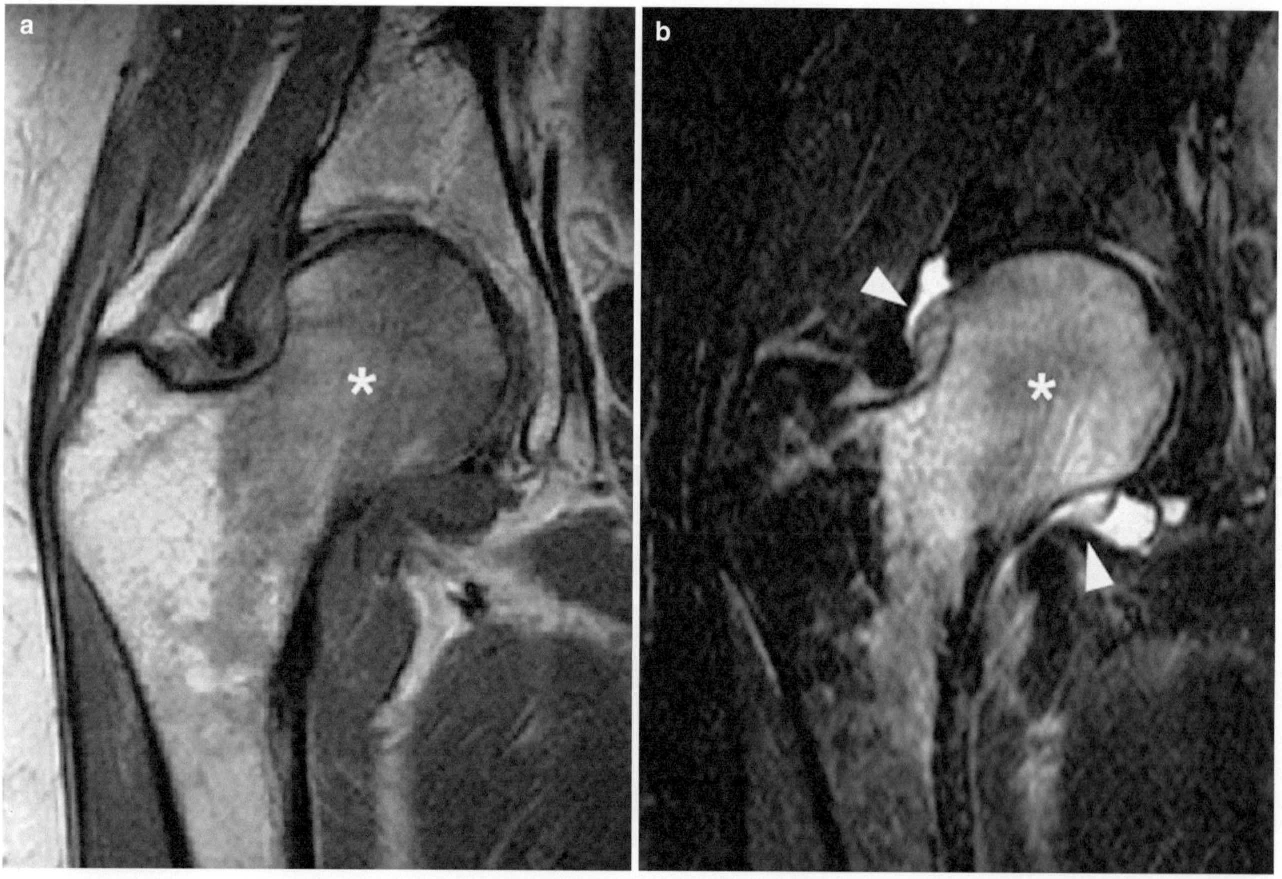

Fig. 3 (**a**, **b**) Transient bone marrow edema syndrome of the hip. (**a**) Coronal T1-weighted TSE image and (**b**) corresponding STIR TSE image show extensive bone marrow edema (*asterisk*) of the proximal femur in the absence of segmental or linear abnormalities of subchondral bone. Note reactive synovitis and joint effusion (*arrowheads*)

Stress Injuries

Subchondral Insufficiency Fracture

Subchondral insufficiency fracture of the femoral head is most often observed in elderly females and renal transplant recipients with osteopenic bone. Patients report a sudden onset of hip pain which is typically worse with weight-bearing. Biomechanical failure occurs in the statically overloaded areas of the femoral head. Histologic examinations show a subchondral fracture with intraosseous callus formation and reactive hypervacularization of surrounding bone marrow. The natural course of the disease is either healing or collapse of the femoral head with consequent joint destruction. It is estimated that SIF of the femoral head accounts for 5–6% of all total hip replacements. The condition is likely to represent the underlying pathology in so-called "rapidly destructive osteoarthritis of the hip" [13–16].

MR imaging shows a hypointense subchondral fracture line as well as bone marrow edema in the femoral head and neck (Fig. 4). In the majority of cases the fracture is located in the anterior segment of the femoral head and runs parallel to the joint surface. In contrast to AVN, the bone marrow between the fracture and the articular cartilage enhances after intravenous contrast application. Cartilage defects, synovitis and joint effusion are typical associated findings [13, 14, 17]. With collapse of subchondral bone progressive loss of signal intensity, entrance of fluid and cyst formation might be seen.

Initial findings indicating a poor clinical prognosis include lateral location, non-parallel course and great extent of the fracture, large cartilage defects, bone marrow edema on both sides of the joint, and high patient age [13–15, 17].

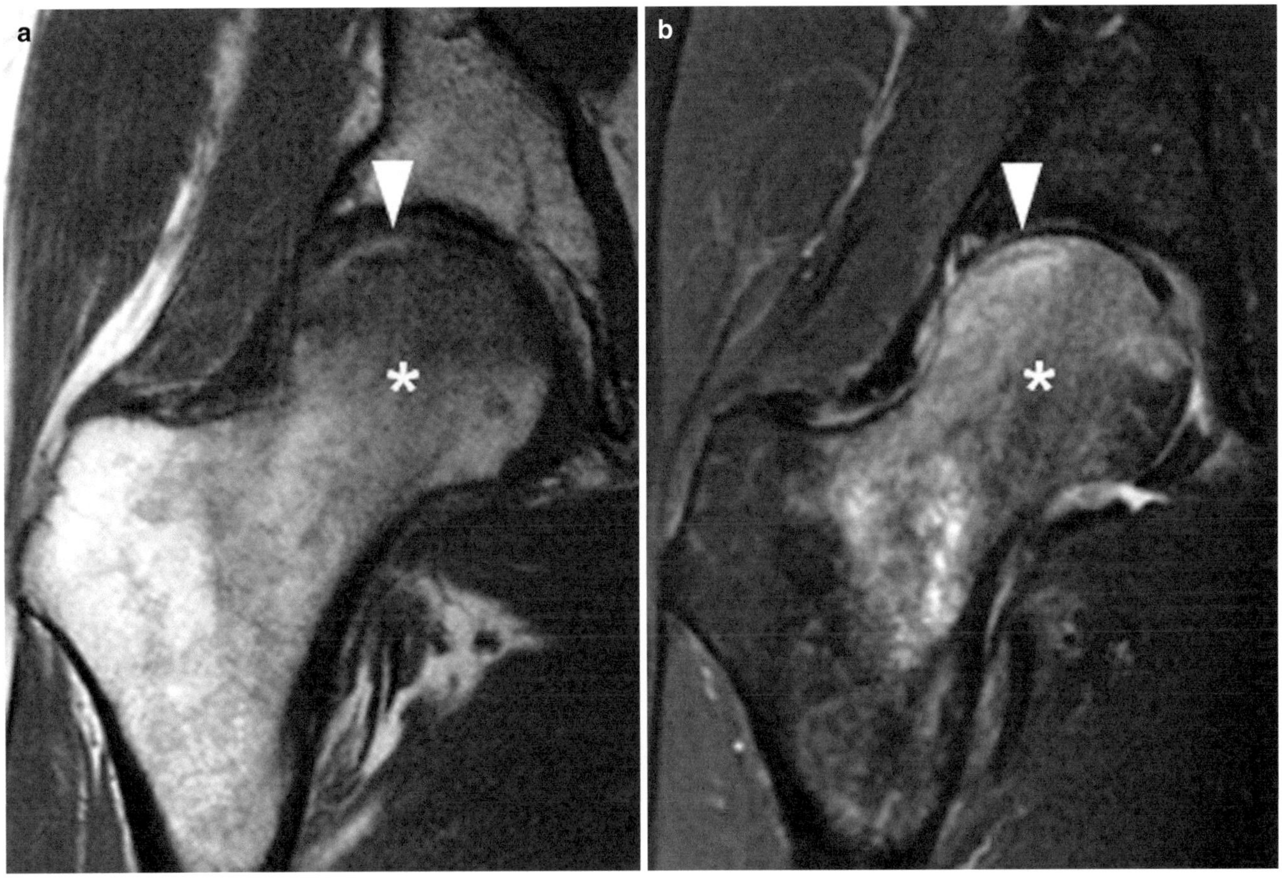

Fig. 4 (**a**, **b**) Subchondral insufficiency fracture (SIF) of the femoral head. Coronal (**a**) T1-weighted TSE image, (**b**) intermediate weighted TSE image with fat suppression and (**c**) contrast-enhanced T1-weighted TSE image with fat suppression show a hypointense subchondral fracture line (*arrow*) oriented parallel to the surface of the femoral head with associated bone marrow edema (*asterisk*). Note contrast enhancement of the bone segment proximal to the fracture

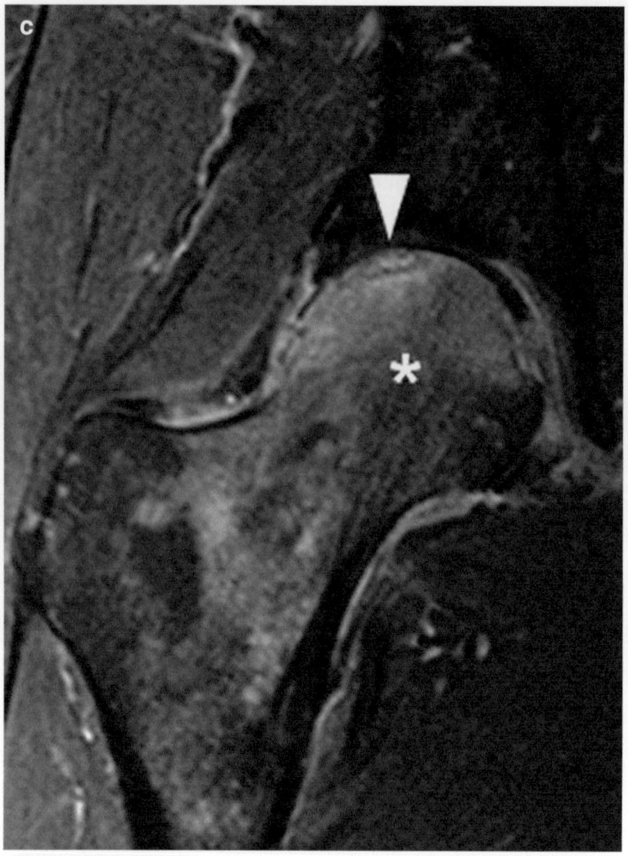

Fig. 4 (continued)

Fatigue Fracture

Fatigue fractures of the femoral head and neck typically occur in runners and military recruits with the femoral neck representing the most common location at the hip. In runners, stress injuries of the femoral neck are usually the sequel of a changed regimen or an increased frequency or intensity of training. Patients complain about groin or anterior hip pain with loading rather than at rest. The clinical symptoms are however unspecific and may mimic a labral tear or a muscle injury. Whereas fatigue fractures at the inferomedial (basicervical) aspect of the femoral neck due to compression forces usually have an uncomplicated course and can be treated conservatively, superolateral (subcapital) fractures represent distraction injuries that bear a higher risk for dislocation and thus, might require surgery [18, 19].

Stress reactions are precursor lesions of fatigue fractures which are distinguished from the latter by the absence of a distinct fracture line.

Radiographs are not very sensitive in depicting stress injuries of bone. The first radiographic signs are the “grey cortex sign” (circumscribed cortical osteopenia) and a lamellar periosteal reaction, which might later transform into solid bone production. In the femoral neck, superficial new bone formation is however often minimal or absent. With a frank fatigue fracture a horizontal line of increased density might become visible. On MR imaging (Fig. 5), stress reactions of

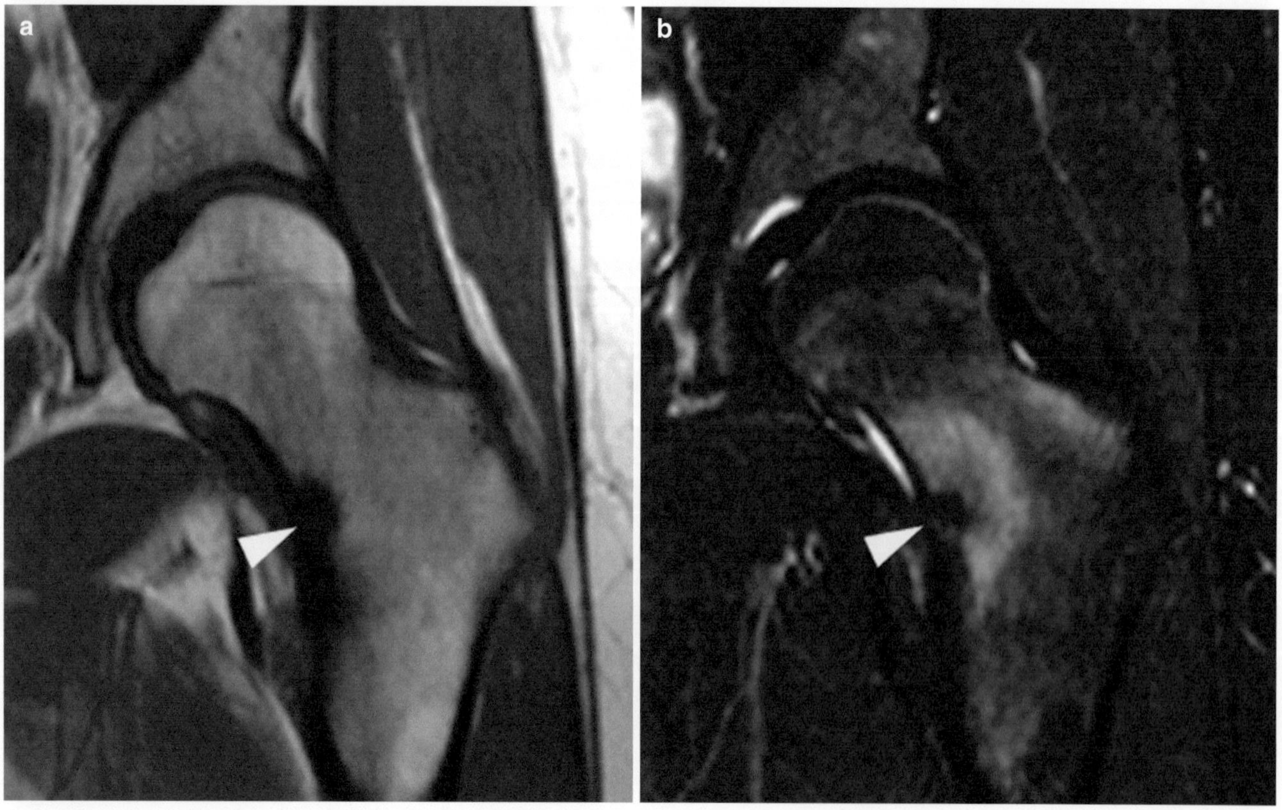

Fig. 5 (**a**, **b**) Inferomedial fatigue fracture of the femoral neck. (**a**) Coronal T1-weighted TSE image and (**b**) corresponding STIR TSE image show a focal band of low signal intensity (*arrowhead*) perpendicular to the medial cortex surrounded by bone marrow edema

the proximal femur are characterized by bone marrow edema as well as increased T2-weighted signal intensity at the bone surface due to periosteal activation. A fatigue fracture should be diagnosed if a line of low signal intensity perpendicular to the cortex is seen in addition to the latter [18, 20]. In doubtful cases, CT might be helpful in depicting the fracture line or in differentiation of a stress injury from an osteoid osteoma. In the majority of patients with fatigue fractures of the femoral neck, abnormal signal intensity on MR imaging resolves within 6 months of the initial diagnosis. Residual sclerosis or fatty marrow conversion might remain at the former facture site [21].

Articular Anatomy and Pathology

Hip Capsule

Stability of the hip results from its bony anatomy whereby the acetabular socket contains the majority of the femoral head, the labrum that further deepens the acetabular socket, and from the thick capsular ligaments that reinforce the hip capsule. The capsular ligaments of the hip consist of the pubofemoral, ischiofemoral and iliofemoral ligaments that collectively encircle the hip joint [22] The pubofemoral ligament is located inferiorly and the ischiofemoral ligament is located posteriorly. The obturator externus bursa, which normally communicates with the inferior hip joint, arises from the area of the ischiofemoral ligament attachment and may be distended in patients with a hip effusion [23] The zona orbicularis is a compact set of fibers perpendicular to these capsular ligaments further reinforcing the superior, posterior and inferior capsule resulting in a narrow constriction at the femoral neck that is well seen with MR imaging [22].

The iliofemoral ligament is the strongest of the capsular ligaments and reinforces the anterior hip capsule. It has an inverted Y configuration, consisting of a horizontal superior band and a vertical inferior band. The superior band is well seen on axial MR images as it courses from the anterior acetabulum to insert on a tubercle on the anterior femoral neck. Injury to this portion of the iliofemoral ligament is a common finding in patients who have undergone transient posterior hip subluxation, typically occurring near its femoral insertion [24].

Unlike the shoulder, posterior subluxation/dislocation is more common at the hip than anterior instability. Transient posterior hip subluxation typically results from a fall on a flexed and adducted hip and is often clinically misdiagnosed as a hip sprain. Frank hip dislocation is typically the result of significant trauma such as motor vehicle accident, sports related injury or a significant fall. Males are more commonly affected than females. Correct diagnosis of this injury is essential to minimize future hip instability and reduce the risk of avascular necrosis.

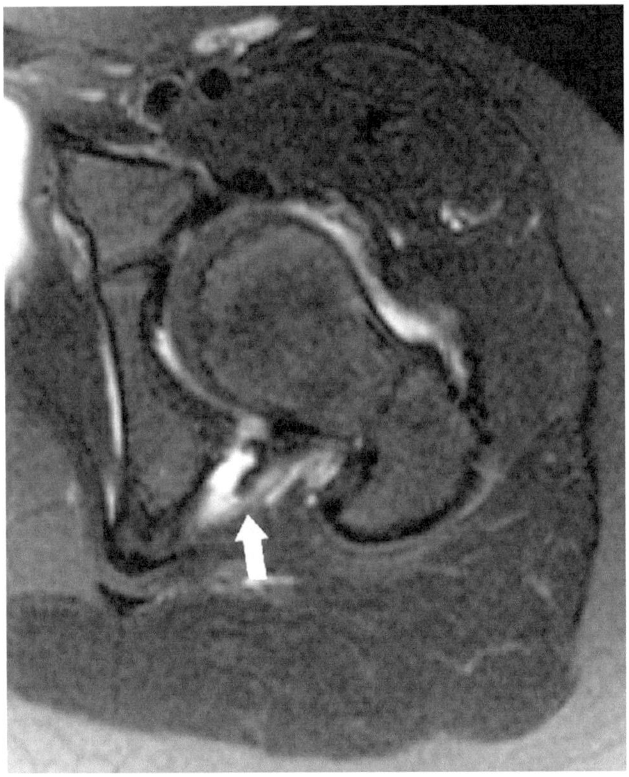

Fig. 6 Posterior hip subluxation. Axial T2-weighted MR image of the left hip in a 9 year old female obtained following a soccer injury demonstrates avulsion of the posterior labrum with overlying soft tissue swelling. (*arrow*) There is also mild edema in the anterior hip capsule within the iliofemoral ligament, consistent with transient hip subluxation

Findings on MR that suggest transient posterior hip subluxation and dislocation include posterior acetabular rim marrow edema or fracture, posterior labral tearing or avulsion, and the presence of a significant effusion and/or hemarthrosis. (Fig. 6) Injury to the anterior and posterior capsule may be present, along with strain of the external rotator muscles, damage to the external rotator tendons, and edema in the fat surrounding the sciatic nerve posterior to the hip capsule [25] Injury to the obturator externus tendon in particular appears to be associated with concurrent damage to the deep branch of the medial circumflex artery to the femoral head and subsequent avascular necrosis [26]

Acetabular Labrum

The acetabular labrum is a poorly-vascularized fibrocartilaginous structure that encircles the majority of the acetabulum, deepening its fossa to help contain and stabilize the femoral head [27]. The acetabular labrum is deficient at the inferior acetabulum, where it is replaced by the transverse ligament. Tearing of the labrum can take place due to degeneration, repetitive trauma or acute injury. Like other fibrocartilaginous structures such as the intervertebral disk, menisci and glenoid labrum, degeneration and tearing are common with aging and are not necessarily symptomatic. In older patients, the labrum may even be absent, presumably due to degeneration/tearing and secondary attrition.

Assessment of labral pathology is challenging with modalities other than MR imaging. MR evaluation of the hip labrum is best performed with high resolution imaging using small field of view focused on the hip. It is thickest superiorly and posteriorly and widest superiorly and anteriorly, appearing as a triangular or less commonly, a rounded low signal structure at the margins of the bony acetabular rim. MR arthrography is widely employed for assessment of the labrum as it helps to visualize the labrum by distending the joint and outlining it with fluid [28]. The increase in accuracy of labral assessment with MR arthrography is less pronounced when there is a native effusion, particularly on 3 T MR systems.

Patients with symptomatic labral pathology typically present with mechanical symptoms of clicking, locking and catching superimposed on variable degrees of hip and groin pain [29]. As in the shoulder, disorders of the labrum can take the form of intrasubstance tearing or detachment of the labrum from its osteochondral attachment. Tearing of the labrum most commonly involves the superior and anterosuperior labrum. Patients with developmental dysplasia, where the labrum experiences greater loading due to lateral acetabular deficiency, are at high risk for labral tears involving the superior and posterosuperior labrum [28].

Tears of the labrum can result in a variety of MR appearances depending on their size, location and orientation. Frank linear fluid within the labral substance, fibrillation of the labral surface and labral displacement may be seen (Fig. 7). Chondrolabral separation results in fluid between the labrum and underlying cartilage. Thickening or thinning of the labrum, disorganized internal labral signal, and blunting of the labral tip can be seen with labral degeneration. A paralabral cyst is a helpful finding indicating the presence of underlying labral pathology, particularly in the absence of joint fluid.

Numerous variants have been emphasized whereby fluid may be interposed between the labrum and adjacent structures. The normal perilabral sulcus is located above the labrum where fluid is interposed between the labrum and the capsule [30]. This normal fluid collection is well-recognized and typically easy to differentiate from a tear. Similarly, normal sulci between the transverse ligament and the far inferior labrum are common and rarely confused with labral tears due to their characteristic far inferior location. Normal sublabral sulci between the cartilage and the remainder of the labrum are however more challenging to differentiate tears. These types of clefts are common, particularly at the posterior labrum. It is important to remember that labral tears are typically located anterosuperiorly and anteriorly. Posterior location, thin fluid, smooth margins and absence of adjacent chondral disease suggests a variant sublabral sulcus rather than a detachment or tear of the labrum [27].

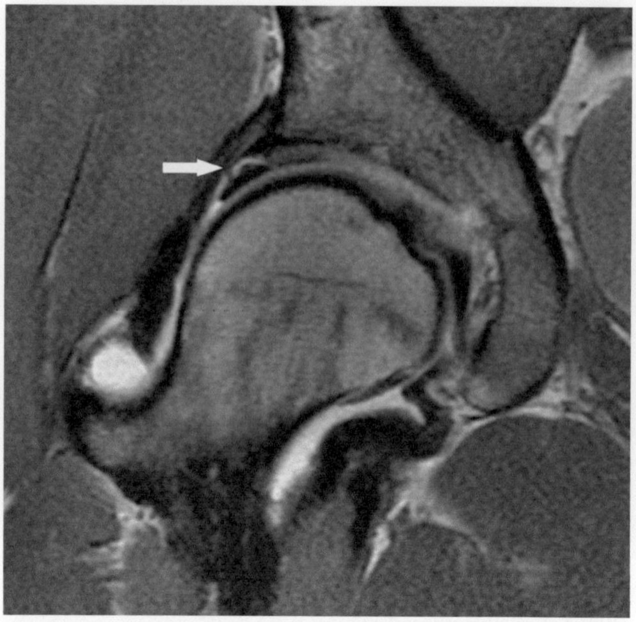

Fig. 7 Labral tear. Small field-of-view coronal T1-weighted MR image of the right hip performed following intra-articular injection of diluted Gd-DTPA shows fluid extending into the substance of the superior hip labrum (*arrow*) indicating a tear

Ligamentum Teres

Unlike the circumferential shoulder labrum, the hip labrum is incomplete inferiorly, where it is replaced by the transverse ligament. The transverse ligament along with the pubic and ischial margins of the acetabulum, gives rise to the triangular ligamentum teres (ligamentum capitis femoris), which narrows as it extends superiorly from a broad inferior base to insert at the fovea of the femoral head [31, 32]. The function of the ligamentum teres remains uncertain; it contributes to femoral head stability and vascularity, but these contributions appear to be minor as it may be excised without causing significant hip dysfunction.

The intraarticular transverse ligament and ligamentum teres are well seen on axial and coronal MR imaging whenever there is an effusion or following hip arthrography. On coronal images, the transverse ligament is seen in cross section at the inferior hip joint and the ligamentum teres appears as a vertical low signal band extending superiorly from it to the fovea where it thickens slightly, separating the medial aspect of the femoral head from the acetabular pulvinar fat. Because it arises from 2 to 3 distinct bundles, thin linear striations may be present within the ligamentum teres, particularly at its inferior aspect [31]. On axial images, the ligamentum teres can be confused with an intraarticular body, but its characteristic ovoid configuration, absence of internal marrow and correlation with the coronal images help avoid this imaging pitfall. While the transverse ligament is well seen on sagittal images, the ligamentum teres is not well evaluated is this plane due to partial volume artifacts.

The spectrum of pathology of the ligamentum teres is similar to that of the anterior cruciate ligament, consisting of degeneration, partial tear, complete tear and avulsion fractures at its insertion [33]. Ligament degeneration is histologically similar to tendon degeneration, resulting in ligament thickening and increased signal due to myxoid, fatty and fibrous deposition [32]. Interstitial tearing of the ligamentum teres may be superimposed on degeneration. In patients with crystal deposition disorders, calcifications may also be present within the ligament, though these are difficult to visualize with MR imaging. Degeneration and degenerative tearing of the ligamentum teres is commonly seen on MR imaging in older patients but the clinical significance of such alterations is difficult to assess because of the frequency of asymptomatic ligament degeneration.

In young patients, ligamentum teres abnormalities are more likely to be traumatic than degenerative. Traumatic tearing of the ligamentum teres usually results from hyperabduction trauma, external rotation twisting injury or following transient hip dislocation. 4–15% of sports-related injuries to the hip involve the ligamentum teres so it should be carefully assessed in patients with hip pain following trauma [31]. Injury can take the form of partial or complete tear of the ligament or an avulsion fracture of the femoral head in its foveal region (Fig. 8). Avulsion fractures of the fovea are uncommon and are seen typically in children, associated with marrow edema at the medial femoral head.

Compete tears of the ligamentum teres usually result from a single episode of significant trauma resulting in a hip effusion and associated transverse ligament, labral and chondral injury. Frank discontinuity of the ligament is seen on MR imaging, occasionally associated with rotation and displacement of the ligament. Patients with partial tears typically present in an insidious fashion with complaints of chronic hip pain. Partial tears typically result in thickening, irregularity and fluid signal within the ligamentum teres. Tearing of the ligamentum teres takes place most commonly near the foveal insertion and may also be associated with marrow edema at the fovea or in chronic cases, foveal enlargement and bony hypertrophy at the foveal margins [31].

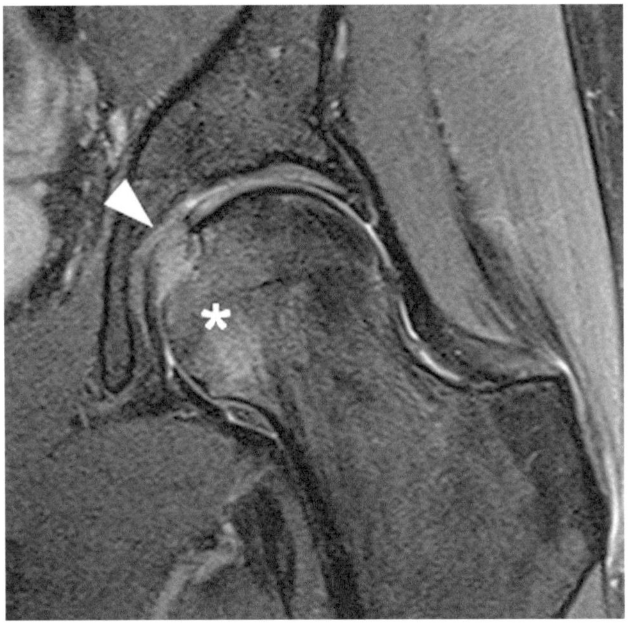

Fig. 8 Ligamentum teres tear. Coronal proton-density-weighted fat-saturated image of the left hip in 24 year old male following twisting injury during sports demonstrates thickening and abnormal increased signal in the ligamentum teres near its foveal attachment (*arrowhead*) related to a high grade partial tear. Note bone marrow edema in the femoral head adjacent to the fovea (*asterisk*) related to tearing of the ligament

Femoroacetabular Impingement

Femoroacetabular impingement (FAI) is a recently emphasized disorder of the hip resulting from abnormal contact between the femoral head and neck with the acetabulum. It has been reported to affect 10–15% of patients with hip pain and be a significant risk factor in the development of premature osteoarthrosis in young, active patients [34]. Patients present with groin and hip pain that is aggravated when the hip is placed in flexion, adduction and internal rotation [34]. Treatment initially consists of analgesics, activity modification, and intraarticular steroid injection, with surgery reserved for recalcitrant cases. The surgical approach to patients with FAI is not trivial, consisting of labral resection/repair, chondral microfracture/repair, and resection of bone from the femoral head neck junction.

Femoroacetabular impingement is subdivided into Cam type associated with atypical morphology of the femoral head/neck junction (Cam type FAI) and Pincer type FAI where the morphologic alterations are at the acetabulum. In many cases, the disorder is mixed whereby both sides of the joint contribute to impingement. Cam type impingement is more common, typically affecting young active adult males and this type is more commonly referred for arthroscopic surgery. Pincer type impingement typically affects older females and is managed similar to conventional osteoarthrosis.

Cam type impingement results from abnormal contact of the anterior and anterosuperior femoral neck with the anterosuperior acetabular rim, resulting in tearing of the labrum and chondral loss at the acetabulum. Radiographic features associated with this disorder include bone proliferation at the femoral head neck junction, resulting in flattening of the normal waist of the femoral neck, referred to as a "pistol-grip deformity", os acetabuli and fibrocystic changes at the femoral head neck junction (Fig. 9). On MR imaging, oblique axial images can be used to quantify the degree of flattening at the femoral head neck junction, using the alpha angle [35]. The alpha angle is constructed by drawing a line along the femoral neck passing through the center of the femoral head and a circle approximating the circumference of the femoral head. The angle between the femoral neck line and the point at which the femoral head circle diverges from the line is typically less than 55–65 degrees [35].

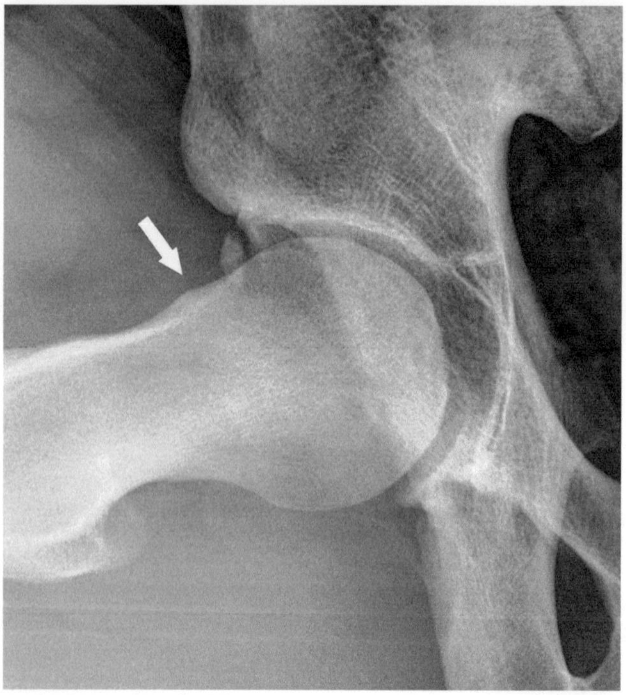

Fig. 9 Cam-type FAI. Frog-leg lateral view of the right hip in a 28 year old male with clinical symptoms of femoracetabular impingement demonstrates bony overgrowth at the anterior femoral head-neck junction (*arrow*). Note small os acetabuli adjacent to the labrum

There are a range of abnormal acetabular morphologies that result in abnormal contact between the posterior femoral head and posterior acetabular rim resulting in pincer type FAI. These include developmental variants of acetabular morphology such as generalized retroversion, focal superior acetabular retroversion, and primary protrusio acetabuli as well a range of conditions resulting in acquired protrusio due to bone softening and arthrosis [36]. Superimposed degenerative changes resulting in acetabular osteophytes and degenerative labral ossification and femoral changes such as coxa magna and posterior femoral head/neck proliferation can further contribute to this syndrome. The cross-over sign, where the superior anterior acetabular rim projects lateral to the posterior acetabular rim, and measurements of acetabular depth on both radiography and MR imaging have been emphasized in establishing this diagnosis [34]. Pincer type FAI results in chondral loss at the posterior acetabulum which can be evaluated on axial and sagittal MR images.

Femoroacetabular impingement is a controversial topic and the role of imaging and surgery continues to evolve [37]. Regarding imaging, recent articles have emphasized that there is poor specificity of the imaging findings that have been described in this disorder. Imaging findings of FAI are commonly present in asymptomatic individuals, with radiographic findings of Cam-type morphology present in 35% of males and 10% of females and Pincer-type morphology in 34% of males and 10% of females [38] The cross-over sign, described as a finding of superior acetabular overcoverage, was present in almost half of asymptomatic teenager [38]. Given the poor specificity of imaging findings, the diagnosis of FAI must be confirmed with clinical symptoms and physical examination, with imaging used to confirm and quantify the diagnosis. Similarly, regarding treatment, there is poor consensus in the orthopedic community about the indications for surgical management [37].

Adverse Reactions to Hip Prosthesis

Hip arthroplasty can be complicated by adverse reactions to wear of several prosthetic components. The two most commonly observed problems are polyethylene induced synovitis following total hip arthroplasty and hypersensiitivity to metallic debris in patients with metal-on-metal prosthesis. Wear disease (particle disease) typically occurs 1–5 years postoperatively and can lead to synovitis, pseudotumor formation and osteolysis [39–41]. The clinical picture shows a wide range from totally asymptomatic to chronic hip pain, limitation of motion, instability, limb shortening, and symptoms caused by compression of nearby soft tissue structures.

On radiographs, osteolysis appear as well-defined geographic radiolucencies adjacent to the prosthetic components (Fig. 10). Lytic bone lesions are more common in polyethylene wear and are best seen on MR images with metal artifact correction. Pseudotumors within the soft tissues might develop from capsular distension and dehiscence as well as involvement of adjacent bursae. Intra- and extraosseous abnormalities reveal intermediate to high signal intensity on T1 weighted images and show hyperintense synovial fluid with debris of low to intermediate signal intensity on images with T2-contrast [40, 41]. The peripheral lining of the lesions is often hypointense and can enhance with intravenous contrast adiministration. Internal enhancement is typically absent (Fig. 10).

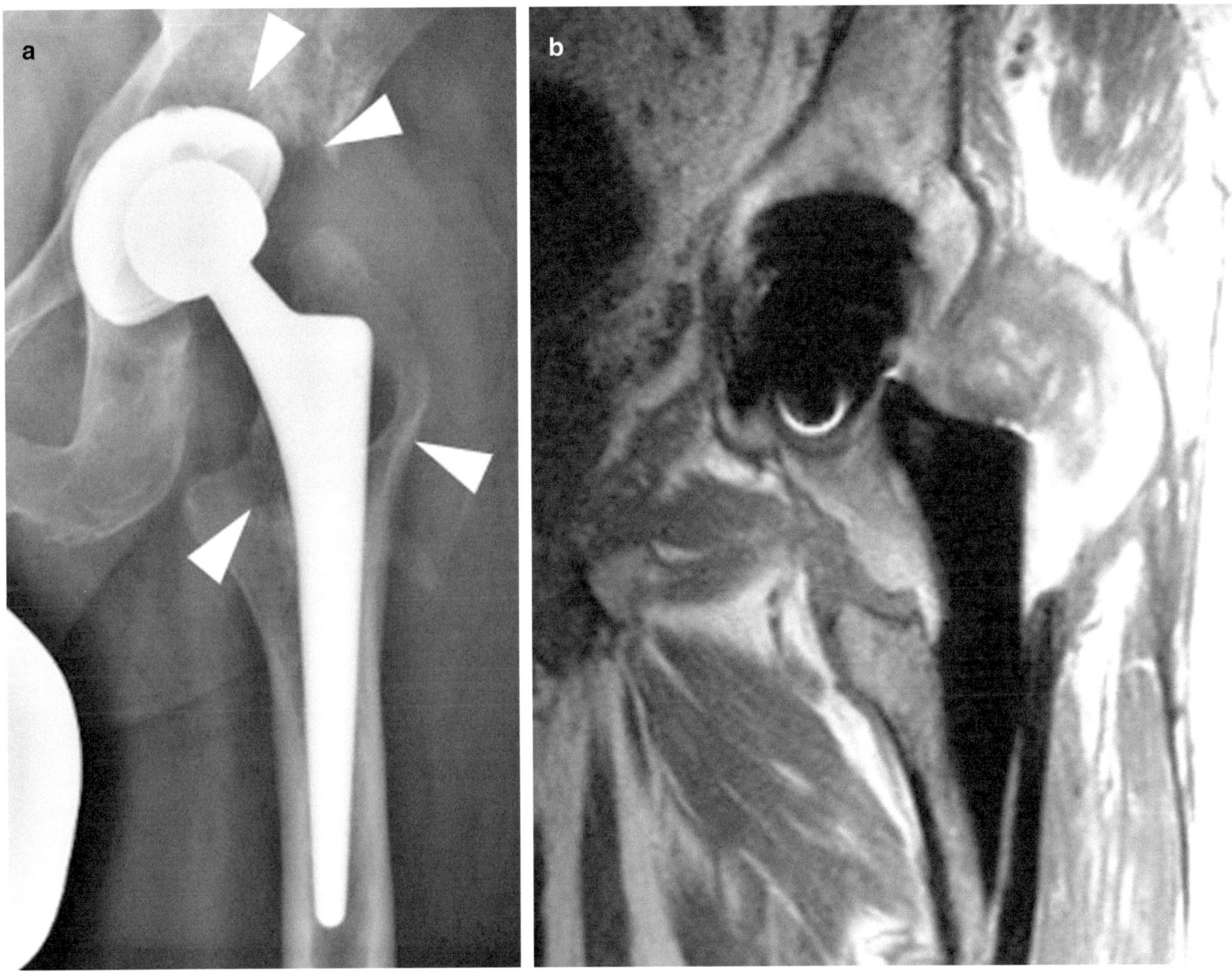

Fig. 10 (**a**–**e**) Wear disease (polyethylene-induced synovitis) following total hip arthroplasty. (**a**) AP radiograph demonstrates osteolyis adjacent to acetabular component and prostetic stem (*arrowheads*). Coronal (**b**) T1-weighted, (**c**) STIR, (**d**) gadolinium subtraction and (**e**) axial T2-weighted TSE images with metal artifact correction show distended pseudocapsule and osteolysis by high-signal-intensity fluid and intermediate-signal-intensity debris. Note hypointensity and contrast enhancement of peripheral lining of pseudotumor

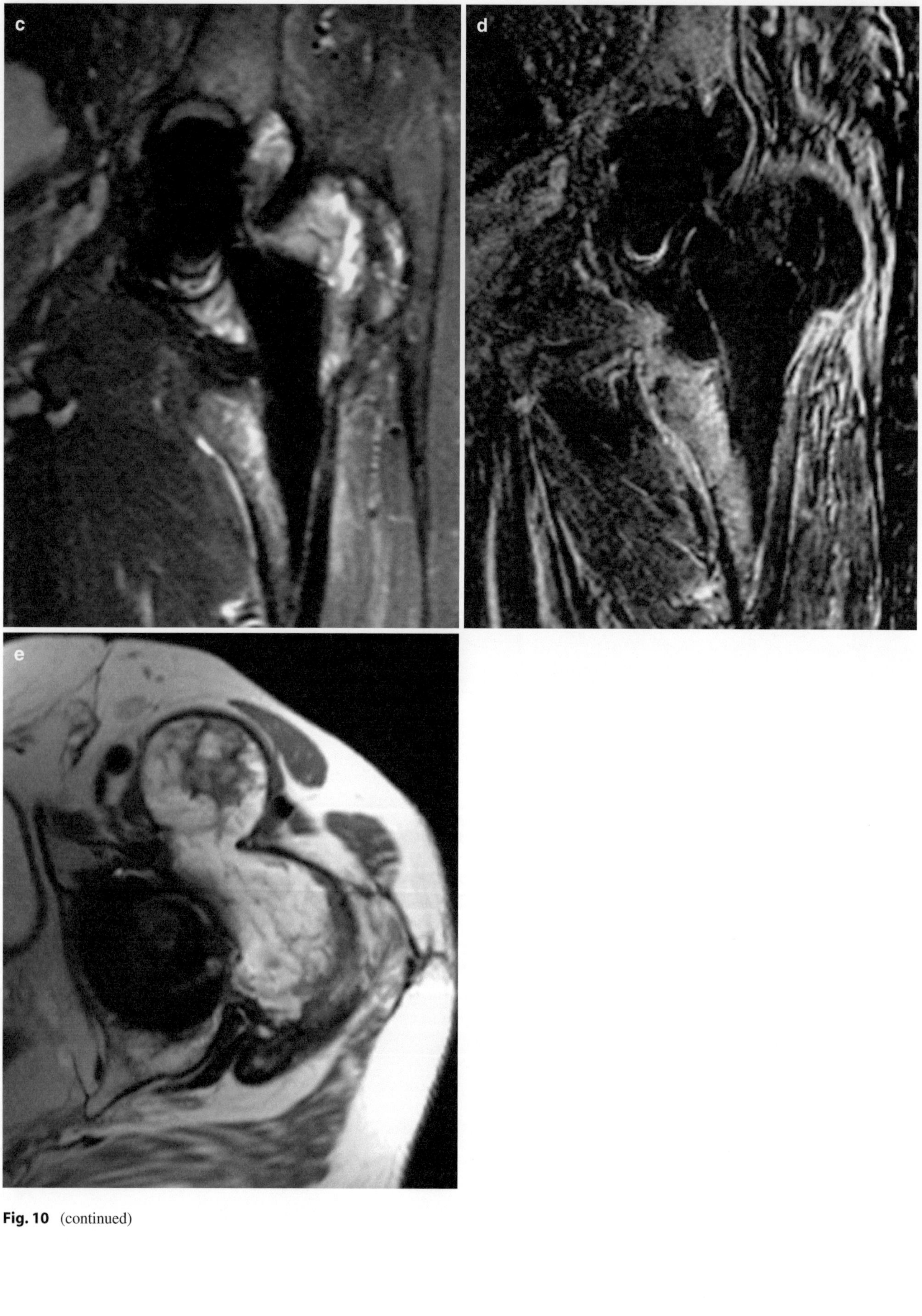

Fig. 10 (continued)

References

1. Watson RM, Roach NA, Dalinka MK (2004) Avascular necrosis and bone marrow edema syndrome. Radiol Clin N Am 42:207–219
2. Fujioka M, Kubo T, Nakamura F et al (2001) Initial changes of non-traumatic osteonecrosis of femoral head in fat suppression images: bone marrow edema was not found before the appearance of band patterns. Magn Reson Imaging 19:985–991
3. Meier R, Kraus TM, Schaeffeler C, Torka S, Schlitter AM, Specht K, Haller B, Waldt S, Rechl H, Rummeny EJ, Woertler K (2014) Bone marrow oedema on MR imaging indicates ARCO stage 3 disease in patients with AVN of the femoral head. Eur Radiol 24:2271–2278
4. Gardeniers JWM (1993) Report of the committee of staging and nomenclature. ARCO News Letter 5:79–82
5. Waldt S, Woertler K (2014) Measurements and classifications in musculoskeletal radiology. Thieme, Stuttgart, New York
6. Vande Berg BC, Malghem JI, Lecouvet FE, Jamart J, Maldague BE (1999) Idiopathic bone marrow edema lesions of the femoral head: predictive value of MR imaging findings. Radiology 212:525–535
7. Mueller D, Schaeffeler C, Baum T, Walter F, Rechl H, Rummeny EJ, Woertler K (2014) Magnetic resonance perfusion and diffusion imaging characteristics of transient bone marrow edema, avascular necrosis and subchondral insufficiency fractures of the proximal femur. Eur J Radiol 83:1862–1869
8. Huang GS, Chan WP, Chang YC, Chang CY, Chen CY, Yu JS (2003) MR imaging of bone marrow edema and joint effusion on patients with osteonecrosis of the femoral head: relationship to pain. AJR 181:545–549
9. Ito H, Matsuno T, Minami A (2006) Relationship between bone marrow edema and development of symptoms in patients with osteonecrosis of the femoral head. AJR 186:1761–1770
10. Kim YM, Oh HC, Kim HJ (2000) The pattern of bone marrow oedema on MRI in osteonecrosis of the femoral head. J Bone Joint Surg Br 82-B:837–841
11. Klontzas ME, Vassalou EE, Zibis AH, Bintoudi AS, Karantanas AH (2015) MR imaging of transient osteoporosis of the hip: an update on 155 hip joints. Eur J Radiol 84:431–436
12. Malizos KN, Zibis AH, Dailiana Z, Hantes M, Karachalios T, Karantanas AH (2004) MR imaging findings in transient osteoporosis of the hip. Eur J Radiol 50:238–244
13. Hackney LA, Lee MH, Joseph GB, Vail TP, Link TM (2016) Subchondral insufficiency fracture of the femoral head: associated imaging findings and predictors of clinical progression. Eur Radiol 26:1929–1941
14. Yamamoto T, Schneider R, Bullough PG (2001) Subchondral insufficiency fracture of the femoral head: histopathologic correlation with MRI. Skelet Radiol 30:247–254
15. Yamamoto T, Bullough PG (2000) The role of subchondral insufficiency fracture in rapid destruction of the hip joint: a preliminary report. Arthritis Rheum 43:2423–2427
16. Boutry N, Christelle P, Leroy X et al (2002) Rapidly destructive osteoarthritis of the hip: MR imaging findings. AJR 179:657–663
17. Iwasaki K, Yamamoto T, Motomura G et al (2016) Common site of subchondral insufficiency fractures of the femoral head based on three-dimensional magnetic resonance imaging. Skelet Radiol 45:105–113
18. Agten CA, Sutter R, Buck FM, Pfirrman CWA (2016) Hip imaging in athletes: sports imaging series. Radiology 280:351–389
19. De Franco MJ, Recht M, Schils J, Parker RD (2006) Stress fractures of the femur in athletes. Clin Sports Med 25:89–103, ix
20. Navas A, Kassarjian A (2011) Bone marrow changes in stress injuries. Semin Musculoskelet Radiol 15:183–197
21. Slocum KA, Gorman JD, Puckett ML, Jones SB (1997) Resolution of abnormal MR signal intensity in patients with stress fractures of the femoral neck. AJR 168:1295–1299
22. Wagner FV, Negrao JR, Campos J et al (2012) Capsular ligaments of the hip: anatomic, histologic, and positional study in cadaveric specimens with MR arthrography. Radiology 263:189–198
23. Robinson P, White LM, Agur A et al (2003) Obturator externus bursa: anatomic origin and MR imaging features of pathologic involvement. Radiology 228:230–234
24. Moorman CT III, Warren RF, Hershman EB et al (2003) Traumatic posterior hip subluxation in American football. J Bone Joint Surg Am 85:1190–1196
25. Stiris MG (2000) MR imaging after sports-induced hip dislocations: report of three cases. Acta Radiol 41:300–302
26. Tannast M, Pleaus F, Bonel H et al (2010) Magnetic resonance imaging in traumatic posterior hip dislocation. J Orthop Trauma 24:723–731
27. Nguyen MS, Kheyfits V, Giordano BD et al (2013) Hip anatomic variants that may mimic abnormalities at MRI: labral variants. AJR 201:W394–W400
28. Blankenbaker DG, De Smet AA, Keene JS et al (2007) Classification and location of acetabular labral tears. Skelet Radiol 36:391–397
29. Petersilge CA (2001) MR arthrography for evaluation of the acetabular labrum. Skelet Radiol 30:423–430
30. Petersilge CA (2005) Imaging of the acetabular labrum. MRI Clin N Am 13:641–652
31. Cerezal L, Kassarjian A, Canga A et al (2010) Anatomy, biomechanics, imaging and management of ligamentum teres injuries. Radiographics 30:1637–1651
32. Sampatchalit S, Barbosa D, Gentili A et al (2009) Degenerative changes in the ligamentum teres of the hip: cadaveric study with magnetic resonance arthrography, anatomical inspection, and histologic examination. J Comput Assist Tomogr 33:927–933
33. Gray AJ, Villar RN (1997) The ligamentum teres of the hip: an arthroscopic classification of its pathology. Arthroscopy 13:575–578
34. Tannast M, Siebenrock KA, Anderson SE Femoroacetabular impingment: radiographic diagnosis—what the radiologist should know. AJR 188:1540–1552
35. Pfirrmann CW, Mengiardi B, Dora C et al (2006) Cam and pincer femoroacetabular impingment: characteristic MR arthrographic findings in 50 patients. Radiology 240:778–785
36. Beall DP, Sweet CF, Martin HD et al (2005) Imaging findings of femoroacetabular impingement syndrome. Skelet Radiol 34:691–701
37. Palmer WE (2010) Femoroacetabular impingement: caution is warranted in making imaging-based assumptions and diagnoses. Radiology 257:4–7
38. Laborie LB, Lehmann TG, Engesaeter IO et al (2011) Prevalence of radiographic findings thought to be associated with femoroacetabular impingement in a population-based cohort of 2081 healthy young adults. Radiology 260:494–502
39. Chang EY, McAnally JL, Van Horne JR et al (2012) Metal-on-metal total hip arthroplasty: do symptoms correlate with MR imaging findings? Radiology 265:848–857
40. Fritz J, Lurie B, Miller TT (2013) Imaging of hip arthroplasty. Semin Musculoskelet Radiol 17:316–327
41. Walde TA, Weiland DE, Leung SB et al (2005) Comparison of CT, MRI, and radiographs in assessing pelvic osteolysis: a cadaveric study. Clin Orthop Relat Res 437:138–144

Infection

William B. Morrison and Apostolos H. Karantanas

Introduction

Diagnosis of infection can be challenging. Radiologic examinations can improve patient care, if applied appropriately early in the disease process. However, misdiagnosis or delayed diagnosis can lead to poor outcomes. This article discusses the advantages and disadvantages of imaging modalities, the imaging appearance of various types and manifestations of infection, as well as complicating factors and pitfalls.

General Principles

Routes of Infection

There are three basic routes for introduction of infection in the body: hematogenous, direct implantation and contiguous spread [1, 2]. Hematogenous spread is the most common cause of osteomyelitis in most areas of the body, including the spine. Direct implantation is relatively common in the hands and feet (i.e., puncture wounds, penetrating trauma) and in various areas of the body as a result of open surgery and percutaneous procedures. Contiguous spread is related to transmission of infection through the skin or from adjacent tissues. The most common clinical scenarios involving contiguous spread of infection include diabetic pedal infection and pelvic osteomyelitis in paralyzed patients.

W.B. Morrison (✉) • A.H. Karantanas
Department of Radiology, Thomas Jefferson University Hospital, 132 S. 10th St. Suite 1079a, Philadelphia, PA 08075, USA

Department of Radiology, University of Crete-University Hospital, Voutes, Heraklion 71110, Greece
e-mail: William.morrison@jefferson.edu; akarantanas@gmail.com

Modalities

Radiography

For patients with clinical suspicion of infection, radiographs are typically the initial radiologic examination obtained [3, 4]. Early infection is seen as soft tissue swelling, representing cellulitis. However, this findings is nonspecific. Septic arthritis is characterized in the early stages by joint effusion. Depending on location (i.e., deep joints), effusion may not be detected radiographically. As the disease progresses, erosions and joint space narrowing representing chondrolysis is observed. Finally, with onset of osteomyelitis, frank bone destruction is seen. Periosteal reaction may be seen in later stages. Radiographic changes of osteomyelitis can be delayed as much as 2 weeks after onset of infection. Overall, radiographs are insensitive to osteomyelitis in early stages and cannot determine the extent of involvement of osseous or soft tissue disease. Therefore, whether negative or positive, additional imaging is necessary. Despite low utility for diagnosing osteomyelitis, the wide availability and excellent overview of anatomy make radiography excellent for follow-up examinations, evaluation of postoperative changes, identification of soft tissue calcification, gas, and foreign bodies, and characterization of the pattern and distribution of arthritis, including neuropathic osteoarthropathy.

Computed Tomography

CT provides similar findings on radiographs but with more anatomic definition [5]. If intravenous contrast medium is administered, soft tissue enhancement reflecting cellulitis and rim enhancing fluid collections indicating abscess formation can be detected. In later stages of infection, as osteomyelitis sets in, periostitis and rarefaction of bone will be seen. Eventually, frank bone destruction ensues. Joint effusion, articular narrowing, and marginal erosions indicate septic arthritis. Determining the extent of involvement within

J. Hodler et al. (eds.), *Musculoskeletal Diseases 2017-2020*, DOI 10.1007/978-3-319-54018-4_7

the bone as well as in the soft tissues remains limited with CT. Given these limitations as well as associated expense, its use as a clinical tool for this purpose is limited. However, if anatomic information is needed and MRI cannot be obtained, or if there are metal implants, CT may be useful [6].

Ultrasonography

Use of a high-frequency transducer offers excellent depiction of soft tissue anatomic detail, and ultrasonography can be useful for answering specific questions, such as whether there is an infected fluid collection in the subcutaneous tissues [7]. Abscesses and effusions are seen as focal regions of hypoechogenicity often with complex internal characteristics. Joint effusions and tendon sheath fluid can be detected, but these findings are common in the absence of infection. Power Doppler can demonstrate hyperemia of the synovium and surrounding tissues, suggestive of inflammation. Although ultrasonography cannot visualize the marrow compartment, a focused examination can demonstrate cortical breakthrough and periosteal elevation. Owing to availability of other modalities that offer a more comprehensive evaluation, use of ultrasonography for this purpose is limited.

Magnetic Resonance Imaging

MRI is the imaging modality of choice for evaluation infection [8, 9]. Soft tissue and bone marrow pathology can be detected with high sensitivity. High contrast between different tissue types as well as inflammatory versus non-inflammatory tissue combined with anatomic definition has made this modality useful to surgeons interested in acquiring a "road map" of pathologic tissue before surgery. Additionally, with intravenous contrast administration it is possible to identify abcesses, extension of phelgmonous tissue and to evaluate areas of devitalization that may require débridement [10, 11].

Nuclear Medicine

Three-phase bone scintigraphy and labeled leukocyte imaging are the most commonly performed radionuclide tests in the evaluation of pedal infection [12, 13]. Although the three-phase bone scan is sensitive for detecting osteomyelitis, many conditions in the diabetic foot demonstrate focal hyperperfusion, hyperemia and bony uptake, mimicking infection, and, consequently, specificity is low. When there is no increased uptake the test is excellent for excluding the presence of osteomyelitis, except in the setting of severe vascular disease. Labeled white blood cell examination has higher specificity and is generally interpreted in conjunction with the three-phase bone scintiscan.

The uptake in three-phase bone scintigraphy using 99mTc-labeled methylene diphosphonate is related to blood flow and osteoblastic activity. Localized bone uptake on the delayed third phase is nonspecific, but if all three phases are positive with clinical suspicion of infection the test is highly sensitive for diagnosis of osteomyelitis. Cellulitis, abscess, and other soft tissue infections show increased uptake on the initial blood flow and second blood pool phases that fails to concentrate in bone on the third phase. Occasionally, and especially in ischemic feet, there is persistent blood pool activity which can be suspected if there is poorly defined tracer distribution. Residual bony uptake on a fourth phase, acquired after 24 h, can help distinguish osteomyelitis from overlying cellulitis in this setting. Severe ischemia results in photopenia or relative lack of uptake and chronic osteomyelitis or partially treated infection may not show characteristic uptake on the first two phases resulting in false negative examinations [12, 13]. Persistent radiotracer uptake may be seen with treated osteomyelitis. Bone turnover and hyperemia caused by neuropathic osteoarthropathy, trauma, recent surgery, or inflammatory arthropathy can appear similar to infection, leading to a false-positive examination. Specificity is lower as a result of vascular insufficiency and complicating neuroarthropathy. In the setting of underlying complicating conditions, where there is nonspecific uptake on the delayed phase, corresponding uptake on a labeled white blood cell scan increases specificity.

White blood cell scanning is based on accumulation of labeled leukocytes in infected tissue with reported sensitivity and specificity ranging from 75 to 100% and 69 to 100% respectively. Combined with three-phase bone scintigraphy, specificity increases to 90 to 100%. Focal uptake in the foot, without appreciable amounts of red marrow, is generally indicative of infection. It may be difficult to separate soft tissue from bone infection, both of which will accumulate leukocytes. Corresponding delayed uptake on a three-phase bone scintiscan can make the diagnosis of osteomyelitis. False negatives may be seen with prior antibiotic treatment and ischemia. Noninfectious inflammatory conditions such as rheumatoid arthritis and hyperemic conditions such as acute neuropathic disease can occasionally show increased uptake, a false positive.

Positron Emission Tomography and Cross Sectional Imaging

18-F-FDG Positron emission tomography (PET) combined with CT (PET/CT) has shown promise for imaging infection, related to increased metabolism of glucose in areas of inflammation [14]. The high resolution of PET is a significant advantage over bone and labeled leukocyte imaging. However, to date, limited data exist to test its efficacy in the diabetic foot and the jury is still out. Hybridization of PET with MRI (PET/MRI) is emerging as a new tool to provide important diagnostic information, with data predominantly limited as of yet, to oncological applications. Perhaps, in the future hybridization techniques may play a useful role in the evaluation of diabetic foot infection.

Imaging Manifestations of Infection

Septic Arthritis

Septic arthritis (SA) results from seeding of microorganisms, usually bacteria, either with direct inoculation or more commonly hematogenously [15]. The risk for joint infections is related to IV drug use, immunocompromised state and diagnostic and therapeutic injections. The earlier the diagnosis the lower is the risk for irreversible destruction of the articular cartilage. The clinical and serologic findings are suggestive of pyogenic SA which is established with drainage and culture. The role of imaging is secondary and is mainly related to suggest a clinically unsuspected SA. Absence of joint effusion on US, shows a high negative predictive value for SA. Normal radiographs cannot exclude a SA. The earliest radiographic findings are soft tissue swelling and joint effusion which lack reproducibility and are non specific. MRI findings suggesting SA include joint effusion, synovial thickening and surrounding soft tissue changes such as fasciitis and myositis (Fig. 1). Contrast administration may show diffuse synovitis and soft tissue abscess formation. Limited subchondral bone marrow edema is usually reactive whereas diffuse marrow edema, particularly if obvious on T1-w images, is suggesting osteomyelitis [16]. Although sensitive, MRI lacks specificity as most of the above described findings may be seen in inflammatory joint disease as well [17].

Tuberculous arthritis (TBa) has a more chronic course compared to pyogenic SA, is common in endemic areas but in developed countries it is seen in immunosuppressed, immigrants, and elderly patients. TBa is considered to occur secondarily to hematogenously induced osteomyelitis, is mostly nonoarticular with the hip being involved up to 15% and if untreated results in joint destruction [18, 19]. Establishment of diagnosis is not possible based on imaging findings alone. The "*Phemister's triad*" refers to the presence of *periarticular osteopenia, peripheral erosions* and *gradual joint space narrowing* on plain radiographs. Minimal subarticular sclerosis, soft tissue swelling, osteolysis and minimal periosteal reaction may also be seen [18, 19]. Joint space will be narrowed late in the course of the disease. Effusion and synovial hypertophy seen on MRI, are

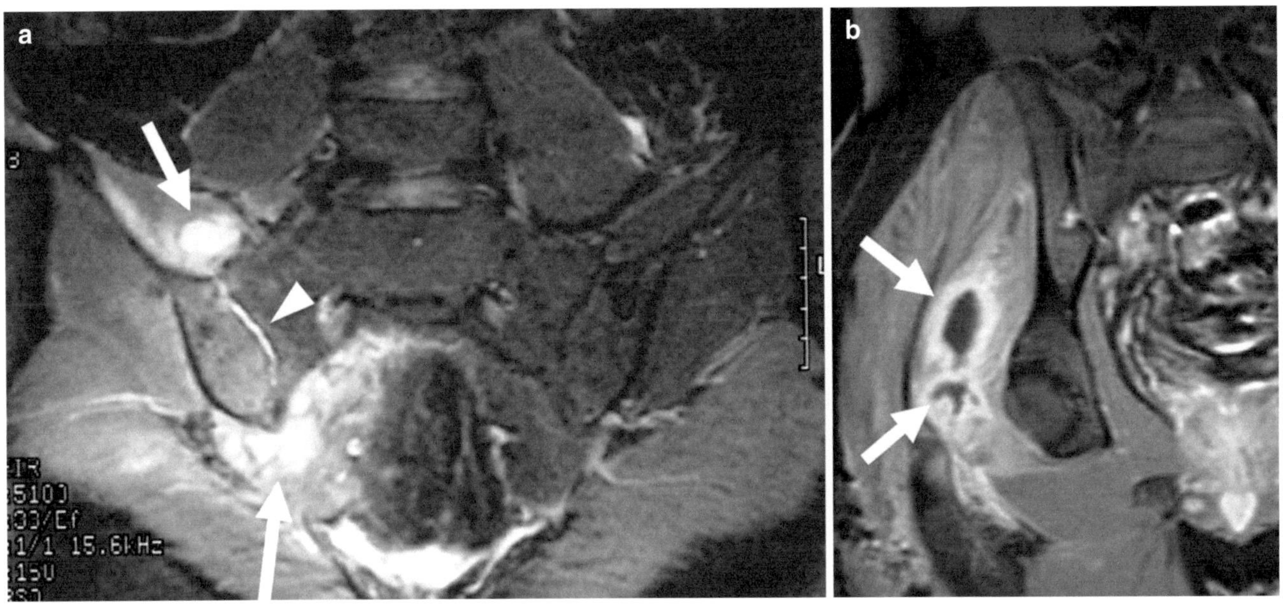

Fig. 1 35-year-old male patient with right lower back pain for 2 weeks; recent onset of right sciatic pain. Low grade fever. Aspiration-proven *Staphylococcus aureus* septic sacroiliitis. Coronal STIR image (**a**) shows fluid signal within the joint (*arrowhead*) with distension of the joint recesses superiorly and inferiorly (*arrows*), the latter extending into the sciatic notch. Note surrounding soft tissue edema representing inflammation. Coronal T1-weighted fat suppressed post-contrast image (**b**) shows rim-enhancing abscesses (*arrows*) in the gluteus musculature

indistinguishable from those seen in other arthritides. Chronic synovitis though, may show minimal on no enhancement at all. Sacroiliac joint involvement may show abscesses, often calcified, and are best appreciated with CT.

In our practice, any patient with joint effusion and clinical suspicion of SA, undergoes image-guided aspiration of the fluid with fluoroscopy, ultrasonography or CT, depending upon the individual joint involvement and the body habitus of the patient.

Cellulitis

Cellulitis is seen as replacement of the normal fat signal in subcutaneous tissues on T1-weighted images, with high signal (though less than fluid) on T2-weighted or STIR images and diffuse enhancement after contrast agent administration. The margins are generally poorly defined. Abscesses appear as a focal collection of signal approximating fluid on T2-weighted or STIR images, with thick rim enhancement on post-contrast T1-weighted images. Sinus tracts are characterized by a thin, discrete line of fluid signal extending through the soft tissues with enhancement of the hyperemic margins. Sinus tracts are visualized as parallel lines of enhancement in a "tram-track" configuration.

Osteomyelitis

Osteomyelitis is characterized by altered bone marrow signal, with low signal (loss of the normal fat signal) on T1-weighted images, edema signal on T2-weighted or STIR images, and enhancement on postgadolinium T1-weighted images (Fig. 2). Other MRI findings in cases of osteomyelitis include cortical disruption and periostitis. Periostitis is seen as a thin, linear pattern of edema and enhancement surrounding the outer cortical margin that will appear thickened if the periostitis is chronic.

Recognition of abnormal bone marrow signal in the appropriate clinical setting results in high sensitivity for diagnosis of osteomyelitis. Other entities can mimic this alteration in signal, including fracture, tumor, active inflammatory arthritis or neuropathic disease, infarction, or recent postoperative change. However, these other processes usually have different morphology than osteomyelitis and recognition of these patterns often enables differentiation. For

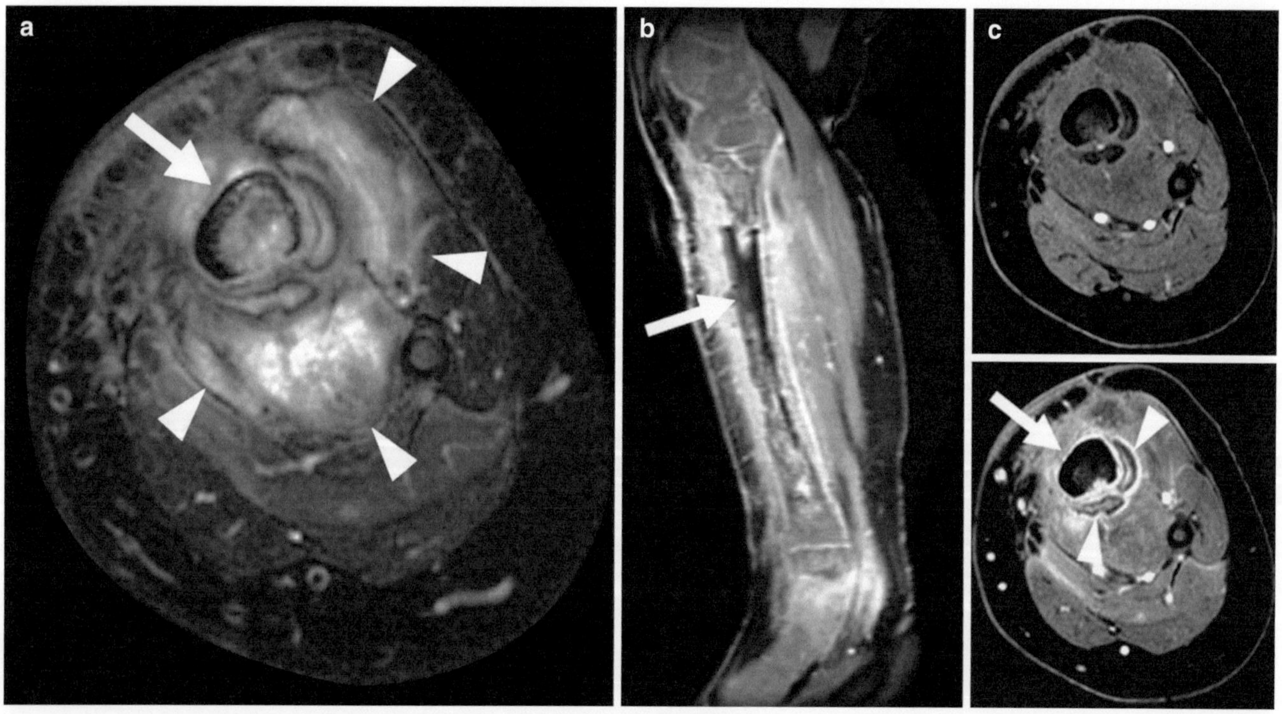

Fig. 2 10-year-old boy with chronic leg pain, fevers. Biopsy-proven osteomyelitis. Axial T2-weighted fat suppressed image (**a**) of the lower leg demonstrates abnormal signal in the tibia (*arrow*) representing osteomyelitis. Note surrounding phlegmonous tissue (*arrowheads*). Sagittal T1-weighted fat suppressed post contrast image (**b**) and axial T1-weighted fat suppressed pre- and post-contrast images (**c**) show non-enhancement of the mid tibial shaft (*arrow*) consistent with devitalization (a sequestrum). A rim of enhancing new bone formation (involucrum, *arrowheads*) is present

example, identification of a fracture line, a discrete lesion, adjacent arthritis or neuropathic disease, or postoperative metal artifact improves specificity. Correlation with radiographs and clinical history is also important. Additionally, over 90% of the time osteomyelitis of the foot and ankle is a result of contiguous spread through the skin1 with the majority of cases demonstrating skin ulceration, cellulitis, soft tissue abscess, or a sinus tract. These findings can be thought of as "secondary signs" of osteomyelitis, recognition of which improves specificity.

Devitalization

Changes related to ischemia should be taken into account when interpreting MRI of the diabetic foot. Documentation of the presence and extent of ischemic and devitalized areas facilitate surgical planning for débridement and limited, foot-sparing amputations. Pre- and postcontrast MR images can detect ischemia and devitalization of the foot as focal or regional lack of soft tissue contrast enhancement. Devitalization, or foot "infarction," is seen as a focal area of nonenhancement with a sharp cutoff with increased enhancement in the surrounding reactive, hypervascular tissue. Only contrast-enhanced images allow reliable recognition of gangrenous tissue because T2- and T1-weighted images reveal uncharacteristic signal alterations.

Underlying infection, including osteomyelitis, cellulitis, and abscess would not be expected to enhance within necrotic areas (Fig. 2). In this setting, signal characteristics on T1- and T2-weighted images should be primarily relied on for diagnosis of soft tissue and osseous infection. If intravenous contrast is provided, the radiologist should be familiar with the appearance of devitalized tissue to reduce false-negative readings for infection.

Evaluation of Extent of Involvement

Extent of infection in soft tissue and bone is fairly well delineated on postcontrast MR images. However, infection does not tend to remain confined by fascial planes and spreads centripetally from the inoculation site across fascial compartments, into and across joints, and through tendons. Soft tissue involvement is often more extensive than the osseous disease, requiring careful examination of the soft tissues proximal to the source of infection. Without proper débridement the patient may fail the foot-sparing procedure and require more extensive amputation.

Spinal Infection

Infectious spondylodiscitis is an inflammatory disorder which involves the osseous structures, vertebral bodies (osteomyelitis) and the discs (discitis). Posterior elements, isolated facet joint infection and paravertebral soft tissue abscesses may also occur. The earlier the diagnosis is made, the better the prognosis is. Since clinical symptoms, physical examination findings and laboratory data are often non specific, imaging has a crucial role in early diagnosis and treatment planning. Spinal infection represents around 3–5% of all cases of osseous infection and is increasing in prevalence due to increased number of mobile population, diabetes mellitus, intravenous drug abuse, immunocompromised patients of any cause, increased number of surgical and diagnostic image guided procedures and higher awareness. Diabetic men in the 5th and 6th decades of life and elderly of both sexes are more commonly afflicted. In about 25% of patients, the organisms cannot be identified. Early diagnosis is associated with good outcome whereas delay in diagnosis may be life threatening. Spinal infection may be caused by bacteria, fungi and parasites.

The routes of infection include *arterial spread* from distal septic foci, *venous spread* through the Batson's plexus from pelvic infections, and *direct extension* from adjacent soft tissue or *implantation*, either iatrogenically or rarely by penetrating injury [20]. The lumbar spine is more commonly involved (50%) followed by thoracic spine (35%) [21]. Septic emboli location depends upon the age group. In children under age 4, end arteries enter the intervertebral disc and thus discitis may be the initial and perhaps the only demonstration due to the rich intraosseous network of arterial anastomoses. In adolescents and adults, the richest arterial network lies beneath the anterior endplate which is the equivalent to long bone metaphysis. Thus, infection appears first in the anterior vertebral body and then spreads through the endplates into the disc and the contiguous vertebral body. Pre/paravertebral and epidural extension may occur via subligamentous route. Epidural abscess formation is an emergency situation and the role of radiologist in prompt diagnosis is crucial [22].

Pyogenic

Pyogenic spondylodiscitis (PS) is the most commonly encountered spine infection. Common causative bacteria are *Staphylococcus aureus* (up to 60%) followed by *Enterobacter* (up to 30%), *Streptococcus*, *Pseudomonas*, *Klebsiella* and *Salmonella*. The course may be acute or chronic and the symptoms are non specific. Elevated ESR, PRC and WBC, are not constant laboratory findings. The primary radiologic finding is destruction of two contiguous vertebral bodies and the intervertebral disc. Plain radiographs are not sensitive in the early stages and become positive 2–4 weeks after onset of symptoms. Progressive osteolysis beneath the anterior endplate and loss of endplate definition, are signs highly suggesting PS (20). A rapid loss of the intervertebral space matched with loss of definition in the opposing endplate and associated osteolysis beneath it, suggest spread to the contiguous vertebral body. As a rule, the presence of gas ("vacuum" in the disc and "cleft" beneath the endplate), rules out infection. CT is more sensitive to earlier changes showing in addition to plain films effacement of paravertebral fat planes and contrast enhancement of paravertebral soft tissue changes. It may be useful when MRI findings are equivocal, by showing the presence of disc "vacuum" sign and the lack of endplate destruction which help to rule out infection. It offers in addition a guidance of the route for diagnostic aspiration. MRI is the method of choice for early detection and accurate diagnosis of PS. Low on T1-weighted and high on fluid sensitive sequences bone marrow edema initially, followed by loss of the "black" outline of the endplate cortex, are the acute phase imaging findings [20, 21]. Bone marrow edema is located underneath the disrupted endplate cortex. Later, high signal on fluid sensitive sequences is seen within the involved disc. Fat suppressed images following contrast medium administration, show enhancement of the bone marrow and the disc, excluding the necrotic areas [20, 21]. Occasionally, depending on the duration of symptoms, a paraspinal or intra-canalicular phlegmon may be seen. A peripheral rim enhancement corresponds to abscess formation, often in thoracic spine. Epidural abscesses result in high morbidity and mortality and may be the initial feature of the disease from a remote underlying infection in cases of extension from facets and retroperitoneum or from hematogenous spread directly to this anatomic location. Subdural abscess is a rare and urgent disorder, suggested on MRI when the shape of the sac and the epidural fat are preserved. Major differential diagnosis of PS should include Modic type I endplate degenerative changes [20–22]. In favor of infection are the high signal of the disc and lack of the normal intranuclear cleft on T2-weighted images as well as presence of disc enhancement. Dialysis-associated destructive spondyloarthropathy, showing sharply demarcated endplate erosions and low T2 signal in the paraspinal lesions, should also be included in the differential diagnosis [20]. Paraspinal edema and enhancement may be seen in axial spondyloarthritis-related enthesopathy. Acute Schmorl's node and aseptic spondylodiscitis, previously known as Andersson's lesion in the context of axial spondylarthropathy, may simulate early infection. A useful sign of PS healing on MRI is the focal return of bone marrow fatty signal on T1-weighted images. However, MRI is not recommended for follow-up as it lags 4–8 weeks behind clinical and serologic improvement in successful treatment [20, 23]. Thus, persistent or worse MRI findings in patients with clinical improvement, do not suggest a failed treatment. Newer techniques, such as diffusion-weighted imaging may show increased diffusivity and drop in the ACD values in PS, often indistinguishable from malignancy [24] but helpful in differentiating infectious from degenerative changes in the endplates, the latter showing lower ADC values [25]. Radionuclide imaging is not currently used routinely as it is limited by false negative results, inability to detect soft tissue involvement and the fact that it remains abnormal during the normal healing phase after resolution of infection [26]. Indeed, it is reserved for cases that MRI findings are inconclusive, for depicting multiple foci and for patients with contraindication for MRI. FDG-PET/CT may be more accurate than MRI in low-grade spondylodiscitis and useful particularly when severe degenerative changes coexist [26].

Postoperative

Postoperative or post-intervention infection is rare, occurs usually from direct implantation of microorganisms and may be located in the body (osteomyelitis), disc (discitis) or both. Recurrent pain in the spine following the initial postoperative clinical improvement and a positive straight leg-raising test are suggesting clinical symptom and finding respectively favoring a diagnosis of PS. A positive CRP which was negative preoperatively is also a reliable test for infection. MRI in the postoperative setting is not as useful because of the presence of hardware-related susceptibility artifacts and normal postoperative changes which persist for months. Thus, discrimination between infection and normal postoperative changes are possible later than 3 weeks after operation and more reliable later than 6 months after surgery. Familiarity with normal postoperative changes regarding individual surgery, is important. In general, absence of endplate and subchondral bone signal changes, rules out spondylodiscitis and thus the major role of MRI in the immediate postoperative state is to exclude infection.

Atypical Infections

The causative microorganisms in nonpyogenic infectious spondylitis, include *Mycobacterium tuberculosis*, *Brucella bacillus*, *fungi* and *parasites*.

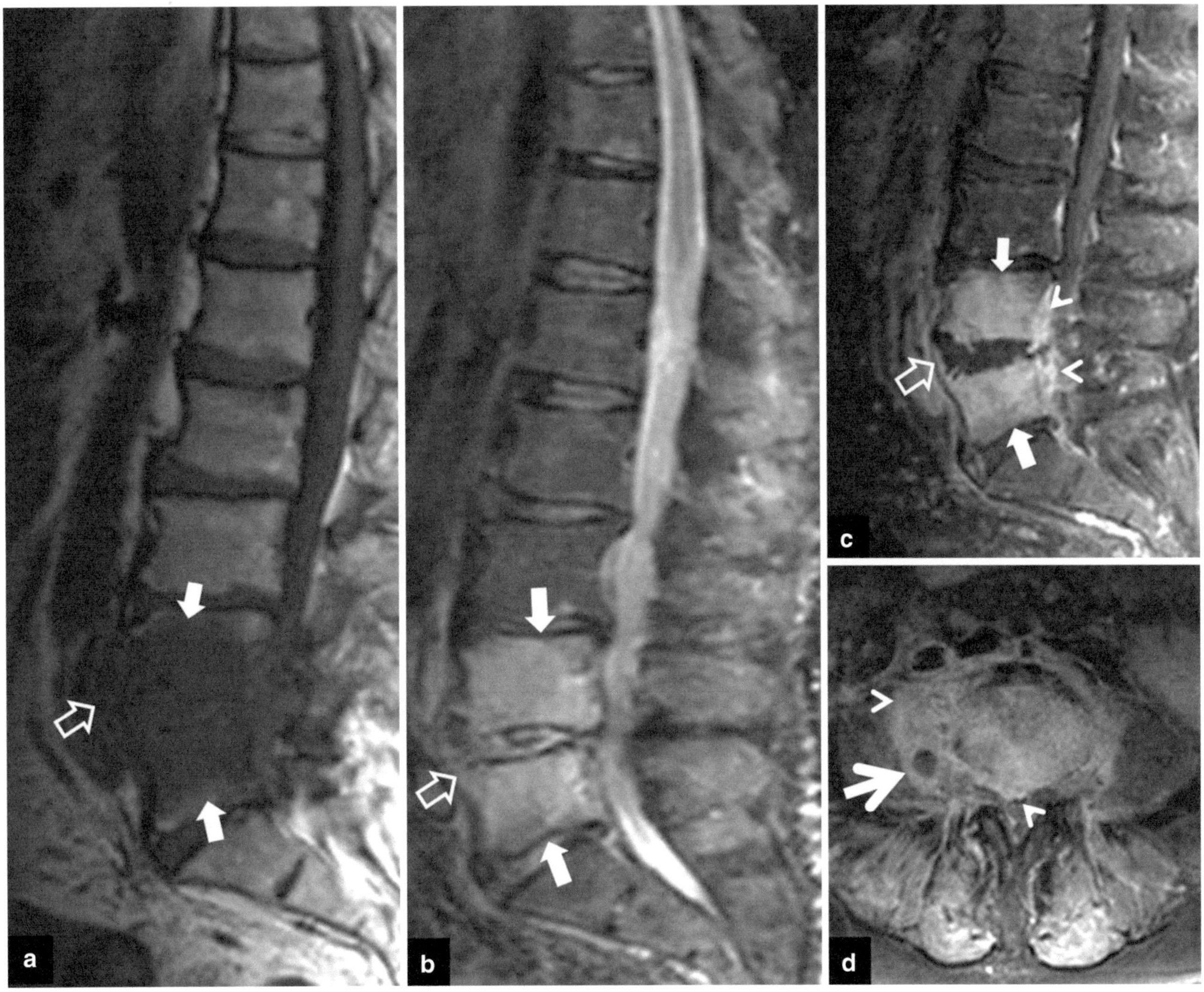

Fig. 3 70-year-old male patient with a history of 5 months of low back pain and a final diagnosis of tuberculous spondylodiscitis. MRI with sagittal T1-weighted (**a**), STIR (**b**), and contrast enhanced fat suppressed T1 on sagittal (**c**) and axial (**d**) planes, show bone marrow edema in the L4 and L5 vertebral bodies (*arrows*), subligamentous spread sparing the disc (*open arrows*), epidural and paraspinal phlegmon (*arrowheads*) and paraspinal abscess formation (*thick arrow*)

Tuberculous spondylitis (TBs), also known as *Pott's* disease, is the most common non pyogenic granulomatous infection of the spine and is increasing due to immigration from endemic areas and HIV patients. The clinical course is indolent and symptoms may last for months before diagnosis is suspected and imaging is performed. TBs is located primarily in the thoracolumbar junction and is the result of hematogenous spread from a foci in the lung parenchyma. The anterior initial focus tends to spread subligamentously in all directions, often skipping the disc space. Late in the course of an undiagnosed TBs, TB meningitis may occur. Plain films are not always able to differentiate between pyogenic and non pyogenic infections. With progression of the TBs, radiographs show vertebral collapse with gibbus formation secondary to anterior wedging. Osteoslcerosis and contiguous vertebra ankylosis indicate healing on plain films. MRI is the method of choice and TBs is indicated when the following are depicted: involvement of a single vertebral body or multiple vertebral bodies with preservation or less severe and late involvement of the intervertebral disc and presence of paravertebral soft tissue abscesses, often large and bilateral [20] (Fig. 3). The presence of calcifications within abscesses is a diagnostic sign. Global spine MRI is necessary because multiple non-contiguous, often asymptomatic lesions, are present in up to 70%.

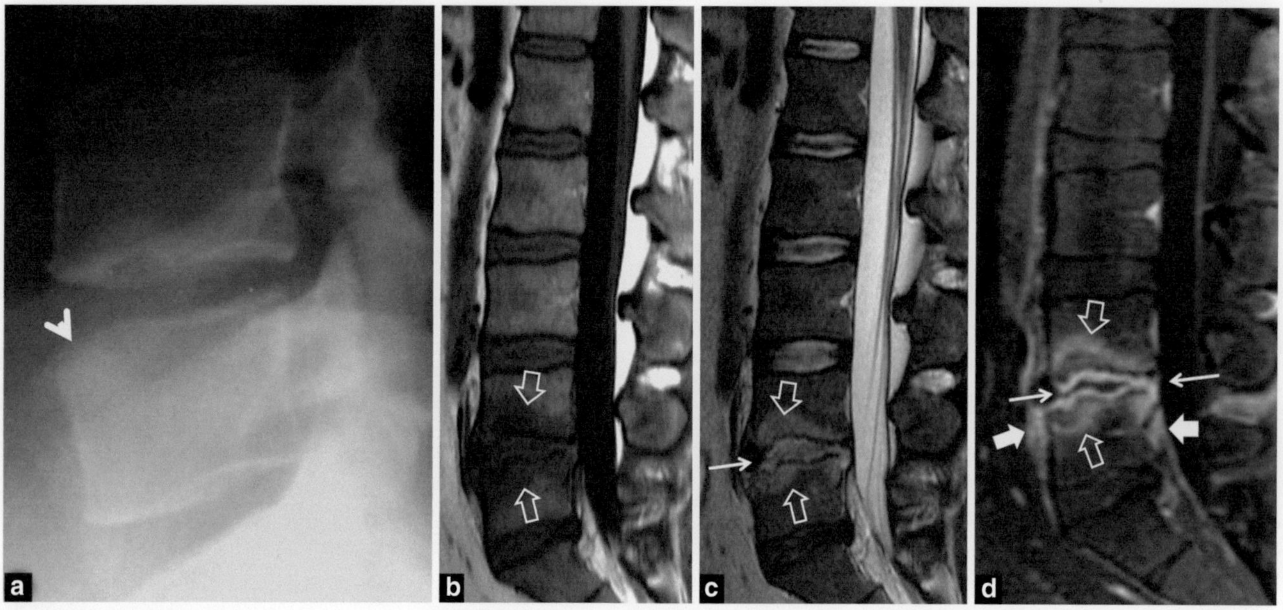

Fig. 4 34-year-old male patient with 2 months of low back pain without sciatica and a final diagnosis of Brucella spondylodiscitis. Lateral radiograph (**a**) shows indistinct anterior superior endplate of L5 vertebral body (*arrowhead*) and subcortical sclerosis. Sagittal T1 (**b**), T2 (**c**) and fat suppressed contrast enhanced T1-weighted (**d**) MR images, show abnormal signal and enhancement in the disc and disc space narrowing (*thin arrows*), bone marrow edema (*open arrows*) and paraspinal and epidural phlegmon (*arrows*)

Brucellosis is a systemic zoonosis which is endemic in the Mediterranean, Central Asia, Central and South American and Arabic countries and results from a gram negative bacillus with various species depending upon the animal involved. *Brucella spondylodiscitis* (Bs) is clinically demonstrated with fever, sweating, malaise, and local spine tenderness. Positive tests in the serum establish the diagnosis. Interestingly, sampling of the involved spinal segments is not usually diagnostic. The most common locations are the sacroiliac joints in the acute form of the disease in young adults and lumbosacral in the subacute and chronic forms in older patients. Multilevel location may be seen [27]. The initial feature on plain radiographs is osteopenia of the involved vertebral body and erosion with sclerosis and osteophyte formation (parrot's beak appearance) of the anterior-superior endplate, often at L4 level, also known as *Pons* sign. Focal anterior or global disc collapse will follow. MRI findings show mainly disc involvement and vertebral body preservation until late in the course of the disease (Fig. 4). Soft tissue abscesses are not a constant findings but peritoneal thickening and paraaortic lymph node enlargement may be seen.

Fungal spondylodiscitis is rare and seen almost exclusively, as an opportunistic infection in immunocompromised or chronically ill patients. Lumbar spine is often involved with sparing of the disc and intranuclear cleft preservation, and no severe vertebral body destruction. Aspergillus and Candida are most frequently the causative species. Limited publications exist on the imaging findings of *Aspergillus spondylodiscitis*. One study showed MRI findings similar to TBs emphasizing skip lesions with normal intervening vertebral bodies and discs, subligamentous extension, a serrated pattern of the endplates and hypointensity on T2-w images of the bone marrow under the endplates [28]. Another report on patients with *Candida spondylodiscitis*, showed contiguous vertebral involvement without disc destruction, small paraspinal abscesses and characteristic low signal on T2-w images of the paraspinal inflammation [29].

Parasitic spondylodiscitis usually results from hematogenous seeding of the subarachnoid space or direct inoculation from soft tissue involvement. *Hydatid* infection is commonly seen in sheepherders in Middle East and Australia. Neurocysticercosis and Schistosomiasis, may initially present with myelitis of the cord. Due to rich blood supply, spine is involved in hydatid osseous disease in more than 50% [30]. MRI findings include presence of high T2 signal coalescent hydatid cysts within the vertebral bodies but also within discs and spinal canal (Fig. 5).

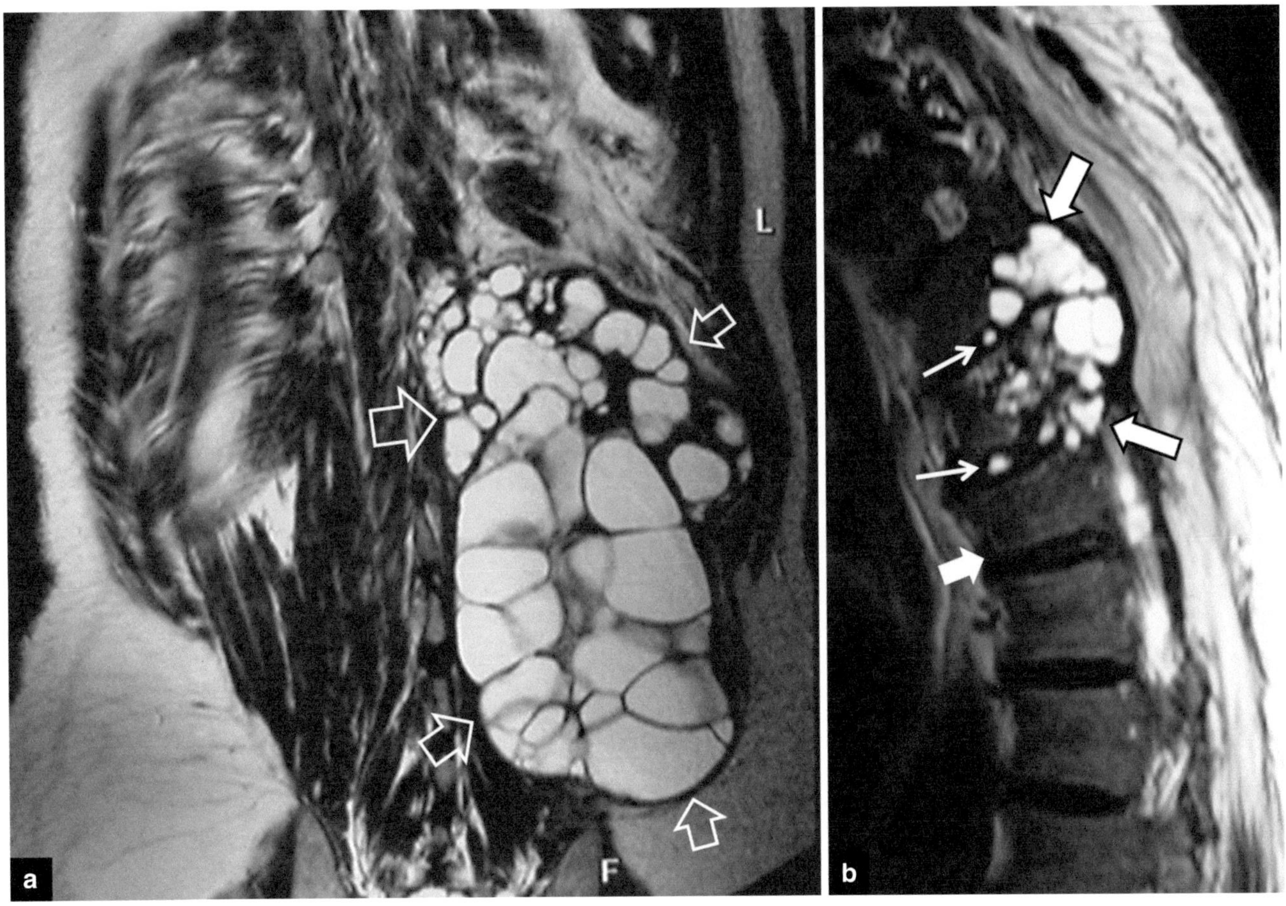

Fig. 5 76-year-old man with previous soft tissue hydatid disease presenting 6 years postoperatively with dorsal back pain and gradually increasing weakness of left leg. (**a**) Coronal T2-weighted MR image shows the initial hydatid soft tissue infection in the left thoracolumbar area (*open arrows*). (**b**) Left parasagittal T2-weighted MR image show hydatid cysts in disks (*thin arrows*) and in the epidural space (*arrows*)

Mimickers of Infection and Complicating Factors: Example—Neuropathic Osteoarthropathy

Differentiation of osteomyelitis and neuropathic osteoarthropathy can be difficult, because both can demonstrate marrow abnormality, joint effusion, and surrounding soft tissue edema [31]. Some rules may be used to help differentiate these entities on MR images. First, the vast majority of cases of osteomyelitis of the foot and ankle are due to contiguous spread. Therefore, a bone marrow abnormality without adjacent skin ulceration, sinus tract, or soft tissue inflammation is less likely to represent infection. This concept is particularly useful when there are extensive bone marrow signal abnormalities and lack of subcutaneous tissue involvement. Second, neuropathic osteoarthropathy is predominantly an articular process manifesting as instability, often with multiple regional joints involved (e.g., the Lisfranc, Chopart, or multiple adjacent metatarsophalangeal joints). This and other articular manifestations of neuropathic disease (subluxation, cysts, necrotic debris) are not as common in infection. Associated neuropathic marrow changes can be extensive (especially at the midfoot) but tend to be centered equally about a joint and at the subarticular bone. Osteomyelitis shows more diffuse marrow involvement, and unless there is a primary septic arthritis the marrow changes are generally greater on one side of the joint. Finally, location of disease is important. Neuropathic osteoarthropathy by far is most common at the Lisfranc and Chopart joints.

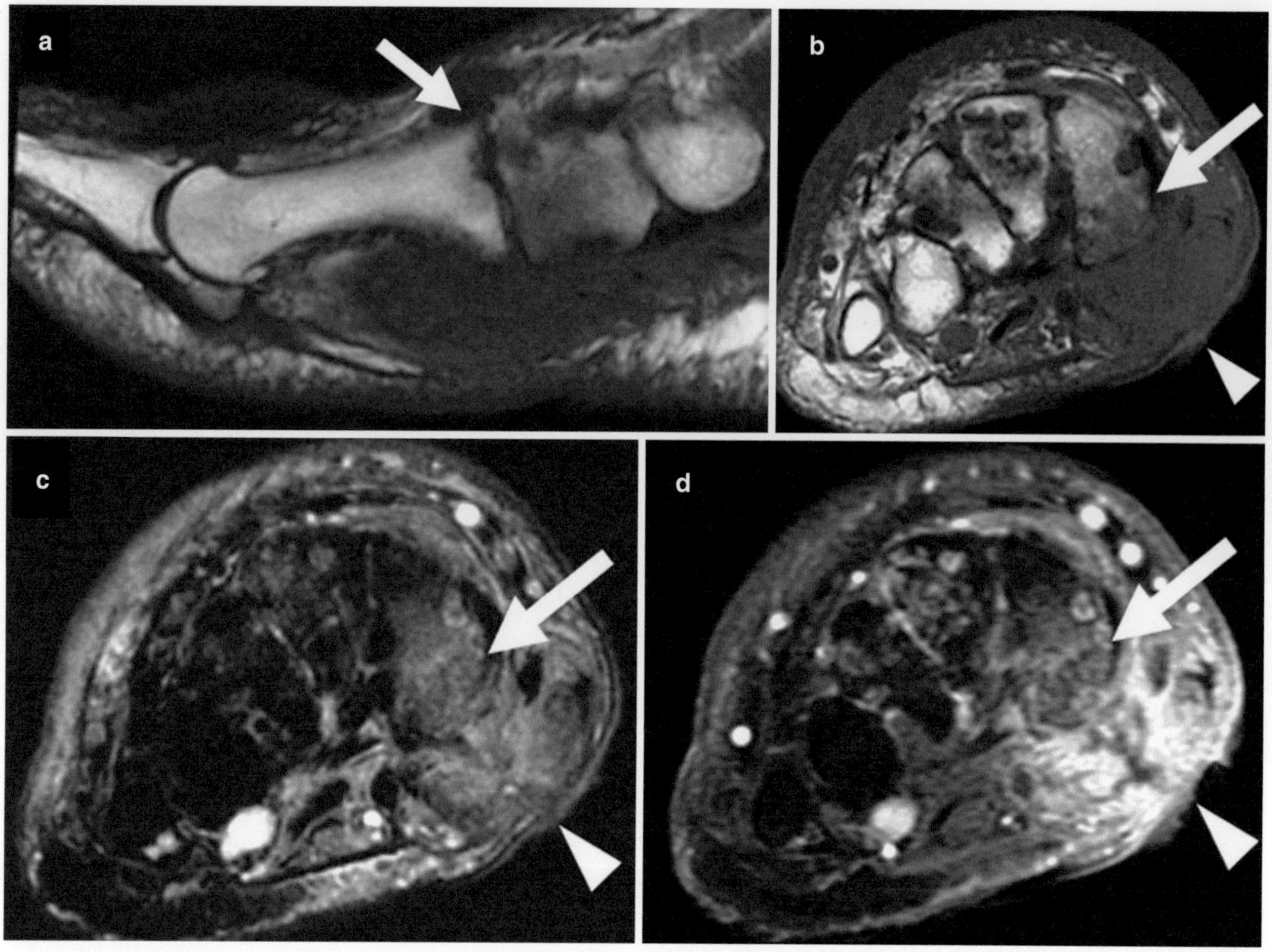

Fig. 6 56-year-old man with neuropathic osteoarthropathy of the midfoot presents with an ulceration and concern for superimposed osteomyelitis. Sagittal T1-weighted image (**a**) shows Charcot arthropathy involving the Lisfranc joint (*arrow*). Coronal T1-weighted (**b**), T2-weighted fat suppressed (**c**) and T1-weighted fat suppressed post-contrast image (**d**) of the midfoot demonstrates ulceration (*arrowheads*) with cellulitis and adjacent sinus tract extending to the medial cuneiform (*arrows*) where marrow signal alteration is consistent with superimposed osteomyelitis

Osteomyelitis occurs predominantly at the metatarsal heads, toes, calcaneus, and malleoli, a distribution that mirrors that of friction, callus, and ulceration. However, contiguous spread of infection can occur at atypical sites if there is a foot deformity (e.g., the cuboid in cases of rocker-bottom deformity) (Fig. 6).

Summary

Radiological examinations play an essential role in diagnosis and management of infection. The practitioner should maintain up-to-date knowledge regarding advantages and limitations of the different imaging modalities to provide the most efficacious care.

References

1. Turecki MB, Taljanovic MS, Stubbs AY, Graham AR, Holden DA, Hunter TB, Rogers LF (2010) Imaging of musculoskeletal soft tissue infections. Skelet Radiol 39(10):957–971
2. Christian S, Kraas J, Conway WF (2007) Musculoskeletal infections. Semin Roentgenol 42(2):92–101
3. Santiago Restrepo C, Giménez CR, McCarthy K (2003) Imaging of osteomyelitis and musculoskeletal soft tissue infections: current concepts. Rheum Dis Clin N Am 29(1):89–109
4. Gold RH, Hawkins RA, Katz RD (1991) Bacterial osteomyelitis: findings on plain radiography, CT, MR, and scintigraphy. AJR Am J Roentgenol 157(2):365–370
5. Ma LD, Frassica FJ, Bluemke DA, Fishman EK (1997) CT and MRI evaluation of musculoskeletal infection. Crit Rev Diagn Imaging 38(6):535–568
6. Fayad LM, Carrino JA, Fishman EK (2007) Musculoskeletal infection: role of CT in the emergency department. Radiographics 27(6):1723–1736

7. Smith SE, Salanitri J, Lisle D (2007) Ultrasound evaluation of soft tissue masses and fluid collections. Semin Musculoskelet Radiol 11(2):174–191
8. Erdman WA, Tamburro F, Jayson HT, Weatherall PT, Ferry KB, Peshock RM (1991) Osteomyelitis: characteristics and pitfalls of diagnosis with MR imaging. Radiology 180(2):533–539
9. Soldatos T, Durand DJ, Subhawong TK, Carrino JA, Chhabra A (2012) Magnetic resonance imaging of musculoskeletal infections: systematic diagnostic assessment and key points. Acad Radiol 19(11):1434–1443
10. Morrison WB, Schweitzer ME, Bock GW et al (1993) Diagnosis of osteomyelitis: utility of fat-suppressed contrast-enhanced MR imaging. Radiology 189:251–257
11. Ledermann HP, Schweitzer ME, Morrison WB (2002) Nonenhancing tissue on MR imaging of pedal infection: characterization of necrotic tissue and associated limitations for diagnosis of osteomyelitis and abscess. AJR Am J Roentgenol 178: 215–222
12. Glaudemans AW, Israel O, Slart RH (2015) Pitfalls and limitations of radionuclide and hybrid imaging in infection and inflammation. Semin Nucl Med 45(6):500–512
13. Vijayanathan S, Butt S, Gnanasegaran G, Groves AM (2009) Advantages and limitations of imaging the musculoskeletal system by conventional radiological, radionuclide, and hybrid modalities. Semin Nucl Med 39(6):357–368
14. Andersen KF, Jensen KE, Loft A (2016) PET/MR imaging in musculoskeletal disorders. PET Clin 11(4):453–463
15. Graif M, Schweitzer ME, Deely D, Matteucci T (1999) The septic versus nonseptic inflamed joint: MRI characteristics. Skelet Radiol 28:616–620
16. Karchevsky M, Schweitzer ME, Morrison WB et al (2004) MRI findings of septic arthritis and associated osteomyelitis in adults. AJR Am J Roentgenol 182:119–122
17. Kompel A, Murakami A, Guermazi A (2016) MRI of non traumatic musculoskeletal emergencies. Magn Reson Imaging Clin N Am 24:369–389
18. Moore SL, Rafii M (2003) Advanced imaging of tuberculosis arthritis. Semin Musculoskelet Radiol 7:143–153
19. De Backer AI, Mortele KJ, Vanhoenacker FM et al (2006) Imaging of extraspinal musculoskeletal tuberculosis. Eur J Radiol 57: 119–130
20. Torres C, Zakhari N (2016) Imaging of spine infection. Semin Roentgenol. http://dx.doi.org/10.1053/j.ro.2016.05.013 (in press)
21. Prodi E, Grassi R, Iacobellis F et al (2016) Imaging in spondylodiscitis. Magn Reson Imaging Clin N Am 24:581–600
22. Diehn FE (2012) Imaging of spine infection. Radiol Clin N Am 50:777–798
23. Kowalski TJ, Layton KF, Berbari EF et al (2007) MR imaging in patients with pyogenic spine infections: lack of correlation with clinical features. AJNR Am J Neuroradiol 28:693–699
24. Khoo MM, Tyler PA, Saiffuddin A et al (2011) Diffusion-weighted imaging (DWI) in musculoskeletal MRI: a critical review. Skelet Radiol 40:665–681
25. Egushi Y, Ohtori S, Yamashita M et al (2011) Diffusion magnetic resonance imaging to differentiate degenerative from infectious endplate abnormalities in the lumbar spine. Spine 36:E198–E202. [Phila Pa 1976]
26. Love C, Palestro CJ (2016) Nuclear medicine imaging of bone infections. Clin Radiol 71:632–646
27. Raptopoulou A, Karantanas AH, Poumboulidis K et al (2006) Brucellar spondylodiscitis: noncontiguous multifocal involvement of the cervical, thoracic, and lumbar spine. Clin Imaging 30:214–217
28. Kwon JW, Hong SH, Choi SH et al (2011) MRI findings of aspergillus spondylitis. AJR Am J Roentgenol 19:W919–W923
29. Lee SW, Lee SH, Chung HW et al (2013) Candida spondylitis: comparison of MRI findings with bacterial and tuberculous causes. AJR Am J Roentgenol 201:872–877
30. Arkun R, Mete BD (2011) Musculoskeletal hydatid disease. Semin Musculoskelet Radiol 15:527–540
31. Ahmadi ME, Morrison WB, Schweitzer ME et al (2006) Neuropathic arthropathy of the foot with and without superimposed osteomyelitis: MR imaging characteristics. Radiology 238:622–631

Imaging of the Knee

Eva Llopis and Lynne S. Steinbach

Introduction

It is important for radiologists to be familiar with many of the imaging abnormalities that afflict the knee joint. Beginning with the obvious and subtle findings on knee radiographs and progressing to more detailed findings on cross-sectional imaging and ultrasound, it is critical to properly interpret the findings. This chapter will cover various aspects of imaging the meniscus, cruciate ligaments, collateral ligaments, and posterolateral corner. We will also discuss various abnormalities associated with instability, patellar dislocation, patellar tendinopathy and chondral lesions with additional focus on osseous injury to the distal femoral condyles.

Imaging Modalities

Conventional radiographs are the first line of imaging for the painful knee. Standard projections are frontal and lateral views, preferably with weight-bearing for the AP view. Additional projections include standing posteroanterior bent knee radiographs for improved detection of joint space narrowing and Merchant or Sunrise views to evaluate the patellofemoral joint for narrowing, tilt, subluxation and dislocation.

MRI is the method of choice for the evaluation of internal derangement using a combination of planes and sequences that includes high-resolution proton density and fluid sensitive sequences that include fat suppression. T1 weighting in one plane is useful for additional evaluation of marrow in combination with the T2-sensitive studies. MR arthrography is occasionally performed with dilute gadolinium in the postoperative setting to assess for meniscal re-tears.

Computed tomography is mainly used for evaluation of intra-articular fracture and surgical planning and follow-up. Studies should include reformatted images in orthogonal planes. Additional three-dimensional surface projections can be useful to the surgeons. If hardware is present, metal reduction techniques can be obtained to limit artifact. Occasionally, CT arthrography is performed to assess internal derangement in patients who are unable to undergo MRI examinations. CT arthrography is also useful to evaluate surface cartilage defects and the postoperative meniscus.

Ultrasound is useful for characterization of adjacent soft tissue abnormalities, including muscle and tendon injury, bursae and other soft tissue masses. Ultrasound can also be utilized for targeted injections.

Meniscus

Anatomy

The menisci are fibrocartilaginous structures comprised mainly of collagen type I fibers in longitudinal and radial orientations [1–3]. The peripheral 10–15% of the meniscus is highly vascularized and is called the "red zone". The larger mesial portion of the meniscus is relatively avascular and is termed the "white zone". A tear in the more vascular peripheral meniscus will respond to surgical repair or heal on it's own more often than an injury in the avascular region, which benefits more from debridement and resection [4, 5]. Menisci have three zones from anterior to posterior. These include the anterior horn, body and posterior horn. The medial meniscus has a C-shape morphology with a wider posterior horn, while the more circular lateral meniscus is more compact and relatively the same size throughout. Both menisci have anterior and posterior roots that anchor them to the tibia. Disruption of the root can lead to displacement of the meniscus and cartilage loss within a short time period and can be an important finding that can be repaired

E. Llopis
Department of Radiology, Hospital Universitario de La Ribera, Paseo Ciudadela 13-15D, Valencia 46003, Spain
e-mail: evallopis@gmail.com

L.S. Steinbach (✉)
Department of Radiology and Biomedical Imaging, University of California San Francisco, 505 Parnassus, Suite M392, San Francisco, CA 94143, USA
e-mail: Lynne.steinbach@ucsf.edu

J. Hodler et al. (eds.), *Musculoskeletal Diseases 2017-2020*, DOI 10.1007/978-3-319-54018-4_8

surgically if it is acute. The medial meniscus is completely attached to the capsule whereas the lateral meniscus has a posterolateral disruption in its attachment to the capsule where the popliteus tendon traverses through the meniscopopliteal ligaments that attach the deficient meniscus to the capsule [1–3]. While menisci are usually low signal intensity on all imaging sequences, the posterior horn of the lateral meniscus can extend 55 degrees to the main magnetic field and is often intermediate signal intensity on shorter TE sequences.

Meniscal Abnormalities

One MR criteria for a meniscal tear is the presence of abnormal intra-meniscal signal that extends to the superior, inferior or mesial articular surface on two or more consecutive planes. The abnormal signal is most often visible on proton density and T1-weighted images. Fluid may track within the tear, producing high signal intensity on T2-weighted images. The other important criterion for a meniscal tear is abnormal morphology with loss of the normal triangular shape or fragmentation of the meniscus.

The sensitivity and specificity of MR diagnosis for meniscal tear is from 90% to 95%, using arthroscopy as the gold standard. Tears of the lateral meniscus are more likely to be missed than those of the medial meniscus [1, 2, 6, 7].

Normal variants should be differentiated from tears. These can include the presence of a meniscal flounce, which represents a wavy meniscus without abnormal signal intensity or fragmentation. The intermediate signal intensity interfaces of ligamentous attachments at the anterior horns of either meniscus created by the transverse meniscal ligament or at the posterior horn of the lateral meniscus, created by the lateral meniscofemoral ligament should not be confused with a tear [3].

The MR report of meniscal tears should include the location, morphology, extent and the presence of an associated parameniscal cyst. Posterior horn tears are the most frequent. Tears can be divided into stable and unstable. Stable is defined when the tear extends only to one articular surface, without displacement [1–3, 6–9].

Horizontal tears (which include oblique tears to one surface) are the most frequent and are usually degenerative in nature. These are most common in the posterior horns of the menisci. Vertical tears extend from the superior to the inferior surface of the meniscus. These types of tears are more often related to trauma and more often require surgical repair or debridement. Displacement of the tear into the intercondylar notch results in a bucket handle tear. On MRI the bucket handle tear can present with fewer bowties on the sagittal image related to displacement of a portion of the meniscus into the notch. The displaced fragment can lie under the posterior cruciate ligament if it is from the medial meniscus or if it originates from the lateral meniscus in the presence of an ACL tear. This is called the "double PCL sign". If the fragment displaces from posterior to anterior, a "double anterior horn sign" can result and this is called a flipped meniscus. Radial tears are vertical tears that extend from the free edge to the periphery of the meniscus (Fig. 1). These are

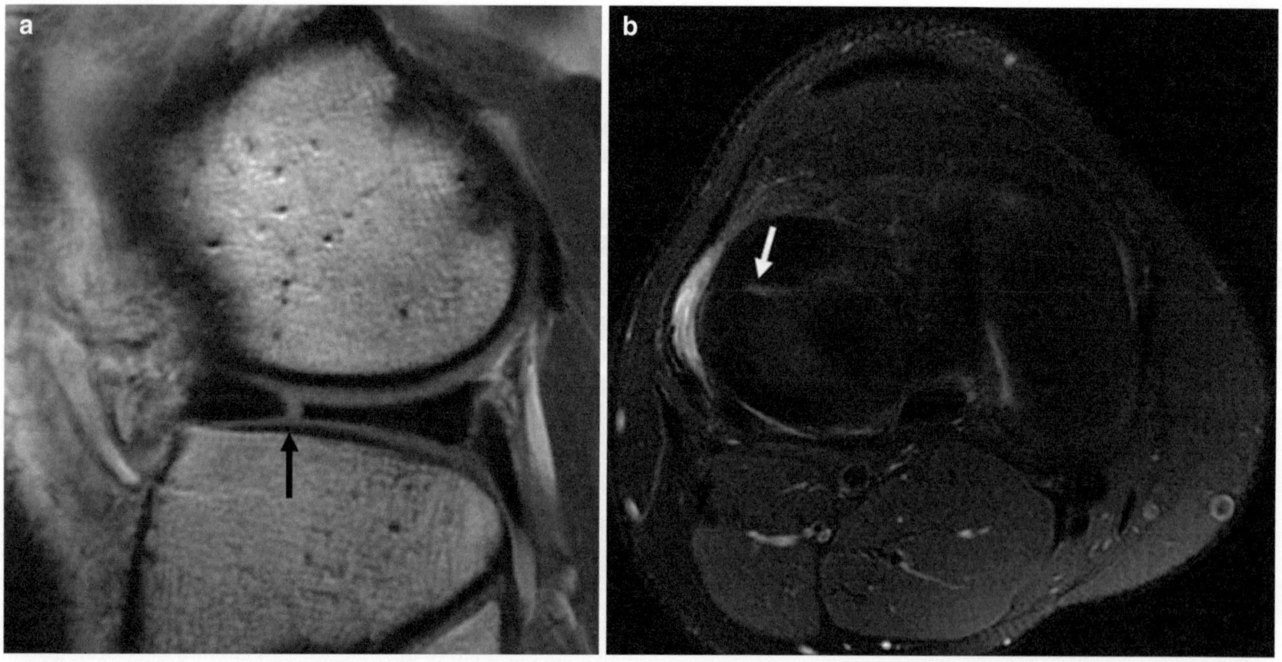

Fig. 1 (**a**) Sagittal proton density MR image demonstrates a radial tear in the body of the lateral meniscus (*arrow*). (**b**) The radial tear is seen as a high signal intensity spoke in the wheel of the lateral meniscus on the axial T2 weighted image (*arrow*)

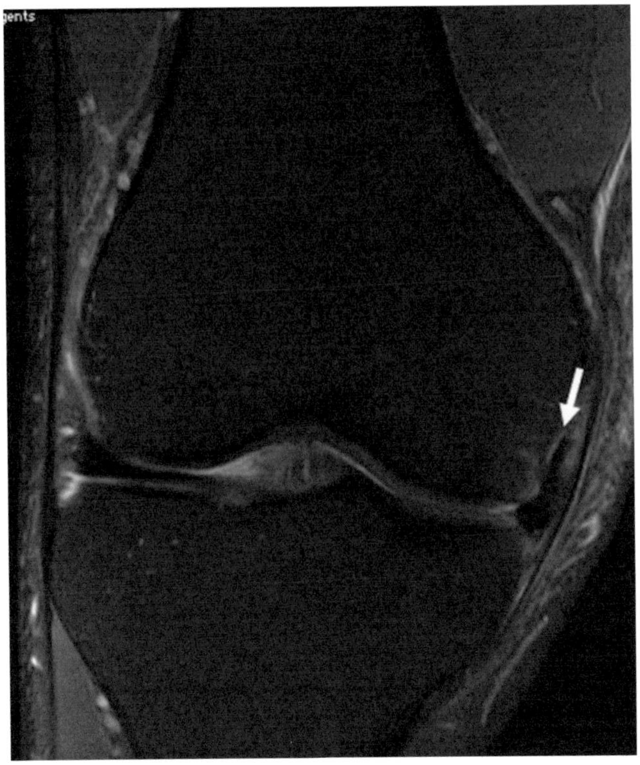

Fig. 2 Flap tear of the body of the medial meniscus extends into the superior gutter adjacent to the medial femoral condyle on this coronal fat suppressed T2-weighted MR image. There is reactive change in the adjacent distal femoral corner

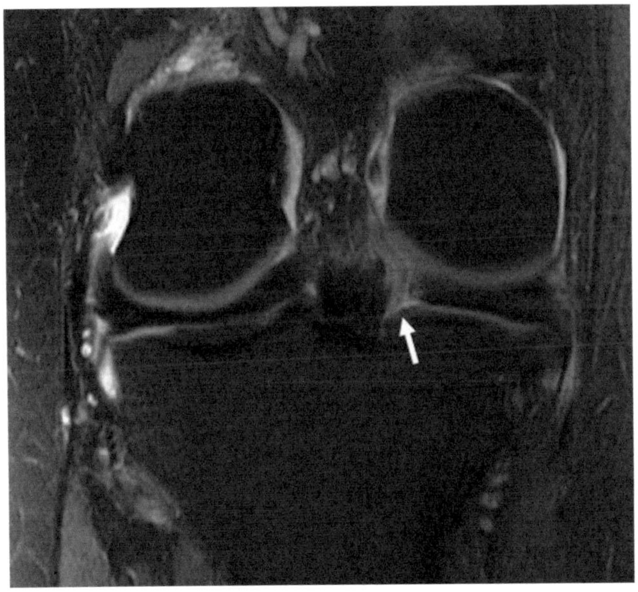

Fig. 3 A coronal fat suppressed T2-weighted MR image demonstrates a defect at the posterior tibial attachment of the medial meniscus consistent with a root tear (*arrow*)

more often degenerative and difficult to repair, and often result in subsequent cartilage loss in the region of the tear. They present with a blunted shape of the free edge or an absent portion called the "ghost meniscus" in planes parallel to the tear. These often occur in the posterior horns or at the junction of the anterior horn or posterior horn with the body of the meniscus. Horizontal and vertical tears can have a portion that displaces but is still connected to the meniscus and is termed a flap tear (Fig. 2). These are often painful and treated surgically with resection of the flap. Tears in the meniscal central attachment are called meniscal root tears (Fig. 3). Root tears are a cause of meniscal extrusion with loss of normal meniscal function, resulting in rapid progression of cartilage loss and osteoarthritis. When acute, root tears are unstable and are often surgically reattached to the tibia. Some tears involve more than one cleavage plane and are classified as complex and unstable [1–3, 6–9].

Cruciate Ligaments

Anterior Cruciate Ligament

The anterior cruciate ligament (ACL) originates from the lateral femoral intercondylar notch and inserts into the tibial spine. It is composed of anteromedial and posterolateral bundles that lie parallel or more vertical to the roof of the intercondylar notch (Blumesaat's line). Because the ACL courses at 55 degrees to the main magnetic field, it is subject to the magic angle phenomenon, especially at the tibial insertion [10]. It also interfaces with the anterior horn of the lateral meniscus which creates an intermediate signal speckled appearance to the meniscus, that can extend to the surface and should not be mistaken for a tear.

ACL tears can be partial or complete. The diagnosis is based upon clinical exam with the aid of imaging. Partial tears may affect one of the two bundles and can be subtle. Complete tears cause disruption of the all of the fibers and are most common within the central tendon but closer to the femoral attachment. Avulsion fractures more commonly occur in children and young adolescents and are usually located distally at the insertion on the tibial plateau.

Depending on the mechanism of injury there will be a different pattern of bone contusions on the MR images. The classic pattern related to valgus stress is associated with contusions of the lateral femoral condyle and posterior lateral tibial plateau, and in some cases there is an additional contusion in the posterior medial tibial plateau [10, 11]. A deepened condylopatellar sulcus in the lateral femoral condyle greater than 2 mm can be the result of impaction with this type of injury and is also visualized on radiographs as a clue to the presence of an ACL injury [11, 12] (Fig. 4). Hyperextension can cause ACL or posterior cruciate ligament (PCL) tears. Contusions associated with this mechanism of injury are located along the anterior aspect of the femur and tibia around the knee joint. A third mechanism of ACL injury is varus stress with an avulsion of the tibia below the plateau,

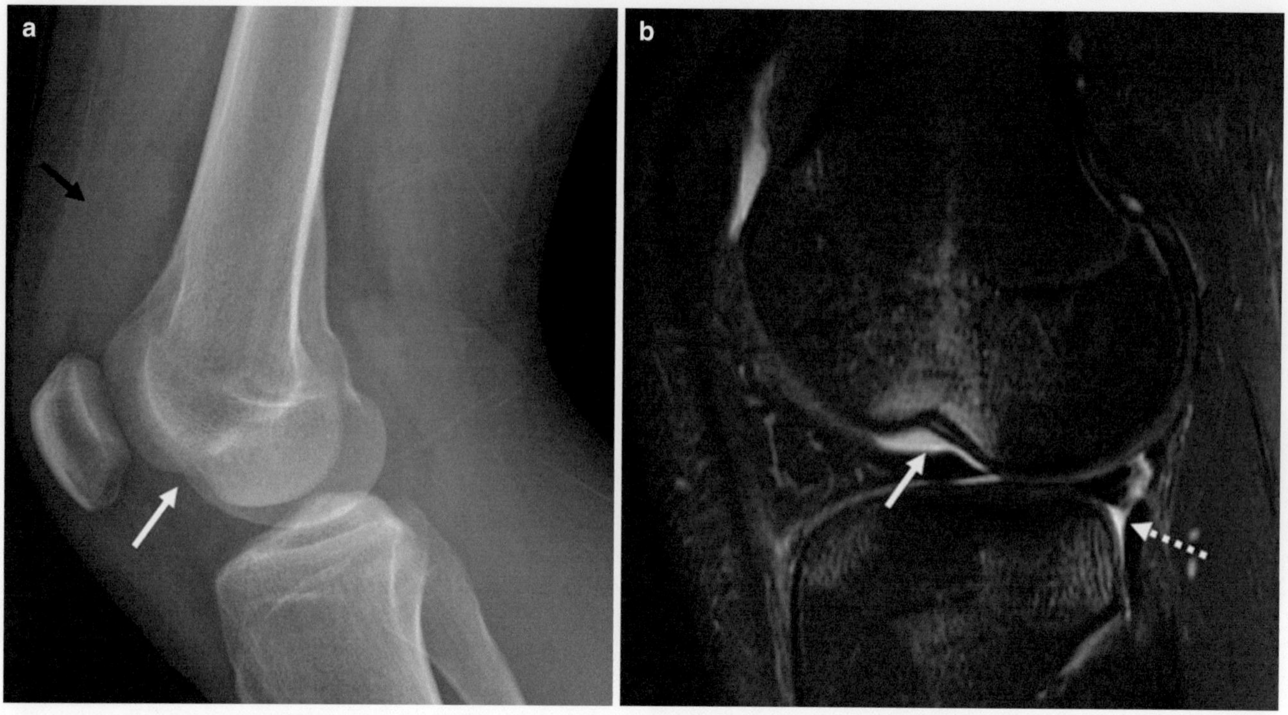

Fig. 4 (**a**) Lateral view of the knee following an acute valgus injury to the knee demonstrates a deep condylopatellar sulcus consistent with an impaction injury related to ACL tear (*white arrow*). There is a large suprapatellar effusion (*black arrow*). (**b**) The corresponding sagittal fat suppressed T2-weighted image shows many of the secondary signs associated with ACL tear including the deep sulcus in the femur with adjacent contusion in the femur (*arrow*) as well as the anterior and posterior aspect of the tibial plateau. There is anterior translation of the tibia as well as uncovering of the posterior horn of the lateral meniscus (*dashed arrow*)

resulting in the Segond fracture. These fractures are easier to see on conventional radiographs but can be found on MRI in the region of the attachment of the iliotibial band and anterolateral ligament on the tibia. Because they are avulsions, there is little reactive marrow change in the tibia.

All three orthogonal planes can compliment each other to evaluate the ACL. Slight external rotation of the knee is favored. Various planes parallel and perpendicular to the ACL have also been suggested in more difficult cases. New 3D volumetric FSE images will allow thin section reconstructions in the desired plane [10, 13].

Disruption with high signal intensity of the normal fibrillar low signal intensity structure of the ACL is the primary MRI sign. The ACL may also lie at a more acute angle or can be displaced anteriorly causing a locked knee. The secondary anterior translation of the knee where the posterior margin of the tibia lies anterior to the posterior margin of the femur can be measured with MR sagittal images at the lateral femoral condyle, and is considered abnormal when it is greater than 5 mm [10]. Partial tears are more difficult to diagnose. It is helpful to follow each bundle in multiple planes. The anteromedial bundle is more often disrupted than posterolateral bundle [14]. In some situations, these partial tears are repaired or reconstructed if there is resultant knee instability.

Chronic ruptures of the ACL may be obvious with an empty notch sign signifying an absent ACL. An old ACL tear might be called if the alignment of the ACL is at an acute angle to the roof of the intercondylar notch. The torn ACL fibers may adhere to the PCL. A thickened ACL or one that lacks striation is a clue to an old injury. On the other hand, sometimes the ACL tear heals with fibrous tissue and may look normal on MRI. Despite a normal MR appearance, the ligament may be associated with laxity resulting in clinically detectable knee instability that requires ACL reconstruction. Anterior translation of the tibia can help to identify some of these cases. Most ACL tears are reconstructed with a patellar or hamstring autograft. In some circumstances the torn ACL will heal without surgery and the patient will be able to return to athletic activity [15].

Posterior Cruciate Ligament (PCL)

The comma-shaped posterior cruciate ligament originates from the medial aspect of the intercondylar notch of the

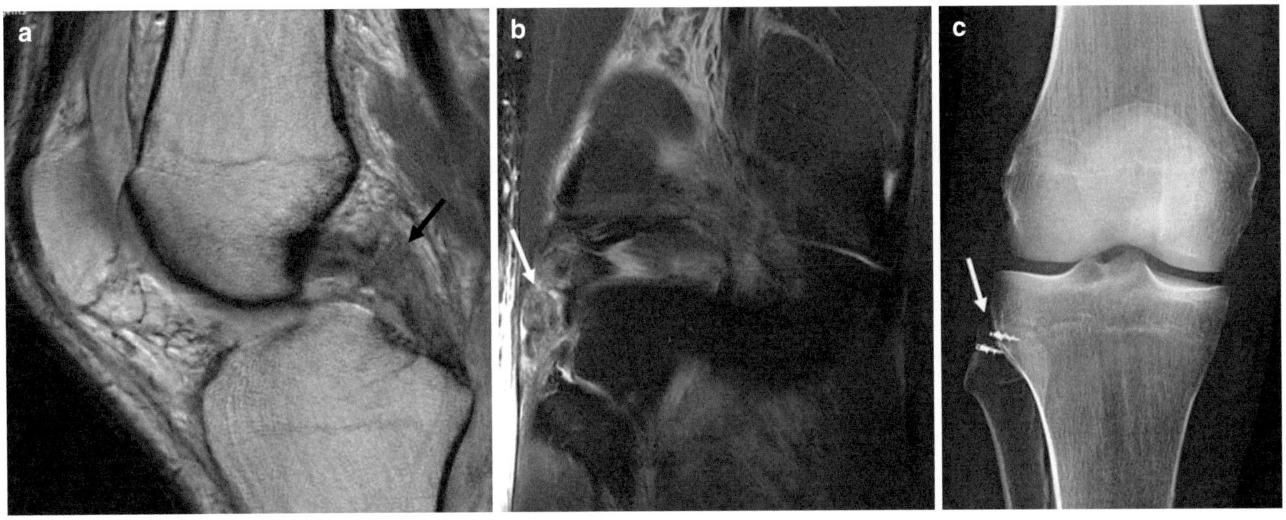

Fig. 5 (**a**) Sagittal proton density MR image demonstrates a PCL tear (*arrow*). (**b**) On the coronal fat suppressed T2 weighted image there is an associated posterolateral corner injury (*arrow*). (**c**) The posterolateral corner was reconstructed with a tendon graft anchored to the fibular head (*arrow*)

femur and inserts into the posterior tibia. Tears are most often seen in the proximal third of the PCL, and can be intrasubstance, partial or complete (Fig. 5). Avulsions of the PCL are also seen at the tibial plateau. The mechanisms of injury of the PCL include a direct anterior force on a flexed knee as may be seen in an auto crash involving a passenger in the front seat. Hyperextension and severe valgus stress may also affect the PCL. The PCL has even greater potential than the ACL to heal spontaneously [10, 16]. The MRI often looks normal in these cases. Thickening of the PCL can be a sign of an old injury.

Collateral Ligaments and the Posterior Corners of the Knee

Medial Structures

Medial ligaments include the medial collateral ligament (MCL) complex and components of the medial retinaculum. There are three layers of tissue that comprise these ligaments. The medial collateral ligament extends from the medial femur to the proximal tibial diaphysis approximately 7 cm below the tibial plateau. The medial patellofemoral ligament (MPFL) is part of a retinacular complex that goes from the patella to the femur, meniscus, and tibia. The MPFL extends from the medial patella to the adductor tubercle of the femur where it blends in with the MCL. The MPFL stabilizes the medial patellofemoral joint. These anteromedial structures have three layers. The superficial component (layer I) is composed of the crural fascia that includes the sartorius and anteriorly is fused with layer II forming the medial retinaculum and the medial patellofemoral ligament. The medial layer, layer II corresponds to the superficial layer of the medial collateral ligament (MCL) and posteriorly is fused with layer III forming the posterior oblique ligament (POL) of the medial collateral ligament complex. The deepest layer (layer III) includes the joint capsule, meniscopatellar ligament and meniscofemoral and meniscotibial (coronary) ligaments. A tibial collateral ligament bursa lies between the superficial and deep layers of the MCL [10, 17–21].

MCL Injury

The MCL is the most commonly injured ligament of the knee. Trauma to this ligament is usually related to valgus stress and external rotation, a mechanism of injury that may also injure the ACL and the posterior horn of the medial meniscus, especially at its meniscocapsular attachment.

The simplest description of MCL sprain and tear involves three different grades. Grade I represents a sprain or small partial tear of the superficial layer of the MCL without knee instability. On MRI there is associated T2 hyperintensity medial to but not involving the ligament. Grade II represents a partial tear produced by moderate valgus instability that involves deep and superficial layers on MRI and demonstrates T2 hyperintensity and morphologic disruption of some of the fibers of the MCL without complete discontinuity or avulsion. Grade III represents a complete tear, with discontinuity of the fibers and instability

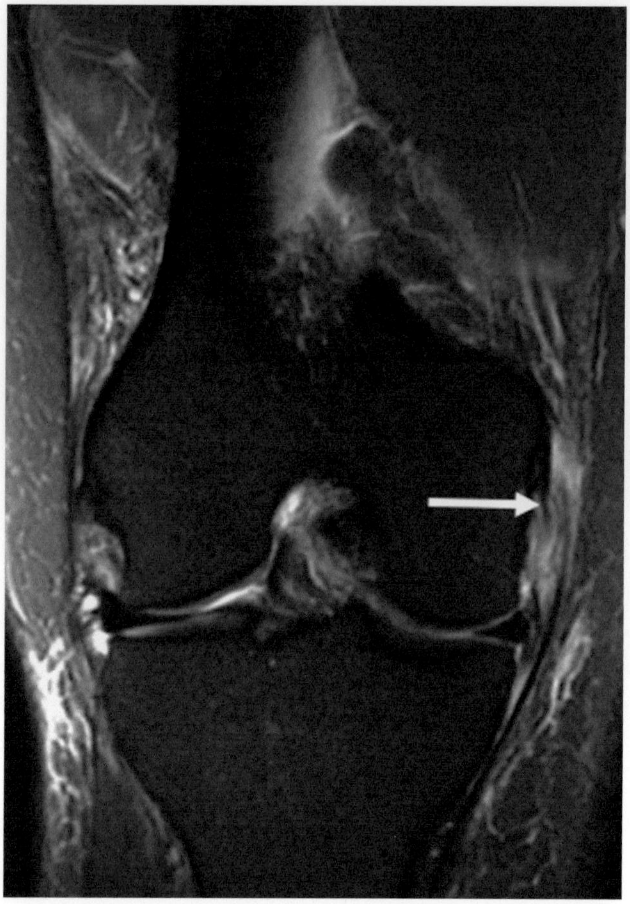

Fig. 6 A full thickness tear in the proximal medial collateral ligament is seen on this fat suppressed T2-weighted coronal MR image (*arrow*)

(Fig. 6). This MR classification system does not completely correlate with surgical findings and is based mainly on the superficial layer of MCL. Treatment of MCL tears is usually conservative. Surgery is considered when there is a complete tear of the MCL, especially if there are associated injuries of the posteromedial corner involving the posterior oblique ligament. Distally the MCL may tear at the tibial attachment and lie superficial to the pes anserine tendons. In this situation, the interposition of the tendons, may block healing of the tear, similar to a Stener lesion of a Gamekeeper's thumb, and would also require surgery. Chronic injuries of the MCL produce thickening of the ligament on MRI. Chronic injury may also be associated with ossification of the ligament that is better seen on radiographs, and has been termed a Pellegrini Stieda lesion [10, 18, 21].

Posteromedial Corner

The posteromedial corner structures are essential for the stability of the medial side of the knee. These are comprised of several components: (1) the posterior horn of the medial meniscus; (2) the posterior oblique ligament (POL is the posterior portion of the MCL); (3) the semimembranosus complex expansions; (4) the oblique popliteal ligament (OPL); and (5) the meniscotibial ligament (distal portion of the deep MCL).

The POL is a component of the MCL that represents a discrete anatomical thickening of the capsule that lies posterior to the MCL proper. POL injuries are strongly associated with instability when complete rupture is present, and are better visualized in the axial and coronal planes.

The semimembranosus tendon has five distal attachments that include a tibial, direct and inferior capsular arm, as well as the expansion to the oblique popliteal ligament. This is the most frequently injured region in the posteromedial corner and abnormalities of the various structures can be difficult to identify on MRI. The oblique popliteal ligament is a band of tissue that extends to the superior lateral posterior part of the knee close to the lateral gastrocnemius [17–21]. It presents as a thickening of the posterior capsule and can be difficult to identify on MRI. Injuries of OPL are seen on axial plane as soft tissue edema and irregularity of the deep posteromedial structures extending laterally [17–21].

Injury to the posteromedial structures lead to anteromedial rotatory instability, and are frequently associated with ACL and PCL rupture. Although controversial, there is growing evidence that surgery is needed when these structures are injured in order to avoid future instability and failure of the ACL graft. It is essential to distinguish between isolated MCL lesions vs. involvement of the posteromedial corner since the former are treated conservatively whereas the latter situation might require surgery [10, 17–21].

Lateral Structures

Lateral structures can be divided by location. They are grouped as anterior, middle and posterolateral. Anterior stabilizers include the lateral retinaculum, the vastus lateralis fibers and the iliotibial band. Posterior to the iliotibial band in the middle compartment is the anterior oblique band, a central vertical and longitudinal thickening of the capsule. The more recently discovered anterolateral ligament also can be found in this region. The anterolateral ligament is sometimes seen on MRI, but not consistently. In the posterolateral corner, the intra- and extra-articular popliteus tendon extends from the popliteus hiatus of the femur to the popliteus muscle that attaches on the posterior tibia. It has a tendon sheath. There are meniscopopliteal fascicles that extend from the posterior horn of the lateral meniscus around this tendon to attach to the capsule. The posterolateral corner also includes a complex network of structures including the fibular collateral ligament and the biceps femoris tendons that combine to form a conjoined attachment to the fibular styloid. There are also smaller but important structures in this area including the popliteofibular, fibulofabellar and arcuate ligaments. These structures are important static and dynamic stabilizers of the knee and they act together to resist posterior translation, varus and external rotation [10, 17, 18, 22–24]. The popliteofibular ligament extends from the fibular styloid to the popliteus tendon.

Iliotibial Band and Anterolateral Ligament

The iliotibial band is a thick fascia that extends proximally from the iliac crest and tensor fascia attaching distally to the anterior lateral tibia at "Gerdy's tubercle". Continuous friction on this structure during flexion due to running and other athletic activities causes anterolateral knee pain. Iliotibial band friction syndrome is a clinical diagnosis and can be confirmed in some cases on MRI which demonstrates soft tissue increased signal intensity on T2 -weighting or bursitis deep to the iliotibial band [25] (Fig. 7). A Segond fracture is an avulsion fracture that occurs along the lateral aspect of the proximal tibia, near to but not at the plateau, that is associated with ACL rupture and meniscal tear. Some believe that it represents an avulsion of the iliotibial tract or/and anterior oblique band. However recently the there has been some discussion of this avulsion being related to the more posterior anterolateral ligament that arises from the lateral femoral condyle close to the popliteus tendon and inserts distally on the lateral tibia between Gerdy's tubercle and the fibular head [10, 17, 18, 26, 27].

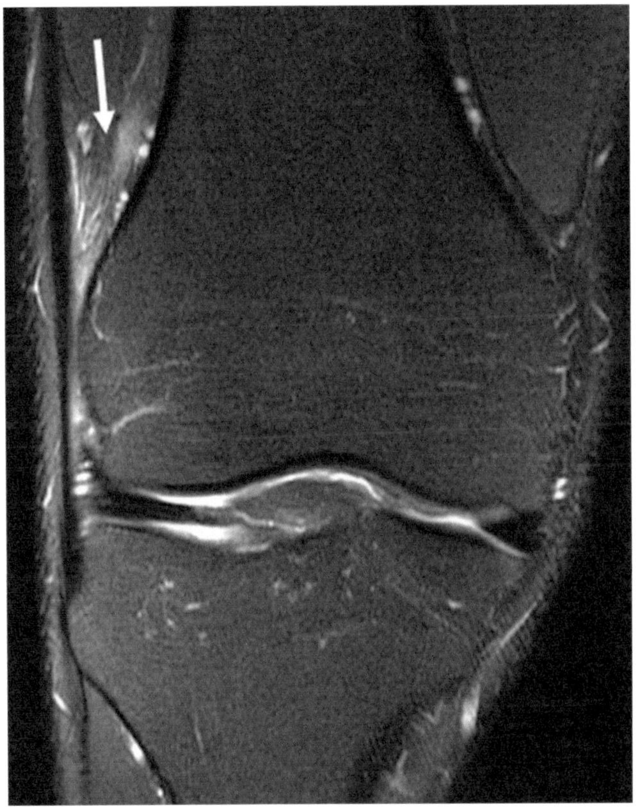

Fig. 7 Coronal fat suppressed T2-weighted image shows increased signal intensity deep to the iliotibial band consistent with iliotibial band friction syndrome (*arrow*)

Posterolateral Structures

The posterolateral stabilizers of the knee are essential for maintaining knee stability, resisting varus and external rotation forces. Their injuries are frequently associated with cruciate ligament injuries (Fig. 5) as well as neurovascular injury. This complex can be divided into static and dynamic structures that act together to maintain stability. Static structures include the fibular (lateral) collateral ligament (LCL), popliteofibular ligament, arcuate ligament complex and the posterolateral capsule. Dynamic structures are the biceps femoris and popliteus tendons. The deep layer has many anatomical variants. The most important structures are the LCL, popliteofibular ligament, popliteal tendon and biceps femoris tendon. Most of these structures take an oblique course and should be carefully followed sometimes facilitated by including tailored oblique planes best obtained with 3D volume imaging [10, 17, 18, 22–24]. Avulsion of the conjoined tendon on the fibular head, the so-called arcuate fracture, or a Segond fracture seen on conventional radiographs are often the first sign of significant internal derangement and should be followed up with MRI to identify the associated injuries [10, 12, 22–24].

Anterior Knee Pain

Anterior knee pain can be secondary to acute trauma, including transient patellar dislocation. Chronic anterior knee pain is related to overuse of the patellofemoral joint, patellar tendon and quadriceps that upsets normal knee homeostasis. Patellofemoral tracking disorders increase the load on anterior structures and therefore lead to problems as well [28–30].

Patellofemoral Instability

Anterior knee alignment and normal tracking of the patella depends on the relationship between the quadriceps tendon, patellar tendon and medial and lateral retinaculum. There are some anatomical features bone and soft tissue that predispose to maltracking and dislocation. Osseous abnormalities such as trochlear dysplasia, patellar facet asymmetry, lateralization of the tibial tuberosity, and femorotibial malrotation cause tracking disorders. Soft tissue abnormalities such as patella alta, generalized laxity or a tight lateral retinaculum can also predispose to maltracking [28–31].

Acute Patellar Dislocation

In the setting of patellofemoral instability or with an acute injury, the patella can dislocate laterally and return to anatomic position anterior to the trochlea. In this setting, the inferomedial aspect of the patella impacts the anterolateral femoral condyle. Sometimes this is transitory and the diagnosis is not obvious. MRI can be useful in this situation as there is a typical bone marrow edema pattern secondary to the contusions of the medial patella and anterior lateral femoral condyle. It is important to make an early and accurate diagnosis because associated lesions in acute patella dislocation might require surgery. Associated findings on MRI include a large effusion, medial patellofemoral ligament rupture, medial collateral ligament tears or sprains, vastus medialis tear, and or osteochondral or chondral fragments, especially off of the medial patella or lateral femoral condyle (Fig. 8).

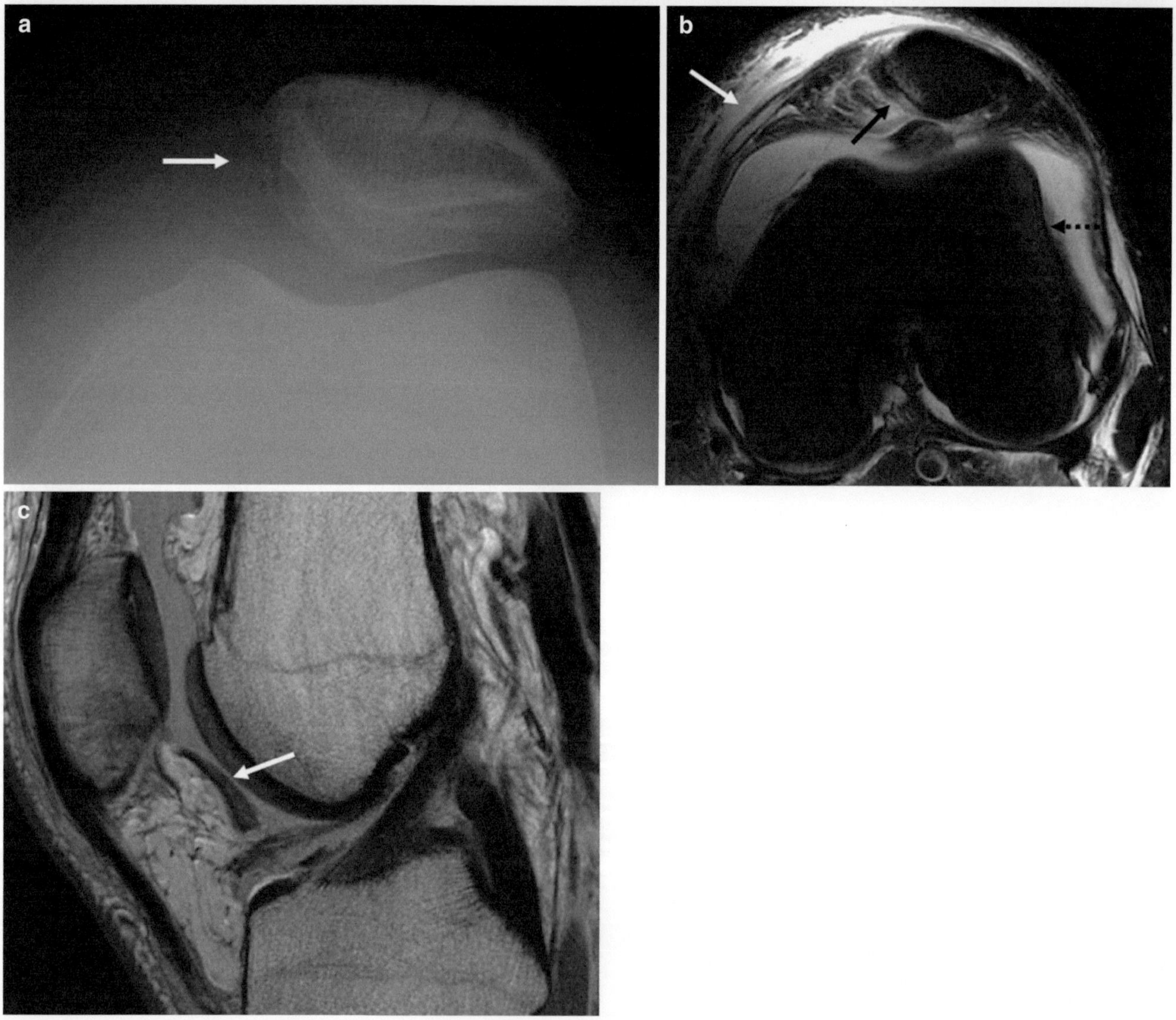

Fig. 8 (**a**) There is a fracture of the medial patella on the Merchant view (*arrow*). (**b**) An axial fat suppressed T2-weighted image shows the typical contusions along the medial patella (*solid black arrow*) and lateral femoral condyle (*dashed black arrow*) consistent with transient lateral patellar dislocation. The medial patellofemoral ligament is torn (*white arrow*) and there is a large suprapatellar effusion. (**c**) An osteochondral fragment lies just behind Hoffa's fat pad (*arrow*)

Patellar Tendinopathy

Patellar tendinopathy is related to repetitive overuse especially from those sports that require knee flexion and extension, such as basketball and volleyball. Tendon tears can also result from repetitive acute contraction of the quadriceps tendon. In addition, patella alta can predispose to patellar tendinopathy. Ultrasound and MRI are useful for demonstrating the findings of tendon thickening in the region of tendinosis with disruptions in areas of focal tearing. Abnormalities of Hoffa's fat pad or distension of the surrounding pre-patellar or deep infra-patellar bursae are often associated with patellar tendinopathy on ultrasound and MRI [27–33].

Patellofemoral Chondrosis

Chondral lesions are a frequent cause of anterior knee pain. Cartilage lesions in the undersurface of the patella are frequent in young adults and related to sports such as running. Lateral lesions are usually related to overuse secondary to friction from patellar tilt and medial sided lesions are often related to maltracking and instability. The modified Outerbridge classification is frequently used to grade these lesions on MRI [27–35]. Trochlear cartilage lesions are often seen as well.

Osteochondral Injury

Osteochondral injury in children and young adults, sometimes termed "osteochondritis dissecans (OCD)" in younger patients, is a common source of knee pain. The cause is probably multifactorial but repetitive microtrauma has been proposed as the most common mechanism. The most frequent location is along the mesial aspect of the medial femoral condyle, followed by lateral femoral condyle, and posterior patella. MR imaging aspires to differentiate between stable and unstable osteochondral fragments since surgery is often performed for unstable injuries. A recent article suggests that MR predictions of stability may not always be successful [36]. The presence of a high signal intensity rim of fluid surrounding the fragment (Fig. 9b), multiple breaks of the subchondral bone plate as well as dislodgement of the fragment from the parent bone are some of the established criteria used to determine stability. The presence of cysts surrounding the lesion is not specific for OCD but if they are multiple or greater than 5 mm helps to determine if the injury is stable or unstable [37, 38]. A differential diagnosis of linear low signal intensity associated with T2 hyperintensity in the distal femoral condylar surfaces includes insufficiency fracture and osteonecrosis.

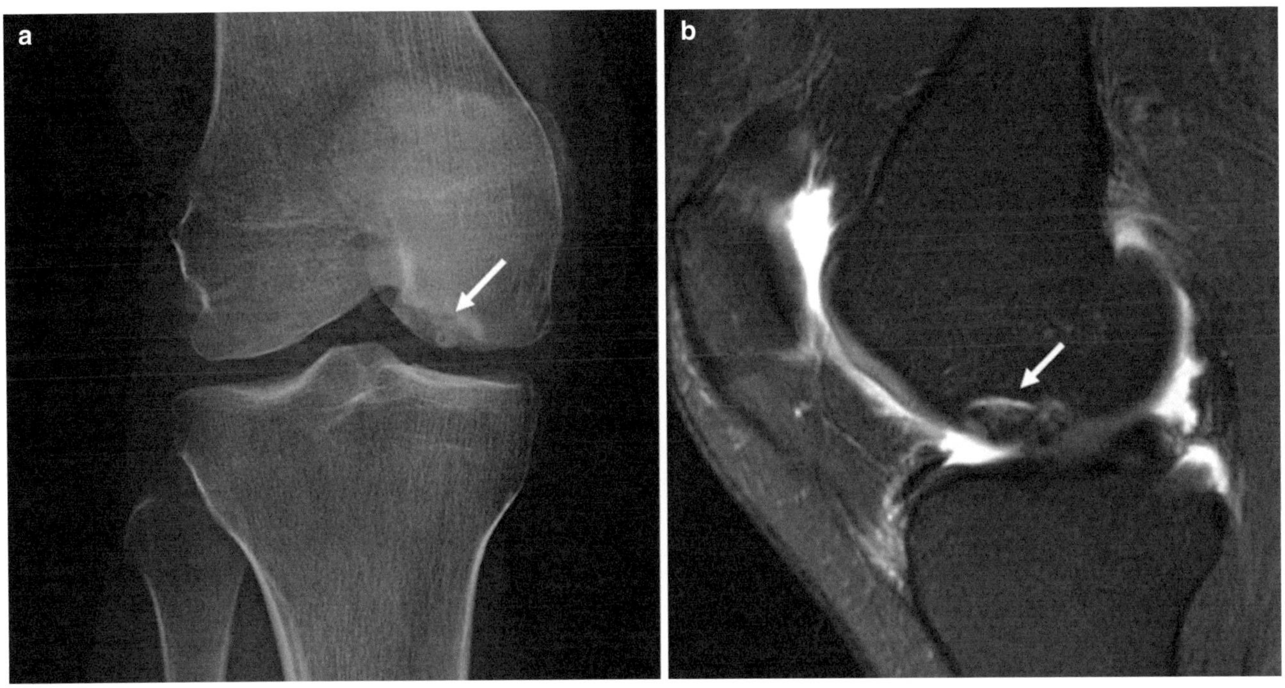

Fig. 9 (**a**) A frontal radiograph reveals an osteochondral injury along the mesial aspect of the medial femoral condyle (*arrow*). (**b**) There is increased signal intensity along the margin of the osteochondral injury with the parent bone on the sagittal T2-weighted MR image, suggesting instability (*arrow*)

References

1. Probyn LJ, White LM (2015) Chapter 26, internal derangement of the knee: meniscal injuries. In: Pope T, Bloem H, Beltran J, Morrison W, Wilson DJ (eds) MRI of the musculoskeletal system, 2nd edn. Elsevier, Philadelphia
2. Tzalonikou M (2012) The meniscus. In: Kramer J (ed) MRI of the Knee, University Publisher, p 97–108
3. Rubin DA, Paletta GA (2000) Current concepts and controversies in meniscal imaging. Magn Reson Imaging Clin N Am 8(2): 243–270
4. Mohankumar R, White LM, Naraghi A (2013) Pitfalls and pearls in MRI of the knee. AJR Am J Roentgenol 203(3):516–530
5. Hauger O, Frank LR et al (2000) Characterization of the "red zone" of knee meniscus: MR imaging and histologic correlation. Radiology 217(1):193–200
6. Gatehouse PD, He T et al (2004) Contrast-enhanced MRI of the menisci of the knee using ultrashort echo time (UTE) pulse sequences: imaging of the red and white zones. Br J Radiol 77(920):641–647
7. De Smet AA, Graf BK (1994) Meniscal tears missed on MR imaging: relationship to meniscal tear patterns and anterior cruciate ligament tears. AJR Am J Roentgenol 162(4):905–911
8. De Smet AA, Mukherjee R (2008) Clinical, MRI, and arthroscopic findings associated with failure to diagnose a lateral meniscal tear on knee MRI. AJR Am J Roentgenol 190(1):22–26
9. Nguyen JC, De Smet AA, Graf BK, Rosas HG (2014) MR imaging-based diagnosis and classification of meniscal tears. Radiographics 34(4):981–999
10. Mc Nally E (2015) Chapter 27, internal derangement of the knee: ligament injuries. In: Pope T, Bloem H, Beltran J, Morrison W, Wilson DJ (eds) MRI of the musculoskeletal system, 2nd edn. Elsevier, Philadelphia
11. Sanders TG, Medynski MA et al (2000) Bone contusion patterns of the knee at MR imaging: footprint of the mechanism of injury. Radiographics. 20 Spec No:S135–51
12. Gottsegen CJ, Eyer BA, White EA et al (2008) Avulsion fractures of the knee: imaging findings and clinical significance. Radiographics 28(6):1755–1770
13. Pass B, Robinson P, Hodgson R et al (2015) Can a single isotropic 3D fast spin echo sequence replace three-plane standard proton density fat-saturated knee MRI at 1.5 T? Br J Radiol. 88
14. Chang MJ, Chang C et al (2013) How useful is MRI in diagnosing isolated bundle ACL injuries? Clin Orthop Relat Res 471(10):3283–3290
15. Costa-Paz M, Ayerza MA et al (2012) Spontaneous healing in complete ACL ruptures. Clin Orthop Relat Res 470:979–985
16. Sonin AH, Fitzgerald SW et al (1995) MR imaging of the posterior cruciate ligament: normal, abnormal, and associated injury patterns. Radiographics 15(3):551–561
17. Geiger D, Chang E, Pathria M et al (2013) Posterolateral and posteromedial corner injuries of the knee. Radiol Clin N Am 51(3):413–432
18. Recondo JA, Salvador E, Villanúa JA, et al (2000) Lateral stabilizing structures of the knee: functional anatomy and injuries assessed with MR imaging. Radiographics 20 Spec No:S91–S102
19. Robinson JR, Sanchez-Ballester J, Bull AM et al (2004) The posteromedial corner revisited. An anatomical description of the passive restraining structures of the medial aspect of the human knee. Bone Joint Surg Br 86(5):674–681
20. Sims WF, Jacobson KE (2004) The posteromedial corner of the knee: medial-sided injury patterns revisited. Am J Sports Med 32(2):337–345
21. Stannard JP (2010) Medial and posteromedial instability of the knee: evaluation, treatment, and results. Sports Med Arthrosc 18(4):263–268
22. Llopis E, Ramiro R, Fernandez E (2012) Posterolateral corner of the knee. In: Kramer J (ed) MRI of the Knee. University Publisher, p 97–108
23. Seebacher JR, Inglis AE, Marshall JL et al (1982) The structure of the posterolateral aspect of the knee. J Bone Joint Surg Am 64(4):536–541
24. Vinson EN, Major NM, Helms CA (2008) The posterolateral corner of the knee. AJR Am J Roentgenol 190(2):449–458
25. Muhle C, Ahn JM, Yeh L et al (1999) Iliotibial band friction syndrome: MR imaging findings in 16 patients and MR arthrographic study of six cadaveric knees. Radiology 212(1):103–110
26. Porrino J Jr, Maloney E, Richardson M et al (2015) The anterolateral ligament of the knee: MRI appearance, association with the Segond fracture, and historical perspective. AJR Am J Roentgenol 204(2):367–373
27. Musahl V, Rahnemai-Azar AA, van Eck CF et al (2016) Anterolateral ligament of the knee, fact or fiction? Knee Surg Sports Traumatol Arthrosc 24(1):2–3
28. Llopis E, Padron M (2007) Anterior knee pain. Eur J Radiol 62(1):27–43
29. Samim M, Smitaman E et al (2014) MRI of anterior knee pain. Skelet Radiol 43:875–893
30. Boric I (2012). Anterior aspect of the knee. In: Kramer J (ed) Imaging of the knee. University Publisher, p 109–138
31. Scheurecker G, Kramer J (2013) Patellofemoral instability. In: Kramer J (ed) Imaging of the knee. University Publisher, Breitenseher p 139–161
32. Draghi F, Ferrozzi G et al (2016) Hoffa's fat pad abnormalities, knee pain and magnetic resonance imaging in daily practice. Insights Imaging 7(3):373–383
33. Miller TT (2013) The patellar tendon. Semin Musculoskelet Radiol 17(1):56–59
34. Gold G, Chen C et al (2009) Recent advances in MRI of articular cartilage. AJR Am J Roentgenol 193(3):628–638
35. Crema MD, Roemer FW et al (2011) Articular cartilage in the knee: current MR imaging techniques and applications in clinical practice and research. Radiographics 31(1):37–61
36. Ellermann JM, Donald B, Rohr S et al (2016) Magnetic resonance imaging of osteochondritis dissecans: validation study for the ICRS classification system. Acad Radiol 23:724–729
37. De Smet AA, Ilahi OA, Graf BK (1996) Reassesment of the MR criteria for stability of osteochondritis dissecans in the knee and ankle. Skelet Radiol 25:159–163
38. Kijowski R, Blankenbaker DG et al (2008) Juvenile versus adult osteochondritis dissecans of the knee: appropriate MR imaging criteria for instability. Radiology 248:571–578

Musculoskeletal Manifestations of Endocrine Disease

J.F. Griffith

Diabetes Mellitus

Diabetes mellitus is a common metabolic disorder with several noteworthy musculoskeletal manifestations seen in patients with chronic disease.

Charcot's neuroarthopathy of the foot is the most severe and best known musculoskeletal consequence of diabetes mellitus. Charcot's neuroarthropathy most likely results from a combination of factors. Neuropathy compromises proprioception and increases pain tolerance which makes the foot prone to repetitive microtrauma during daily activities. Vascular compromise and an excessive inflammatory response to trauma, mediated through pro- inflammatory cytokines, results in poor healing. Neuropathy of the sympathetic nerves increases pedal blood flow which in turn leads to increased osteoclastic activity.

Although Charcot's neuroarthopathy is said to have an initial resorptive phase followed by a hypertrophic reparative phase, these distinctive stages are not usually apparent in clinical practice. Charcot's neuroarthropathy is relatively pain free given the degree of arthropathy present. The disease presents insidiously with mild foot pain, progressive swelling/deformity and with several joints affected on imaging to a variable degree. Classically The classic radiographic, CT or MRI appearances of Charcot's neuroarthropathy are the 6 D's i.e. **d**isorganization, **d**estruction, **d**ebris, **d**ensity preservation, **d**istension of joint, and **d**islocation. CT is excellent at demonstrating the extent of midfoot and hindfoot disease while radiography is sufficient to assess forefoot disease.

Charcot's neuroarthopathy most commonly affects the mid-foot where it always seems to start at the second/third tarsometatarsal joint and thereafter extend in an orderly fashion to involve the navicular, cuboid and the lateral aspect of the midfoot/hindfoot junction (Fig. 1). Mid-foot disease at a late stage involves the hindfoot but does not involve the forefoot. End-stage Charcot's neuroarthropathy of the midfoot leads to a 'rocker bottom deformity'. Charcot's neuroarthropathy is bilateral in 75% of cases though involvement of the less affected foot is often subclinical. Lisfranc fracture-dislocation occurs in 40% and is bilateral in 20%. Tarsal bone fracture occurs in 20% [1].

Much less commonly, hindfoot or ankle neuroarthropathy may develop de novo in the absence of midfoot disease. Similarly forefoot disease may develop de novo and tends to be atrophic in type with bony reabsorption and 'penciling' of the phalanges.

Charcot' neuroarthropathy sometimes needs to be differentiated from osteomyelitis and septic arthritis. Osteomyelitis is uncommon in the absence of cutaneous ulceration since it usually occurs secondary to soft tissue infection.

Helpful imaging features to distinguishing between neuroarthropathy and osteomyelitis are as follows:

1. Charcot's neuroarthropathy is joint centered while osteomyelitis commonly involves the non-articular segments of bone. An inflammatory response not centred on the joint is indicative of osteomyelitis.
2. Charcot's arthropathy has got a classic pattern of progression in the midfoot (Fig. 1) [1]. If this pattern is not followed then one should strongly consider osteomyelitis. If for example, one sees cuboid destruction in the absence of arthropathy on the medial aspect of the tarsus, then this would strongly favour osteomyelitis.
3. Continuity of any inflammation with cutaneous ulceration favours osteomyelitis. Osteomyelitis usually occurs at pressure sites prone to soft tissue injury and ulceration such as the first and fifth metatarsophalangeal joints, distal phalanx of the big toe, the posterior aspect of the calcaneum, or the base of the midfoot with 'rocker bottom deformity' consequent on end-stage Charcot's neuroarthropathy.
4. Soft tissue fluid collections on ultrasound, CT or MRI examination favour infection. These collections may be aspirated under image guidance.

J.F. Griffith
Department of Imaging and Interventional Radiology,
The Prince of Wales Hospital, The Chinese University of Hong Kong,
Shatin, Hong Kong
e-mail: griffith@cuhk.edu.hk

J. Hodler et al. (eds.), *Musculoskeletal Diseases 2017-2020*, DOI 10.1007/978-3-319-54018-4_9

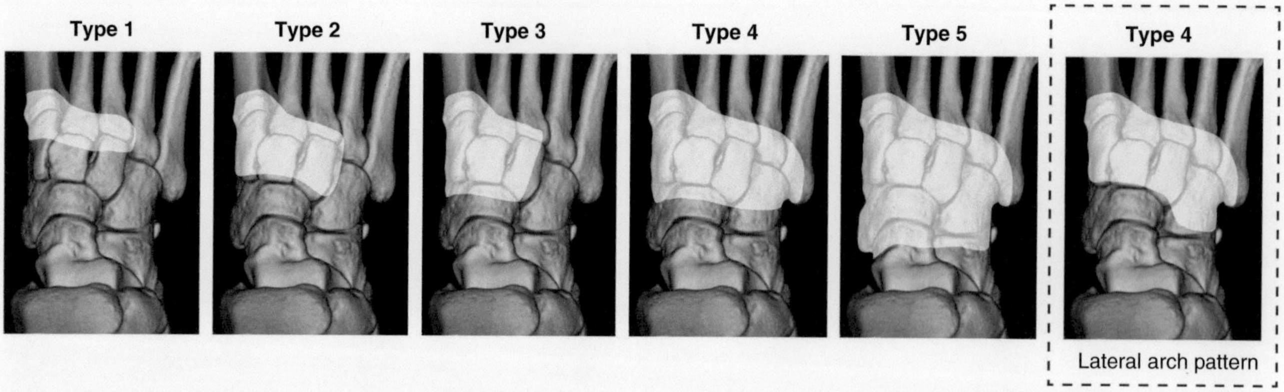

Fig. 1 Schematic diagram showing orderly progression of neuroarthropathic changes across the midfoot [1]. **Type 1**. Changes limited to medial three tarsometatarsal joints and adjacent inter-cuneiform joints. **Type 2**. Additional involvement of the 4th tarsometatarsal joint. **Type 3**. Additional involvement of the cuneiform-navicular joints. **Type 4**. Additional involvement of the 5th tarsometatarsal and peri-cuboid joints. Type 4 (lateral) is relatively greater involvement of cuboid than navicular bone. **Type 5**. Additional involvement of the hindfoot

5. Severe localised osteolysis or progressive osteolysis favours osteomyelitis. Review of any prior imaging studies is helpful.
6. Identification of osseous or soft tissue sinus tracts on CT or MRI is also indicative of osteomyelitis.
7. Positive indium-111 labelled leucocyte scintigraphy scan favours osteomyelitis.
8. 18-F flourodeoxy glucose positron emission tomography-computed tomography (PET-CT) imaging is more specific than three-phase bone scintigraphy and also probably more specific than indium-111 labelled leucocyte scintigraphy though has not been directly compared with the latter in the diabetic foot [2–4].

Diabetes mellitus is also associated with an increased prevalence of musculoskeletal manifestations related to increased tissue fibrosis. These include:

Diabetic cheiroarthropathy (*cheiros* = hand in Greek) is a quite common complication said to effect at least 10% with both insulin-dependent and non-insulin-dependent diabetes. It is marked by hand stiffness (hence also known as 'stiff hand syndrome' or 'limited joint mobility syndrome") and mainly affects persons with poorly controlled diabetes, particularly if a smoker. It is characterised by thick, waxy skin on the dorsum of the fingers and hands with flexion contractures of the metacarpophalangeal and interphalangeal joints [5]. Skin changes in the absence of joint problems can be found. Arterial calcification is a quite common accompaniment.

Clinically it can be similar to scleroderma though the absence of Raynaud's phenomen, calcinosis, cutaneous telangiectasia, dermal atrophy, and autoantibodies allows distinction between diabetic cheiroarthropathy and scleroderma.

Although common in diabetes mellitus, diabetic cheiroarthropathy is not often encountered in radiology departments as it is a clinical diagnosis that does not require imaging confirmation. The classic clinical signs are the 'prayer sign' and 'table top sign' when the patient is not able to extend the fingers fully in a prayer position or to lie the fingers flat on the table top (Fig. 2) [5].

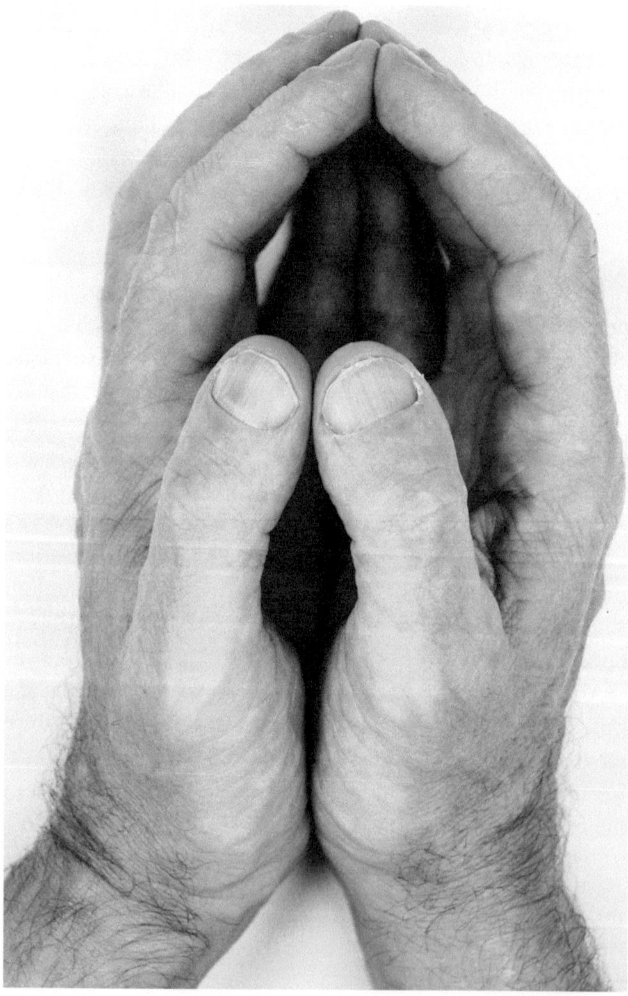

Fig. 2 Prayer sign were the fingers are held in slight palmar flexion limiting the ability to hold the fingers in a prayer position

Dupuytren's disease affects 1% of patients with diabetes mellitus. In the early stages of Dupuytren's disease, contracture may be present and palmar nodular thickening may be the only clinical manifestation without finger contraction. Ultrasound can help at this early stage of the diagnosis when the clinical signs are not clear-cut. Peripheral hypoxia results in increased free radicles which stimulate fibroblasts [5].

Trigger Finger

A similar aetiology lies behind the development of trigger finger. Trigger finger results from thickening of the A1 pulley usually with restricted movement of the underlying flexor digitorum tendons. The normal thickness of the A1 pulley measured at 10 or 2 o'clock is <0.5 mm (Fig. 3). Trigger finger is said to affect 5% of patients with diabetes mellitus. It usually affects the ring and middle fingers as well as the thumb. In routine clinical patients, if more than three fingers are affected, then diabetes mellitus should be actively excluded [5].

A condition closely related to trigger finger is deQuervain's disease. This is associated with thickening of the extensor retinaculum of the first compartment extensor tendons. It is particularly common in postpartum women ('babies thumb') though in this context is not usually associated with diabetes mellitus.

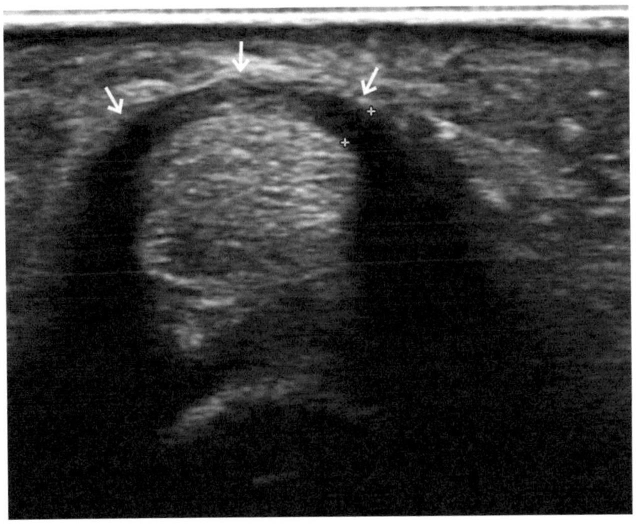

Fig. 3 Transverse ultrasound of the middle finger metatarsophalangeal region in a patient with clinically apparent trigger finger. The A1 pulley (*arrows*) is markedly thickened (1.2 mm) as shown by the electronic calipers at the 2 o'clock position. Normal thickness of the A1 pulley is <0.5 mm. This is consistent with trigger finger

Carpal Tunnel Syndrome

Carpal tunnel syndrome also occurs with increased frequency in diabetes mellitus though it is not clear whether this association is due to increased fibrosis of the transverse retinaculum and/or the coexistence of obesity and diabetes mellitus. Carpal tunnel syndrome is diagnosed clinically supported by nerve conduction tests or ultrasound examination. Ultrasound examination is almost as sensitive as nerve conduction test for confirming carpal tunnel syndrome. Various ultrasound parameters are used. In our department, a cross-sectional area of the median nerve just proximal to the tunnel inlet, at the tunnel inlet, at the tunnel outlet, or just distal to the tunnel outlet of >14 mm^2 is considered diagnostic of carpal tunnel syndrome. A CSA of <10 mm^2 at all of these locations is considered normal. If any measurement is >10 mm^2 but <14 mm^2, this is considered suggestive of but not diagnostic [6]. Different MRI criteria can also be applied to diagnose carpal tunnel syndrome.

Adhesive capsulitis affects about 10% of patients with diabetes mellitus compared to about 2% of control subjects [5]. Adhesive capsulitis is characterised by limitation of shoulder movement. During the initial inflammatory stage, the disease is very painful, especially during movement and when lying on the affected shoulder. Later, during the fibrotic stage, the pain subsides and limitation of movement, particularly external rotation, becomes the predominant feature. Finally, slow progressive improvement in the degree of shoulder movement occurs until complete resolution. The entire process, from initiation to resolution, lasts about 3–4 years.

Histologically there is synovitis and capsular proliferation of fibroblasts. MRI is an excellent modality to determine the existence of, severity of and type of (inflammatory or fibrotic) adhesive capsulitis. Synovial/capsular thickening can be seen in the subcoracoid recess, along the coracohumeral ligament, in the rotator cuff interval, along the glenohumeral ligaments, and at the axillary recess particularly the anterior limb of the inferior glenohumeral ligament.

Adhesive capsulitis seems to develop earlier in diabetic patients and non-diabetic patient i.e. before the age of 40 years of age. It seems to be associated with the duration but not with the type of diabetes.

Other Manifestations of Diabetes Mellitus

Diabetic Muscle Infarction

This is a relatively uncommon condition usually seen in end-stage diabetes mellitus and therefore in association with nephropathy, retinopathy, neuropathy and arteriopathy. It presents as painful muscle swelling. Onset is both acute and severe. The thigh muscles are most commonly affected followed by the gluteal and calf muscles. Creatinine kinase levels may be slightly elevated. It may present clinically as a soft tissue sarcoma. On imaging, one usually sees an area of nodular fibrotic-type swelling thickening in the centre of the muscle with surrounding muscle oedema. Both the ultrasound and MRI appearances are quite characteristic allowing the diagnosis to be made with confidence in the appropriate clinical setting and with no need for percutaneous biopsy [7]. Classically, ultrasound shows no surrounding hyperaemia in the early stages followed by progressive hyperaemia as repair occurs. Similarly, on MRI examination, one sees an area of muscle haemorrhage/oedema with peripheral hyper-perfusion (Fig. 4a–c). The lesion tends to become progressively smaller and more nodular/fibrotic in nature with healing. It is associated with a poor overall prognosis in that patient's usually succumb to the other manifestations of diabetes within 1–2 years of developing diabetic muscle infarction [7].

Diffuse idiopathic skeletal hyperostosis (DISH) with flowing intervertebral ossification is also more common in diabetes mellitus. The definition of DISH requires the presence of flowing ossification between four adjoining vertebral bodies. DISH results from ossification of the anterior longitudinal ligament. DISH mainly affects the thoracic spine though can also affect the lumbar and cervical spine. The reason for the association between DISH and diabetes mellitus is unknown. It may have a vascular aetiology. It may also be related to obesity and hence the association with diabetes. Growth hormone levels and inflammatory-like growth factor I (IGFI) are increased in patient with DISH. This may stimulate soft tissue ossification through osteoblastic proliferation and/or activation.

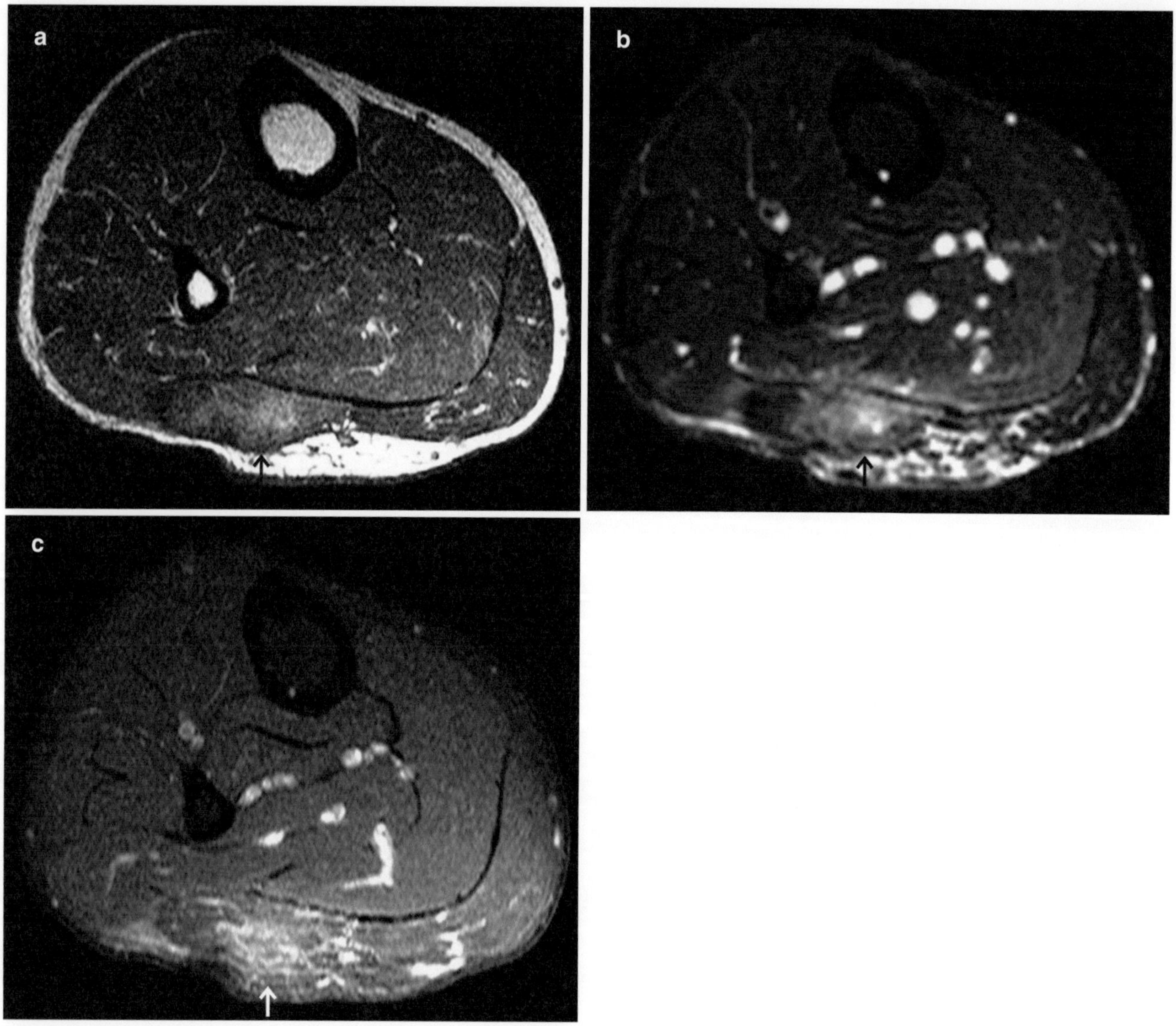

Fig. 4 Typical appearances of diabetic muscle infarction (**a**) T1-weighted axial MR image of the calf showing T1 hyperintensity within lateral belly gastrocnemius muscle (*arrow*) as a result of intramuscular haemorrhage. (**b**) T2-weighted fat-suppressed axial images at the same level as Fig. 4a, showing marked oedema within lateral belly gastrocnemius muscle (*arrow*). (**c**) T1-weighted fat-suppressed axial image post-contrast at the same level showing marked enhancement within lateral belly of the gastrocnemius muscle (*arrow*)

DISH is associated with hypertrophic osteoarthritis as well as ligamentous and tendon ossification. DISH is frequently accompanied by ossification of the posterior longitudinal ligament (OPLL). Whilst many patients with DISH may be asymptomatic, it can be, as expected be associated with spinal stiffness.

Osteoporosis

Diabetes mellitus is associated with osteoporosis. Both type I and type 2 diabetes are at increased risk of insufficiency fracture secondary to osteoporosis. On DXA examination, insulin-dependent diabetics classically show reduced bone density while non-insulin-dependent diabetics tend to show normal or increased bone mineral density, particularly in the lumbar spine, as a result of obesity and increased degenerative change. Insufficiency fractures seen in diabetes are similar to those of senile osteoporosis.

Osteoarthritis

Obesity in diabetes mellitus is associated with osteoarthritis, particularly of the knees.

Gout

Diabetes mellitus, through its association with metabolic syndrome, is associated with hyperuricaemia and gout.

Calcium Pyrophostate Deposition Disease

Diabetes mellitus is also probably associated with calcium prior phosphate deposition disease (CPPD).

Calcific tendinitis of the rotator cuff tendons is also thought to be more common in diabetes mellitus (Fig. 5a). It is characterized by hydroxyapatite deposition disease (HADD) within the rotator cuff tendons, most commonly the supraspinatus tendon though also the other tendons and the long head of biceps tendon. This can be associated with severe peri-calcific inflammation (Fig. 5b).

Rheumatoid arthritis is associated with an increased risk of diabetes mellitus but this risk appears to be limited only to those RA patients with positive cyclic citrullinated peptide (CCP) antibodies. This is most likely related to a specific allele being part of a common pathway for both of these autoimmune diseases (diabetes and rheumatoid arthritis).

Renal Osteodystrophy

Diabetes mellitus, through its association with chronic renal failure, can be associated with the varied musculoskeletal manifestations of chronic renal insufficiency [8].

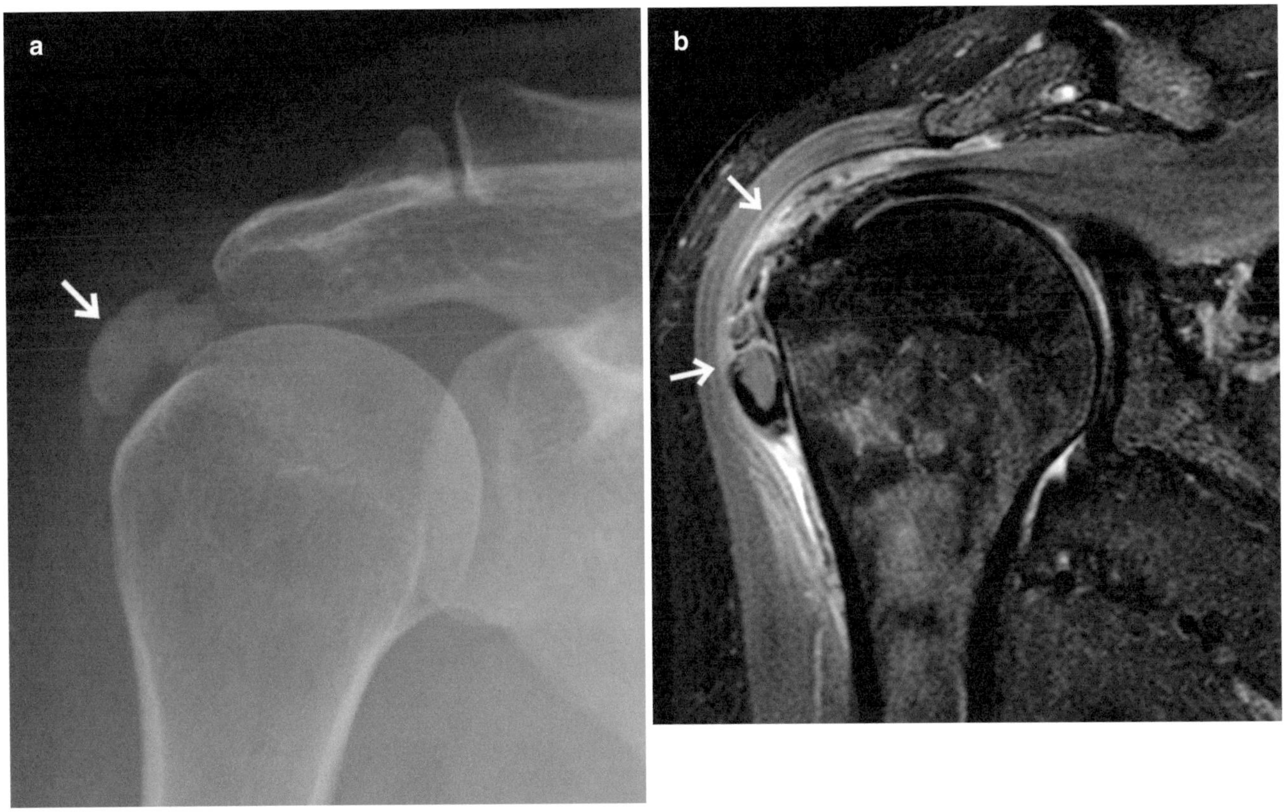

Fig. 5 (**a**) Frontal radiograph of the shoulder showing dense calcification (*arrow*) in the region of the supraspinatus tendon superficial to greater trochanter. (**b**) T2-weighted gradient-echo oblique coronal image three weeks later, shows that the calcification now lies within the subacromial-subdeltoid bursa as well as within the superficial fibres of the tendon (*arrows*). There is marked surrounding soft tissue oedema with ascites

These include the following:

- Secondary hyperparathyroidism
- Osteomalacia
- Osteoporosis
- Soft tissue and vascular calcification
- Tumoural calcinosis
- Amyloidosis, including amyloid spondyloarthropathy
- Aluminium toxicity leading to adynamic bone disease/ increased fracture risk
- Tendinopathy
- Osteonecrosis
- Spinal and other infections

Diabetic amyotrophy typically occurs in well-controlled recently diagnosed type 2 diabetes mellitus patients. It is due to a diabetic lumbosacral plexopathy akin to the mononeuritis multiplex. Presentation is one of acute onset proximal leg pain followed by muscle weakness. It is usually unilateral at presentation though tends to become bilateral at a later date. Ischemic neural injury due to microvasculopathy is the most likely etiology. The lateral history is one of a self-limiting course with spontaneous resolution within months though muscular weakness or pain may persists. Imaging is typically normal.

Acromegaly

A benign pituitary adenoma is present in >90% of cases with growth hormone hypersecretion. The remaining cases are due to hypothalamic adenomas, pancreatic islet cell tumour or carcinoid tumour. The skeletal manifestation of growth hormone hypersecretion varies depending on whether this is present prior to or after skeletal maturity. Prior to skeletal maturity, excessive growth hormone leads to physeal stimulation with gigantism. Following skeletal maturity, growth hormone hypersecretion leads to more generalized stimulation of bone formation. This gives rise to the typical imaging appearances of acromegaly (Fig. 6). This comprises coarse facial features and cortical hyperostosis associated with:

- Calvarial thickening, enlarged sinuses, frontal bossing and mandibular prognathism
- Spade-like terminal tufts and widened phalanges ('spade phalanx sign').
- Mild joint space widening (hands & feet)
- Premature osteoarthritis ('acromegalic arthropathy')
- Soft tissue hypertrophy (heel pad thickening of >25 mm, carpal tunnel syndrome, trigger finger)

Hypercortisolism

Adrenocorticotrophic hormone (ACTH) produced by the anterior pituitary stimulates the renal cortex to secrete cortisol. ACTH-dependent causes of hypercortisolism include ACTH-secreting pituitary adenomas (i.e. Cushing syndrome), and, less commonly, ectopic production of ACTH such as in small cell lung carcinoma and carcinoid tumours. ACTH-independent forms of Cushing syndrome include adrenal adenoma, adrenal cortical carcinoma, and adrenal hyperplasia. Nevertheless, the most common cause of Cushing syndrome is excessive therapeutic use of glucocorticoids. Hypercortisolism leads to

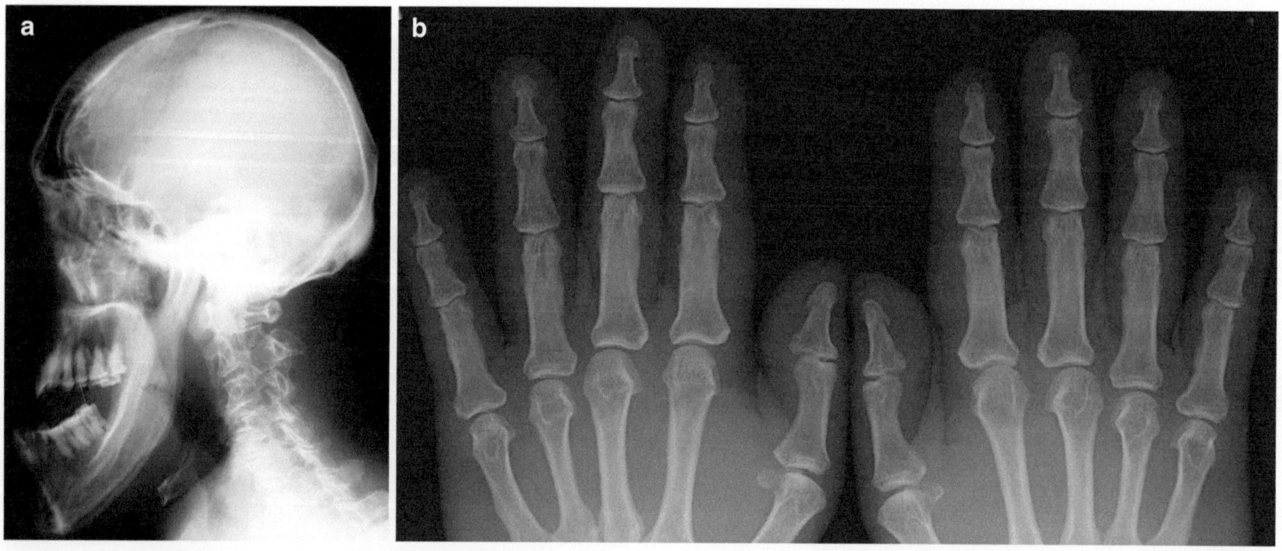

Fig. 6 (**a**) Lateral radiograph of the skull and facial bones showing calvarial thickening, mild frontal bossing, enlarged frontal sinus and markedly prognathic jaw in acromegaly. (**b**) Frontal radiograph of the fingers showing hypertrophied terminal phalangeal tufts and "spade appearance" of digits ('spade phalanx sign')

reduced bone density and osteoporosis, insufficiency fractures, particularly of the vertebral bodies, and avascular necrosis.

Glucocorticoid-induced osteoporosis is a biphasic process with an early rapid bone loss phase possibly mediated by osteoclastic hyperactivity and a later, slower progressive impaired bone formation phase [9]. Long-term glucocorticoid excess is associated with decreased osteoblast formation and activity as well as increased osteoblast apoptosis, while osteoclast number and activity is maintained [10]. Glucocorticoid also induces apoptosis of osteocytes, which serve as mechanosensors for bone metabolism [11]. These features contrast with the increased bone formation and resorption characteristic of postmenopausal osteoporosis and hyperparathyroidism and indicate how bone microstructural deterioration underlying glucocorticoid therapy is different to that of other osteoporosis.

Thyroid Disorders

Hyperthyroidism needs to increased bone reabsorption. There effect is more pronounced in cortical bone than trabecular bone. The manifestations are osteopenia, a lattice-like appearance to the long bones, and insufficiency fractures particularly of the vertebrae, the femoral neck and the distal radius. Other manifestations are dermopathy, myopathy and thyroid acropachy.

Thyroid Dermopathy or Pretibial Myxedema

The chronological sequence is thyroid dysfunction, then opthalmopathy, then dermopathy, and finally acropachy. Of hyperthyroid patients with opthalmopathy, 5% will have dermopathy (pretibial myxedema). Ultrasound demonstrates localised dermal thickening typically in the pretibial region with focal areas of hypoechogenicity due to proteoglycan deposition (Fig. 7). Skin biopsy demonstrates typical features of fibroblast activation and glycosaminoglycan deposition.

Thyroid acropachy is uncommon but is pathognomonic of hyperthyroidism. It is seen in treated hyperthyroidism. It is seen as digital clubbing, swelling and periosteal new bone formation of the extremities, often in an asymmetric pattern [12]. The bony changes include lacy periosteal new bone formation in the diaphysis of the tubular bones of the hands more than the feet (Fig. 8). Of patients with dermopathy (pretibial myxedema), 20% will have acropachy.

Most cases of acropachy therefore will have opthalmopathy and dermopathy allowing the distinction from hypertropic pulmonary osteoarthropathy (HPOA) to be made [9]. The latter is also associated with pulmonary disease, predominant involvement of the long bones in a symmetric pattern. These are not features of acropachy and therefore helpful to distinguish between thyroid acropathy and HPOA. Also in throid acropachy, there is a subperiosteal, frothy, lacy pattern while in HPOA, the periosteal reaction is lamellar [12].

Hypothyroidism in young patients leads to delayed skeletal maturation. There is delayed appearances of the physes as well delayed closure of the skull sutures. Decreased growth of the skull leads to brachycephaly and hypoplasia of the paranasal sinuses and mastoid air cells. Physeal development is also abnormal with irregular or stippled epiphyses, particularly of the femoral or humeral capital epiphysis. In adult patients, the manifestations of hypothyroidism include proximal myopathy, carpal tunnel syndrome and Dupuytren's contracture.

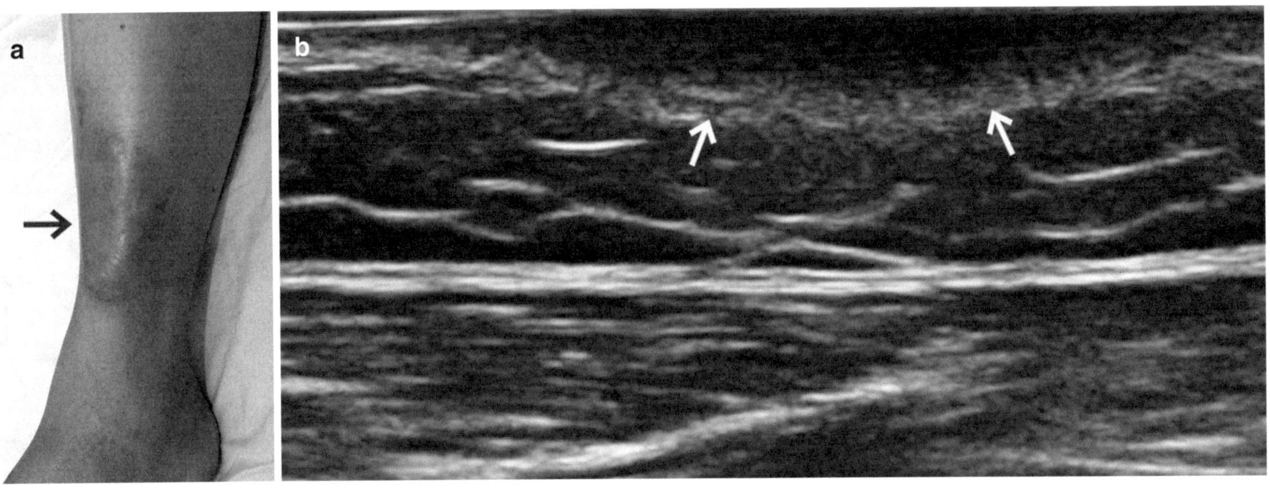

Fig. 7 Diabetic dermopathy. (**a**) Clinical photograph showing area of waxy skin thickening in the pretibial region (*arrow*) consistent with pretibial oedema. (**b**) Ultrasound of same area showing marked dermal thickening with a localised area of subdermal hypoechogenicity (*arrows*) due to focal proteoglycan accumulation

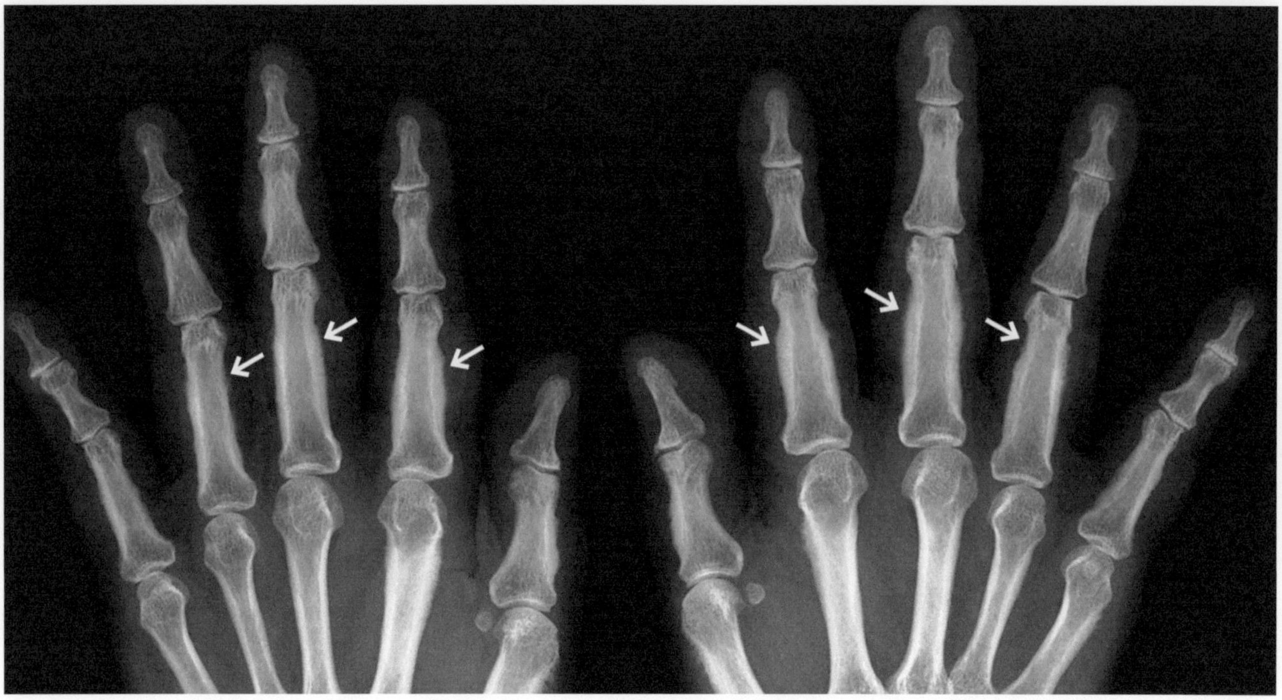

Fig. 8 Thyroid acropachy. Frontal radiograph of the hands showing prominent lacy periosteal reaction bilaterally along the diaphyses of the index, middle, and ring fingers (*arrows*). For this example, the disease is quite symmetric though this is not invariably the case

Parathyroid Disorders

Hyperparathyroidism

Hyperparathyroidism is caused by excessive secretion from the parathyroid glands usually due to a parathyroid adenoma. The most common form of hyperparathyroidism seen in clinical practice is secondary hyperparathyroidism as a result of sustained serum hypocalcaemia usually due to chronic renal failure. Tertiary hyperparathyroidism results from hyperplasia or adenoma of the parathyroid gland due to chronic secondary hyperparathyroidism and is associated with elevated serum calcium and phosphate levels.

The osseous manifestations of hyperparathyroidism are bone reabsorption and brown tumours. Bone reabsorption is most notable in a subperiosteal location, especially along the radial aspect of the middle phalanges of the index and middle fingers. The distal tufts of the phalanges are also commonly affected ('acro-osteolysis') as well as the medial aspects of the tibial, humeral and femoral metaphysis. Cortical bony reabsorption can lead to the intracortical tunneling (Fig. 9a). Patchy bone reabsorption leads to osteopenia and a 'pepper pot' appearance of the skull (Fig. 9b). Subchondral reabsorption is seen around joints (particularly the sternoclavicular, acromioclavicular and pubic symphysis) and at the lateral end of the clavicle. Subligamentous and subtendinous reabsorption occurs at the femoral trochanters, the ischial and humeral tuberosities.

Brown tumours are osteoclastomas which appear as a mildly expansile lytic areas with well-defined margins. The margin is classically non-sclerotic. Brown tumours occur particularly in the pelvis, the radius, clavicles and the metaphyses of the long bones (Fig. 10a, b). Calcium deposition and particularly chondrocalcinosis, due to calcium pyrophosphate deposition disease (CPPD) is a common accompaniment of hyperparathyroidism. The hallmark of CPPD is calcification of fibrocartilage tissue, particularly the articular disc of the triangular fibrocartilaginous complex (TFCC) and the meniscus.

The most common form of hyperparathyroidism is secondary hyperparathyroidism associated with chronic renal disease. In addition to bony reabsorption, brown tumours and chondrocalcinosis, one also sees the radiological changes of chronic renal disease with osteosclerosis and a 'rugger-jersey' spine. Tumoural calcinosis ('metastatic calcification'), due to elevated levels of both calcium and phosphate, may occur with large periarticular calcific masses often with calcium-fluid levels (Fig. 11a, b).

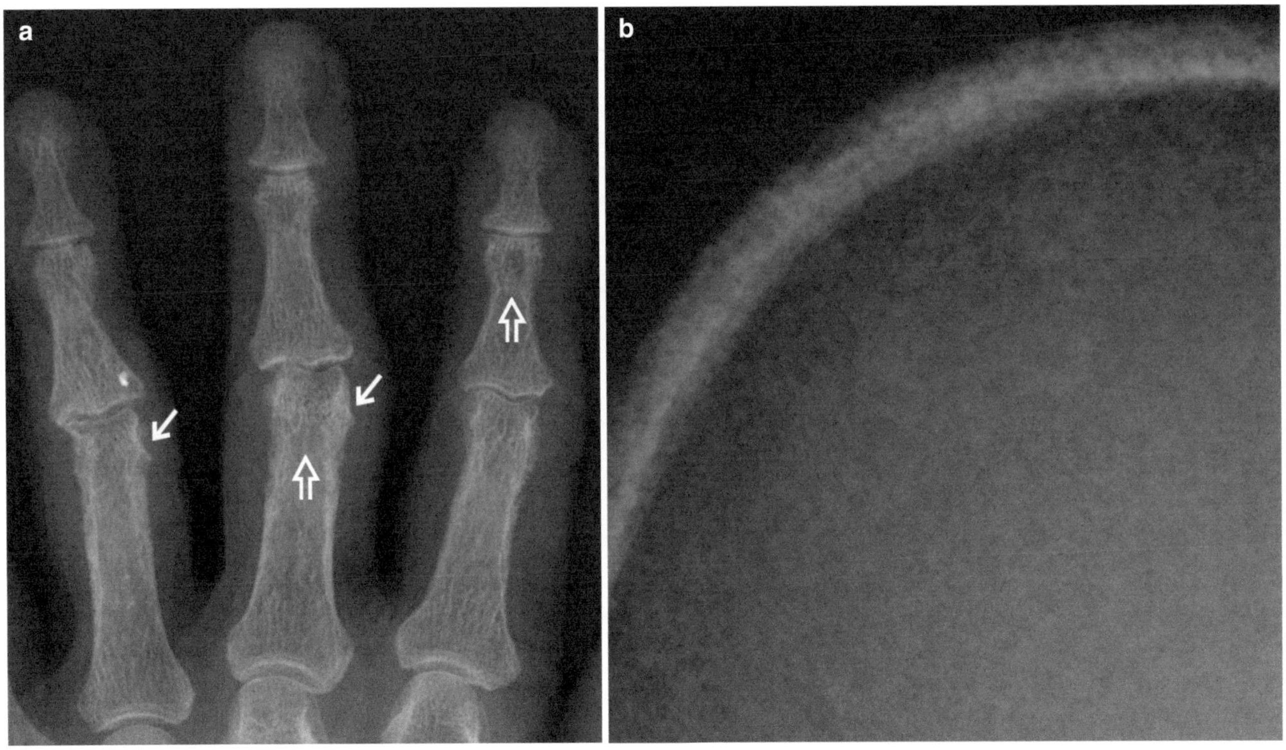

Fig. 9 Hyperparathyroidism. (**a**) Detail from frontal hand radiograph showing marked subperiosteal bony reabsorption particularly of the proximal phalanges (*arrows*). There is moderate generalised osteopenia with small cystic areas ('osteitis fibrosis cystica') (*open arrows*). (**b**) Detail from lateral skull radiograph showing 'pepper pot' appearance due to multiple lytic foci within the calvarium

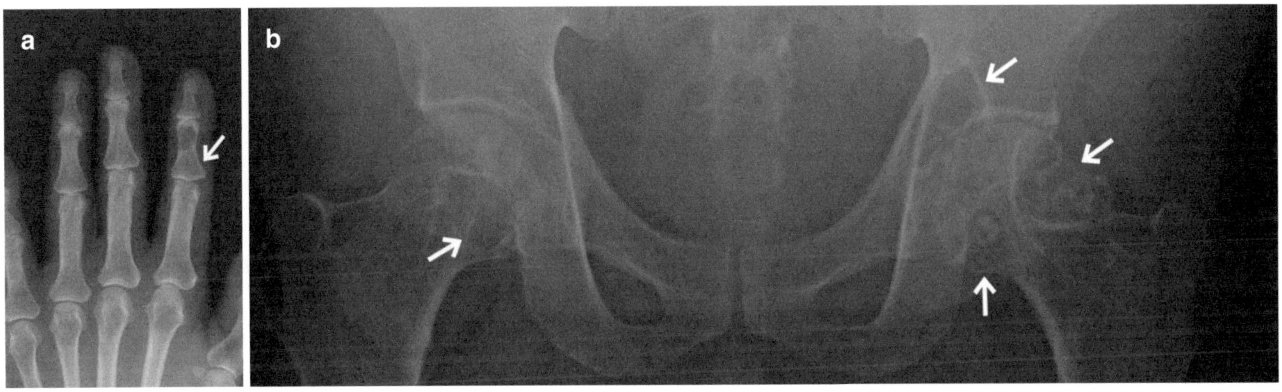

Fig. 10 Hyperparathyroidism with brown tumours. (**a**) Detail from frontal hand radiograph showing medium-sized brown tumour in the middle phalanx of the index finger (*arrow*). No generalised intracortical tunneling with poor definition of the cortices. (**b**). Frontal radiographs of both hips showing large osteolytic areas in both proximal femora and in the left acetabulum (*arrows*). Most of these lesions have a sclerotic rim with mild matrix mineralisation. These were histologically proven brown tumours. A sclerotic rim and matrix mineralisation can be seen with healing

Hypoparathyroidism

Hypoparathyroidism most commonly result from iatrogenic injury or removal of the parathyroid glands during surgery. There can also be an end-organ insensitivity to parathyroid hormone ('pseudohypoparathyroidism'), where the clinical features of hypoparathyroidism are seen but the parathyroid level is normal. The radiological features of pseudohypoparathyroidism are shortening of the metatarsal and metacarpal bones, (normally of the ring and little fingers) shortening of the middle and distal phalanges, coned epiphyses of the hands and feet as well as widening of the metacarpal and metatarsal bones. In addition, there is short stature, rounded facies, central obesity and mild mental retardation.

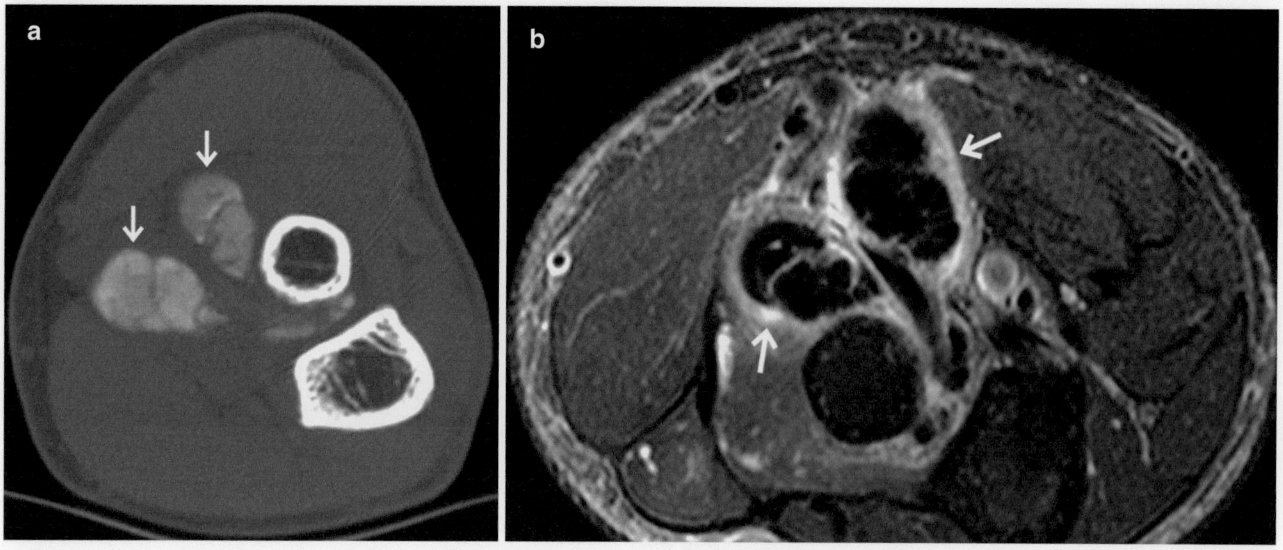

Fig. 11 Tumoural calcinosis. (**a**) CT showing tumoural calcinosis (*arrows*) of the radiobicipital bursa in patient with chronic renal failure. (**b**) T2-weighted fat-suppressed image of the same patient showing the degree of bursitis and soft tissue inflammation (*arrows*) associated with this uraemic tumoural calcinosis

Conclusion

The imaging appearances of endocrine disease are diverse and interesting. Knowing these imaging manifestations enables one to appreciate in greater depth the varied pathology associated with these diseases and, in some instances, allows the radiologist to identify the underlying endocrine disorder before it is clinically appreciated.

References

1. Griffith J, Davies AM, Close CF, Nattrass M (1995) Organized chaos? Computed tomographic evaluation of the neuropathic diabetic foot. Br J Radiol 68(805):27–33
2. Leone A, Cassar-Pullicino VN, Semprini A, Tonetti L, Magarelli N, Colosimo C (2016) Neuropathic osteoarthropathy with and without superimposed osteomyelitis in patients with a diabetic foot. Skelet Radiol 45(6):735–754
3. Shagos GS, Shanmugasundaram P, Varma AK, Padma S, Sarma M (2015) 18-F flourodeoxy glucose positron emission tomography-computed tomography imaging: a viable alternative to three phase bone scan in evaluating diabetic foot complications? Indian J Nucl Med 30(2):97–103
4. Meller J, Köster G, Liersch T, Siefker U, Lehmann K, Meyer I, Schreiber K, Altenvoerde G, Becker W (2002) Chronic bacterial osteomyelitis: prospective comparison of (18)F-FDG imaging with a dual-head coincidence camera and (111)In-labelled autologous leucocyte scintigraphy. Eur J Nucl Med Mol Imaging 29(1): 53–60
5. Boswell SB, Patel DB, White EA, Gottsegen CJ, Forrester DM, Masih S, Matcuk GR Jr (2014) Musculoskeletal manifestations of endocrine disorders. Clin Imaging 38(4):384–396
6. Wong SM, Griffith JF, Hui AC, Tang A, Wong KS (2002) Discriminatory sonographic criteria for the diagnosis of carpal tunnel syndrome. Arthritis Rheum 46(7):1914–1921
7. Chow KM, Szeto CC, Griffith JF, Wong TY, Li PK (2002) Unusual muscle pain in two patients with diabetic renal failure. Hong Kong Med J 8(5):368–371
8. Lim CY, Ong KO (2013) Various musculoskeletal manifestations of chronic renal insufficiency. Clin Radiol 68(7):e397–e411
9. Canalis E, Bilezikian JP, Angeli A, Giustina A (2004) Perspectives on glucocorticoid-induced osteoporosis. Bone 34(4):593–598
10. Weinstein RS, Jilka RL, Parfitt AM, Manolagas SC (1998) Inhibition of osteoblastogenesis and promotion of apoptosis of osteoblasts and osteocytes by glucocorticoids. Potential mechanisms of their deleterious effects on bone. J Clin Invest 102(2):274–282
11. O'Brien CA, Jia D, Plotkin LI, Bellido T, Powers CC, Stewart SA et al (2004) Glucocorticoids act directly on osteoblasts and osteocytes to induce their apoptosis and reduce bone formation and strength. Endocrinology 145(4):1835–1841
12. Gutch M, Sanjay S, Razi SM, Gupta KK (2014) Thyroid acropachy: frequently overlooked finding. Indian J Endocrinol Metab 18(4): 590–591

Metabolic Bone Diseases with Emphasis on Insufficiency Stress Fractures

Bruno Vande Berg, Charbel Mourad, Vasiliki Perlepe, Souad Acid, Thomas Kirchgesner, and Frédéric Lecouvet

Any component of the musculo-skeletal system can be involved by metabolic disorders as a resultant of endocrinological diseases, genetic alterations and environmental or nutritional aspects (Table 1). Metabolic disorders are generally indolent; their initial clinical manifestations may be due to complications. Early detection of these disorders is crucial because of the availability of efficient therapies. This chapter provides an overview on imaging features observed in metabolic bone disorders with emphasis on insufficiency stress fractures (ISF).

Table 1 Metabolic disorders of the musculoskeletal system

Muscles	Sarcopenia, drug-induced myopathies (statins.), necrosis (diabetes mellitus), fat atrophy (steroids)
Tendons	Chondrocalcinosis, hypercholesterolemia, hyperuricemia, hypervitaminosis A, drug-induced (quinolones)
Cartilage	Chondrocalcinosis, hyperuricemia, recurrent haemorrhage, hemochromatosis, ochronosis
Synovium	Hyperuricemia, amyloidosis
Bone	Osteopenia, osteoporosis, rickets, osteomalacia, renal osteodystrophy, hyperparathyroidism, thyroid acropachy, acromegaly, drug-induced disorders
Bone marrow	Hemosiderosis, aplasia, anemias, serous atrophy, fatty atrophy, drug-induced disorders

B. Vande Berg (✉) • C. Mourad • V. Perlepe • S. Acid
T. Kirchgesner • F. Lecouvet
Department of Radiology, Cliniques Universitaires Saint-Luc, IREC Institut de Recherche Clinique, Université Catholique de Louvain, Louvain Academy, 10 Avenue Hippocrate, Brussels 1200, Belgium
e-mail: bruno.vandeberg@uclouvain.be

Normal Bone Metabolism

Bone is a specialized connective tissue made up of a matrix of collagen fibers, mucopolysaccharides and inorganic crystalline mineral matrix (calcium hydroxyapatite) that is distributed along the length of the collagen fibers. Bone remains metabolically active throughout life (bone turnover) with bone being constantly resorbed by osteoclasts (osteoclastic activity) and accreted by osteoblasts (osteoblastic activity) [1, 2]. Since bone turnover mainly takes place on bone surface, trabecular bone which has a greater surface to volume ratio than compact bone, is consequently some eight times more metabolically active than cortical bone. The strength of bone is related not only to its hardness and other physical properties but also to its size, shape, and architectural arrangement of the compact and trabecular bone.

Bone formation and bone resorption are linked in a consistent sequence under normal circumstances. Percursor bone cells are activated at a particular skeletal site to form osteoclast, which erode a flairly constant amount of bone. After a period of time, the bone resorption ceases and osteoblasts are required to fill the eroded space with new bone tissue. This coupling of osteoblastic and osteoclastic activity constitutes the basal multi-cellular unit (BMU) of bone and is normally in balance, with the amount of bone eroded being replaced with amount of new bone in about 3–4 months. At any one time, there are numerous BMUs throughout the skeleton at different stages of this cycle. The amount of bone in the skeleton at any moment is entirely dependent on peak bone mass attained during puberty and adolescence and on the balance between bone resorption and formation. Bone turnover is under the influence of general factors including age and hormones but is also locally modified by many factors such as physical forces.

J. Hodler et al. (eds.), *Musculoskeletal Diseases 2017-2020*, DOI 10.1007/978-3-319-54018-4_10

Osteoporosis

Definition

Osteoporosis, by far the most common metabolic disease in western countries, is a systemic skeletal disease with quantitative abnormality of bone whereas, in rickets/osteomalacia, there is qualitative abnormality of bone (Fig. 1). Osteoporosis is characterized by reduction in bone mass (amount of mineralized bone per volume unit) and by altered trabecular structure due to a loss of trabeculae interconnectivity with a consequent increase in bone fragility (decrease in biomechanical strength) and susceptibility to fracture (insufficiency fractures) [3] (Fig. 2).

Prevalence of Osteoporosis

In the western world, osteoporosis is reported to affect 1 in 2 women and 1 in 5 men older than the age of 50 years in their life time [4]. The risk of fracture increases with advancing age and progressive loss of bone mass and varies with the population being considered. The incidence of hip fracture has doubled over the past three decades and is predicted to continue to grow beyond what one would predicted from increased longevity. At 1 year after hip fracture, 40% patients are unable to walk independently, 60% have difficulty with one essential activity of life, 80% are restricted in other leaving activity, and 27% will be admitted to a nursing home for the first time [4].

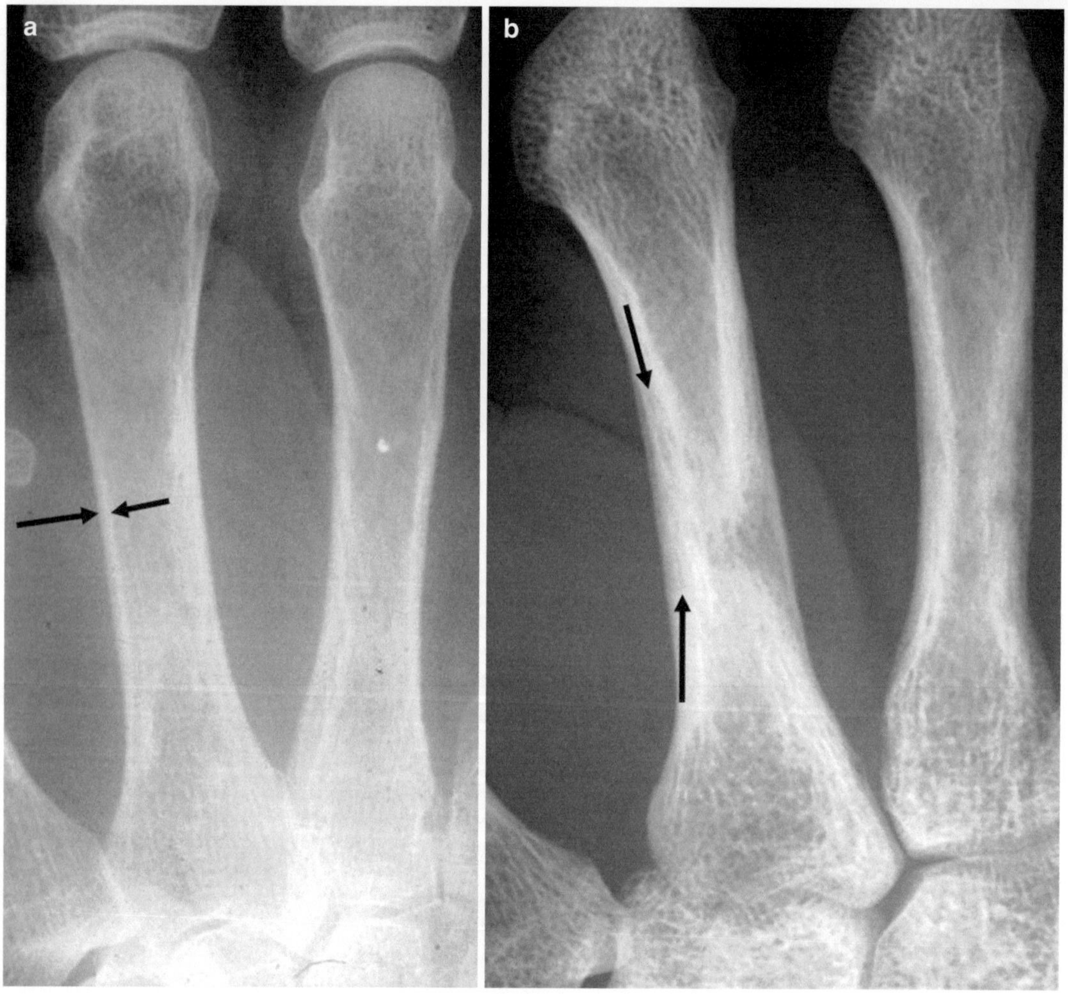

Fig. 1 Osteopenia and osteomalacia. (**a**) Osteopenia is characterized by quantitative bone abnormality with decreased bone density and cortical thinning (*arrows*). (**b**) Osteomalacia is characterized by qualitative bone abnormality with intracortical lucencies (*arrows*)

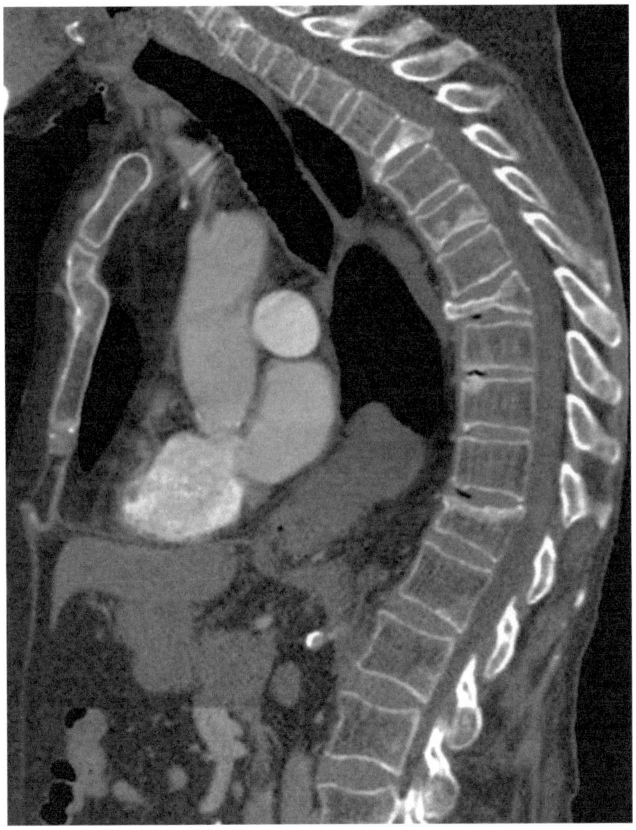

Fig. 2 Osteoporosis. Presence of multiple vertebral fractures with thoracic kyphosis. Sclerosis in fractured vertebral bodies corresponds to bone callus. Note the sternal fracture associated with thoracic kyphosis

Clinical Presentation and Etiology

Generalized osteoporosis is the end-stage of several diseases and can be either primary or secondary (Tables 2 and 3). Clinical significance of osteoporosis is limited until fractures develop. Vertebral fractures are the most commonly occurring osteoporotic fractures (Fig. 2). They occur as an acute event related to minor trauma or spontaneously. Vertebral fractures cause disability and limited spinal mobility and are associated within increased morbidity but symptoms generally resolve spontaneously over 6–8 weeks. They are powerful predictors of future fracture with a 12% increased risk of a future vertebral fracture within 12 months if a single vertebral fracture is present (22% increased risk in the presence of multiple fractures) [2]. Questionnaires are also available to evaluate fracture risk (FRAX). Consequently, the accurate identification and clear reporting of vertebral fracture by radiologists have a vital role to play in the diagnosis and appropriate management of patient with, or at risk of, osteoporosis.

Table 2 Causes of primary osteoporosis

Idiopathic juvenile osteoporosis: self-limited (2–4 year duration) form of osteoporosis in pre-pubertal children. Acute course of the disease with growth arrest and fractures. Mild to severe forms. Differential diagnosis: osteogenesis perfecta or other forms of juvenile osteoporosis. Cortisolism and leukaemia
Post-monopausal (type I) osteoporosis: Onset at the time of menopause but important bone loss during first 4 years after the menopause related to reduction in blood oestrogen. Clinically significant in women 15–20 years after the menopause. Fractures in bones with high trabecular cortical ratio (vertebral bodies and distal forearm)
Senile (type 2) osteoporosis: men and women 75 years or older due to age-related bone loss (age-related impaired bone formation associated with secondary hyperparathyroidism as a consequence of reduced calcium absorption from the intestine secondary to decreased production of the active metabolic vitamine D in the kidney). Reduction in both cortical and trabecular bone. Fractures in vertebrae but also in bones with low trabecular cortical ratio (tibia, humerus and pelvis)
Osteogenesis imperfecta: congenital disorders due to gene mutation associated with osteoporosis of variable severity. Blue sclerae and occasional dental involvement

Table 3 Causes of secondary osteoporosis

Endocrine: glucocorticoid excess, oestrogene/testosterone deficiency, hyperthyroidism, hyperparathyroidism
Nutritional: intestinal malabsorption, chronic alcoholism, chronic liver disease, partial gastrectomy, vitamine C deficiency
Hereditary: homocystineuria, Marfan syndrome, Heler-Danlos syndrome
Hematologic: sickle-cell disease, thalassemia, Gaucher disease, multiple myeloma
Others: rheumatoid arthritis, hemochromatosis, long-term heparin therapy

Imaging Findings in Osteoporosis

Radiography is relatively insensitive in detecting early bone loss and 30–40% loss of bone tissue usually remain occult on radiographs. Radiographic bone density is also affected by patient characteristics and technical parameters used to obtain the radiographs. The subjectivity of visual judgement of bone density on conventional radiographs supports the value of modern quantitative techniques such as bone densitometry.

The main radiographic features of generalized osteoporosis include cortical thinning and disappearance of the trabecular network. Resorption and thinning of trabeculae initially affect secondary trabeculae that are parallel to the biomechanical stresses and the primary trabeculae that are perpendicular to the biomechanical stresses may appear more prominent because they are affected at a later stage (Fig. 3).

Cortical thinning occurs as a result of endosteal, periosteal, or intra-cortical (cortical tunnelling) bone resorption. Endosteal

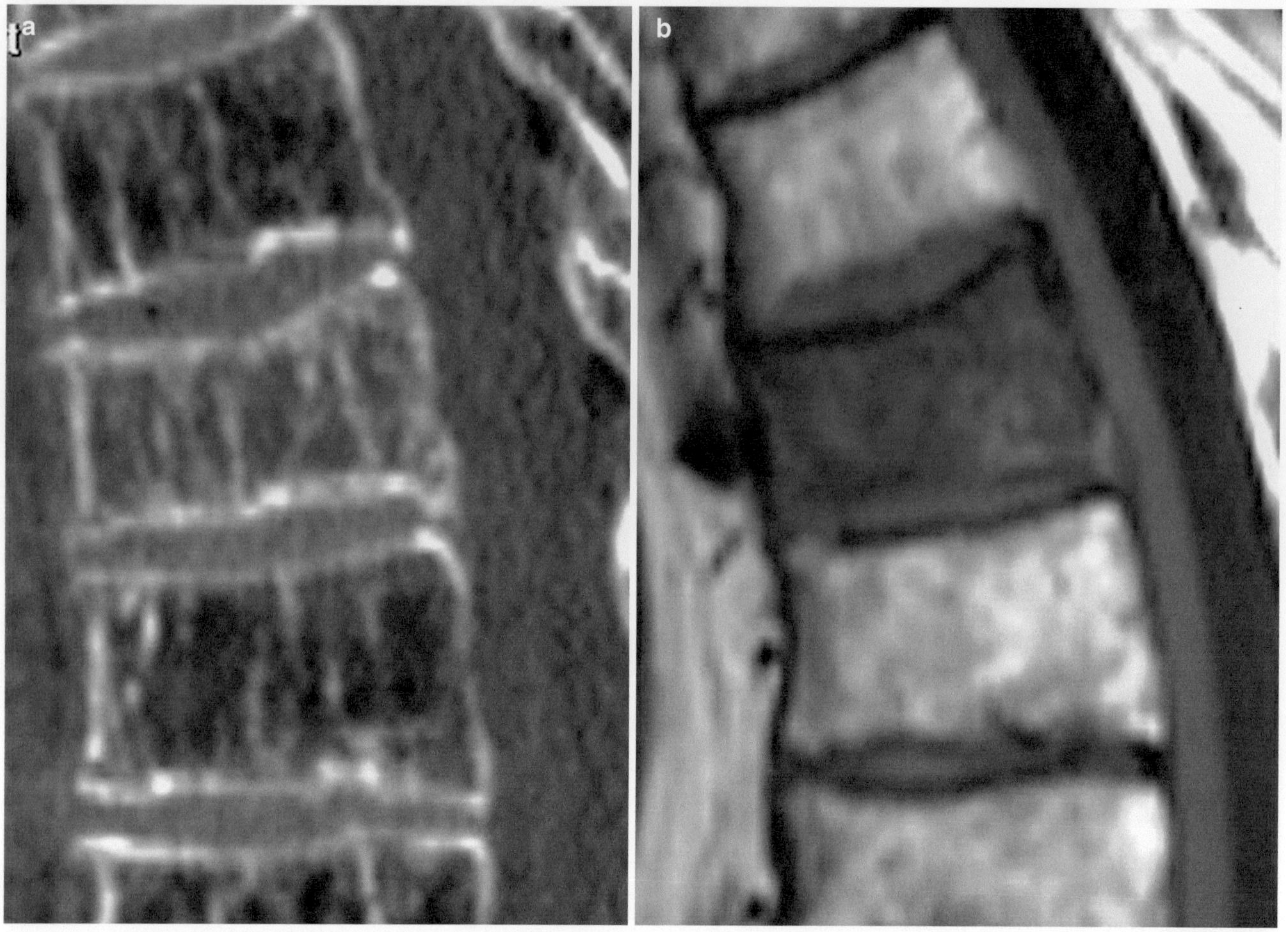

Fig. 3 Osteoporosis and vertebral fracture. (**a**) A sagittal CT reformat of the thoracic spine shows reduced trabecular bone density and a vertebral fracture. (**b**) The corresponding sagittal T1-w SE image shows decreased signal intensity in the fractured vertebral body (recent fracture). Altered trabecular bone pattern seen on CT is not visible on routine MR images

resorption is the least specific radiographic finding because it may be evident in metabolic disorders, including osteoporosis but also in marrow disorders. Intra-cortical tunnelling is more specific occurring mainly in disorders with rapid bone turnover such as diffuse osteoporosis and reflex sympathetic osteodystrophy. Subperiosteal resorption is the most specific finding, being diagnostic of hyperparathyroidism.

Osteoporosis remains occult on MR images (Fig. 3) although a relationship between trabecular bone density and marrow fat has been reported. The presence at spine MRI of multiple vertebral fractures including acute (marrow edema) and healed (marrow fat) fractures suggests increased bone fragility and, hence, osteoporosis.

Quantification of Osteoporosis

Several quantitative techniques including Dual energy X-ray absorptiometry (DXA), quantitative computed tomography (QCT), and quantitative ultrasonography (QUS) have been developed to enable accurate and precise assessment of mineral bone density [2]. Several methods have been used in the past to standardize measurements of cortical thickness (radiogrametry), trabecular pattern (Singh index), and vertebral deformity (morphometry) from radiographs (Table 4). These measurements lack accuracy or predictive value but they remain worth reporting when present on radiographs.

Table 4 Radiographic quantitative methods for osteoporosis

Radiogrametry involves the measurement of cortical thickness of various bones on radiographs and the most frequently used bone is the second metacarpal bone of the non dominant hand. The metacarpal index corresponds to the ratio between the mid diaphyseal diameter of the bone (from each periosteal surface) and the medullary cavity (distance between endosteal surface)
Trabecular pattern was assessed by using the Singh index which takes into account the number, thickness and arrangement of trabeculae in the femoral neck. Texture analysis of that area could be of interest
Vertebral morphometry according to various methods have been proposed to standardize a subjective visual assessment vertebral fracture and to quantitate alteration in vertebral height and shape. Vertebral fractures are defined as endplate, wedge or crush. Changes in shape of the vertebrae are generally defined by the six points methods, in which the anterior, mid- and posterior points of the superior and inferior endplates of the vertebral body are identified, to measure anterior, mid, and posterior height. The change in shape can be graded (mild, moderate, severe) for each pattern on deformity (wedge, biconcave, crush)

Rickets and Osteomalacia

Rickets and osteomalacia are similar metabolic bone disorders characterized by inadequate or delayed mineralization of osteoid in cortical and trabecular bone in children and in adults, respectively [5].

Pseudofracture or looser's zone is the radiological hallmark of osteomalacia as it represents cortical fracture without a mineralized callus. Looser's zone corresponds to a linear cortical lucency frequently perpendicular to the cortex of the bone without periosteal reaction (Fig. 4). It typically involves the ribs, the superior and inferior pubic rami, and the inner margins of the proximal femora or lateral margin of the scapula. Widened physeal growth plate and metaphyseal cupping and fraying are the radiological signs of rickets that are best seen at rapidly growing ends of bone such as distal femur and radius or anterior ends of ribs. Additional radio-

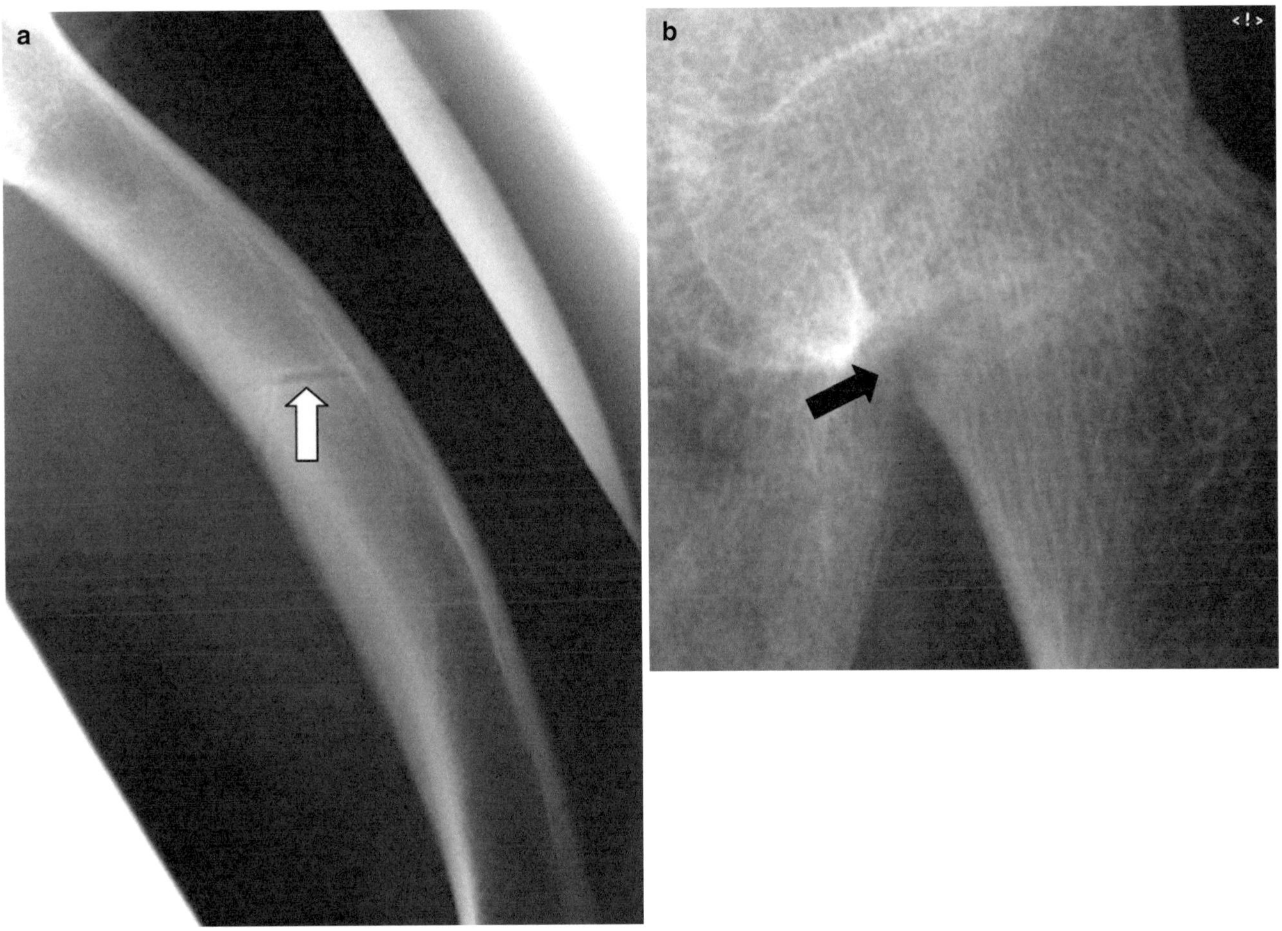

Fig. 4 Osteomalacia. (**a**) A lateral radiograph of a femur from a patient with osteomalacia demonstrates anterior bowing of the femoral shaft and a lucent line corresponding to a fracture (*white arrow*). (**b**) A close-up radiograph of a femoral neck in another patient with osteomalacia demonstrates cortical discontinuity and bone resorption (*black arrow*) corresponding to a chronic fracture or Looser's zone

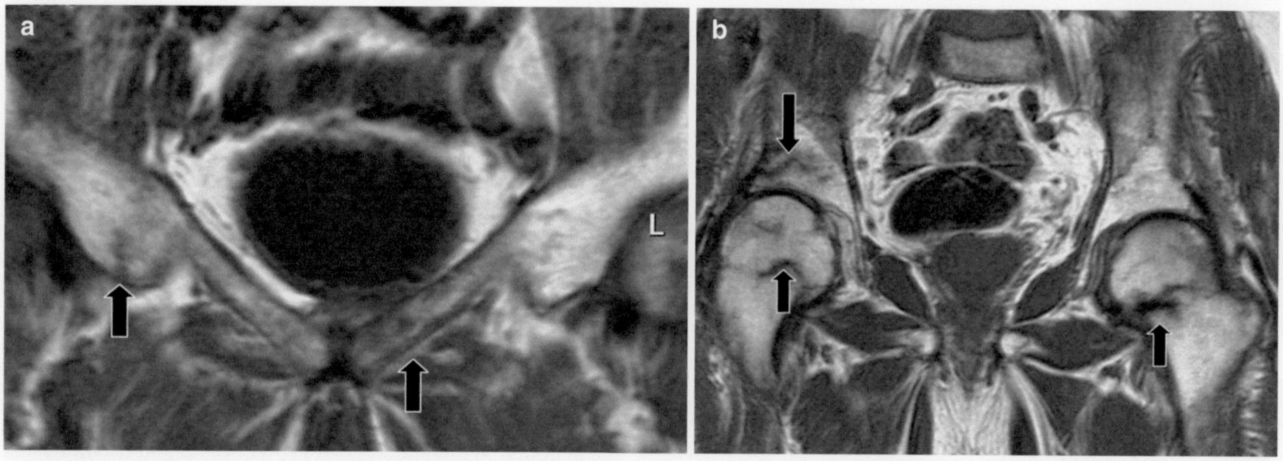

Fig. 5 Osteomalacia. (**a**, **b**) Coronal T1-weighted images of the pelvis of a patient with osteomalacia demonstrate multiple trabecular bone fractures (*arrows*)

logical findings of rickets/osteomalacia include bone deformities, osteopenia or a coarsened pattern of the cancellous bone [5].

There is no hallmark of osteomalacia at MR imaging because cortical fractures with deficient healing (Looser's zones) are difficult to detect on MR images. However, the presence of multiple trabecular bone fractures with variable appearance on fluid-sensitive sequences should suggest osteomalacia. This variability could reflect the deficient healing process associated with osteomalacia [6, 7] (Fig. 5).

Renal Osteodystrophy and Hyperparathyroidism

The term renal osteodystrophy relates to all musculoskeletal manifestations of chronic renal failure [5]. Traditionally, renal osteodystrophy encompassed osteoporosis, osteomalacia, secondary hyperparathyroidism and soft tissue calcifications. The radiographic signs of hyperparathyroidism are subperiosteal bone resorption on the radial side of the finger phalanges and/or exclusive phalangeal tuft resorption (Fig. 6). The hand is the earliest and most sensitive site for detection of hyperparathyroidism but bone resorption can also be seen at the end of the clavicle, at the sacro-iliac joints or on periosteal surfaces of the proximal humeri or proximal femora. Marginal erosions in small joints can also develop most likely due to traction at capsular insertions. They are usually discrete and joint space is preserved.

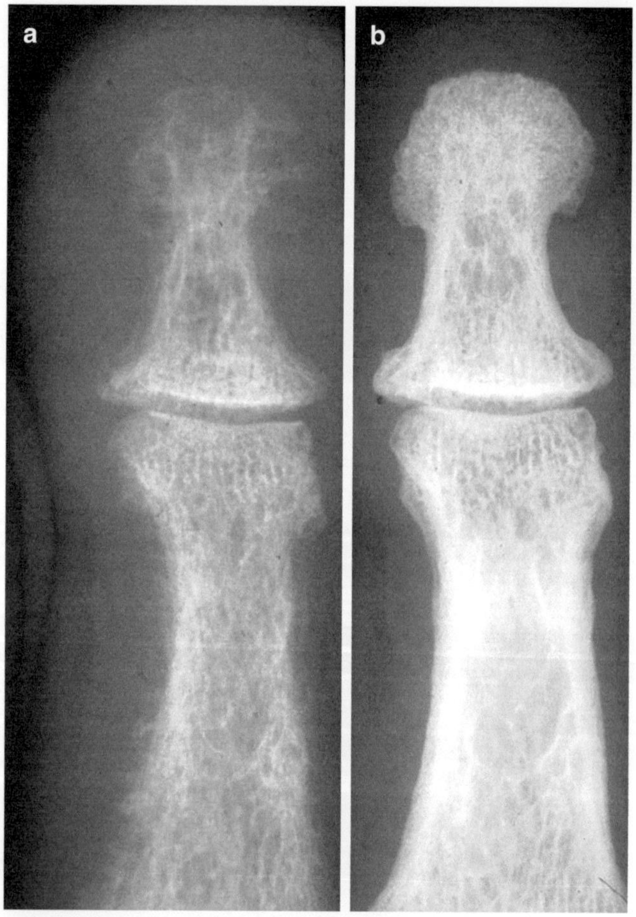

Fig. 6 Hyperparathyroidism. (**a**) Radiographic signs of hyperparathyroidism include subperiosteal bone and phalangeal tuft resorption. (**b**) After successful treatment, reappearance of woven bone

Osteosclerosis may also be encountered in renal osteodystrophy. It is commonly appreciated in vertebrae, pelvis, ribs and metaphyses of long tubular bones. In vertebrae, sclerosis is frequently confined to the end-plates, producing a characteristic appearance of alternating bands of different density (the "rugger jersey" spine).

Soft tissue calcifications may develop anywhere, in the vessel walls but also in the muscles and tendons. Massive amorphous calcification can develop in the soft tissue around articulations and probably reflect poorly controlled renal osteodystrophy. Presence of chondrocalcinosis (knees and wrists) in patient younger than 50 years of age should raise the possibility of hypercalcemia but hemochromatosis may also present with osteoporosis and chondrocalcinosis.

Primary hyperparathyroidism (generally related to the presence of a solitary adenoma in the parathyroïd gland) and the classic radiographic changes of hyperparathyroidism are largely historical because of the routine evaluation of serum calcium levels in the population. Osteoclastoma or brown tumors are lytic bone lesions associated with chronic hyperparathyroidism.

Insufficiency Stress Fractures

Classifications of Fractures

In general, fractures are classified according to the bone status before the fracture and to the applied forces (Table 5). Traumatic fractures result from an acute increase in biomechanical stress on normal bone. Fatigue fractures result from a chronic repetitive increase in biomechanical stresses on normal bone. Insufficiency stress fracture (ISF) result from a normal or slightly increased stress on diffusely weakened bones. Pathological fractures result from normal forces applied on locally weakened bone due to an underlying, generally lytic, lesion. Medical imaging plays a crucial role in the diagnosis of insufficiency and pathological fractures because of the lack of a suggestive clinical history [8–10]. The distinction between these two conditions can be challenging or even impossible as in patients with multiple myeloma.

Table 5 Classification of fractures

	Bone strength	Applied forces	Clinical clues
Traumatic fracture	Normal	Increased, acute	History
Fatigue fracture	Normal	Increased, chronic	History
Insufficiency fracture	Diffuse decrease	Normal	None
Pathological fracture	Focal decrease	Normal	None

Imaging of Insufficiency Stress Fractures

The spectrum of radiographic and MR findings observed in ISF largely depends on the predominantly involved bone (trabecular or cortical) and on the time delay between fracture and imaging (acute, subacute, chronic). Trabecular bone fractures will merely involve the vertebral bodies, the sacrum and acetabulum, the femoral head, neck and condyles, the tibial epiphyses and the small bones of the feet. Cortical fractures will develop in the pubic rami, the femoral neck and the diaphysis of the femur, tibia and metatarsal bones.

On radiographs, early diagnosis of ISF is difficult because of poor conspicuity of bone interruption and of limited bone deformity in the absence of external forces (no trauma) (Table 6). At a later stage, callus formation and periosteal bone formation can be detected on radiographs. Trabecular callus is typically linear and perpendicular to the dominant trabecular network because trabecular insufficiency fractures generally result from compressive forces.

At MR imaging, trabecular ISF include marrow edema and intramedullary low signal intensity bands (impaction fractures) (Table 7). The distinction between stress-induced and fracture-related marrow changes is unclear and marrow edema may also occur in response to increased biomechanical stress without definite fracture. Low signal intensity bands within the medullary cavity are important to recognize because of their specificity. Their conspicuity on the different MR sequences varies according to poorly understood parameters in an unpredictable manner. Some other imaging

Table 6 Radiologic appearance of trabecular and cortical insufficiency stress fracture (ISF)

Radiographs/CT	Acute ISF	Chronic ISF	Healed ISF
Trabecular bone	Normal	Mild sclerosis	Normal
Cortical bone	Cortical interruption	Periosteal reaction	Cortical thickening

Table 7 MR appearance of trabecular and cortical insufficiency stress fracture (ISF)

MR imaging	Acute ISF	Chronic ISF	Healed ISF
Trabecular bone	Extensive edema	Band, edema	Normal
Cortical bone	Subtle marrow and soft tissue edema	Subtle marrow and soft tissue edema, periosteal callus	Normal

features may also be associated with fracture including altered bone shape, cortical interruption, and periosteal reaction. In case of cortical ISF, cortical interruption is barely visible on routine MR images. Extensive edema within the adjacent medullary cavity or soft tissues is frequently seen. It can suggest other condition such as tumors or infection if the cortical fracture is not recognized.

Topographic Approach of ISF

ISF of the Spine

ISF predominantly involve the thoraco-lumbar spine but do not occur in the cervical spine. The anterior and central mid-portion of the vertebral body withstand compression forces less well than the posterior and outer ring element of the vertebrae, resulting in wedge or endplate fractures or, less commonly, crush fractures. A good radiographic technique is required when imaging the spine, particularly in the lateral projection. The spine must be parallel to the radiographic table to prevent the vertebrae appearing to have an apparent biconcave endplate, which is an artefact due to tilting of the vertebrae or the divergence of the X-ray beam (beam cam effect). Scheuermann's disease also causes vertebral body deformities. Endplate irregularity, most commonly in the thoracic spine, involving several adjacent vertebrae generally enables the differentiation between vertebral fracture and growth-related bone deformities.

Typically, spinal ISF involves one or several vertebral bodies of the thoraco-lumbar junction. Anterior wedge-shaped deformity is the most frequent pattern. Extensive bone marrow edema on MR images generally spares the posterior arch and the vertebral body opposite to the fractured vertebral end plate (differential diagnosis from disc-related marrow changes) (Fig. 7). The medullary low signal bands are parallel to and located a few millimeters from the involved vertebral end plate.

ISF of the Pelvic Bones

ISF of the pelvic ring involve pubic and ischiatic rami, supraacetabular area and lateral aspects of sacrum (Fig. 5) [11]. There is an increased prevalence of these lesions in patients with previous radiation therapy (importance of differential diagnosis with metastases). Radiographs are rarely diagnostic except in pubic bones (cortical fractures). CT may contribute to the diagnosis by demonstrating cortical interruption or callus formation in trabecular bone (sacrum). MR imaging is the best imaging modality for sacral and supra-acetabular fractures (Fig. 8).

ISF of the Femur

Early recognition of femoral ISF is extremely important because of possible progression to displaced fracture and subsequent possible complications in elderly patients. They may involve the femoral neck or the proximal femoral diaphysis. Femoral neck ISF are frequently occult on radiographs as cortical interruption when present is subtle and trabecular bone fracture is barely visible. MR imaging better displays associated marrow edema with intramedullary low signal intensity bands (Fig. 9).

Insufficiency stress fracture of the femoral shaft has gained particular attention as they occur in patients with untreated osteoporosis but also in patients with long-standing bisphosphonate therapy for osteoporosis (Fig. 10) [12]. On radiographs, they appear as transverse cortical lucencies, occasionally multiple and almost always located on the lateral aspect of the femur. Because of their chronicity, periosteal new bone formation is associated that leads to a beak appearance. In case of overt fracture, the fracture line may extend longitudinally. These lesions are more easily detected on radiographs or CT than on MRI because of the lack of edema given their chronicity and the limited conspicuity of cortical changes at MRI [13]. It is recommended to obtain radiographs of both femurs because these lesions are

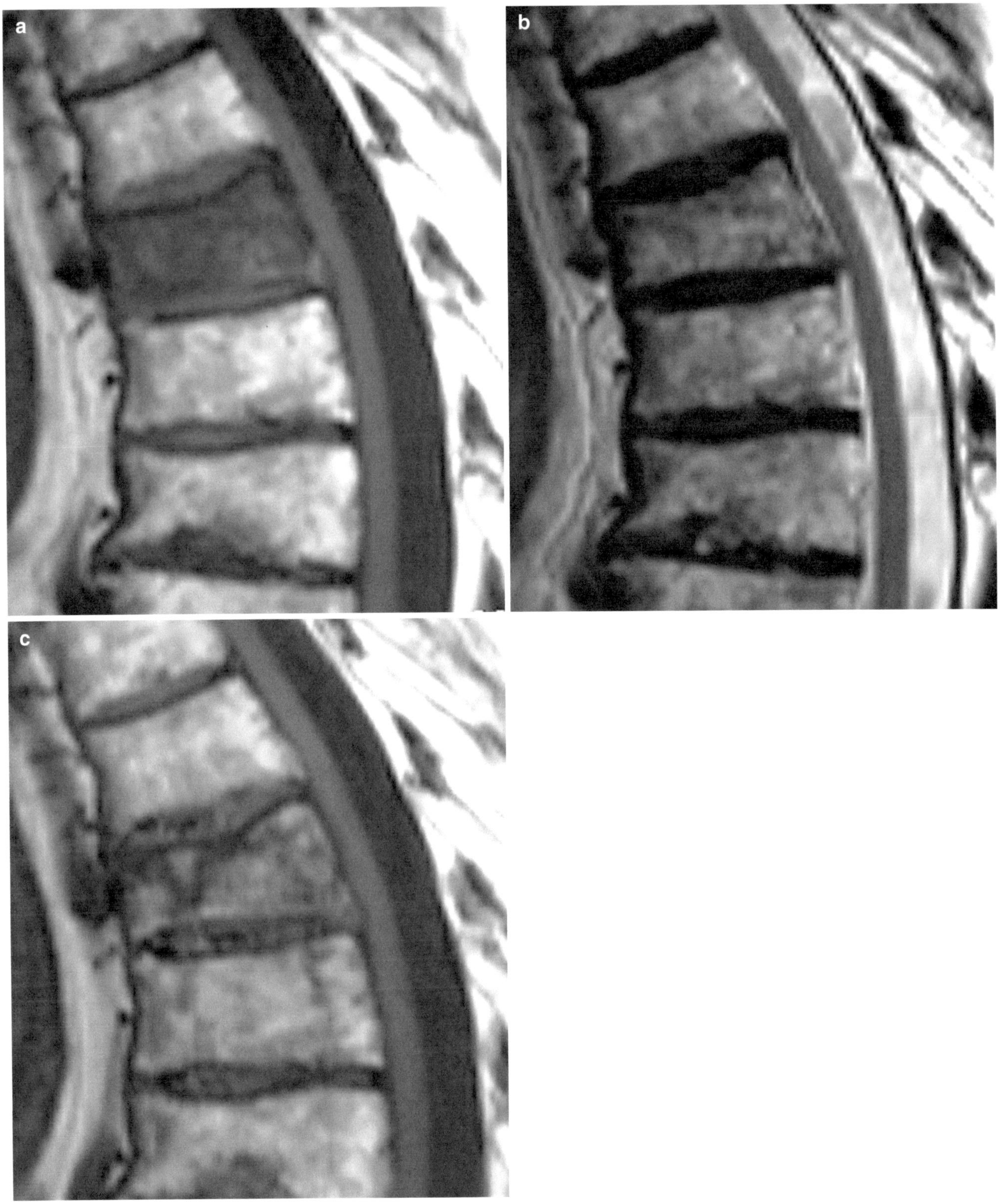

Fig. 7 Spontaneous ISF of a thoracic vertebral body. (**a**) A sagittal T1-weighted image of the thoracic spine demonstrates a vertebral body with decreased signal intensity. (**b**) On the corresponding T2-weighted SE image, the vertebral body shows intermediate signal. (**c**) On the follow-up T1-weighted SE image obtained 2 months later, there is partial regression of the lesion with appearance of intra-vertebral lines of low signal intensity

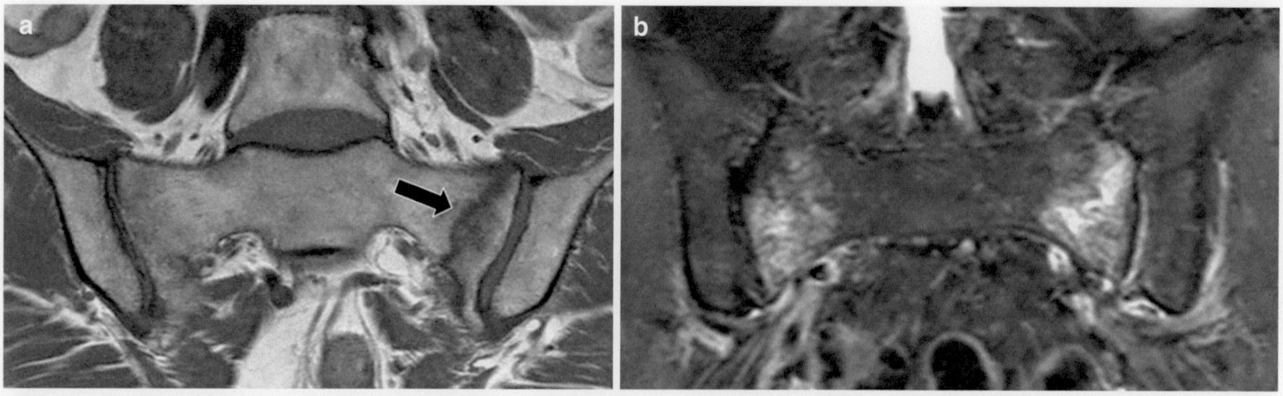

Fig. 8 Bilateral ISF of the sacrum. (**a**) A coronal T1-weighted image of the sacrum demonstrates a low signal intensity line (*arrow*) in left sacrum with adjacent marrow edema. (**b**) A coronal STIR image demonstrates bilateral extensive edema in sacrum

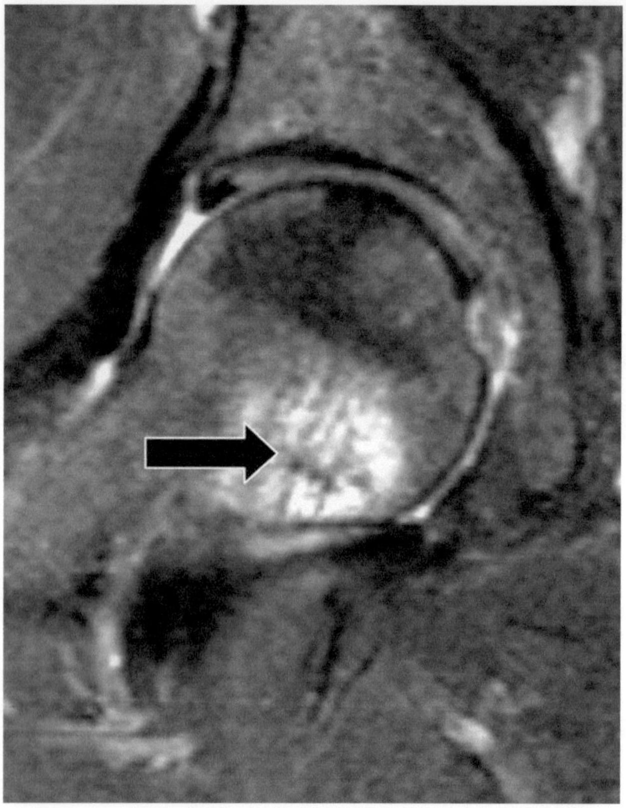

Fig. 9 Femoral neck ISF in a patient with osteoporosis. A coronal fat-saturated IW image of the *right hip* shows an area of increased signal in the medullary cavity. A low signal intensity line (*arrow*) indicates trabecular bone fractures within the area of marrow edema

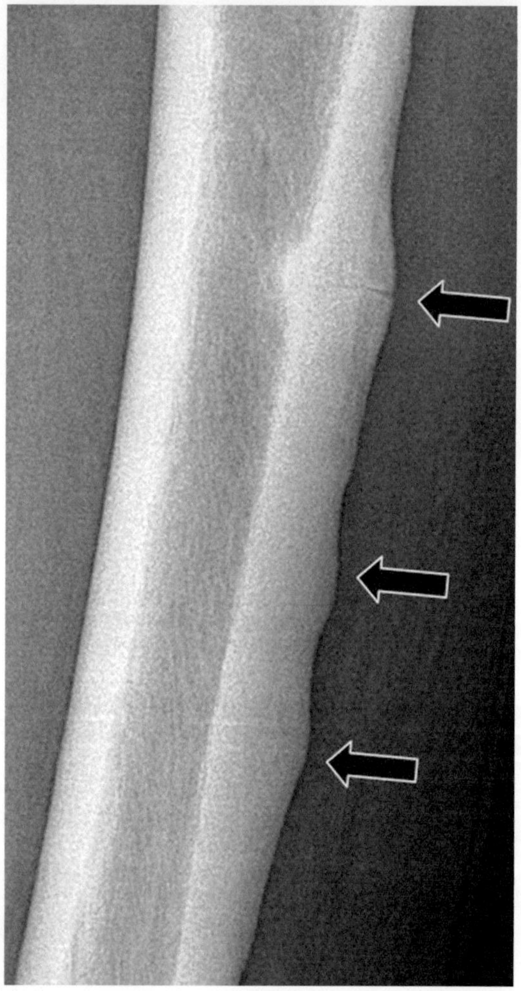

Fig. 10 A radiograph of the left femur of a 80-year-old woman on bisphosphonate therapy since 12 years demonstrates multiple transverse partial cortical fractures (*arrows*)

occasionally bilateral and preventive nailing of the femur with these fractures has been recommended to prevent overt fracture [14]. Similar fractures occur in the lateral or anterior aspect of the diaphysis in femurs with Paget's disease, also. In osteomalacia, cortical fractures tend to involve the medial aspect of the cortex and lack mineralized callus.

Cortical insufficiency stress fractures are usually transverse or slightly oblique. Rarely, the fracture line has a longitudinal orientation and it may involve the tibia but also the femur and metatarsal bones [15]. They are associated with extensive edema in the adjacent medullary cavity and soft tissues (Fig. 11). Cortical interruption is not visible on long axis images and short axis MR or better CT images are mandatory to demonstrate cortical break and callus formation (importance of bone settings window at CT) [15]. The lesion may be confused with infection or tumor at MR imaging because of the longitudinal extent of marrow infiltration [16] (Fig. 11).

Epiphyseal ISF

Until the early 90s, epiphyseal ISF remained underdiagnosed and almost all spontaneous (non-traumatic) epiphyseal fractures were considered to be due to underlying osteonecrosis. The concept of spontaneously resolutive epiphyseal bone lesions corresponding presumably to non traumatic fractures (fatigue or insufficiency) emerged progressively [9]. It has become a widely accepted concept.

Epiphyseal ISF involve convex weight-bearing epiphyses such as the femoral head, the femoral condyles and metatarsal heads [9, 17–19] (Fig. 12). Concave epiphyses such as the tibial epiphyses are less frequently involved. Radiographs are generally normal but may show subtle subchondral sclerosis. MR imaging reveals extensive marrow edema and low signal intensity bands located at a few millimeters from the subchondral bone plate that is generally not altered.

Insufficiency Stress Fractures of the Tarsal Bones

ISF of the tarsal bones frequently involves the greater tuberosity of the calcaneus, the talar dome and neck and the cuboid bone. Imaging features are similar to those observed

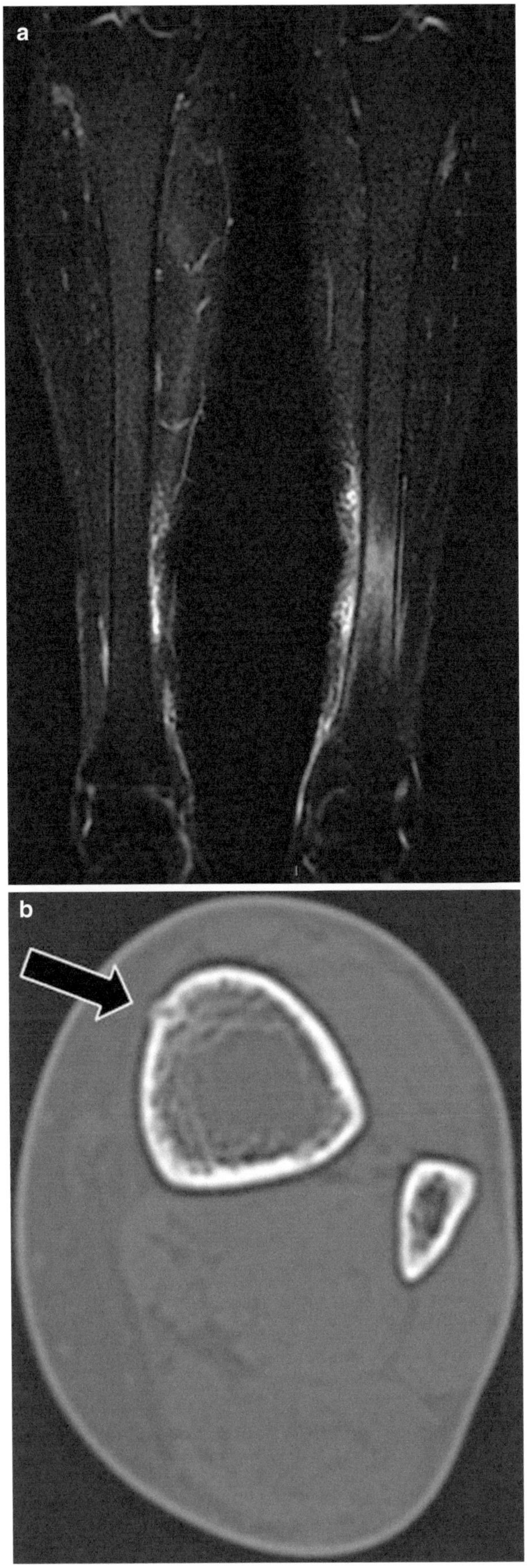

Fig. 11 Longitudinal ISF of the left tibia. (**a**) A coronal STIR image of both tibias demonstrates oedema in the medullary cavity and adjacent soft tissues of the left tibia. (**b**) A CT image of the left tibia shows a cortical fracture with periosteal and endosteal callus (*arrow*)

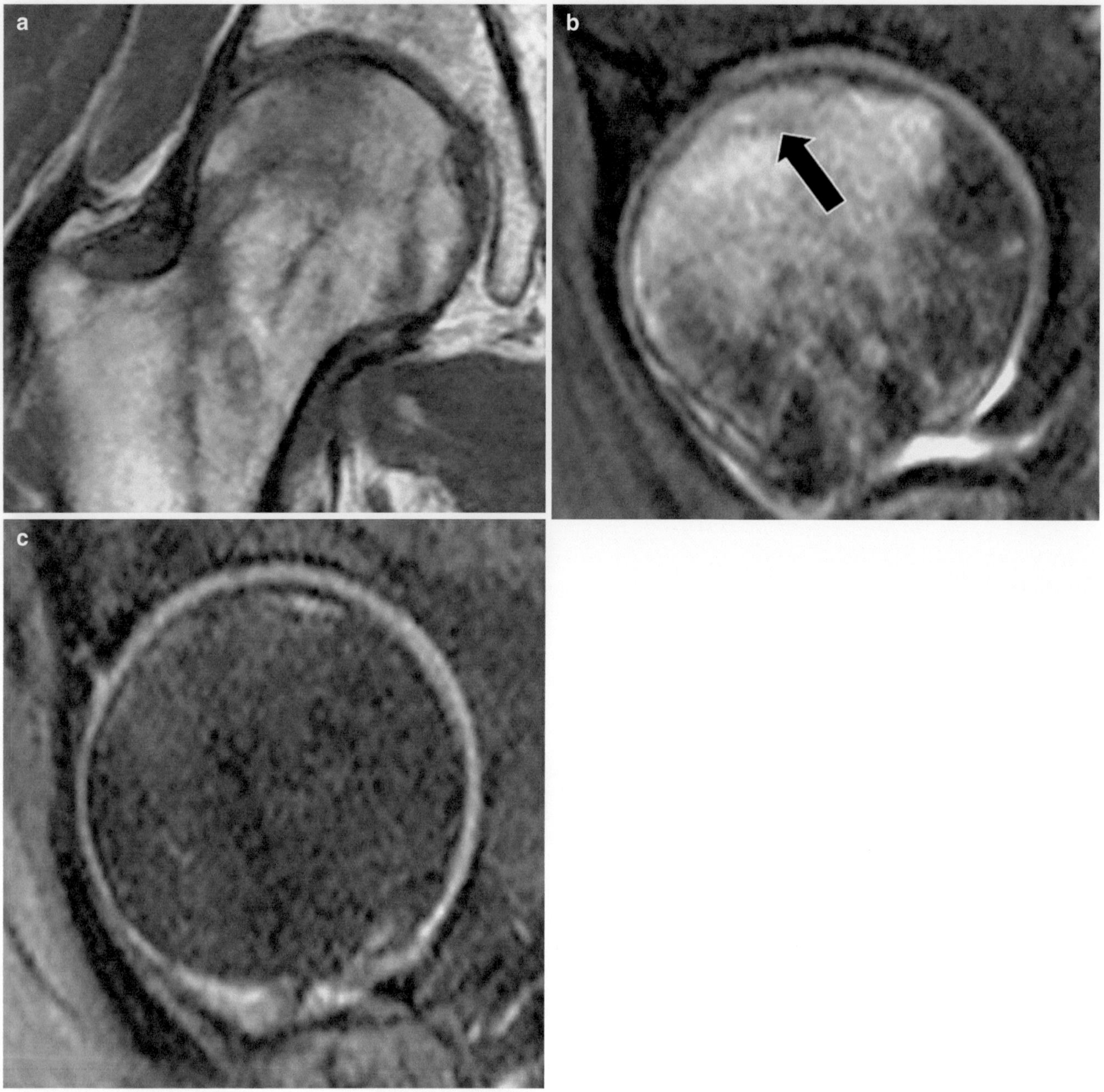

Fig. 12 ISF of the femoral head in a 47-yo male with severe osteoporosis. (**a**) A coronal SE T1-weighted image of the right hip shows an ill-delimited area of marrow oedema in the femoral head. (**b**) On a sagittal proton-density-weighted image, the lesion shows high signal intensity. A low signal intensity line (*arrow*) indicates a trabecular bone fracture. This line is thin, located at a few millimetres from the subchondral bone plate and there is oedema all around it. (**c**) Almost complete regression of the lesion at 2-months follow-up on a sagittal fat-saturated PD image

in the vertebral bodies because fractures involve the trabecular network and result from compressive stress. The female athlete triad is worth mentioning and it consists of disordered eating, amenorrhea, and osteoporosis [20]. Long-distance runners and ballet dancers are most frequently concerned. Foot fractures are common and represent fatigue (overuse) and insufficiency (bone weakening) fractures.

Complications of ISF

Complications of Trabecular ISF

Predominantly trabecular ISFs usually heal normally with appropriate conservative therapy. Secondary displacement rarely occurs because these fractures result from normal stress that is compressive stress. Sequellae due to bone deformity may occur, mainly in the spine. Delayed union and subsequent non-union of trabecular ISF may occur if immobilization is difficult to achieve, if vasculature is sparse (epiphyseal ISF) or if the bone metabolism is altered (radiation therapy, steroids) [21] (Table 8). In such a case of altered healing process, progressive collapse may occur.

In the past literature, epiphyseal ISF that progressed to bone collapse were considered to represent osteonecrosis: vertebral osteonecrosis (Fig. 13) and spontaneous osteonecrosis of the medial femoral condyle (SONK) (Fig. 14) are the most well-known conditions [18, 22]. This complication may also be observed in femoral and metatarsal heads. Early recognition of these conditions is important: in the spine, vertebral osteonecrosis may lead to spinal cord compression, an uncommon feature in vertebral ISF. In pelvic ring fractures, abnormal healing may lead to the formation of lytic bone lesions mimicking malignant fractures. In the proximal and distal epiphyses of the femur, delayed-union may lead to progressive epiphyseal collapse and subsequent osteoarthritis. Several imaging features may contribute to the recognition of lesions with poor prognosis that are likely to progress to irreversible fracture and collapse [23–26].

Table 8 Causes of abnormal healing in ISF

Local causes	Distraction stress (scaphoid), persistent mechanical stress (pubis, epiphysis, rib)
Regional causes	Radiation therapy Vascular disorders
Diffuse causes	Metabolic bone diseases (osteomalacia, steroid, fluor therapy) Altered threshold of pain (steroid, alcohol, neuropathy)

Complications of Cortical ISF

Cortical ISF of the long bones may progress to overt displaced fractures if not recognized in part because the causative stresses (torsion, compression, traction) favor displacement.

Take Home Points

1. Metabolic disorders of the musculo-skeletal system may involve the bones, the marrow, the muscles, the tendons, the cartilage and the synovium. Metabolic disorders are usually clinically silent until complications do occur including mechanical failure (bone fracture, tendon tear) and inflammation (arthritis).
2. Radiographs, CT and MRI have limited value in the quantification of metabolic bone disorders but accurate reporting of incidental findings such as old vertebral fracture on chest radiographs or CT is important.
3. ISF of the thoraco-lumbar spine and lower limb bones are the most frequent complications of metabolic bone disorders. Medical imaging plays an important role in their diagnosis in the absence of suggestive clinical history (lack of trauma or of repetitive activity). Imaging findings depend on many parameters and vary according to the time delay from fracture.
4. Bone marrow edema is a predominant but non-specific MR feature observed in ISF. Presence of low signal intensity bands or lines indicates impaction fracture of the trabeculae. In cortical ISF, cortical discontinuity is best appreciated on CT than on MR images.
5. Overt displaced fracture may complicate cortical ISF (femur, tibia). Delayed-union may complicate trabecular SIF and may occasionally lead to marked deformity (vertebral body, long bone epiphyses).

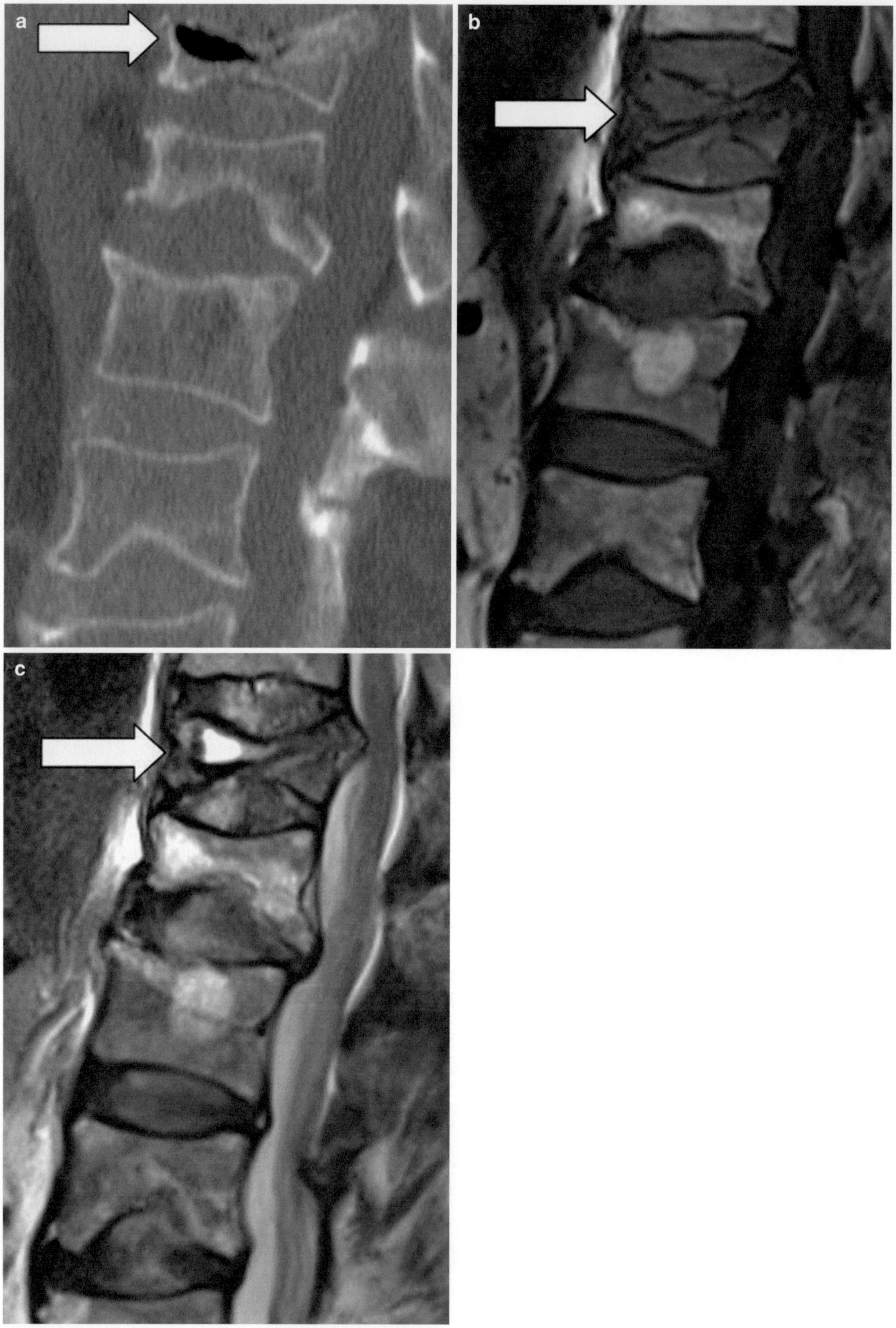

Fig. 13 Vertebral osteonecrosis in a 71-yo male. (**a**) A sagittal CT reformat of the lumbar spine demonstrates fracture of L1 with intravertebral vacuum phenomenon (*arrow*). Note posterior displacement of the vertebral wall and healed fractures in L1 and L3. (**b**, **c**) On the corresponding SE T1- and T2-weighted images, a fluid-collection (*arrow*) is seen in L1

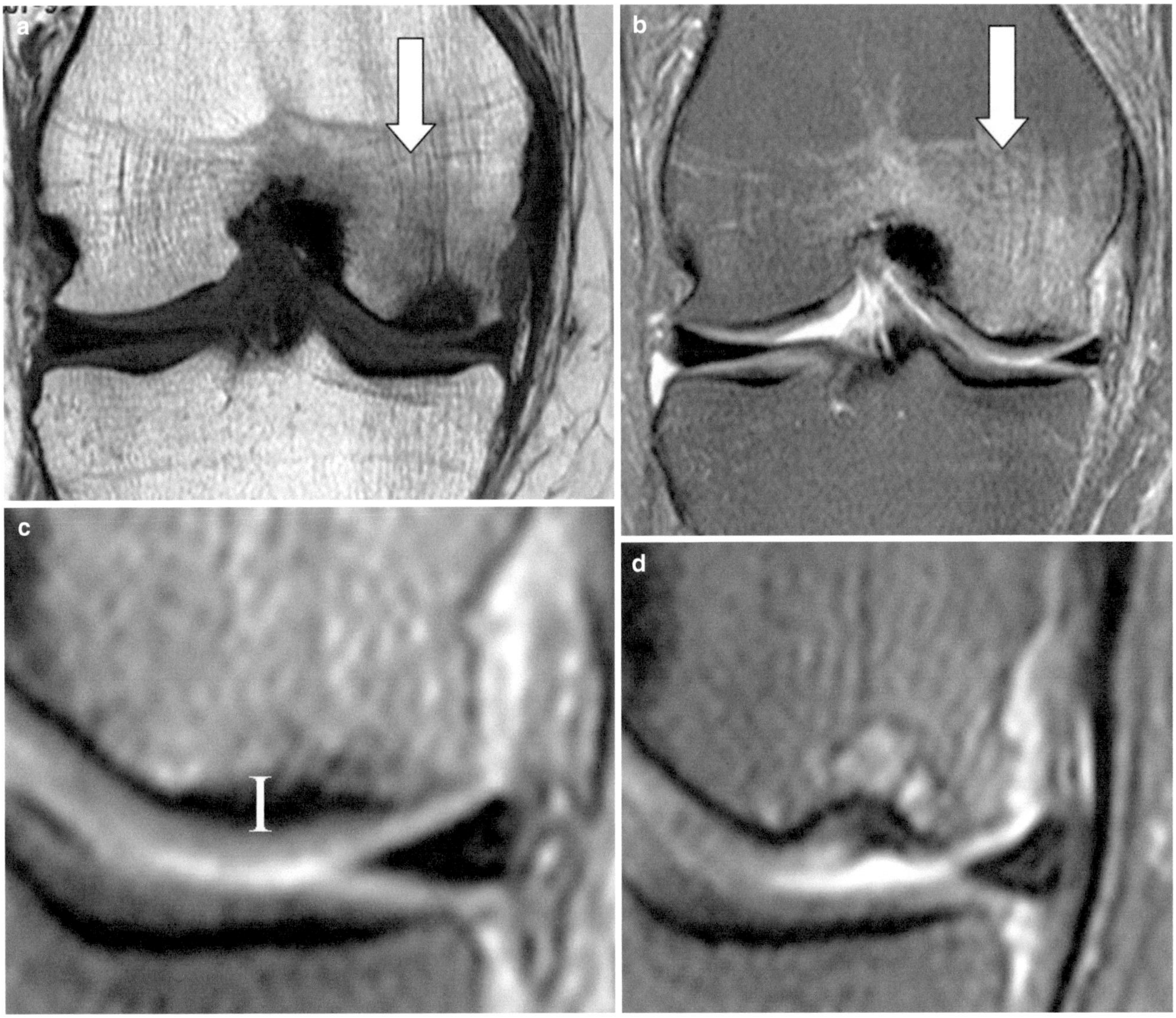

Fig. 14 ISF of the medial condyle and subsequent « spontaneous » osteonecrosis in a 65-yo woman. (**a**, **b**) Initial coronal SE T1 and fat-saturated proton-density images of the right knee demonstrate extensive marrow edema in medial condyle (*arrow*) with more pronounced decrease in signal in subchondral marrow. (**c**) On a magnified view of **b**, there is a thick area of low signal intensity signal (*vertical bar*) that indicates a poor prognosis as it corresponds to necrotic tissue. (**d**) A follow-up MR image obtained 6 months later demonstrates focal deformity of the subchondral bone plate (*arrow*) and adjacent geodes indicative of fragment mobility. This lesion is known as "spontaneous osteonecrosis of the knee" in the literature

References

1. Resnik, N (1988) Diagnosis of bone and joint disorders, vol 4, 2nd edn. WB Saunders Company, Philadelphia PA, p. 1983–1987; 2096–2099
2. Adams J (2008) In: Thomas Lee Pope et al (eds) Osteoporosis in Imaging of the musculoskeletal system, 1st edn. Saunders, Philadelphia PA, p. 1489–1508
3. Bouxsein ML, Karasik D (2006) Bone geometry and skeletal fragility. Curr Osteoporos Rep 4:49–56
4. Sambrook P, Cooper C (2006) Osteoporosis. Lancet 367:2010–2018
5. Sundaram M, Schils J (2008) In: Thomas Lee Pope et al (eds) Hyperparathyroidism, Renal osteodystrophy osteomalacia and rickets in Imaging of the musculoskeletal system, 1st edn. Saunders, p. 1509–1523
6. Kanberoglu K, Kantarci F, Cebi D, Yilmaz MH, Kurugoglu S, Bilici A, Koyuncu H (2005) Magnetic resonance imaging in osteomalacic insufficiency fractures of the pelvis. Clin Radiol 60(1): 105–111
7. Ohashi K, Ohnishi T, Ishikawa T, Tani H, Uesugi K, Takagi M (1999) Oncogenic osteomalacia presenting as bilateral stress fractures of the tibia. Skelet Radiol 28(1):46–48
8. Soubrier M, Dubost JJ, Boisgard S, Sauvezie B, Gaillard P, Michel JL, Ristori JM (2003 Jun) Insufficiency fracture. A survey of 60 cases and review of the literature. Joint Bone Spine 70(3):209–218
9. Vande Berg BC, Malghem J, Goffin EJ, Duprez TP, Maldague BE (1994) Transient epiphyseal lesions in renal transplant recipients: presumed insufficiency stress fractures. Radiology 191(2):403–407
10. Vande Berg BC, Malghem J, Lecouvet FE, Maldague B (2001) Magnetic resonance imaging and differential diagnosis of epiphyseal osteonecrosis. Semin Musculoskelet Radiol 5(1):57–67

11. Cabarrus MC, Ambekar A, Lu Y, Link TM (2008 Oct) MRI and CT of insufficiency fractures of the pelvis and the proximal femur. AJR Am J Roentgenol 191(4):995–1001
12. Shane E, Burr D, Ebeling PR et al (2010) Atypical subtrochanteric and diaphyseal femoral fractures: report of task forces of the American Society for Bone and Mineral Research. J Bone Miner Res 25:2267–2294
13. Chan SS, Rosenberg ZS, Chan K, Capeci C (2010) Subtrochanteric femoral fractures in patients receiving long-term alendronate therapy: imaging features. AJR Am J Roentgenol 194:1581–1586
14. Haworth AE, Webb J (2012) Skeletal complications of bisphosphonate use: what the radiologist should know. Br J Radiol 85(1018):1333–1342
15. Feydy A, Drapé J, Beret E, Sarazin L, Pessis E, Minoui A, Chevrot A (1998) Longitudinal stress fractures of the tibia: comparative study of CT and MR imaging. Eur Radiol 8(4):598–602
16. Craig JG, Widman D, van Holsbeeck M (2003) Longitudinal stress fracture: patterns of edema and the importance of the nutrient foramen. Skelet Radiol 32(1):22–27. Epub 2002 Nov 23
17. Yamamoto T, Schneider R, Bullough PG (2001) Subchondral insufficiency fracture of the femoral head: histopathologic correlation with MRI. Skelet Radiol 30:247–254
18. Yamamoto T, Bullough PG (2000) Spontaneous osteonecrosis of the knee: the result of subchondral insufficiency fracture. J Bone Joint Surg Am 82(6):858–866
19. Torriani M, Thomas BJ, Bredella MA, Ouellette H (2008) MRI of metatarsal head subchondral fractures in patients with forefoot pain. AJR Am J Roentgenol 190(3):570–575
20. Nattiv A, Kennedy G, Barrack MT, Abdelkerim A, Goolsby MA, Arends JC, Seeger LL (2013) Correlation of MRI grading of bone stress injuries with clinical risk factors and return to play: a 5-year prospective study in collegiate track and field athletes. Am J Sports Med 41(8):1930–1941
21. Kwon JW, Huh SJ, Yoon YC, Choi SH, Jung JY, Oh D, Choe BK (2008) Pelvic bone complications after radiation therapy of uterine cervical cancer: evaluation with MRI. AJR Am J Roentgenol 191(4):987–994
22. Malghem J, Maldague B, Labaisse MA, Dooms G, Duprez T, Devogelaer JP, Vande Berg B (1993) Intravertebral vacuum cleft: changes in content after supine positioning. Radiology 187(2):483–487
23. Vande Berg BC, Malghem JJ, Lecouvet FE, Jamart J, Maldague BE (1999) Idiopathic bone marrow edema lesions of the femoral head: predictive value of MR imaging findings. Radiology 212(2):527–535
24. Geith T, Niethammer T, Milz S, Dietrich O, Reiser M, Baur-Melnyk A (2016) Transient bone marrow edema syndrome versus osteonecrosis: perfusion patterns at dynamic contrast-enhanced MR imaging with high temporal resolution can allow differentiation. Radiology 1:152665. [Epub ahead of print]
25. Lecouvet FE, Vande Berg BC, Maldague BE, Lebon CJ, Jamart J, Saleh M, Noël H, Malghem J (1998) Early irreversible osteonecrosis versus transient lesions of the femoral condyles: prognostic value of subchondral bone and marrow changes on MR imaging. AJR Am J Roentgenol 170(1):71–77
26. Plett SK, Hackney LA, Heilmeier U, Nardo L, Yu A, Zhang CA, Link TM (2015) Femoral condyle insufficiency fractures: associated clinical and morphological findings and impact on outcome. Skelet Radiol 44(12):1785–1794

Muscle Imaging

David A. Rubin and Theodore T. Miller

MR imaging and ultrasound are exquisitely sensitive for a variety of disorders affected striated (skeletal) muscles, including those due to various types of trauma, nerve insults, and diseases of inflammatory, congenital, metabolic, infectious, and neoplastic etiologies. Often MR imaging provides complimentary or superior information to clinical assessment and other ancillary procedures such as serologic testing or electromyography.

Technique

On ultrasound, the angle of the transducer affects the apparent echogenicity of muscle due to its inherent anisotropy [1]. The examiner should position the transducer as perpendicular as possible to the long axis of the muscle and insonate all muscles in two approximately orthogonal planes to minimize errors. Normal muscle fibers are separated by the relatively hyperechoic fibroadipose septa of the perimysium. Edematous muscle demonstrates fibers that are more hypoechoic than normal, sometimes with enlargement of the muscle. Muscle fiber echogenicity is increased when there is fatty infiltration, with decreased muscle bulk in severe cases [2, 3]. Side-to-side ultrasound comparison—keeping transducer frequency, gain, and depth constant—may aid diagnosis when atrophy, hypertrophy, or altered echogenicity is subtle. Sonography is also a useful technique for guiding percutaneous needle placement, whether for diagnostic muscle biopsy or aspiration, or to administer a therapeutic agent [4, 5].

D.A. Rubin (✉)
Department of Radiology, Washington University School of Medicine, Mallinckrodt Institute of Radiology, 510 South Kingshighway Blvd., Saint Louis, MO 63110, USA
e-mail: rubinda@wustl.edu

T.T. Miller
Department of Radiology and Imaging, Hospital for Special Surgery, 535 E. 70th Street, New York, NY 10021, USA
e-mail: millertt@hss.edu

The signal intensity of normal muscle is lower than that of fat on T1- and T2-weighted images. On T1-weighted images, fat between fiber bundles in normal muscle produces a "marbled" texture [6]. Adipose in the fascial layers between muscles separates one from another. Much muscular pathology results in an increase in the extracellular water content, causing a prolongation of T1 and T2 relaxation times. The conspicuity of muscle lesions is increased on fat-suppressed images, and especially on short-TI inversion recovery (STIR) images, where T1 and T2 effects are additive [7]. T1-weighted images are still crucial, however, to demonstrate anatomic detail, hemorrhage, and fatty atrophy. Imaging protocols should include images obtained in both the short-axis (axial) and long-axis (sagittal or coronal) of the muscle(s) being investigated. Comparison with the unaffected limb can be useful to show atrophy, hypertrophy, and normal variants [6].

Muscle Injury

Muscles are commonly injured, affecting everyone from the non-athlete to the "weekend warrior" to the professional athlete. Reasons to image the patient include confirmation of the clinical diagnosis, determination of the extent of injury, monitoring of healing, and assessment of risk of recurrent injury. The physical examination may be unreliable due to the subjective nature of pain, guarding by the patient, or masking by the patient [8]. The extent of the injury has implications for what treatment is undertaken (e.g., conservative, percutaneous, surgical) and implications for return to play. Patients with persistent pain may not be healing, and the presence of scar tissue in a healed muscle may place the patient at risk for recurrent muscle tear [9]. MR imaging, by virtue of its large field of view and excellent soft tissue contrast, is uniquely suited to evaluate muscle injuries.

J. Hodler et al. (eds.), *Musculoskeletal Diseases 2017-2020*, DOI 10.1007/978-3-319-54018-4_11

Strain

Acute, non-contact muscle injury usually occurs during sprinting or acceleration. Risk factors for tear are: muscles with high content of type two fibers because these fast twitch fibers cause powerful muscle contraction; muscles with two heads because of the complex biomechanics of these muscles; muscles that cross two joints because of their complex biomechanics; muscles that are fatigued because they are stiff and less able to absorb the energy of eccentric contractions; and muscles with a preexisting injury [10–13]. The quadriceps muscles, the hamstring muscles, and the gastrocnemius muscles fit these criteria and are most commonly injured [14, 15].

The majority of muscle tears occur at the myotendinous junction, with the remainder occurring at the myofascial junction. Remember that the myotendinous junction is not only where the tendon emerges from the muscle belly, but also along the central tendon within the muscle belly [16].

Several different classifications of muscle injury have been described, using ultrasound and MR imaging [17–19]. Grade 1 injuries are the most minor, consisting of interstitial blood (seen as feathery high signal intensity on T2 weighted images) without architectural distortion (Fig. 1). Grade 2 injuries are partial tears with varying amounts of architectural disruption of the muscle. Thin, high signal intensity blood may be seen in the adjacent fascial plane and there may be an intramuscular hematoma. A Grade 3 injury is rupture of the muscle, with or without retraction. Given the wide spectrum of severity in the Grade 2 partial tears, it is often best to describe the extent of the injury in addition to grading it.

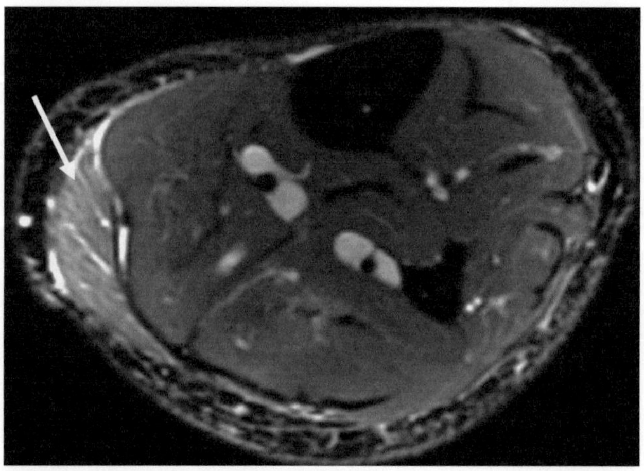

Fig. 1 Grade 1 strain. Axial fat-suppressed T2WI through the leg shows feathery edema (*arrow*) in the medial gastrocnemius muscle

Tears are graded because the severity of the injury has implications for return to play, and not surprisingly the greater the injury, the longer it takes to recover. A study of professional soccer players with acute hamstring pain found that players with normal MR imaging examinations had an average of 8 days to return to play, players with Grade 1 injuries had an average of 17 days to return, Grade 2 injuries had 22 days to return, and Grade 3 had 73 days to return [19]. The length and area of involvement on MR are the best predictors of time to return to play [20].

Intramuscular hematomas have variable appearances, partly influenced by the time course. Acute hematomas may be low to isointense to muscle on T1WI, and high signal intensity on T2WI. After several days, they may show intermediate to high signal intensity on T1WI due to proteins and methemoglobin. Both acute and subacute hematomas may have heterogeneous signal intensity. After several weeks they may appear more like fluid, with a low signal intensity rim due to deposition of hemosiderin [9, 21].

The optimum outcome for healing of muscle tears is a return to normal architecture and signal intensity, but low signal intensity fibrosis may occur at the site of healed tear. An area of scar or fibrosis in the muscle may place the muscle at risk for recurrent tear because the fibrosis is stronger than the adjacent normal muscle and acts as a stress riser [9] but a recent study of athletes with and without fibrosis following initial hamstring injuries found no statistical difference in rate of recurrent tear [22].

Fascial Herniation

Traumatic tears of the myofascia or regions of fascial weakness may allow the muscle to focally herniate. The lower extremity is the most common site of muscle hernias [9, 15, 23]. The herniation usually presents as a painless bulge that the patient can reproduce with muscle contraction, but occasionally the herniation may be tender or painful. On imaging, the muscle looks normal at rest. Dynamic scanning is usually necessary to demonstrate the herniation, and sonography, by virtue of its real-time nature, is well suited to visualize these abnormalities [23–26].

Myositis Ossificans

Myositis ossificans refers to the development of heterotopic ossification in skeletal muscle. Common causes include contusion, surgery, burns, and paralysis, but in up to 40% of cases the patient is not able to recall a precipitating

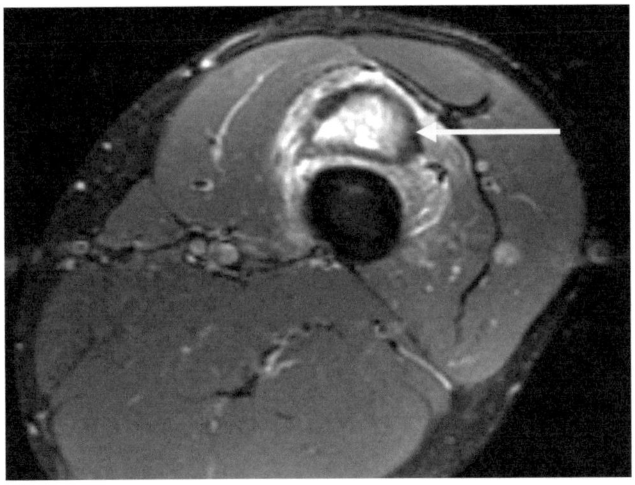

Fig. 2 Myositis ossificans. Axial fat-suppressed T2WI through the thigh shows the low signal intensity zonal ossification (*arrow*) in the vastus intermedius muscle with surrounding high signal intensity muscle edema

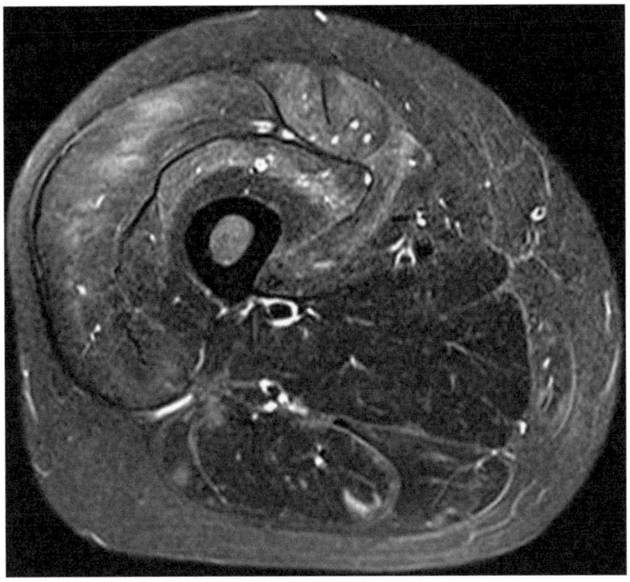

Fig. 3 Delayed onset muscle soreness. Axial fat-suppressed T2WI through the thigh in a woman 2 days after doing lunges in the gym for the first time. There is patchy hyperintense edema predominantly in the quadriceps muscles, and to a lesser extent in the hamstrings

event [27]. The patient typically presents with pain and swelling. MR imaging in this acute phase will show extensive muscle edema surrounding a poorly defined mass. Although a soft tissue sarcoma might be considered in the imaging differential, the extensive soft tissue edema is much more suggestive of myositis ossificans [9, 15]. Over the course of several weeks the edema will subside and a zone of peripheral ossification will develop (Fig. 2). This mineralization may be detected earlier with CT than with MR imaging. The more mature heterotopic ossification will exhibit areas of T1 hyperintensity reflecting marrow [9, 15, 27]. The maturing focus may incite periosteal reaction in an adjacent bone, and may eventually become incorporated into the adjacent bone [27].

Delayed Onset Muscle Soreness

Delayed onset muscle soreness (DOMS) is the term to describe muscle pain and swelling occurring a day or two after intense eccentric muscle contractions, especially in a non-conditioned muscle. It is an over-use injury that demonstrates feathery or patchy T2 signal hyperintensity in the affected muscle or muscles, similar to a Grade 1 muscle strain (Fig. 3). Clinical history and symptomatic relief over the ensuing week help to differentiate DOMS from a Grade 1 strain [9, 15, 28]. Sonography of DOMS shows muscle enlargement with diffuse well-defined hyperechogenicity of the muscle representing edema, and hyperemia using color or power Doppler sonography [29].

Compartment Syndrome

Compartment syndrome is swelling of a muscle in a closed anatomic compartment with resultant elevated pressure causing a disturbance in the muscle's microcirculation, which in turn can lead to muscle ischemia [15, 28, 30]. Acute compartment syndrome is usually due to fracture or less commonly a muscle contusion (direct blow) or strain, and is a surgical emergency requiring fasciotomy. It is a clinical diagnosis, based on severe pain out of proportion to the initial injury, pain to palpation and passive stretching, and increased direct intracompartmental pressure measurements. MR imaging is usually not indicated in acute compartment syndrome, as time is of the essence. Delayed or missed diagnosis will lead to irreversible muscle ischemia and necrosis with eventual fibrosis (Volkmann's contracture) [15].

Chronic exertional compartment syndrome refers to exercise-related or activity-related pain due to elevated intramuscular pressure and transient ischemia, which resolves when the offending activity is stopped [15, 30]. The leg is the most common site of involvement, affecting the anterior compartment most commonly, followed by the deep posterior, lateral, and superficial posterior compartments [30]. Post-exertional MR imaging shows T2 hyperintensity in the affected muscle [30, 31]. Longstanding cases may exhibit fascial thickening, muscle atrophy, and fibrosis [15, 28].

Denervation

A predictable series of events occurs when the peripheral nerve supply to skeletal muscle is abruptly interrupted (say by a complete laceration or experimental sectioning) [32]. For the first week, the muscle maintains its normal gross and microscopic appearance. Additionally, electromyography of the affected muscles is relatively insensitive in the acute setting [33]. No morphologic changes initially occur on MR or ultrasound during this period [34]; nevertheless, early shifts of fluid from the intracellular to the extracellular spaces in the muscle can be detected with MR diffusion techniques [35, 36].

After approximately two weeks, subacute denervation will become apparent on standard MR images. Specifically, increased extracellular fluid results in prolongation of both T1 and T2 values in muscle [37], which will be most conspicuous on STIR images [34]. This edema pattern will involve the entire muscle belly relatively homogeneously (an exception is in muscles that have a dual nerve supply) and does not affect the fascia (a distinguishing characteristic from traumatic and many inflammatory muscle etiologies). However, what best distinguishes muscle denervation from other conditions is its distribution: denervation will involve the muscles supplied by the affected motor nerve (Fig. 4) [38]. Thus mapping the muscles involved and those spared, can predict the location of a lesion in the neuroaxis [39]. At that point, electrophysiology or imaging studies can be directed to that area for diagnosis of extrinsic nerve compression (due to a tunnel syndrome or a mass like a ganglion cyst, for example) or intrinsic nerve lesions (e.g., a nerve sheath tumor).

This approach of predicting the location of a nerve insult based on the pattern of muscle involvement works for single peripheral nerve lesions as well as more complex injuries [38]. Insults to the spinal cord (Guillain-Barré syndrome or transverse myelitis, for example), limb nerve supply (polio, traumatic nerve root avulsions), brachial or lumbar plexus (Parsonage-Turner syndrome, radiation plexopathy), individual nerve roots (disc herniation), and even peripheral nerve branches (nerve lacerations) will produce predictable distributions of muscle involvement. Similarly, diseases that cause polyneuritis or mononeuritis multiplex will involve several motor nerve distributions.

If reinnervation does not occur, after several months chronic denervation sets in. The muscles become atrophic with decreased bulk and replacement of the muscle fibers by fat, which is recognizable as high signal intensity tissue, isointense to subcutaneous fat, on T1-weighted and other short-TE MR sequences [34]. It is important not to rely on an MR protocol that consists entirely of fat-suppressed sequences (which is not uncommon in some practices for MR arthrograms), because fat-replaced and normal muscle appear essentially identical on these images. On ultrasound, fatty replacement is characterized by generalized increased echogenicity of the muscles compared to spared muscles and compared to the internal septa [3]. Note that fatty muscle atrophy is a common end-stage process in multiple conditions including following complete ruptures of either the myotendinous junction or the tendon attaching the muscle to bone, for example in chronic rotator cuff tears. End-stage ischemia, inflammatory, and myopathic disorders also lead to fatty replacement (see below). In most cases replaced muscle will be decreased in bulk, but there are circumstances where fatty infiltration is so great that the muscle appears enlarged, a condition called pseudohypertrophy [40–42]. However, as is the case for muscle edema due to denervation, denervation atrophy is recognizable because it occurs in a given nerve distribution.

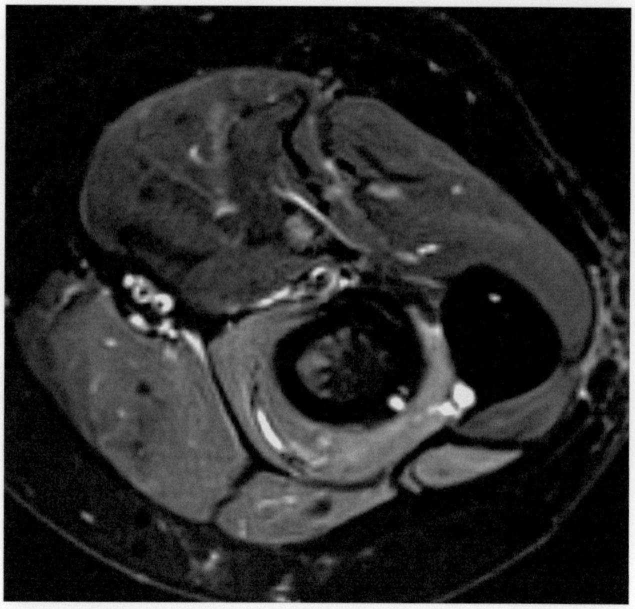

Fig. 4 Subacute denervation in a 47 year-old woman. A fat-suppressed T2-weighted image shows high signal intensity throughout the forearm extensor muscles and the supinator, corresponding to the radial nerve distribution. Note the lack of fascial edema. Compression of the nerve was found proximally, at the lateral intermuscular septum or the triceps

In reality, the transition from subacute to chronic denervation is not always predictable. Most nerve lesions do not act like acute, complete lacerations. Nerve compression due to a tunnel syndrome or mass occurs gradually over time and may affect the peripheral motor neurons in a nerve earlier and more severely than the central ones. Stretching injuries occur on a spectrum that includes partial or complete disruption of the myelin, endoneurium, axon, and epineurium in varying combinations [43]. Viral, drug, metabolic, nutritional, radiation, ischemic, and other insults can involve different nerves to varying degrees and with an unpredictable time course. And each of these conditions has different potential for nerve healing, either spontaneously or following removal of the causative agent or nerve repair. Thus, muscle changes of subacute and chronic denervation often coexist on a single imaging study. Research shows that the calculated T2 value of the affected muscles correlates with the severity and reversibility of the nerve insult [44]. Furthermore, sequential MR examinations are useful for predicting the success or failure of interventions like nerve repair, and have added value compared with clinical and electrophysiological monitoring [44, 45]. Specifically, normalization of muscle signal on STIR sequences before fatty infiltration occurs is a sign of successfully reinnervation [46, 47].

Inflammatory Myositis

Inflammatory myositis describes a group of related diseases that are characterized by autoimmune inflammation affecting skeletal muscle, and in some subtypes, other tissues including skin, fascia, cardiac muscle, and lung [48]. Clinically the conditions all share muscle weakness as a cardinal symptom. Age-of-onset, time course, distribution, serologic markers, and extra-muscular involvement differ among the various disorders [49, 50].

There are four or five major categories of inflammatory myositis, several with recognized subtypes [48]. The main types are dermatomyositis, juvenile dermatomyositis, polymyositis, immune-mediated necrotizing myopathy, and sporadic inclusion body myositis. In addition to the clinical and serologic differences among them, each also carries a different prognosis and treatment regimen, making positive identification a key tenet in management [50, 51]. As discussed below, exact diagnosis usually requires muscle biopsy.

Dermatomyositis includes skin involvement, with several possible rashes, most commonly a violaceous discoloration of the eyelids [52]. Proximal thigh weakness usually develops over a course of weeks. Women are affected more often than men. Disease onset may be a harbinger of a carcinoma in the body (with an overall increase risk of 3×) that presents in the first few years after dermatomyositis is recognized [53]. An amopathic form has the typical skin findings without overt muscle weakness. Juvenile dermatomyositis has onset before age 18 [54]. In the juvenile form, skin and subcutaneous involvement may be clinically occult, or may take the form of cutaneous calcification with or without ulceration [55]. Vasculitis in the gastrointestinal tract is also a prevalent feature of juvenile dermatomyositis [54]. Polymyositis is less common than (and lacks the skin findings of) dermatomyositis. Compared to dermatomyositis, it occurs in an older age group, and usually has a more insidious, slower onset. Symmetric weakness of both the proximal upper and lower extremity muscles is typical of polymyositis [49, 50]. The risk of associated cancer is lower in polymyositis compared to dermatomyositis [53].

Sporadic inclusion body myositis is more common than dermatomyositis and polymyositis after age 50 [48]. It has a much slower onset (often years) than the other conditions and is more likely to present asymmetrically and involve the distal extremity muscles early in the disease. There is evidence that buildup of tau and amyloid proteins in the muscle occurs in this condition, analogous to Alzheimer's disease in the brain [56]. Immune-mediated necrotizing myopathy occurs after a triggering event, like viral infection or drug (including statin) administration [57].

Because of overlap in symptoms and serologic markers (which are only present in 50% of patients), it is frequently impossible to distinguish the various inflammatory myositis conditions from each other [51]. Furthermore, many other conditions—which have different treatments and prognoses—are also characterized by insidious onset muscle weakness. The differential diagnosis is broad and includes metabolic conditions, endocrinopathies (e.g., disorders of thyroid hormone), infectious causes (viral, parasitic, and bacterial pyomyositis), some muscular dystrophies and mitochondrial myopathies, and collagen-vascular conditions like scleroderma [50]. While some of these disorders can be diagnosed or excluded based on clinical, laboratory, and electromyographic criteria, muscle biopsy is always required for a certain diagnosis and classification of inflammatory myositis [51]. A prompt biopsy-derived diagnosis is especially important because institution of specific immunosuppressive therapy early in the disease course can prevent severe, often irreversible muscle damage and weakness in conditions like dermatomyositis and polymyositis [58, 59]. However, because histologic involvement of specific muscles is inconsistent and difficult to predict with certainty, biopsies that are directed at muscles based on clinical weakness are falsely negative in approximately 25% of cases [60–63].

Imaging has three important roles in patients with suspected or confirmed inflammatory myositis. At presentation, MR (or less commonly ultrasound) can guide biopsy to muscles that are most likely to yield diagnostic pathologic findings. Second, once a diagnosis is established and treatment has begun, imaging may be used to monitor the disease for response. Third, in longstanding myositis when a patient develops increasing weakness the clinical dilemma is to distinguish whether they are having a flare of their active inflammation (in which case an increase in medication may be warranted), or whether the disease has progressed to the chronic, burned-out stage, in which case more aggressive medical therapy is not indicated. The key observation in each of these scenarios is whether active or chronic myositis is present.

During the active inflammatory phase of myositis, regardless of the subtype, imaging shows edema in the affected muscles. On ultrasound, edematous muscle fibers are more hypoechoic than usual compared to the hyperechoic septa [2, 3]. However, this ultrasound appearance is neither specific for diagnosis of myositis nor its subtype [64]. Use of an ultrasound contrast agent to separate inflammation from other causes of edema has been suggested to improve specificity [65, 66]. MR is more sensitive than ultrasound for identifying active disease, even with the use of ultrasound contrast agents [51, 65]. Active myositis on MR appears as increased signal intensity in the affected muscles on water-sensitive sequences, especially STIR or chemically fat-suppressed T2-weighted sequences (Fig. 5) [67–69]. High signal intensity in the superficial and deep fascia may be present early in the course of dermatomyositis, including in the amyopathic form [70]. The use of intravenous contrast for MR is controversial: while it does not appear to increase sensitivity compared to STIR imaging, contrast enhancement may increase diagnostic confidence and specificity, allowing distinction of inflammatory conditions from metabolic and neurodegenerative ones [62, 71]. Conversely, in chronic, burned-out disease, fatty atrophy is the predominant imaging finding. Atrophied muscles on ultrasound are increased in echogenicity and decreased in size [66]. On MR, muscle atrophy appears as decreased bulk and replacement of muscle tissue with high signal intensity fat on T1-weighted images, without edema on water-sensitive sequences [67, 72].

In all forms of inflammatory myositis, muscle involvement—whether in the active or burned-out stages—is patchy in distribution, with some muscles involved and some spared in individual cases. While certain patterns of involvement may be more characteristic of one disease subtype or another, no pattern is characteristic enough to eliminate the need for biopsy [73]. For example, involvement of the vastus lateralis, rectus femoris, and biceps femoris with sparing of the vastus intermedius is frequent in immune-mediated necrotizing myopathy [74, 75], but can be encountered conditions as well. Similarly, disease preferentially affecting the anterior compartment musculature of the thighs and calves but sparing of the rectus femoris, or involving the flexor digitorum profundus muscle in the forearms is characteristic of inclusion body myositis, but not pathognomonic [76, 77]. One exception is in dermatomyositis: edema in the skin and/or subcutaneous tissues in addition to some skeletal muscles suggests dermatomyositis or juvenile dermatomyositis, and in the latter condition, the cutaneous involvement may be clinically occult [55]. Additionally, superficial and deep fasciitis present on MR in the first few months of disease—with or without muscle involvement—appears to be a typical feature of dermatomyositis not shared by the other subtypes [70].

At presentation, the most important role of imaging is to direct muscle biopsy. Because of the patchy nature of these conditions, the false negative rate of a non-imaging-directed muscle biopsy is approximately 23%; this rate can be reduced to 6% by using MR imaging to target a high-yield biopsy target [78]. Muscles most likely to provide diagnostic material in inflammatory myositis are those that are edematous but not fatty infiltrated on MR imaging, and which are close to the surface and easily accessible [78, 79].

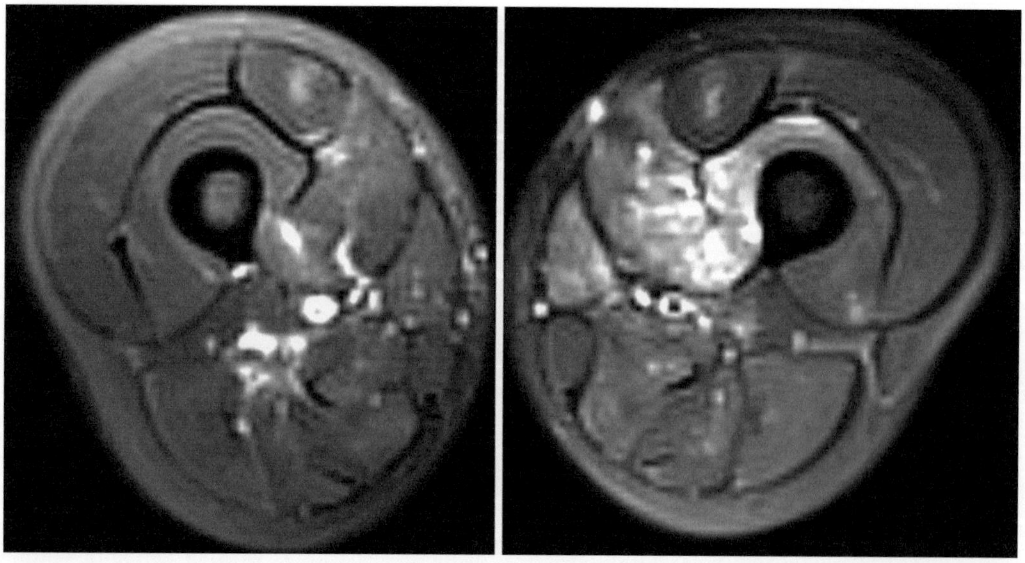

Fig. 5 Active polymyositis in a 19-year-old man. There is asymmetric, patchy edema of the muscles of both thighs on this fat-suppressed T2-weighted image. Based on the MR findings, biopsy of the left vastus medialis muscle was performed, leading to the diagnosis

Using MR to guide initial muscle biopsies may be cost effective as well [60].

Once treatment has begun, the extent of edema in the thigh muscles on STIR images correlates with serum creatine kinase levels and clinical assessments of disease activitly [80]. Compared with repeat muscle biopsy, MR findings correlate better with clinical response after 2–6 months of treatment [81]. Some investigators have advocated whole body MR—either using a body coil or multiple smaller coils in an array—to better gauge overall disease activity in inflammatory myositis [63, 73, 82, 83]. A relatively fast screening examination for active disease can be done with large field-of-view, low resolution fast (turbo) spin echo STIR images alone [82]. Adding T1-weighted images and contrast-enhanced images prolongs the study but may add specificity; some of the excess time can be regained by not including the trunk muscles, which does not seem to increase sensitivity [71]. Nevertheless, in clinical practice, a screening examination of just the thighs and calves (or the shoulder girdles, if weakness is much more profound in the upper extremities) probably suffices.

Several experimental MR techniques have been investigated as potential adjuncts in the evaluation of inflammatory myositis. These procedures include diffusion MR imaging, diffusion tensor imaging, MR elasticity, and MR spectroscopy [80, 84–88]. While each has promise, it is unclear whether any currently has added value over morphologic imaging using STIR technique. More recent studies suggest that using MR to calculate T2 measurements and fat fractions in affected muscles might be a way to quantify the subjective information gained from STIR and T1-weighted images, respectively [89].

Congenital Muscle Disorders

Genetic mutations are responsible for myriad congenital myopathies, muscular dystrophies, and metabolic disorders affecting skeletal muscle, each with varied clinical manifestations. In the last decade, researchers have applied modern DNA sequencing and protein synthesis techniques to better sort and characterize these conditions, which now probably number in the hundreds. Management, prognostication, and genetic counseling depend on making the most accurate and specific diagnosis possible. While phenotype analysis, family history, and genetic testing are now the mainstays of the work-up, imaging can play a role in some conditions by limiting the differential diagnosis to streamline laboratory testing. A second emerging role of imaging is in follow-up of the disease course to track severity, response to treatment, and planning of physical therapy.

The hallmark imaging finding for most congenital muscle disorders is fatty infiltration of (selected) muscles groups, identified as replacement of muscle tissue by fat on T1-weighted MR sequences (Fig. 6) or echogenic material on ultrasound [90–92]. Characteristically, many disorders also predictably spare certain muscle groups, which will appear normal or may even show compensational hypertrophy on imaging studies. Pseudohypertrophy of the affected muscles may occur when the amount of fatty infiltration enlarges the girth of the muscle [41, 42]. Clinically, pseudohypertrophy may be difficult to separate from true hypertrophy, but the distinction is trivial with cross-sectional imaging. Much less commonly, muscle edema—easiest to appreciate on STIR images—may be a minor finding in some congenital conditions, or may transiently occur before fatty infiltration.

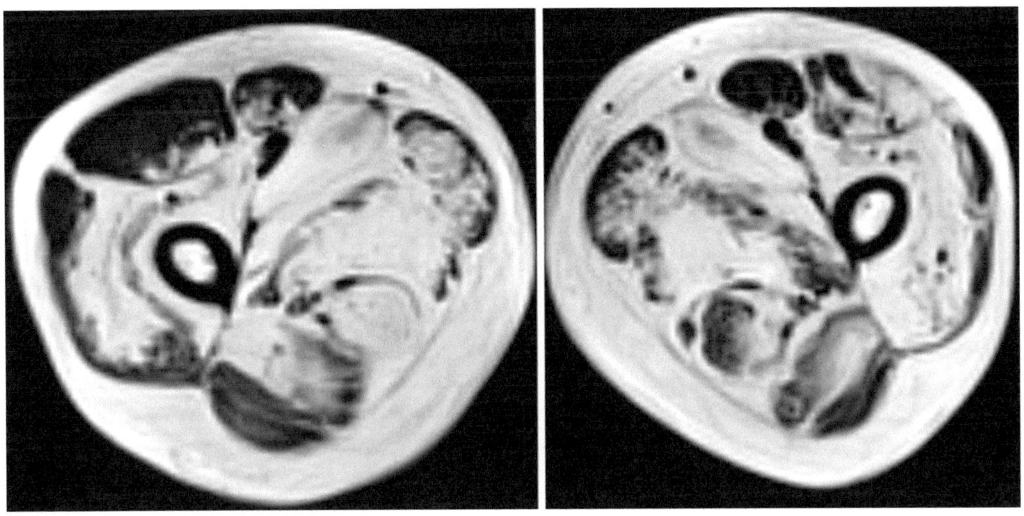

Fig. 6 Limb-girdle muscular dystrophy in a 28-year-old man. The T1-weighted image of both thighs shows profound fatty infiltration of multiple muscle groups, most severe in the adductor compartment. There is relative sparing of the rectus femoris muscles

Congenital myopathies usually present at or near birth with weakness and hypotonia, but don't progress or progress very slowly over time; they are most typically classified according to the pattern of morphological muscle abnormality seen microscopically [93]. At least 35 different genes are implicated in the myopathies, with several different mutations in one gene, or combinations of mutations in several genes leading to more than 35 distinct diseases. Muscular dystrophies are characterized by muscle wasting pathologically (in the absence of histologic evidence of another muscle or nerve disorder) [94]. They progress throughout life and are frequently fatal. Dystrophies are grouped according to the incorrectly coded protein complex (at least seven main subgroups exist), with at least 25 responsible genes identified thus far. Inborn errors of metabolism can also negatively affect the function (primarily energy metabolism) in skeletal muscle, usually resulting in some degree of exercise intolerance. These metabolic myopathies include glycogen storage disorders like Pompe disease, conditions where mitochondria do not function correctly including those where the mitochondrial DNA is faulty, and syndromes where proteins involved in oxidative metabolism are faulty; at least eight enzymes and 25 responsible genes have been identified as culprits [95].

For reasons that are not clear, many of the metabolic conditions have particular patterns of muscles that are severely involved, variably involved, and spared [41, 91, 92, 96]. For example, in Duchenne muscular dystrophy—a relatively common X-linked recessive disease due to a mutated gene coding for the dystrophin protein complex [97]—the gluteus and adductor magnus muscles are affected earliest and most severely, other thigh and calf muscles are involved to a lesser degree, and the gracillis is always spared (and frequently hypertrophied) [98, 99]. Other myopathies, dystrophies, and metabolic conditions will characteristically target other sets of muscle groups, often varying with the disease phenotype [100–103].

While whole body MR has been advocated as potentially useful in specific conditions [104], much information can be gained by a simple MR examination of both thighs for most conditions. As is the case for inflammatory myositis, relatively thick-section transverse T1-weighted and STIR sequences usually suffice. The roles that imaging plays in congenital muscle disorders are expanding. Before final diagnosis, demonstrating a characteristic pattern of involvement can suggest specific genetic testing to complement biopsy results [92]. Subtle muscle edema on STIR images may be a sign of very early disease (before fatty infiltration occurs) in some diseases like limb-girdle and Duchenne muscular dystrophy, at a stage where medical therapy may have a greater chance of success [91, 98]. Similarly, in late-onset Pompe disease, enzyme replacement therapy seems to prevent disease progression best when treating patients who show little-to-no fatty muscle infiltration before therapy [105]. In disorders that affect muscles selectively and asymmetrically, MR or ultrasound can direct muscle biopsy [42, 99]. Additionally, progression or remission on sequential imaging studies may be more sensitive than (or at least complementary to) clinical functional assessments [99, 104]. Last, physical therapy can be tailored to strengthening muscles that are shown to be spared on imaging studies [42].

Diabetic Muscle Ischemia

Diabetic muscle ischemia—also known as diabetic muscle infarction—is a relatively rare muscle condition occurring in some patients with long-standing, poorly controlled diabetes. Both type I and type II diabetics can be affected [106]. More than half the patients have nephropathy and neuropathy, and approximately one-third also have diabetic retinopathy [107]. The condition presents with acute-onset intense pain in the thigh, or less commonly the calf [107, 108]. There may be associated swelling, but usually no fever or systemic symptoms. Serum creatinine kinase and erythrocyte sedimentation rate are usually normal or only slightly elevated [109]. In part because the condition is uncommon, and in part because much of the available literature consists of isolated case reports in subspecialty journals, many primary caregivers are unfamiliar with diabetic muscle ischemia. Thus, when patients present their physicians are often more impressed by the presence of a "mass" rather than the history of acute-onset pain. Regardless of the reasons, it is not unusual for these patients to be referred for cross sectional imaging to evaluate for a potential tumor or infection [108].

Areas of ischemic muscle appear enlarged and hypoattenuating on CT examinations performed with or without contrast. Ultrasound examination will show a defined hypoechoic region within the affected muscle with enhanced through transmission, through usually without an anechoic collection. Linear hyperechoic streaks (likely representing muscle fibers) running though this region are an important clue that a mass displacing or destroying muscle is not present [110]. On MR, the affected muscles may be swollen or have mildly increased signal intensity on T1-weighted images [107, 111]. Regions of geographic edema on water sensitive images represent the ischemic zones. Fascial edema and subcutaneous edema frequently accompany the muscle findings and help differentiate diabetic ischemia from inflammatory myositis (other than dermatomyositis, which can also show subcutaneous and fascial edema) [107, 109]. The distinction from myositis is relevant because diabetic muscle ischemia may be multifocal and/or bilateral, with patchy asymmetric involvement (similar to myositis) [108, 112].

Intravenous contrast administration is not necessary for diagnosis [113], but if contrast is given the affected muscles show homogeneous or peripheral enhancement [109]. In some cases central areas of nonenhancement—representing macroscopic muscle infarction—will also be present. The enhancement is an indicator that ischemia rather than infarction is the predominant insult, probably explaining why spontaneous resolution is the rule [107].

While the etiology is uncertain, most researchers favor spontaneous atherosclerotic thrombosis of small arteries rather than embolism [107, 114]. Biopsy is diagnostic showing coagulative muscle necrosis and microangiopathy without an inflammatory infiltrate [107, 115]. However, recognizing the typical MR pattern in combination with the classic history of a poorly controlled diabetic presenting with acute-onset pain probably obviates the need for confirmatory biopsy [106, 116]. Often it will be the radiologist who first recognizes the constellation of findings and suggests the diagnosis. Making the diagnosis without the need for biopsy is desired because treatment consists of analgesia, rest, and immobilization (early ambulation or physical therapy may increase the risk of bleeding and iatrogenic complications) [109]. Resolution takes 6 weeks to several months [114]. Recurrences, including in the contralateral limb, occur in about half of the patients [108]. Suffering an episode of diabetic muscle ischemia is a prognosticator of poor overall outcomes: 10% of patients will die from diabetic complications in the following two years [113].

Muscle Masses

Certain intramuscular masses have a specific imaging appearance. On ultrasound, simple cysts like ganglia are encapsulated, homogeneous and anechoic, with enhanced through transmission [117]. An intramuscular mass on MR images composed of tissue that is isointense to fat on all pulse sequences, with or without interspersed muscle fibers and thin supporting septa, is a lipoma [118]. A hemangioma can be diagnosed with certainty if an intramuscular mass has interspersed fat, contains vascular channels, and demonstrates low-signal-intensity phleboliths (Fig. 7) [119]. Similarly, an ovoid mass that is mildly hyperintense compared to muscle on T1-weighted images, very hyperintense on water sensitive images, and with target morphology (a bright outer rim on water-sensitive or contrast-enhanced images) represents a benign nerve sheath tumor on MR images [120]).

Still other intramuscular masses may have sufficiently characteristic MR appearances so that together with a classic clinical history, a near certain diagnosis can be made without biopsy. Common examples would include some disorders already discussed like diabetic muscle ischemia or myositis ossificans, specific entities like intramuscular myxomas and proliferative myositis, and muscles that are enlarged due to associated conditions such as deep venous thrombosis [121–123]. And sometimes a specific feature in a given clinical scenario would highly favor a particular diagnosis. An example might be a high signal intensity penumbra on T1-weighted images surrounding a peripherally enhancing intramuscular mass, which makes an abscess much more likely than a necrotic tumor [124, 125].

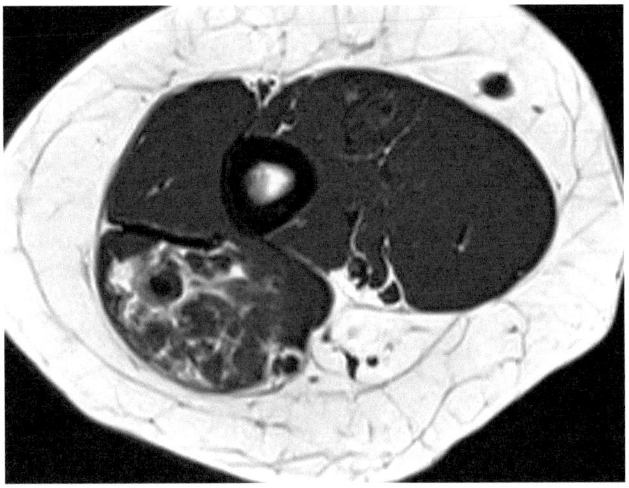

Fig. 7 Intramuscular hemangioma in a 42 year-old woman. A T1-weighted image of the arm shows a mass within the long head of the triceps muscle composed of lobules and tubular structures interspersed with fat. An oval, black structure within a lobule represents a phlebolith

However, in the majority of cases, the MR (or ultrasound) appearance of a muscle mass will not be specific enough for diagnosis. Many benign tumors, malignant primary tumors, lymphomas, metastases, complicated cysts, infections, or even sarcoidosis cannot be distinguished from each other [126–129]. In these cases the role of imaging is to confirm the presence or absence of a clinically-suspected mass, guide biopsy (we tend to target a viable, enhancing part of the mass), and stage the extent of a lesion once its etiology is known. Even the presence of subacute blood products (which are very bright on T1-weighted images) does not guarantee the diagnosis of a simple hematoma: intralesional bleeding after minor trauma is a common presentation of preexisting primary and secondary tumors [130, 131]. Thus intramuscular hematomas found on MR images that occur in the absence of severe trauma and/or over-anticoagulation require follow-up to document resolution, if excisional biopsy is not performed.

References

1. Reimers CD, Finkenstaedt M (1997) Muscle imaging in inflammatory myopathies. Curr Opin Rheumatol 9:475–485
2. Reimers CD, Fleckenstein JL, Witt TN et al (1993) Muscular ultrasound in idiopathic inflammatory myopathies of adults. J Neurol Sci 116:82–92
3. Peetrons P (2002) Ultrasound of muscles. Eur Radiol 12:35–43
4. O'Sullivan PJ, Gorman GM, Hardiman OM et al (2006) Sonographically guided percutaneous muscle biopsy in diagnosis of neuromuscular disease: a useful alternative to open surgical biopsy. J Ultrasound Med 25:1–6
5. Dave RB, Stevens KJ, Shivaram GM et al (2014) Ultrasound-guided musculoskeletal interventions in American football: 18 years of experience. AJR Am J Roentgenol 203:W674–W683
6. Nguyen B, Brandser E, Rubin DA (2000) Pains, strains, and fasciculations: lower extremity muscle disorders. Magn Reson Imaging Clin N Am 8:391–408
7. Fleckenstein JL, Weatherall PT, Bertocci LA et al (1991) Locomotor system assessment by muscle magnetic resonance imaging. Magn Reson Q 7:79–103
8. Reiman MP, Loudon JK, Goode AP (2013) Diagnostic accuracy of clinical tests for assessment of hamstring injury: a systematic review. J Orthop Sports Phys Ther 43:223–231
9. Blankenbaker DG, Tuite MJ (2010) Temporal changes of muscle injury. Semin Musculoskelet Radiol 14:176–193
10. Robinson P, White LM (2005) The biomechanics and imaging of soccer injuries. Semin Musculoskelet Radiol 9:397–420
11. Koulouris G, Connell D (2006) Imaging of hamstring injuries: therapeutic implications. Eur Radiol 16:1478–1487
12. Opar DA, Williams MD, Shield AJ (2012) Hamstring strain injuries: factors that lead to injury and re-injury. Sports Med 42 :209–226
13. Wangensteen A, Tol JL, Witvrouw E et al (2016) Hamstring reinjuries occur at the same location and early after return to sport: a descriptive study of MRI-confirmed reinjuries. Am J Sports Med 44:2112–2121
14. May DA, Disler DG, Jones EA et al (2000) Abnormal signal intensity in skeletal muscle at MR imaging: patterns, pearls, and pitfalls. Radiographics 20 Spec No:S295–S315
15. Boutin RD, Fritz RC, Steinbach LS (2002) Imaging of sports-related muscle injuries. Radiol Clin N Am 40:333–362, vii
16. Brukner P, Connell D (2016) 'Serious thigh muscle strains': beware the intramuscular tendon which plays an important role in difficult hamstring and quadriceps muscle strains. Br J Sports Med 50:205–208
17. Grassi A, Quaglia A, Canata GL et al (2016) An update on the grading of muscle injuries: a narrative review from clinical to comprehensive systems. Joints 4:39–46
18. Hamilton B, Valle X, Rodas G et al (2015) Classification and grading of muscle injuries: a narrative review. Br J Sports Med 49:306
19. Ekstrand J, Healy JC, Walden M et al (2012) Hamstring muscle injuries in professional football: the correlation of MRI findings with return to play. Br J Sports Med 46:112–117
20. Connell DA, Schneider-Kolsky ME, Hoving JL et al (2004) Longitudinal study comparing sonographic and MRI assessments of acute and healing hamstring injuries. AJR Am J Roentgenol 183:975–984
21. Lee YS, Kwon ST, Kim JO et al (2011) Serial MR imaging of intramuscular hematoma: experimental study in a rat model with the pathologic correlation. Korean J Radiol 12:66–77
22. Reurink G, Almusa E, Goudswaard GJ et al (2015) No association between fibrosis on magnetic resonance imaging at return to play and hamstring reinjury risk. Am J Sports Med 43:1228–1234
23. Mellado JM, Perez del Palomar L (1999) Muscle hernias of the lower leg: MRI findings. Skelet Radiol 28:465–469
24. Khaladkar SM, Kondapavuluri SK, Kamal A et al (2016) Detection of myofascial herniation on dynamic sonography and magnetic resonance imaging. Case Rep Radiol 2016:4245189
25. Cormier DJ, Gellhorn AC, Singh JR (2016) Soleus muscle herniation with MRI and ultrasound correlation in a female long distance runner: a case report. PM R
26. Rho NK, Kim WS, Kim YJ et al (2008) The use of dynamic ultrasonography for the confirmation of lower leg muscle herniation. Ann Dermatol 20:190–192
27. Tyler P, Saifuddin A (2010) The imaging of myositis ossificans. Semin Musculoskelet Radiol 14:201–216
28. Shelly MJ, Hodnett PA, MacMahon PJ et al (2009) MR imaging of muscle injury. Magn Reson Imaging Clin N Am 17:757–773, vii
29. Longo V, Jacobson JA, Fessell DP et al (2016) Ultrasound findings of delayed-onset muscle soreness. J Ultrasound Med 35:2517–2521
30. McDonald S, Bearcroft P (2010) Compartment syndromes. Semin Musculoskelet Radiol 14:236–244
31. Ringler MD, Litwiller DV, Felmlee JP et al (2013) MRI accurately detects chronic exertional compartment syndrome: a validation study. Skelet Radiol 42:385–392
32. Ha DH, Choi S, Kang EJ et al (2015) Diffusion tensor imaging and T2 mapping in early denervated skeletal muscle in rats. J Magn Reson Imaging 42:617–623
33. Feinberg J (2006) EMG: myths and facts. HSS J 2:19–21
34. Fleckenstein JL, Watumull D, Conner KE et al (1993) Denervated human skeletal muscle: MR imaging evaluation. Radiology 187:213–218
35. Yamabe E, Nakamura T, Oshio K et al (2007) Line scan diffusion spectrum of the denervated rat skeletal muscle. J Magn Reson Imaging 26:1585–1589
36. Holl N, Echaniz-Laguna A, Bierry G et al (2008) Diffusion-weighted MRI of denervated muscle: a clinical and experimental study. Skelet Radiol 37:1111–1117
37. Polak JF, Jolesz FA, Adams DF (1988) Magnetic resonance imaging of skeletal muscle. Prolongation of T1 and T2 subsequent to denervation. Investig Radiol 23:365–369
38. Uetani M, Hayashi K, Matsunaga N et al (1993) Denervated skeletal muscle: MR imaging. Work in progress. Radiology 189: 511–515
39. Kim SJ, Hong SH, Jun WS et al (2011) MR imaging mapping of skeletal muscle denervation in entrapment and compressive neuropathies. Radiographics 31:319–332
40. Petersilge CA, Pathria MN, Gentili A et al (1995) Denervation hypertrophy of muscle: MR features. J Comput Assist Tomogr 19:596–600
41. Chan WP, Liu GC (2002) MR imaging of primary skeletal muscle diseases in children. AJR Am J Roentgenol 179:989–997
42. Schreiber A, Smith WL, Ionasescu V et al (1987) Magnetic resonance imaging of children with Duchenne muscular dystrophy. Pediatr Radiol 17:495–497
43. Mitchell CH, Brushart TM, Ahlawat S et al (2014) MRI of sports-related peripheral nerve injuries. AJR Am J Roentgenol 203: 1075–1084
44. Yamabe E, Nakamura T, Oshio K et al (2008) Peripheral nerve injury: diagnosis with MR imaging of denervated skeletal muscle—experimental study in rats. Radiology 247:409–417
45. Kikuchi Y, Nakamura T, Takayama S et al (2003) MR imaging in the diagnosis of denervated and reinnervated skeletal muscles: experimental study in rats. Radiology 229:861–867
46. Viddeleer AR, Sijens PE, van Ooijen PM et al (2016) Quantitative STIR of muscle for monitoring nerve regeneration. J Magn Reson Imaging 44:401–410
47. Viddeleer AR, Sijens PE, van Ooyen PM et al (2012) Sequential MR imaging of denervated and reinnervated skeletal muscle as correlated to functional outcome. Radiology 264:522–530
48. Dalakas MC (2015) Inflammatory muscle diseases. N Engl J Med 372:1734–1747

49. Dalakas MC, Sivakumar K (1996) The immunopathologic and inflammatory differences between dermatomyositis, polymyositis and sporadic inclusion body myositis. Curr Opin Neurol 9: 235–239
50. Ernste FC, Reed AM (2013) Idiopathic inflammatory myopathies: current trends in pathogenesis, clinical features, and up-to-date treatment recommendations. Mayo Clin Proc 88:83–105
51. Carstens PO, Schmidt J (2014) Diagnosis, pathogenesis and treatment of myositis: recent advances. Clin Exp Immunol 175: 349–358
52. Rider LG, Miller FW (2011) Deciphering the clinical presentations, pathogenesis, and treatment of the idiopathic inflammatory myopathies. JAMA 305:183–190
53. Hill CL, Zhang Y, Sigurgeirsson B et al (2001) Frequency of specific cancer types in dermatomyositis and polymyositis: a population-based study. Lancet 357:96–100
54. Feldman BM, Rider LG, Reed AM et al (2008) Juvenile dermatomyositis and other idiopathic inflammatory myopathies of childhood. Lancet 371:2201–2212
55. Kimball AB, Summers RM, Turner M et al (2000) Magnetic resonance imaging detection of occult skin and subcutaneous abnormalities in juvenile dermatomyositis. Implications for diagnosis and therapy. Arthritis Rheum 43:1866–1873
56. Griggs RC, Askanas V, DiMauro S et al (1995) Inclusion body myositis and myopathies. Ann Neurol 38:705–713
57. Liang C, Needham M (2011) Necrotizing autoimmune myopathy. Curr Opin Rheumatol 23:612–619
58. Dalakas MC, Hohlfeld R (2003) Polymyositis and dermatomyositis. Lancet 362:971–982
59. Mastaglia FL, Garlepp MJ, Phillips BA et al (2003) Inflammatory myopathies: clinical, diagnostic and therapeutic aspects. Muscle Nerve 27:407–425
60. Schweitzer ME, Fort J (1995) Cost-effectiveness of MR imaging in evaluating polymyositis. AJR Am J Roentgenol 165: 1469–1471
61. Kuo GP, Carrino JA (2007) Skeletal muscle imaging and inflammatory myopathies. Curr Opin Rheumatol 19:530–535
62. Park JH, Olsen NJ (2001) Utility of magnetic resonance imaging in the evaluation of patients with inflammatory myopathies. Curr Rheumatol Rep 3:334–345
63. O'Connell MJ, Powell T, Brennan D et al (2002) Whole-body MR imaging in the diagnosis of polymyositis. AJR Am J Roentgenol 179:967–971
64. Lovitt S, Marden FA, Gundogdu B et al (2004) MRI in myopathy. Neurol Clin 22:509–538, v
65. Weber MA, Jappe U, Essig M et al (2006) Contrast-enhanced ultrasound in dermatomyositis- and polymyositis. J Neurol 253:1625–1632
66. Weber MA (2009) Ultrasound in the inflammatory myopathies. Ann N Y Acad Sci 1154:159–170
67. Adams EM, Chow CK, Premkumar A et al (1995) The idiopathic inflammatory myopathies: spectrum of MR imaging findings. Radiographics 15:563–574
68. Schulze M, Kotter I, Ernemann U et al (2009) MRI findings in inflammatory muscle diseases and their noninflammatory mimics. AJR Am J Roentgenol 192:1708–1716
69. Hernandez RJ, Keim DR, Chenevert TL et al (1992) Fat-suppressed MR imaging of myositis. Radiology 182:217–219
70. Yoshida K, Kurosaka D, Joh K et al (2010) Fasciitis as a common lesion of dermatomyositis, demonstrated early after disease onset by en bloc biopsy combined with magnetic resonance imaging. Arthritis Rheum 62:3751–3759
71. Filli L, Maurer B, Manoliu A et al (2015) Whole-body MRI in adult inflammatory myopathies: do we need imaging of the trunk? Eur Radiol 25:3499–3507
72. Sanner H, Kirkhus E, Merckoll E et al (2010) Long-term muscular outcome and predisposing and prognostic factors in juvenile dermatomyositis: a case-control study. Arthritis Care Res (Hoboken) 62:1103–1111
73. Cantwell C, Ryan M, O'Connell M et al (2005) A comparison of inflammatory myopathies at whole-body turbo STIR MRI. Clin Radiol 60:261–267
74. Zheng Y, Liu L, Wang L et al (2015) Magnetic resonance imaging changes of thigh muscles in myopathy with antibodies to signal recognition particle. Rheumatology (Oxford) 54:1017–1024
75. Grable-Esposito P, Katzberg HD, Greenberg SA et al (2010) Immune-mediated necrotizing myopathy associated with statins. Muscle Nerve 41:185–190
76. Cox FM, Reijnierse M, van Rijswijk CS et al (2011) Magnetic resonance imaging of skeletal muscles in sporadic inclusion body myositis. Rheumatology (Oxford) 50:1153–1161
77. Weihl CC, Pestronk A (2010) Sporadic inclusion body myositis: possible pathogenesis inferred from biomarkers. Curr Opin Neurol 23:482–488
78. Van De Vlekkert J, Maas M, Hoogendijk JE et al (2015) Combining MRI and muscle biopsy improves diagnostic accuracy in subacute-onset idiopathic inflammatory myopathy. Muscle Nerve 51:253–258
79. Connor A, Stebbings S, Anne Hung N et al (2007) STIR MRI to direct muscle biopsy in suspected idiopathic inflammatory myopathy. J Clin Rheumatol 13:341–345
80. Barsotti S, Zampa V, Talarico R et al (2016) Thigh magnetic resonance imaging for the evaluation of disease activity in patients with idiopathic inflammatory myopathies followed in a single center. Muscle Nerve 54:666–672
81. Tomasova Studynkova J, Charvat F, Jarosova K et al (2007) The role of MRI in the assessment of polymyositis and dermatomyositis. Rheumatology (Oxford) 46:1174–1179
82. Elessawy SS, Abdelsalam EM, Abdel Razek E et al (2016) Whole-body MRI for full assessment and characterization of diffuse inflammatory myopathy. Acta Radiol Open 5:2058460116668216
83. Malattia C, Damasio MB, Madeo A et al (2014) Whole-body MRI in the assessment of disease activity in juvenile dermatomyositis. Ann Rheum Dis 73:1083–1090
84. Ai T, Yu K, Gao L et al (2014) Diffusion tensor imaging in evaluation of thigh muscles in patients with polymyositis and dermatomyositis. Br J Radiol 87:20140261
85. McCullough MB, Domire ZJ, Reed AM et al (2011) Evaluation of muscles affected by myositis using magnetic resonance elastography. Muscle Nerve 43:585–590
86. Park JH, Olsen NJ, King L Jr et al (1995) Use of magnetic resonance imaging and P-31 magnetic resonance spectroscopy to detect and quantify muscle dysfunction in the amyopathic and myopathic variants of dermatomyositis. Arthritis Rheum 38:68–77
87. Qi J, Olsen NJ, Price RR et al (2008) Diffusion-weighted imaging of inflammatory myopathies: polymyositis and dermatomyositis. J Magn Reson Imaging 27:212–217
88. Cea G, Bendahan D, Manners D et al (2002) Reduced oxidative phosphorylation and proton efflux suggest reduced capillary blood supply in skeletal muscle of patients with dermatomyositis and polymyositis: a quantitative 31P-magnetic resonance spectroscopy and MRI study. Brain 125:1635–1645
89. Yao L, Yip AL, Shrader JA et al (2016) Magnetic resonance measurement of muscle T2, fat-corrected T2 and fat fraction in the assessment of idiopathic inflammatory myopathies. Rheumatology (Oxford) 55:441–449
90. Dock W, Happak W, Grabenwoger F et al (1990) Neuromuscular diseases: evaluation with high-frequency sonography. Radiology 177:825–828
91. Degardin A, Morillon D, Lacour A et al (2010) Morphologic imaging in muscular dystrophies and inflammatory myopathies. Skelet Radiol 39:1219–1227
92. Wattjes MP, Kley RA, Fischer D (2010) Neuromuscular imaging in inherited muscle diseases. Eur Radiol 20:2447–2460

93. North KN, Wang CH, Clarke N et al (2014) Approach to the diagnosis of congenital myopathies. Neuromuscul Disord 24:97–116
94. Bönnemann CG, Wang CH, Quijano-Roy S et al (2014) Diagnostic approach to the congenital muscular dystrophies. Neuromuscul Disord 24:289–311
95. Olpin SE, Murphy E, Kirk RJ et al (2015) The investigation and management of metabolic myopathies. J Clin Pathol 68:410–417
96. Mercuri E, Clements E, Offiah A et al (2010) Muscle magnetic resonance imaging involvement in muscular dystrophies with rigidity of the spine. Ann Neurol 67:201–208
97. Biggar WD, Klamut HJ, Demacio PC et al (2002) Duchenne muscular dystrophy: current knowledge, treatment, and future prospects. Clin Orthop Relat Res 401:88–106
98. Marden FA, Connolly AM, Siegel MJ et al (2005) Compositional analysis of muscle in boys with Duchenne muscular dystrophy using MR imaging. Skelet Radiol 34:140–148
99. Liu GC, Jong YJ, Chiang CH et al (1993) Duchenne muscular dystrophy: MR grading system with functional correlation. Radiology 186:475–480
100. Klein A, Jungbluth H, Clement E et al (2011) Muscle magnetic resonance imaging in congenital myopathies due to ryanodine receptor type 1 gene mutations. Arch Neurol 68:1171–1179
101. Quijano-Roy S, Carlier RY, Fischer D (2011) Muscle imaging in congenital myopathies. Semin Pediatr Neurol 18:221–229
102. Olsen DB, Langkilde AR, Orngreen MC et al (2003) Muscle structural changes in mitochondrial myopathy relate to genotype. J Neurol 250:1328–1334
103. Diekman EF, van der Pol WL, Nievelstein RA et al (2014) Muscle MRI in patients with long-chain fatty acid oxidation disorders. J Inherit Metab Dis 37:405–413
104. Horvath JJ, Austin SL, Case LE et al (2015) Correlation between quantitative whole-body muscle magnetic resonance imaging and clinical muscle weakness in Pompe disease. Muscle Nerve 51:722–730
105. Gruhn KM, Heyer CM, Guttsches AK et al (2015) Muscle imaging data in late-onset Pompe disease reveal a correlation between the pre-existing degree of lipomatous muscle alterations and the efficacy of long-term enzyme replacement therapy. Mol Genet Metab Rep 3:58–64
106. Huang BK, Monu JU, Doumanian J (2010) Diabetic myopathy: MRI patterns and current trends. AJR Am J Roentgenol 195: 198–204
107. Jelinek JS, Murphey MD, Aboulafia AJ et al (1999) Muscle infarction in patients with diabetes mellitus: MR imaging findings. Radiology 211:241–247
108. Aboulafia AJ, Monson DK, Kennon RE (1999) Clinical and radiological aspects of idiopathic diabetic muscle infarction. Rational approach to diagnosis and treatment. J Bone Joint Surg Br 81: 323–326
109. Kattapuram TM, Suri R, Rosol MS et al (2005) Idiopathic and diabetic skeletal muscle necrosis: evaluation by magnetic resonance imaging. Skelet Radiol 34:203–209
110. Delaney-Sathy LO, Fessell DP, Jacobson JA et al (2000) Sonography of diabetic muscle infarction with MR imaging, CT, and pathologic correlation. AJR Am J Roentgenol 174: 165–169
111. Sharma P, Mangwana S, Kapoor RK (2000) Diabetic muscle infarction: atypical MR appearance. Skelet Radiol 29:477–480
112. Habib GS, Nashashibi M, Saliba W et al (2003) Diabetic muscular infarction: emphasis on pathogenesis. Clin Rheumatol 22: 450–451
113. Parmar MS (2009) Diabetic muscle infarction. BMJ 338:b2271
114. Damron TA, Levinsohn EM, McQuail TM et al (1998) Idiopathic necrosis of skeletal muscle in patients who have diabetes. Report of four cases and review of the literature. J Bone Joint Surg Am 80:262–267
115. Chebbi W, Jerbi S, Klii R et al (2014) Multifocal diabetic muscle infarction: a rare complication of poorly controlled diabetes mellitus. Intern Med 53:2091–2094
116. Baker JC, Demertzis JL, Rhodes NG et al (2012) Diabetic musculoskeletal complications and their imaging mimics. Radiographics 32:1959–1974
117. Bianchi S, Zwass A, Abdelwahab IF et al (1995) Sonographic evaluation of intramuscular ganglia. Clin Radiol 50:235–236
118. Murphey MD, Carroll JF, Flemming DJ et al (2004) From the archives of the AFIP: benign musculoskeletal lipomatous lesions. Radiographics 24:1433–1466
119. Griffin N, Khan N, Thomas JM et al (2007) The radiological manifestations of intramuscular haemangiomas in adults: magnetic resonance imaging, computed tomography and ultrasound appearances. Skelet Radiol 36:1051–1059
120. Bhargava R, Parham DM, Lasater OE et al (1997) MR imaging differentiation of benign and malignant peripheral nerve sheath tumors: use of the target sign. Pediatr Radiol 27:124–129
121. Bancroft LW, Kransdorf MJ, Menke DM et al (2002) Intramuscular myxoma: characteristic MR imaging features. AJR Am J Roentgenol 178:1255–1259
122. Kransdorf MJ, Meis JM, Jelinek JS (1991) Myositis ossificans: MR appearance with radiologic-pathologic correlation. AJR Am J Roentgenol 157:1243–1248
123. Parellada AJ, Morrison WB, Reiter SB et al (2006) Unsuspected lower extremity deep venous thrombosis simulating musculoskeletal pathology. Skelet Radiol 35:659–664
124. McGuinness B, Wilson N, Doyle AJ (2007) The "penumbra sign" on T1-weighted MRI for differentiating musculoskeletal infection from tumour. Skelet Radiol 36:417–421
125. Fleckenstein JL, Burns DK, Murphy FK et al (1991) Differential diagnosis of bacterial myositis in AIDS: evaluation with MR imaging. Radiology 179:653–658
126. Williams JB, Youngberg RA, Bui-Mansfield LT et al (1997) MR imaging of skeletal muscle metastases. AJR Am J Roentgenol 168:555–557
127. Chun CW, Jee WH, Park HJ et al (2010) MRI features of skeletal muscle lymphoma. AJR Am J Roentgenol 195:1355–1360
128. Otake S (1994) Sarcoidosis involving skeletal muscle: imaging findings and relative value of imaging procedures. AJR Am J Roentgenol 162:369–375
129. Gordon BA, Martinez S, Collins AJ (1995) Pyomyositis: characteristics at CT and MR imaging. Radiology 197:279–286
130. Gomez P, Morcuende J (2004) High-grade sarcomas mimicking traumatic intramuscular hematomas: a report of three cases. Iowa Orthop J 24:106–110
131. Taieb S, Penel N, Vanseymortier L et al (2009) Soft tissue sarcomas or intramuscular haematomas? Eur J Radiol 72: 44–49

Pediatric Musculo-Skeletal Trauma: What is Unique and What Not to Miss

Rutger A.J. Nievelstein and Simon G.F. Robben

Introduction

Children are not small adults. The pediatric musculoskeletal system differs from the adult musculoskeletal system in many ways. These differences account for many unique features in pediatric musculoskeletal imaging:

Anatomical differences: Growth plates, epiphyses and metaphyses are unique for the pediatric skeleton, as well as the diseases that accompany these (unique) structures. Growth plates are vulnerable to acute (Salter-Harris fractures) and chronic (slipped capital femoral epiphysis) stress. Premature closure of a growth plate can be caused by traumatic events, and will result in growth arrest and deformity. The younger the child, the more severe the final deformity. Moreover, growth plates may simulate (avulsion) fractures. The joint capsule and ligaments that insert at the metaphyseal rim are responsible for the classic metaphyseal fractures during strain in child abuse. Epiphyses are prone for ischemic necrosis, e.g. Perthes disease, which may simulate trauma (subchondral fractures, fragmentation).

The Haversian canals in pediatric bones are relatively larger and more extensive compared to adults.

Biomechanical differences: The pediatric skeleton consists of more porous bone than adults and tolerates greater deformation. That is why in children bending without breaking can occur, whereas failure of the bone is mainly caused by extensive compression or tension. The physis is the weakest part of bone and least resistant to torsion. It is particularly breakable at the transition zone with the metaphysis. Finally, the periosteum in children is thicker, stronger, and less firmly attached to the (diaphyseal) bone. It is less frequently torn after trauma and, likewise, can act as a stabilizing factor in case of a fracture.

Physiological differences: The increased metabolism causes metaphyses to appear as hot spots on isotope bone scans, simulating trauma or obscuring them. Adults do not have metaphyses anymore. Physiological subperiosteal new bone formation may simulate callus formation in infants.

Psychological differences: If children have pain, they experience the uncomfortable sensation but they are not worried by it, and do not seek medical attention themselves. Instead they try to relief the pain by crying, limping or disuse, which is noted by the parents. Moreover, young children cannot give an appropriate history resulting in "veterinary" medicine, especially when the trauma is not witnessed by the parents.

Other differences: Many inborn errors of metabolism and skeletal dysplasias manifest themselves in childhood. Some can simulate trauma by pseudofractures (metaphyseal dysplasia) or simulate healing occult fractures by subperiosteal new bone formation (e.g. gangliosidosis). Prostaglandin E1 therapy in infants with congenital heart disease also causes subperiosteal new bone formation.

Some skeletal dysplasias and metabolic disorders are prone to develop fractures, e.g. osteogenesis imperfecta.

Finally, "referred pain" is more often seen in children than in adults: it is important to remember that pain in the knee may be the result of referred pain from the distal tibia (e.g. toddler fracture) or from the hip (e.g. Perthes' disease).

These differences between the pediatric and adult musculoskeletal system can cause differences in clinical and radiological presentation. In this chapter on pediatric musculo-skeletal trauma we will focus on (a) typical pediatric fractures, (b) non-accidental injury (child abuse) and (c) diseases that may simulate trauma. Trauma of the skull and vertebral column will not be covered in this chapter.

R.A.J. Nievelstein
Department of Radiology and Nuclear Medicine,
University Medical Center Utrecht, Heidelberglaan 100,
Utrecht, The Netherlands
e-mail: r.a.j.nievelstein@umcutrecht.nl

S.G.F. Robben (✉)
Department of Pediatric Radiology, Maastricht University
Medical Center, P. Debyelaan 25, Maastricht, The Netherlands
e-mail: s.robben@maastrichtuniversity.nl

J. Hodler et al. (eds.), *Musculoskeletal Diseases 2017-2020*, DOI 10.1007/978-3-319-54018-4_12

Table 1 The frequency of the most common fractures in children [1]

Fracture site	Percentage
Distal forearm	25
Hand, Phalanges	19
Carpal-metacarpal	8
Clavicle	8
Ankle	6
Tibia, diaphysis	5
Tarsal-metatarsal	4
Foot, phalanges	3
Radius-ulna diaphysis	3
Supracondylar humerus	3
Proximal humerus	2
Facial skeleton	2
Skull	2
Femoral shaft	2
Radial neck	1
Vertebral fracture	1

Epidemiology of Pediatric Fractures [1]

Fractures constitute 10–25% of all pediatric injuries. They are more common in boys and after the age of 13 years even twice as common in boys than in girls. The incidence of fractures is high in childhood and the chance that a child sustaines a fracture from birth to the age of 16 is 42% in boys and 27% in girls.

The most common injury is a fracture of the distal radius whereas femoral neck and trochanteric fractures are amongst the least common fractures.

The frequency of the most common fracture sites is given in Table 1.

Typical Pediatric Fractures (General)

The relatively large and more extensive Haversian canals, together with the increased elasticity of the pediatric skeleton often result in the so-called incomplete fractures:

Torus or buckle fractures are caused by axial load compression forces. This results in kinking, buckling or notching of the cortex. The metaphyseal region is most vulnarable because the cortex is relatively thin.

Greenstick fractures are caused by axial loading forces and bending when the bone is bent beyond the point that spontaneous recovery is possible. This results is an incomplete fracture at the tension side of the bone whereas the cortex at the compression side remains intact.

Lead-pipe deformity is a combination of a greenstick fracture and a buckle fracture. At the tension side the cortex is ruptured and on the compression side the cortex is buckled (Fig. 1).

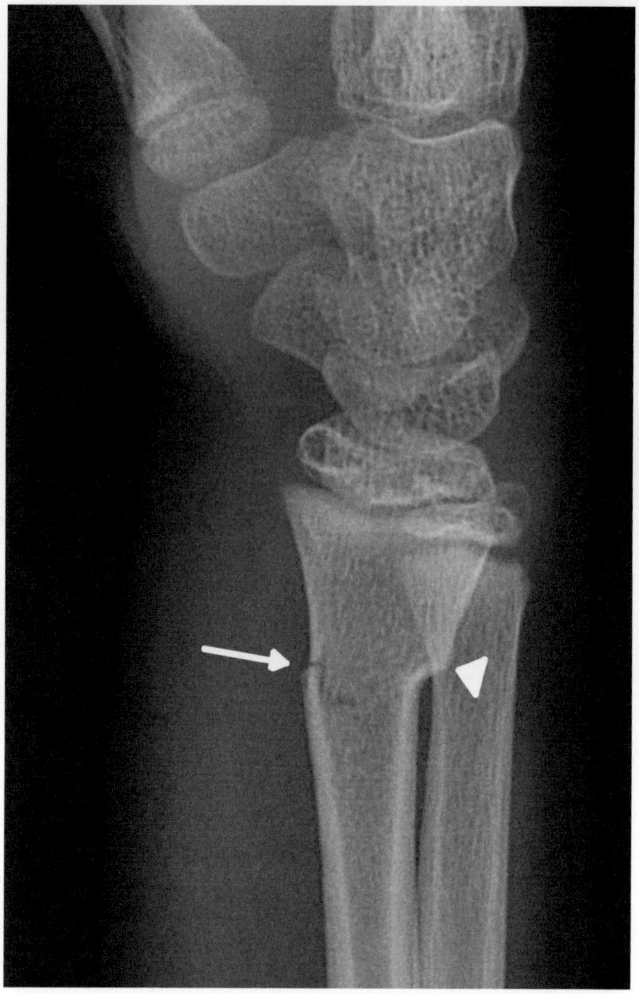

Fig. 1 A 10-year-old girl with a leadpipe deformity: rupture of the cortex at the ventral side (*arrow*) and a buckle fracture on the dorsal side (*arrowhead*)

Plastic bending/bowing fractures are also caused by axial loading forces and bending. They can be considered as a "forme fruste" of the greenstick fracture in which the bone is bent beyond its physiological limits but without visible rupture of the cortex. These fractures can be very subtle and sometimes comparison with the contralateral bone is helpful. Bowing fractures are common in the forearm.

CAST (Childhood Accidental Tibial Spiral fracture) or Toddler fracture is a nondisplaced spiral hairline fracture of the tibial shaft, often difficult to recognize on the radiograph [2]. It is caused by relatively mild rotational forces that occur when a todder stumbles and falls or tries to extricate its foot from between bars of a playpen or portable crib [3].

Typical Pediatric Fractures (Growth-Plate Related)

The growth plate is unique for children. Therefore all fractures that have some relation to the growth plate also are unique for children. Amongst these fractures are Salter-Harris fractures and the epiphyseal transitional fractures (triplane fractures and Tillaux fractures). All growth plate-related fractures are at risk for focal epiphysiodesis (premature focal closure of the growth plate).

Salter-Harris Fractures [4–6] (Fig. 2)

Type I follows the growth plate, separating the metaphysis and epiphysis. The growth plate remains attached to the epiphysis and usually there is no damage to the growth plate. Type I is seen in particular in young children. Relative incidence is 8.5%.

Type II runs through the metaphysis and (in part) the growth plate along the metaphyseal transition zone. It is the most common type (relative incidence 73%), generally in children >10 years of age. Type II heals fast.

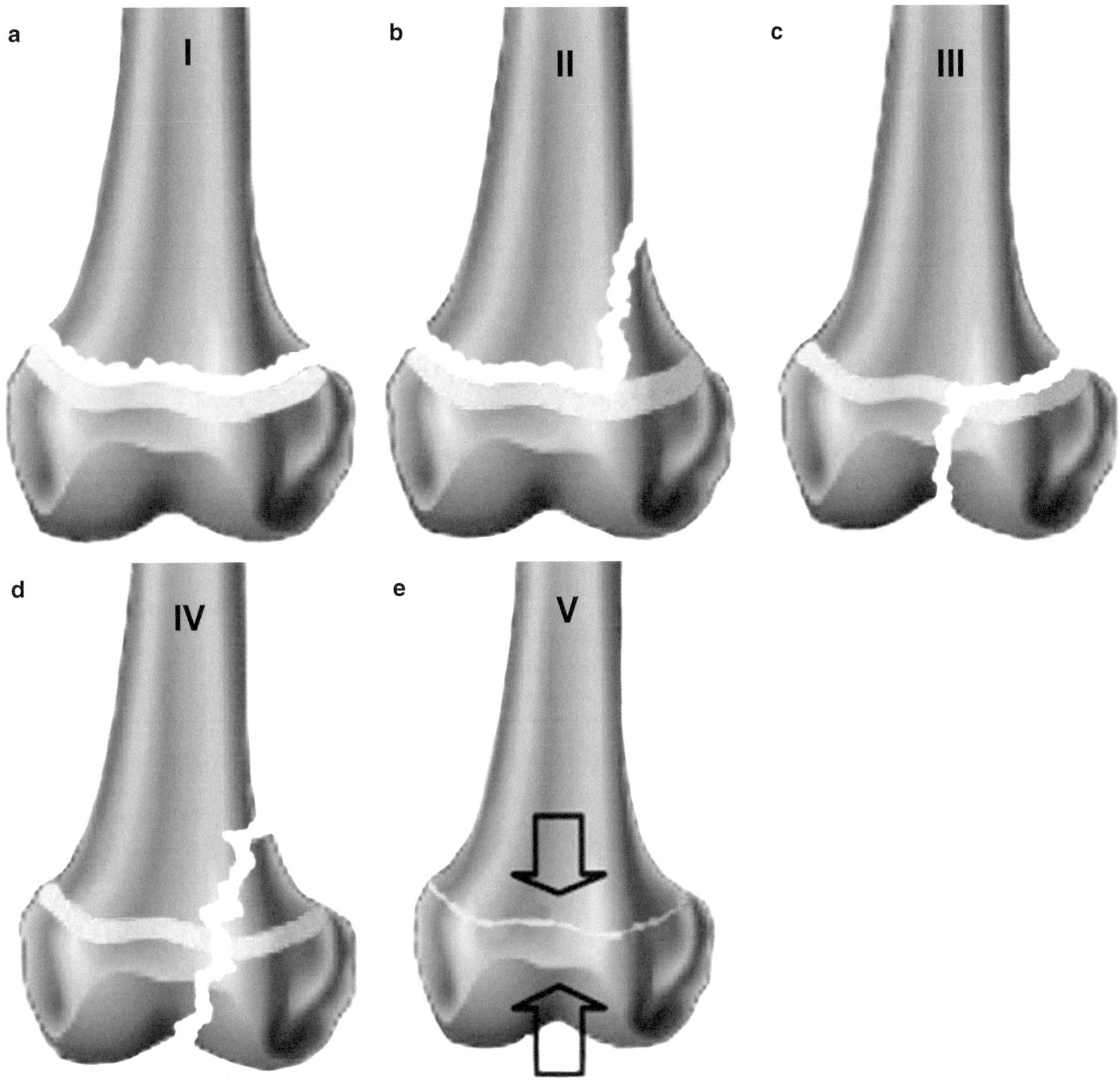

Fig. 2 The Salter-Harris classification

Type III runs through the epiphysis and (in part) the growth plate. It is quite rare (6.5%) and often seen at the lower legs in children in whom the growth plate is partially fused.

Type IV runs across the epiphysis, growth plate and metaphysis. The relative incidence is 12%. The risk for focal epiphysiodesis is substantial and treatment is typically surgical rather than conservative.

Type V is a compression fracture due to axial loading, commonly seen in knee and ankle. It is rare (<1%) and usually occult on initial imaging. The risk for focal epipysiodesis is high.

Epiphyseal Transitional Fractures [7, 8]

These fractures typically occur in the distal tibia during the 18-month period of closure of the growth plate between the ages 12 and 15 years. Closure of the distal tibial growth plate starts centrally and medially before progressing laterally. This partial closure leaves the ankle vulnerable to these types of fracture, especially during external rotation.

The triplane fracture configuration consists of (1) a fracture line along the coronal plane through the posterior metaphysis, (2) a fracture line along the sagittal plane through the epiphysis and (3) a fracture line along the transverse plane through the growth plate. The fracture may consist of 2–4 fragments. The triplane fracture appears as a Salter-Harris type II on lateral radiographs and as a Salter-Harris type III on AP radiographs. CT has a definite impact on fracture classification, displacement and treatment [7, 9]. A gap of >2 mm is considered by some authors as the threshold between conservative and surgical treatment [10]

The Tillaux fracture occur in adolescents within 1 year of complete physeal closure. At that time only the anterolateral part of the growth plate is open and vulnerable to injury. This results in a Salter-Harris type III fracture of this anterolateral part of the epiphysis (the Tillaux fragment).

Apophyseal Injuries

An apophysis can be considered as a nonarticular epiphysis that serves as attachment for muscles or tendons (e.g. trochanter, coracoid process, tibial tuberosity, anterior iliac spines, epicondyles of humerus). Injury of apophyses can be acute or chronic. Acute injury results in an avulsion fracture through the subjacent growth plate. Chronic injury is caused by repetitive microtrauma that exceeds the rate of repair. Apophyseal injuries are age-dependent:

Acute pelvic avulsions: 14–25 years of age
Medial epicondyle avulsions: 9–14 years of age
Tibial tuberosity avulsions: 13–16 years of age
Osgood Schlatter disease: 10–15 years of age.

Pelvic avulsions can be classified as Type I (not displaced), Type II (<2 cm displacement), type III (>2 cm displacement) and type IV (symptomatic nonunion or exostosis) [11].

Conventional radiographs show displacement, ossific irregularity, fragmentation, heterotopic ossification and soft tissue swelling. CT demonstrates the displacement and heterotopic ossification to a better extent whereas MRI is superior in demonstrating bone marrow- and soft tissue edema.

Typical Pediatric Fractures (Anatomy Related) [12–14]

Elbow fractures are not uncommon in children and sometimes difficult to detect because of the complicated anatomy with many epiphyses and apophyses that have a specific ossification pattern:

Capitellum starts to ossify at 1–2 years of age
Radial head: 3–6 years
Internal (medial) epicondyle: 4–6 years
Trochlea: 8 years
Olecranon: 6–12 years
External (lateral) epicondyl: 10–11 years

CRITOE is a mnemonic to memorize the chronological order of visibility of these ossification centres. For instance, if the ossification center of the internal (medial) epicondyle is not visible in a child with a visible trochlear ossification center, this is suspect of a traumatic displacement of the apophysis of the medial epicondyle when the child sustained a trauma to the elbow.

The supracondylar humeral fracture is the most common pediatric elbow fracture caused by a fall onto an extended forearm. Mean age is 5–7 years. In subtle cases a positive posterior fat pad sign may be the only sign of a fracture and also the anterior humeral line is helpful in detecting occult fractures: this line should extend through the middle 1/3 of the capitellum (Fig. 3).

Lateral condylar fractures are typically Salter-Harris IV fractures and account for 10–20% of pediatric elbow fractures, best seen on an internal oblique radiograph. Peak age is 6 years (mean 5–10 years). Fractures with >2 mm displacement are most commonly treated surgically.

Medial epicondylar fractures are apophyseal avulsion fractures (see also paragraph on apophyseal injuries). It is the 3th most common elbow fracture (10%). Displacement >5 mm needs surgical treatment.

A Monteggia fracture dislocation is a fracture of the ulnar shaft and a luxation of the radial head. If an ulnar fracture is present, no matter what type, one should look at the head of the radius for dislocation. The radiocapitellar line, drawn

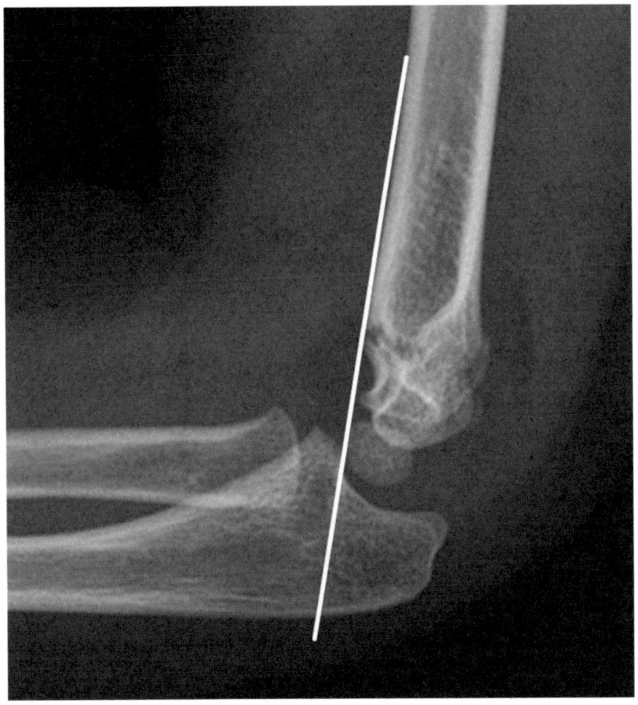

Fig. 3 Supracondylar humeral fracture in a 4-year-old girl who fell from a table. The anterior humeral line does not pass through the middle 1/3 of the capitellum because of dorsal displacement of the capitellum. Note the fracture line and both anterior and posterior fat pad signs

along the center of the radial shaft, should always pass the capitellum on the AP ánd lateral view in normal situations.

A *Galeazzi fracture dislocation* is a fracture of the radial shaft in combination with a dislocation of the distal radioulnar junction. The radial fracture typically involves the middle or distal third of the radius.

Non-accidental Injury (Child Abuse) [15–17]

Radiology plays an important role in the diagnosis of non-accidental injury because it can visualize objective sequela of child abuse, e.g. fractures, subdural hematomas and brain lesions. A radiologist may be asked to report on a skeletal survey in a child that is suspect for abuse, but a radiologist also may be the first to raise suspicion for child abuse when he finds an abnormality in a child that had a radiograph for unrelated reasons, e.g. healing rib fractures on a chest radiograph in a child with fever. Missing the diagnosis of child abuse can turn out to be a fatal mistake. On the other hand, wrongfully accusing parents or caretakers of child abuse can also have dramatic consequences on the social life of these persons.

Therefore the radiological diagnosis of child abuse needs to have a high sensitivity (not to miss the diagnosis) ánd a high specificity (no false positives). That is why it is important to:

- know the specific radiological features of child abuse (Table 2). Moreover, the younger the child the higher the suspicion. Also the suspicion increases if there is a discrepancy between the findings and the history.
- know the radiological features that may simulate child abuse (Table 3).
- perform an adequate skeletal survey (Table 4) [18].

Table 2 Specificity of radiological findings for child abuse

High specificity
Classic metaphyseal lesions
Rib fractures
Scapular fractures
Spinous process fractures
Sternal fractures
Moderate specificity
Multiple fractures, especially bilateral
Fractures of different ages
Epiphyseal separations
Vertebral body fractures
Digital fractures
Complex skull fractures
Pelvic fractures
Common, but low specificity
Subperiosteal new bone formation
Clavicular fractures
Long bone shaft fractures
Linear skull fractures

Table 3 Diseases that may simulate child abuse

Diseases with increased incidence of fractures
Osteogenesis imperfecta
Pycnodysostosis
Osteopetrosis
Rickets
Diseases with periosteal reaction simulating healing fracture
Physiological subperiosteal new bone formation
Caffey's disease (infantile cortical hyperostosis)
Prostaglandin E1 therapy (in congenital heart disease)
Hypervitaminosis A
Congenital infections (e.g. syphilis)

Table 4 Skeletal survey for child abuse

Skull AP and lateral
Cervical spine lateral
Lumbosacral spine lateral
Pelvis AP
Thorax 4 views: AP, lateral, right and left oblique (all bone technique)
Humeri AP
Forearms AP
Hand PA
Femurs AP
Lower legs AP
Feet AP

Post-Traumatic Myositis Ossificans [19]

Posttraumatic myositis ossificans is a benign condition of heterotopic non-neoplastic bone formation that arises after a single direct blow or repeated minor trauma. It most commonly occurs in adolescents or young adults, rarely under the age of 10 years. Common locations are the brachial and quadriceps muscles. Clinical findings include pain, local heat, a palpable mass and limited range of motion.

Conventional radiographs show flocculated densities 3–4 weeks after the injury. Typically the maximum opacity is in the peripheral zone and the central zone is relatively radiolucent. This zoning pattern of peripheral maturation is an important diagnostic feature indicating its benign character. At 6–8 weeks a lacy pattern with circumscript borders evolves (egg shell appearance). Eventually a dense ossified mass is formed.

Scintigraphy is very sensitive in early detection, but lacks specificity. CT is the best imaging technique to visualize the typical zonal pattern of ossification. US and MRI show the soft tissue mass to a good advantage, but the zonal pattern is more difficult to detect.

Radiographic diagnosis is important because biopsy may show proliferating cells with mitotic figures, necrosis and hemorrhage, simulating osteosacroma.

Other trauma-related soft tissue masses are hematomas and fat necrosis.

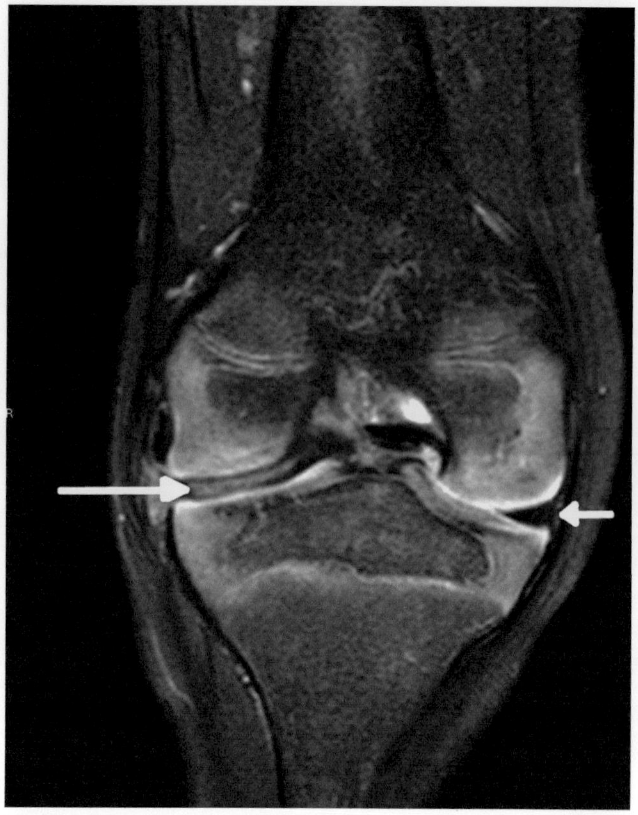

Fig. 4 T2-weighted fatsat MRI shows a discoid lateral meniscus in a 6-year-old boy with a snapping knee. The lateral meniscus (*large arrow*) crosses the whole lateral compartment. The high signal intensity represents degeneration and/or increased vascularity. Note the normal medial meniscus for comparison (*small arrow*)

Ligaments and Menisci [20, 21]

In general, MRI is the modality of choice for trauma of cartilage, ligaments and mensici. MRI features of ligamentous and meniscal injuries are more or less similar to those of adults although in children tears of the anterior cruciate ligament are more frequent in boys, have associated meniscal lesions in 60–79% of cases and collateral ligament injury in 26% of cases [22]. Moreover, meniscal tears are usually vertical in children [23]. Stress along the anterior cruciate ligament that would have resulted in a tear of the ligament in adults may instead avulse the tibial eminence in children and adolescents.

Developmental variants may be potential pitfalls when evaluating ligaments and meniscal injuries.

A discoid mensicus is an congential abnormality where the meniscus covers the weight-baring part of the knee joint [24] (Fig. 4). It occurs more often at the lateral side and is bilateral in 20% of cases. A discoid mensicus is vulnerable to trauma and degeneration and a large torn displaced meniscal fragment may cause diagnostic problems.

Also menisci are richly vascularized in childhood causing high signal intensity that may resemble tears and/or degeneration. Moreover, in children the posterior cruciate ligament is more horizontally orientated than in adults [25].

Articular Cartilage Injuries [21, 26]

Acute trauma may cause chondral injury, especially after acute knee trauma. The injury can involve the articular cartilage alone or can extend into the subchondral bone. In a study of Oeppen et al. the most common injury as a result of acute trauma to the immature knee are chondral. In patients with open growth plates, chondral lesions were more prevalent than anterior cruciate ligament and mensical injuries [27].

The juvenile form of osteochondritis dissecans is a more chronic variety of osteochondral injury and is probably due to repetitive microtrauma, most frequently seen in boys between 10–15 years of age. In the knee most often the lateral side of the medial femoral condyle is affected. Other common sites are the talus and capitellum.

Variants that May Simulate Trauma [28, 29]

Many normal variants may simulate disease, especially in pediatric radiology.

Some growth plates have an undulating or angular course that does not run completely parallel to the x-ray beam. At these sites some parts of the growth plates project distant from the growth plate and simulate fractures e.g. distal tibia en proximal humerus.

But also "simple" growth plates can produce confusing radiographs when they are not optimally projected (Fig. 5).

Another confusing bony entity is the irregular mineralization that may occur in some epiphyses that simulates fragmentation, e.g. the distal femoral epiphysis and trochlea of the elbow.

Also the mineralization centers of apophyses may appear as avulsion fractures especially when the radiograph is taken after a trauma. Well known examples are the epiphyses and apophyses around the elbow and the apophysis at the base of the fifth metatarsal (Fig. 6).

The small physiological offset of the distal fibular epiphysis might be mistaken for a Salter-Harris type I fracture, espedially in spoke wheel bicycle accidents.

Because of all these variants, the book of Keats ("Normal variants that may simulate disease" [29]) is indispensable in a radiology department. However, a sound knowledge of these variants and good clinical judgement are necessary because one should always realize there is another book, with the same number of pages and even the same images with the title: "Diseases that may simulate normal variants".

MRI is useful to discriminate between normal variants and pathology, e.g. is a fragmented epiphysis a normal variant or pathologic (fractured, infarcted, infected), especially in patients who experience pain at the site of an apparent normal variant. In these questionable cases marrow edema, soft tissue edema and joint effusion favor pathology.

Conclusion

The pediatric musculoskeletal system differs from the adult musculoskeletal system in many ways. These differences account for many unique features in pediatric musculoskeletal imaging. Awareness of these differences and good knowledge of normal variants is important to prevent missing fractures that may lead to lifelong disability.

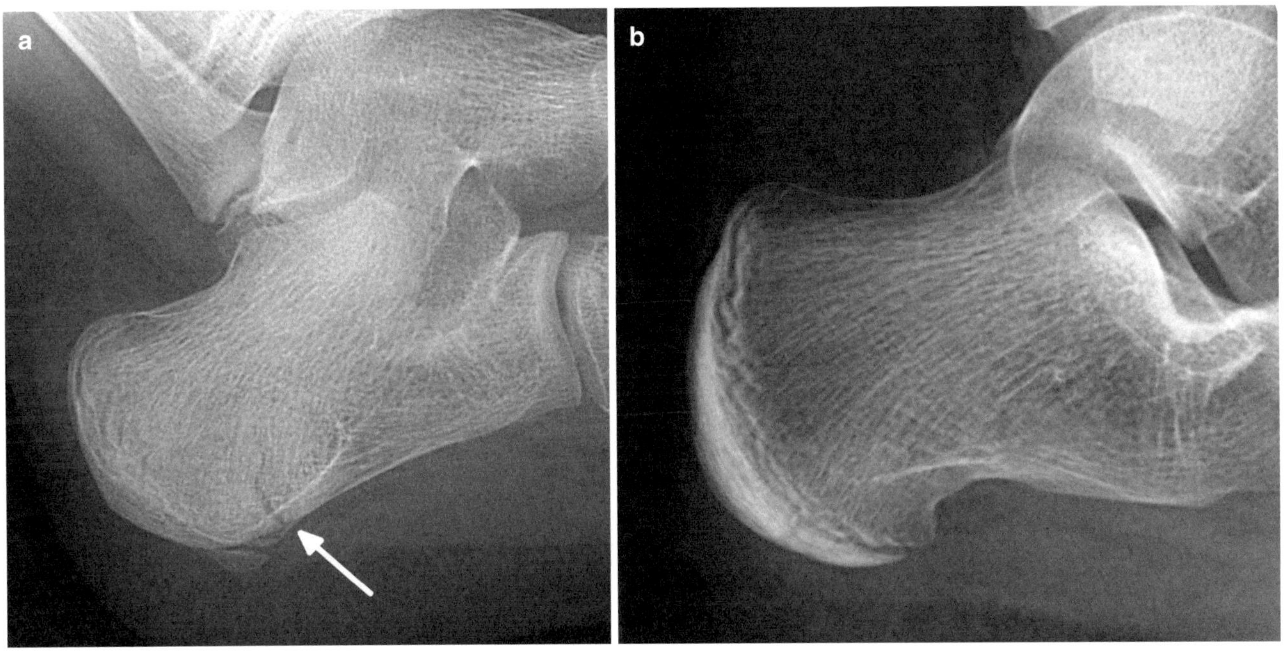

Fig. 5 12-year-old girl. (**a**) The apophyseal growth plate (*arrow*) on the oblique view of the calcaneus simulates a fracture. (**b**) The lateral view shows the growth plate of the calcaneal apophysis to a good advantage. Moreover, the oblique view of the contralateral foot showed identical findings

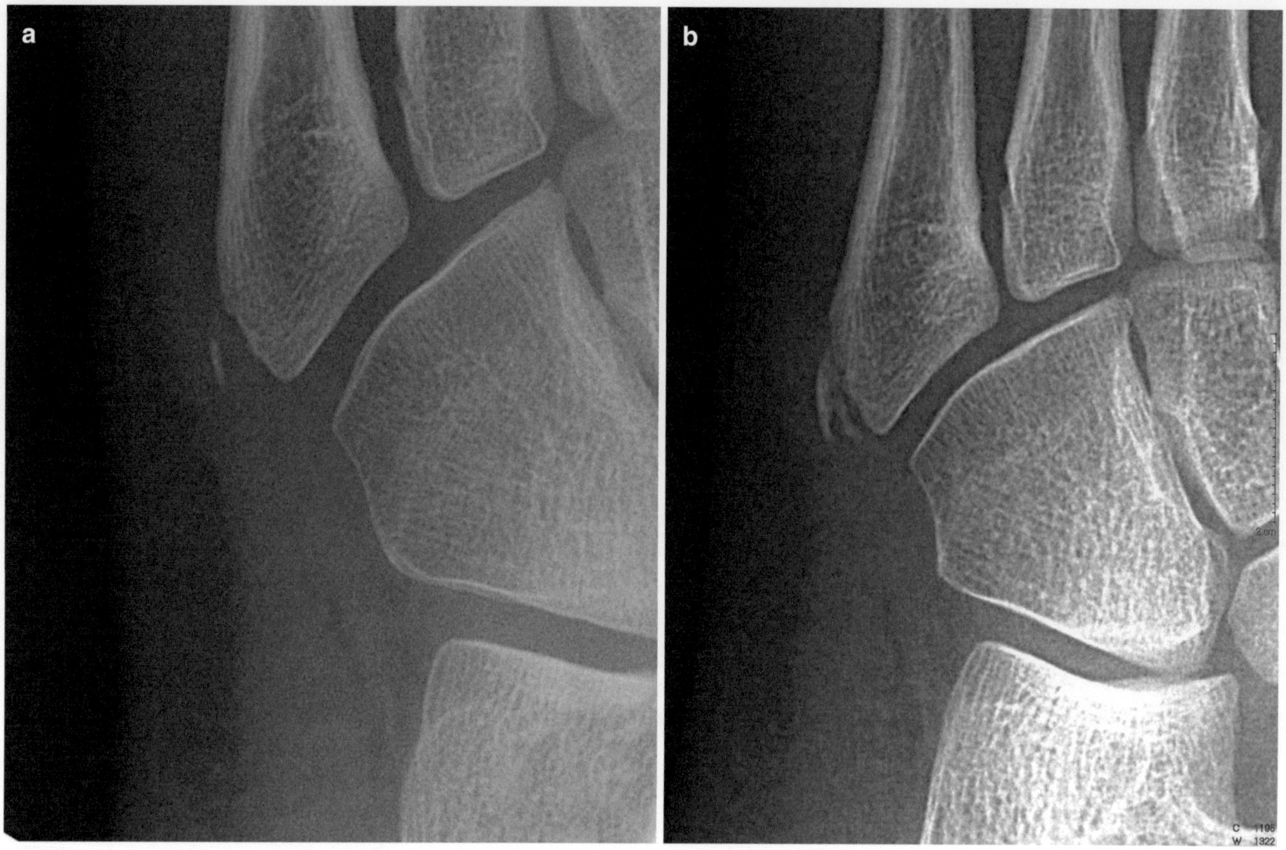

Fig. 6 11-year-old boy, no trauma. The radiograph was taken for other reasons. (**a**) The ossification center of the apophysis of the 5th metatarsal simulates a avulsion fracture. (**b**) One year later the progression of mineralization shows the whole apophysis

References

1. Landin LA (1997) Epidemiology of children's fractures. J Pediatr Orthop B 6:79–83
2. Mellick LB, Milker L, Egsieker E (1999) Childhood accidental spiral tibial (CAST) fractures. Pediatr Emerg Care 15:307–309
3. John SD, Moorthy CS, Swischuk LE (1997) Expanding the concept of the toddler's fracture. Radiographics 17:367–376
4. Donnelly LF (2012) Diagnostic imaging pediatrics: Amirsys.
5. Little JT, Klionsky NB, Chaturvedi A et al (2014) Pediatric distal forearm and wrist injury: an imaging review. Radiographics 34: 472–490
6. Rogers LF, Poznanski AK (1994) Imaging of epiphyseal injuries. Radiology 191:297–308
7. Nenopoulos A, Beslikas T, Gigis I et al (2015) The role of CT in diagnosis and treatment of distal tibial fractures with intra-articular involvement in children. Injury 46:2177–2180
8. Rosenbaum AJ, DiPreta JA, Uhl RL (2012) Review of distal tibial epiphyseal transitional fractures. Orthopedics 35:1046–1049
9. Eismann EA, Stephan ZA, Mehlman CT et al (2015) Pediatric triplane ankle fractures: impact of radiographs and computed tomography on fracture classification and treatment planning. J Bone Joint Surg Am 97:995–1002
10. Crawford AH (2012) Triplane and Tillaux fractures: is a 2 mm residual gap acceptable? J Pediatr Orthop 32(Suppl 1):S69–S73
11. McKinney BI, Nelson C, Carrion W (2009) Apophyseal avulsion fractures of the hip and pelvis. Orthopedics 32:42
12. Ellington MD, Edmonds EW (2016) Pediatric elbow and wrist pathology related to sports participation. Orthop Clin North Am 47:743–748
13. Emery KH, Zingula SN, Anton CG et al (2016) Pediatric elbow fractures: a new angle on an old topic. Pediatr Radiol 46:61–66
14. Moyer JE, Brey JM (2016) Shoulder injuries in pediatric athletes. Orthop Clin North Am 47:749–762
15. Bilo R, van Rijn RR, Robben SGF (2009) Forensic aspects of pediatric fractures. Springer, Berlin and Heidelberg
16. Kleinman PK (2015) Diagnostic imaging of child abuse. Cambridge University Press, Cambridge, UK
17. Offiah A, van Rijn RR, Perez-Rossello JM et al (2009) Skeletal imaging of child abuse (non-accidental injury). Pediatr Radiol 39:461–470
18. Barber I, Perez-Rossello JM, Wilson CR et al (2015) The yield of high-detail radiographic skeletal surveys in suspected infant abuse. Pediatr Radiol 45:69–80
19. Parikh J, Hyare H, Saifuddin A (2002) The imaging features of post-traumatic myositis ossificans, with emphasis on MRI. Clin Radiol 57:1058–1066
20. Fabricant PD, Kocher MS (2016) Anterior cruciate ligament injuries in children and adolescents. Orthop Clin North Am 47:777–788
21. Gans I, Bedoya MA, Ho-Fung V et al (2015) Diagnostic performance of magnetic resonance imaging and pre-surgical evaluation in the assessment of traumatic intra-articular knee disorders in children and adolescents: what conditions still pose diagnostic challenges? Pediatr Radiol 45:194–202

22. Prince JS, Laor T, Bean JA (2005) MRI of anterior cruciate ligament injuries and associated findings in the pediatric knee: changes with skeletal maturation. AJR Am J Roentgenol 185:756–762
23. Major NM, Beard LN Jr, Helms CA (2003) Accuracy of MR imaging of the knee in adolescents. AJR Am J Roentgenol 180:17–19
24. Kramer DE, Micheli LJ (2009) Meniscal tears and discoid meniscus in children: diagnosis and treatment. J Am Acad Orthop Surg 17:698–707
25. Kim HK, Laor T, Shire NJ et al (2008) Anterior and posterior cruciate ligaments at different patient ages: MR imaging findings. Radiology 247:826–835
26. Cruz AI Jr, Shea KG, Ganley TJ (2016) Pediatric knee osteochondritis dissecans lesions. Orthop Clin North Am 47:763–775
27. Oeppen RS, Connolly SA, Bencardino JT et al (2004) Acute injury of the articular cartilage and subchondral bone: a common but unrecognized lesion in the immature knee. AJR Am J Roentgenol 182:111–117
28. Berko NS, Kurian J, Taragin BH et al (2015) Imaging appearances of musculoskeletal developmental variants in the pediatric population. Curr Probl Diagn Radiol 44:88–104
29. Keats TE (2013) Atlas of normal roentgen variants that may simulate diasease. Saunders, Philadelphia

PELVIS and GROIN

William Palmer and Christian Pfirrmann

Common Hamstring Tendon

The common hamstring tendon is comprised of biceps femoris (long head), semitendinosus and semimembranosus [1]. At the ischial attachment site, semitendinosus and biceps femoris (BF-ST) form a conjoined tendon with a common osseous origin from the ischium. The semimembranosus (SM) tendon originates separately, contiguous with the conjoined tendon.

The common hamstring tendon has predictable anatomical relationships to the ischium and sacrotuberous ligament [2]. Less predictable are its relationships to the proximal femur. Anatomical variations in femoral or pelvic morphology, acquired conditions such as trauma-related deformity, and functional disorders such as spinal imbalance, can predispose to ischiofemoral impingement [3]. Chronic impingement can lead to hamstring injury due to entrapment of the common hamstring tendon between the femur and ischium.

The sacrotuberous ligament (STL) is visualized in 100% of pelvis MR examinations as it passes from the sacrum to ischial tuberosity [2]. The STL has both osseous (static) and myotendinous (dynamic) attachments. Proximally, the STL bridges and reinforces the sacroiliac joint while providing an expansive insertion site for gluteus maximus. Distally, the STL fibers converge into a thin cable that partially attaches to the ischial tuberosity and partially merges with the conjoined tendon of BF-ST [4, 5].

Therefore, the STL plays both static and dynamic stabilizing roles. The STL stabilizes the sacroiliac joint passively by bridging the joint and limiting its motion. Active stabilization results from its proximal and distal myotendinous attachments. Gluteus maximums and BF-ST generate forces that are transmitted through the STL to the pelvis, thereby contributing neuromuscular control over the sacroiliac joint. This kinematic chain is understood in the context of evolutionary models that equate the STL with the vestigial remnant of biceps femoris, which originated from the sacrum in lower mammals and evolved to secure itself to the ischium in humans [4, 5].

Hamstring Tendon Injury

Both the hamstring and quadriceps groups cross two joints, increasing susceptibility to myotendinous strain. The hamstring group, which is strained more frequently than quadriceps, functions to extend the hip and flex the knee. The typical noncontact mechanism involves eccentric hamstring contraction with the hip flexed and the knee extended, as occurs in long jumping and hurdling.

In athletes, hamstring strain usually involves muscle at the myotendinous junction [6, 7]. Some activities, such as water skiing, predispose to tendon avulsion due to sudden, forced hip flexion in full knee extension [8]. Although tendon ruptures are rare in adult athletes, they are important to recognize because they are more likely to be repaired surgically than myotendinous strains, which are managed nonoperatively. MRI helps to distinguish tendon tear from muscle strain and to grade the severity of injury [6, 7].

In non-athletes and older individuals, the hamstring tendon becomes prone to injury at the osseous attachment site to ischium [9]. With age and lack of exercise or stretching, the tendon loses compliance. Stiffness leads to

W. Palmer
Department of Radiology, Massachusetts General Hospital, 55 Fruit Street, YAW 6030, Boston, MA 02114, USA
e-mail: wpalmer@mgh.harvard.edu

C. Pfirrmann (✉)
Department of Radiology, Balgrist University Hospital, University of Zurich, Forchstrasse 340, Zurich, Switzerland
e-mail: christian.pfirrmann@balgrist.ch

J. Hodler et al. (eds.), *Musculoskeletal Diseases 2017-2020*, DOI 10.1007/978-3-319-54018-4_13

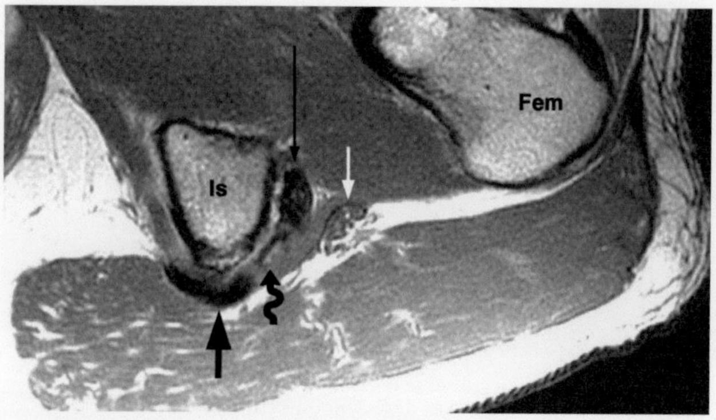

Fig. 1 High-grade tear of hamstring tendon in 51-year-old squash player with increasing pain. Axial proton density-weighted MR image shows semimembranosus tendon (*thin straight black arrow*), sacrotuberous ligament (STL) (*thick straight black arrow*) and sciatic nerve (*white arrow*) at level of ischial tuberosity (Is) and proximal femur (Fem). In expected location of semitendinosus-biceps femoris (ST-BF), ossific focus (*wavy black arrow*) indicates chronic tendinopathy and high-grade tear. Tendon retraction was limited because the STL remained continuous with ST-BF (not shown)

tendinosis and attritional partial tears that lower the threshold for spontaneous tendon rupture. Another common injury pattern is the stripping of BF-ST along the ischium. BF-ST can strip completely from its osseous footprint but remain attached to bone through a tenoperiosteal anchor [2].

The STL reinforces BF-ST at its osseous origin. Because it can remain attached to BF-ST despite high-grade tear and detachment of the conjoined tendon from bone, the extent of hamstring retraction depends on STL continuity with BF-ST (Fig. 1). When intact, the STL prevents or limits distal tendon retraction despite BF-ST stripping or avulsion from the ischium [2, 4, 9]. When the STL is discontinuous, the conjoined tendon is free to retract distally. Therefore, hamstring rupture and tendon retraction are associated with STL discontinuity. The greatest degree of hamstring retraction occurs when BF-ST and SM ruptures are combined with STL discontinuity. In chronic hamstring avulsions with tendon retraction, scarring and fibrotic bands can compress and tether the sciatic nerve resulting in the sciatic syndrome. This syndrome may be treated by hydrodissection or surgical neurolysis.

Ischiofemoral Impingement

Ischiofemoral impingement (IFI) syndrome results from narrowing of the space between the femur and the ischial tuberosity [10–12]. Clinical symptoms and signs are often nonspecific and require correlation with MR findings.

Numerous factors may predispose to IFI. Developmental etiologies include coxa valga, lesser trochanteric prominence, abnormal femoral torsion and variation in pelvic morphology. Acquired etiologies include hip instability, postural imbalances, extreme hypermobility, post-traumatic deformity and ossific enthesopathy.

The distance between the lesser trochanter and ischium depends on patient positioning, which is difficult to standardize during MR imaging. This distance is narrowed when the hip is adducted, internally rotated and extended, but widened when the hip is abducted, externally rotated and flexed. Because of variations in patient positioning, distance measurements in IFI diagnosis remain unvalidated. Asymmetric narrowing of the ischiofemoral space improves specificity when the left and right hips have identical positioning.

Besides narrowing of the ischiofemoral space, major MR findings associated with IFI include edema of quadratus femoris muscle, fatty atrophy of quadratus femoris muscle, edema or bursal fluid involving ischiofemoral fat, and elongated, hook-shaped lesser trochanter (Fig. 2). Less specific findings include hamstring tendon tear, bony proliferative change at ischial tuberosity, and unbalanced adductor-abductor musculature (e.g. asymmetric atrophy of gluteal musculature and tensor fascia lata).

Diagnostic injection can help to confirm the diagnosis of IFI. Using CT or US guidance, a needle is inserted into the ischiofemoral space for administration of anesthetic (with or without corticosteroid). A positive injection test occurs when concordant symptoms are produced during needle placement, or post-injection symptoms are substantially decreased.

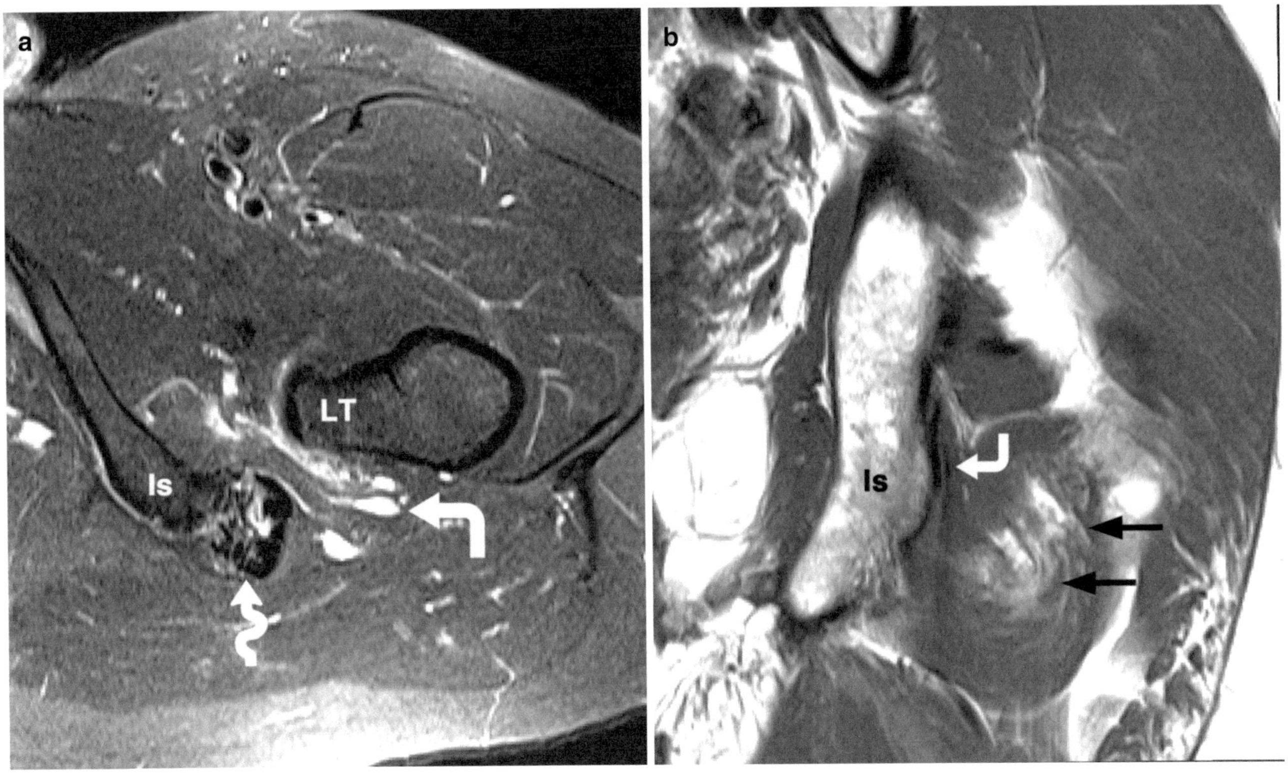

Fig. 2 Ischiofemoral impingement (IFI) in 48y-year-old female with long-standing posterior hip pain. (**a**) On axial T2-weighted MR image, the lesser trochanter (LT) shows close approximation to common hamstring tendon (*wavy white arrow*) at level of ischium (Is). Hamstring tendinopathy and partial tear are present. In the ischiofemoral space, quadratus femoris muscle shows edema and fluid that extends posteriorly (*angled white arrow*). (**b**) Coronal T1W MR images demonstrates fatty changes of quadratus femoris muscle (*black arrows*) adjacent to hamstring tendon (*angled white arrow*) at attachment site to ischium (Is)

Athletic Pubalgia

Athletic pubalgia results from overuse activity. The prevelance of athletic pubalgia is greatest in sports that require rapid changes in speed and direction such as soccer, American football, ice hockey, fencing and certain track and field events.

Groin pain is common in athletes and poses diagnostic challenges because of numerous, complicated etiologies [13]. In clinical practice, patients with athletic pubalgia complain of the insidious onset of exertional pain and tenderness over the pubic, inguinal and adductor regions. Structural abnormalities include adductor longus tear, common adductor-rectus abdominis dysfunction, osteitis pubis and inguinal wall disruption (Sportsman's hernia).

On MR images, functionally related structures include the pubis and pubic symphysis, rectus abdominis, adductor longus, adductor brevis and gracilis [14, 15]. The sheath of rectus abdominis passes over the pubis and pubic symphysis, forming a thick aponeurosis. This aponeurosis creates a prepubic aponeurotic complex (P-PAC) by providing a common adductor longus-rectus abdominis attachment site that also anchors the posterior wall of the inguinal canal.

In athletic pubalgia, MR abnormalities typically involve the adductor longus tendon at the pubic and P-PAC attachment sites. Adductor longus enthesopathy may be associated with adjacent bone marrow edema in the pubis. As the tendons strip away from bone, enthesopathy progresses to a fluid-filled tear best characterized in the coronal or sagittal plane. The secondary cleft sign indicates communication between the adductor tear and the symphyseal joint space (Fig. 3). Adductor tears may propagate along the P-PAC into the attachment site of rectus abdominis.

The spectrum of athletic pubalgia includes altered mechanics, P-PAC insufficiency, symphyseal instability and osteitis pubis characterized by bone marrow edema on MR images. MR signs of chronic instability include fatty infiltration of bone marrow, thickening of the superior pubic ligament, and degenerative changes such as symphyseal sclerosis and subchondral cysts.

Just as pre-existing hamstring tear predisposes to spontaneous tendon rupture, pre-existing adductor tear and symphyseal instability predispose to the avulsion of common adductors, gracilis and rectus abdominis. They also lower the threshold for acute myotendinous strain of parasymphyseal musculature, including pectineus, obturator externus and

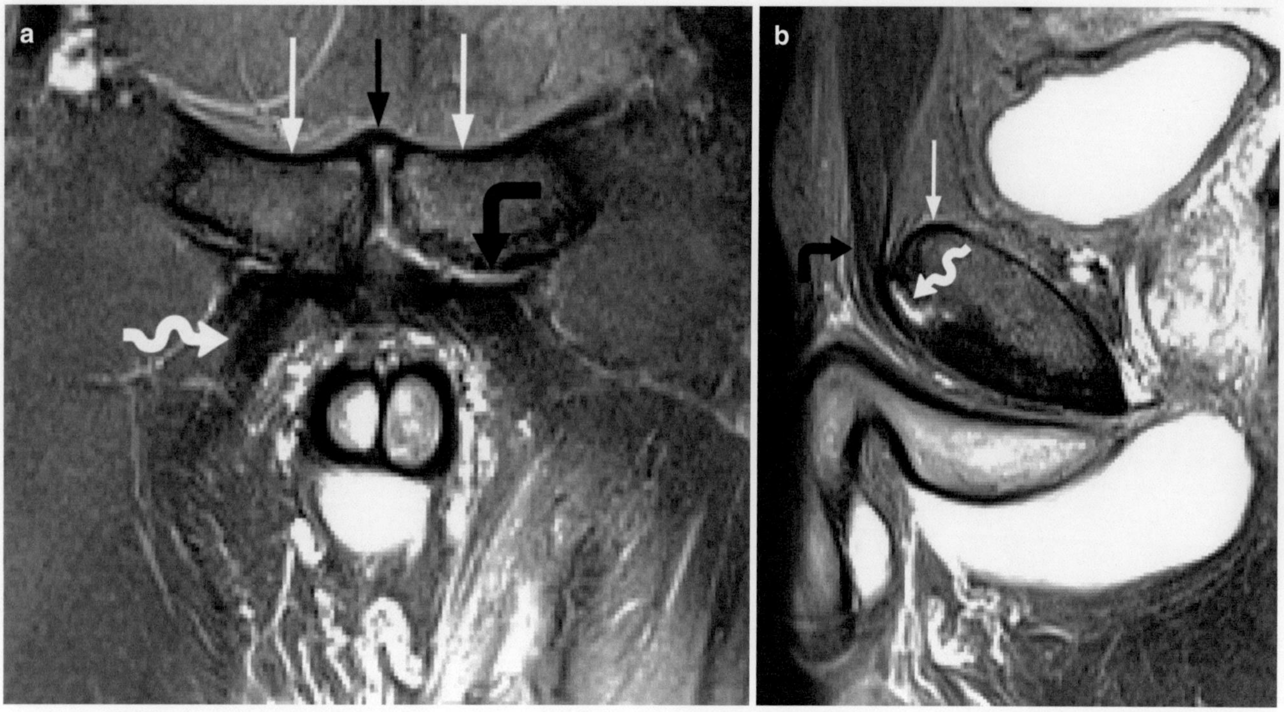

Fig. 3 Partial tear of adductor longus and pre-pubic aponeurosis (P-PAC) in 34-year-old hockey player with athletic pubalgia. (**a**) Coronal fat-suppressed T2-weighted MR image demonstrates the superior pubic ligament (*straight black arrow*), pubic bones (*straight white arrows*), and right adductor longus tendon (*wavy white arrow*). At osseous attachment site of left adductor longus tendon, linear fluid (*angled black arrow*) extends into the symphyseal joint space (secondary cleft sign). (**b**) On sagittal fat-suppressed T2-weighted MR image, linear fluid (*wavy white arrow*) indicates tear extension into the P-PAC at attachment site of rectus abdominis (*black arrow*) to pubis (*straight white arrow*)

adductors. Once the first strain occurs, weakened muscle is susceptible to repeated injury.

The condition called Sportsman's hernia encompasses two distinct inguinal pathologies [13] and insertional fascial deficiencies. In posterior inguinal wall deficiency, the posterior wall of the inguinal canal is weakened due to tearing of the conjoint tendon and transversalis fascia. In Gilmore's groin, the anterior wall and superficial ring of the inguinal canal are weakened due to tearing of the external oblique aponeurosis. No hernia is present in either condition. MR imaging findings are minimal or absent unless the injury is acute, in which case edema and hemorrhage may be detectable in the inguinal canal [14, 15]. Skilled operators may be able to identify subtle inguinal defects using ultrasound.

Greater Trochanter and Abductor Tendons

The surface of the greater trochanter consistently shows four distinct facets—the anterior, lateral, posterior and postero-superior facet [16]. All these facets serve as tendon attachments (anterior, lateral, and postero-superior facet) or are covered by a bursa (posterior facet).

The gluteus medius tendon is a tendon which has attachments all around the greater trochanter. The strong main tendon attaches to the postero-superior facet. The lateral part of the gluteus medius tendon attaches to the lower portion of the lateral facet. The anterior part of the gluteus medius tendon is a muscular attachment onto the gluteus minimus tendon.

In contrast to the gluteus medius tendon, the gluteus minimus tendon is a purely anterior structure. The lateral part attaches to the peripheral areas of the anterior facet, the medial part attaches onto the hip joint capsule.

There are several bursae around the greater trochanter. The bursae are variable and the number and size increase with age. The largest and most important bursa is the trochanteric bursa, which covers the posterior facet. Underneath the lateral part of the gluteus medius tendon and underneath the lateral part of the gluteus minimus tendon a small bursa is present, which covers the parts of the facets which are not used by the tendon attachment [16].

Trochanteric pain syndrome is mainly caused by abnormalities involving abductor tendons. Often a trochanteric bursitis is visible. However detection of high T2 signals in the trochanteric bursa or around the greater trochanter is not a reliable predictor of trochanteric pain syndrome since these

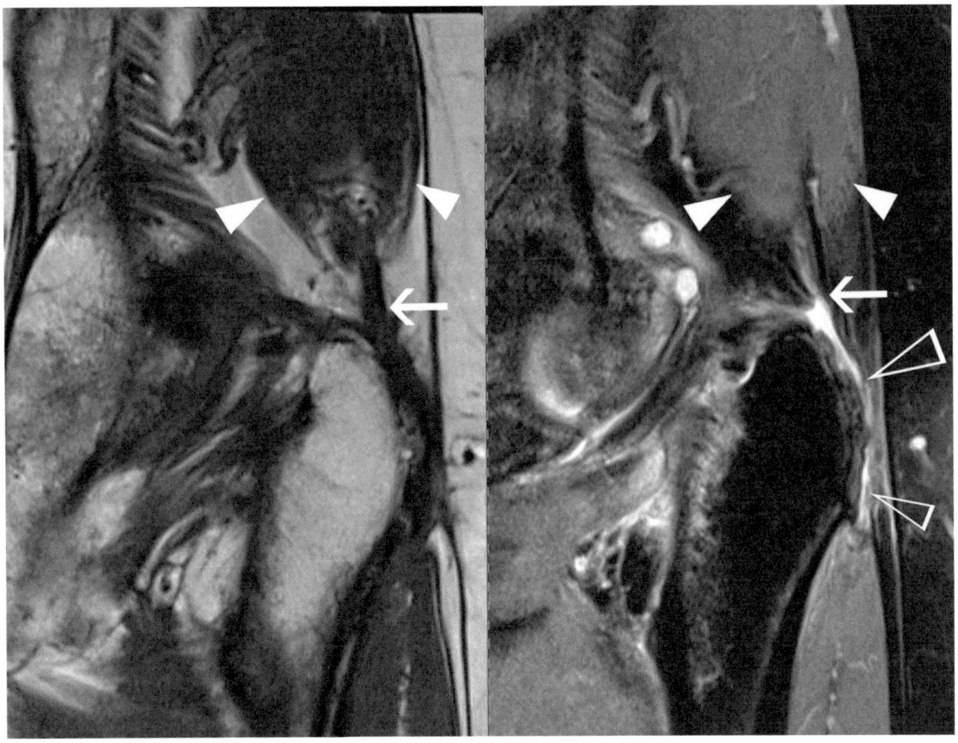

Fig. 4 Full thickness tear of the gluteus medius tendon in a 69-year-old woman. On the T1-weighted (*left image*) and the PD fat sat MR image (*right image*) the tendon of the gluteus medius (*arrow*) and the musculotendinous junction (*arrowhead*) are retracted. Note osseous irregularities at the greater trochanter and fluid collection around the greater trochanter (*open arrows*)

findings are prevalent also in patients without trochanteric pain [17]. The most commonly affected portion of the abductor tendons is the antero-lateral area (gluteus minimus and medius). Quite often partial tears or even full thickness tears are seen (Fig. 4). Bony surface irregularities larger than 2 mm have a very high positive predictive value for a tendon abnormality [18]. Most commonly elderly women are affected. Detachments of the gluteus minimus may be difficult to detect, because there is continuity between the tendons of the gluteus minimus and the vastus lateralis. A complete detachment from the greater trochanter may therefore be present without retraction of the tendon.

It is important to address the contour and the muscle quality of the abductors. Usually the muscle belly of the gluteus medius tendon reaches the tip of the greater trochanter. This is a valuable marker to judge the degree of retraction after a tear. Fatty infiltration of the gluteus medius muscle is a bad prognostic factor. However fatty infiltration of the anterior part of the gluteus minimus seems to be a normal phenomenon, not necessary linked to tears.

Anterior Hip Tendons

The iliopsoas tendon originates from two muscle bellies, the psoas and the iliacus. Therefore, the tendon may have a longitudinal division as an anatomic variant even lower in its course which should not be misdiagnosed as a longitudinal tear [19]. The iliopsoas tendon courses over the anterior edge of the acetabulum and then runs over the hip joint capsule and attaches to the lesser trochanter. Because of this course over the eminence of the femoral head, this may be a cause for a snapping hip [20]. After total hip replacement, irritation and degeneration of the iliopsoas tendon may occur. The typical site is the anterior edge of the acetabular component of the prosthesis, especially if the acetabular component is positioned with reduced anteversion or is not covered with bone. This can be accompanied by a bursitis of the iliopectineal bursa.

The rectus femoris has two parts. The pars recta attaches directly to the anterior inferior iliac (AIIS) spine. The reflected part runs slightly laterally to the main tendon and runs lateral along the upper border of the hip joint capsule. In the adolescent patients the most common lesion is an avulsion of the apophysis of the AIIS (Fig. 5). This usually heals uneventfully with rest. However, a higher degree of displacement may occur. This can lead to a too long AIIS after healing (Fig. 6), which may later interfere with hip flection. This in known by the term “subspine impingement” [21]. In the adult tears of the rectus generally tend to be more distal; proximal lesions are more commonly affecting the pars reflecta of the iliopsoas tendon [22].

The iliocapsularis muscle originates from the AIIS and the anterior hip joint capsule and attaches to the lesser

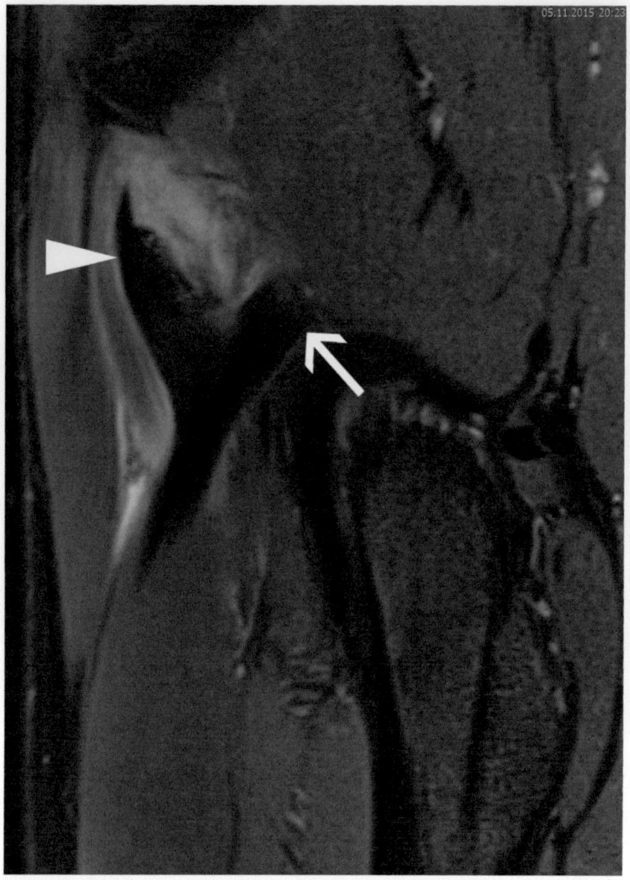

Fig. 5 Avulsion of the AIIS in a 15-years-old soccer player. The sagittal PD fat sat image shows the avulsed apophysis with the straight head of the rectus femoris (*arrowhead*), surrounded by fluid. The reflected head of the rectus femoris curves posteriorly (*arrow*)

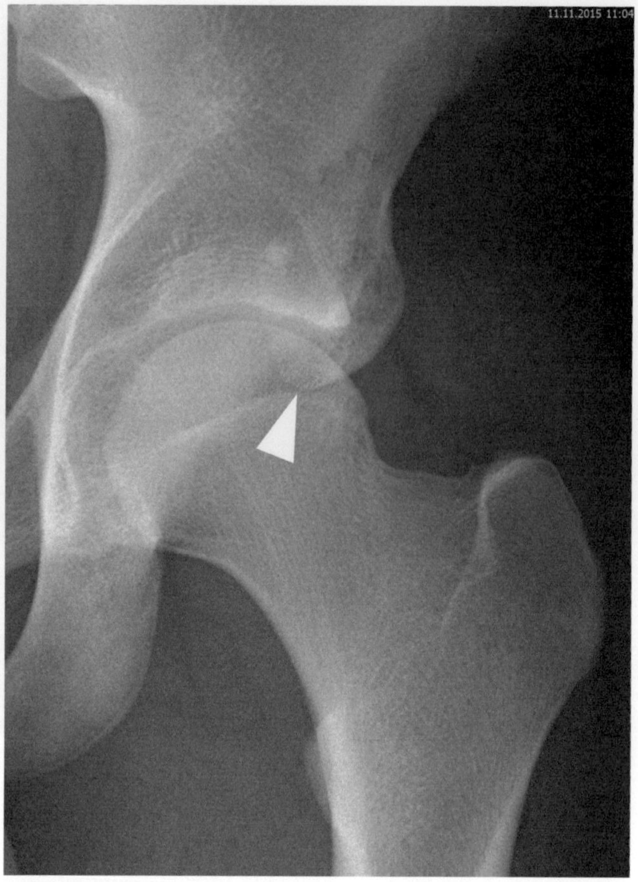

Fig. 6 AP radiography of the left hip in a 24-years-old patient with subspine impingement. The AIIS (*arrowhead*), is enlarged and reaches too far distal

trochanter. The iliocapsular muscle is variable. This muscle is a stabilizer for the femoral head especially in dysplastic hips with a deficient anterior acetabulum. In these cases, a hypertrophy of the muscle may be seen [23].

The tensor fascia lata is located within the fascia lata at the anterolateral aspect of the hip. The origin is the anterior superior iliac spine and the anterior iliac crest, the insertion is the ilitibial band. In patients with insufficient abductor tendons, a hypertrophy of the tensor fasciae latae may be observed [24]. Occasionally this hypertrophy may raise clinical suspicion for a tumor. The hypertrophy of the tensor fascia lata is a compensatory mechanism (Fig. 7).

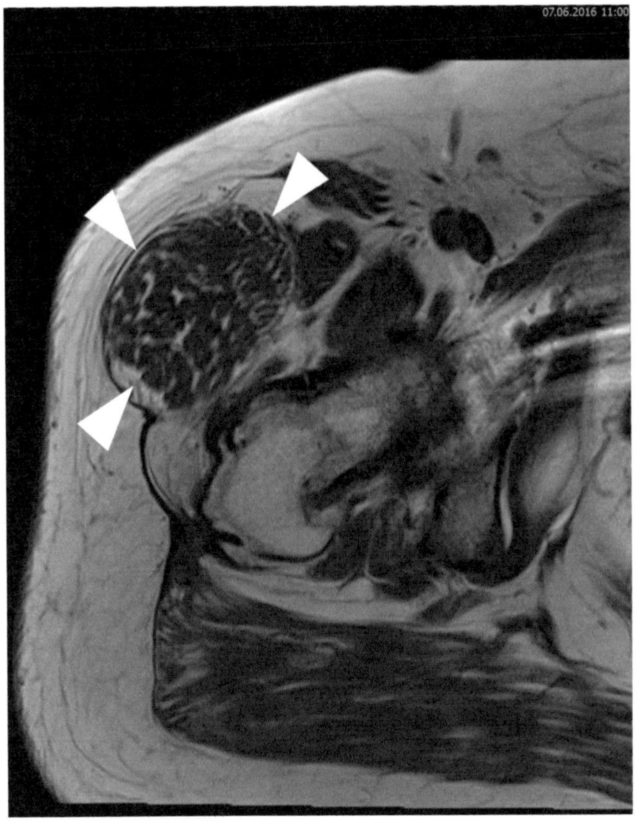

Fig. 7 Hypertrophy of the tensor fasciae latae (*arrowheads*) in a 73-years-old woman with abductor tendon insufficiency

References

1. Martin BF (1968) The origins of the hamstring muscles. J Anat 102(Pt 2):345–352
2. Bierry G, Simeone J, Borg-Stein JP, Clavert P, Palmer WE (2014) Sacrotuberous ligament: relationship to normal, torn, and retracted hamstring tendons on MR images. Radiology 271(1):162–171
3. Hernando MF, Cerezal L, Perez-Carro L, Canga A, Gonzalez RP (2016) Evaluation and management of ischiofemoral impingement: a pathophysiologic, radiologic and therapeutic approach to a complex diagnosis. Skelet Radiol 45(6):771–787
4. van Wingerden JP, Vleeming A, Snijders CJ, Stoeckart R (1993) A functional-anatomical approach to the spine-pelvis mechanism: interaction between the biceps femoris muscle and the sacrotuberous ligament. Eur Spine J 2(3):140–144
5. van Wingerden J, Vleeming A, Kleinrensink G, Stoeckart R (1997) The role of the hamstrings in pelvic and spinal function. In: Vleeming A, Mooney V, Snijders CJ, Dorman TA, Stoeckart R (eds) Movement, stability and low back pain. The essential role of the pelvis. Churchill Livingstone, Edinburgh, pp 207–210
6. Koulouris G, Connell D (2003) Evaluation of the hamstring muscle complex following acute injury. Skelet Radiol 32(10):582–589
7. De Smet AA, Best TM (2000) MR imaging of the distribution and location of acute hamstring injuries in athletes. Am J Roentgenol 174(2):393–399
8. Sallay PI, Friedman RL, Coogan PG, Garrett WE (1996) Hamstring muscle injuries among water skiers. Functional outcome and prevention. Am J Sports Med 24(2):130–136
9. De Smet AA, Blankenbaker DG, Alsheik NH, Lindstrom MJ (2012) MRI appearance of the proximal hamstring tendons in patients with and without symptomatic proximal hamstring tendinopathy. Am J Roentgenol 198(2):418–422
10. Torriani M, Souto SC, Thomas BJ, Ouellette H, Bredella MA (2009) Ischiofemoral impingement syndrome: an entity with hip pain and abnormalities of the quadratus femoris muscle. Am J Roentgenol 193(1):186–190
11. Stafford GH, Villar RN (2011) Ischiofemoral impingement. J Bone Joint Surg (Br) 93-B(10):1300–1302
12. Bredella MA, Azevedo DC, Oliveira AL, Simeone FJ, Chang CY, Stubbs AJ, Torriani M (2015) Pelvic morphology in ischiofemoral impingement. Skelet Radiol 44(2):249–253
13. Gilmore OLA (1991) Gilmore's groin: ten years experience of groin disruption. Sports Med Soft Tissue Trauma 3:5–7
14. Koulouris G (2008) Imaging review of groin pain in elite athletes: an anatomic approach to imaging findings. Am J Roentgenol 191:962–972
15. Omar IM, Zoga AC, Kavanagh EC, Koulouris G, Bergin D, Gopez AG et al (2008) Athletic pubalgia and "sports hernia": optimal MR imaging technique and findings. Radiographics 28:1415–1438
16. Pfirrmann CW, Chung CB, Theumann NH, Trudell DJ, Resnick D (2001) Greater trochanter of the hip: attachment of the abductor mechanism and a complex of three bursae—MR imaging and MR bursography in cadavers and MR imaging in asymptomatic volunteers. Radiology 221:469–477
17. Blankenbaker DG, Ullrick SR, Davis KW, De Smet AA, Haaland B, Fine JP (2008) Correlation of MRI findings with clinical findings of trochanteric pain syndrome. Skelet Radiol 37:903–909
18. Steinert L, Zanetti M, Hodler J, Pfirrmann CW, Dora C, Saupe N (2010) Are radiographic trochanteric surface irregularities associated with abductor tendon abnormalities? Radiology 257:754–763
19. Philippon MJ, Devitt BM, Campbell KJ, Michalski MP, Espinoza C, Wijdicks CA, Laprade RF (2014) Anatomic variance of the iliopsoas tendon. Am J Sports Med 42:807–811
20. Deslandes M, Guillin R, Cardinal E, Hobden R, Bureau NJ (2008) The snapping iliopsoas tendon: new mechanisms using dynamic sonography. AJR Am J Roentgenol 190(3):576–581
21. Larson CM, Kelly BT, Stone RM (2011) Making a case for anterior inferior iliac spine/subspine hip impingement: three representative case reports and proposed concept. Arthroscopy 27(12):1732–1737
22. Ouellette H, Thomas BJ, Nelson E, Torriani M (2006) MR imaging of rectus femoris origin injuries. Skelet Radiol 35(9):665–672
23. Haefeli PC, Steppacher SD, Babst D, Siebenrock KA, Tannast M (2015) An increased iliocapsularis-to-rectus-femoris ratio is suggestive for instability in borderline hips. Clin Orthop Relat Res 473(12):3725–3734
24. Sutter R, Kalberer F, Binkert CA, Graf N, Pfirrmann CW, Gutzeit A (2013) Abductor tendon tears are associated with hypertrophy of the tensor fasciae latae muscle. Skelet Radiol 42(5):627–633

Peripheral Nerve Imaging

Gustav Andreisek and Christopher F. Beaulieu

Introduction

Despite the tremendous advances in cross-sectional imaging modalities from the 1980's to the present, peripheral nerves have often been ignored as unimportant or too small to be reliably seen. However today, ultrasound and magnetic resonance imaging scanners allow high quality depictions of peripheral nerves and the many disorders that may be encountered. While high frequency ultrasound is very useful in the analysis of some peripheral nerves, magnetic resonance nerve imaging has emerged into a more comprehensive and dedicated examination, often referred to as magnetic resonance neurography (MR neurography or MRN) [1]. This term was introduced by Filler and Howe et al. and includes high-resolution morphologic imaging of the peripheral nerves as well as functional imaging based on diffusion weighted imaging (DWI) and diffusion tensor imaging (DTI) [2, 3]. The concept of magnetic resonance neurography is somewhat like magnetic resonance angiography where the visualization of the vascular system is enhanced by suppressing the signal from the surrounding soft tissue. Similarly, the signal from the surrounding tissue is may be suppressed in magnetic resonance neurography for better visualization of small peripheral nerves. Advances in pulse sequences for magnetic resonance neurography are being increasingly adopted by scanner manufacturers for dedicated magnetic resonance neurography.

G. Andreisek (✉)
Department of Radiology, Kantonsspital Muensterlingen, Spitalcampus 1, 8596, Muensterlingen, Switzerland
e-mail: gustav@andreisek.de

C.F. Beaulieu
Stanford University Medical Center, Radiology S-056, 300 Pasteur, Stanford, CA 94305, USA
e-mail: beaulieu@stanford.edu

Dedicated clinical programs in magnetic resonance neurography are currently available at relatively few centers around the world, however, interest in the techniques and clinical indications is spreading rapidly. With increasing availability, outside of dedicated imaging centers, there is an increasing need for training of radiologists as well as technicians to establish and maintain high clinical value of these special techniques. In some centers where MRN techniques are well established, it may make up to 10–20% of the daily musculoskeletal magnetic resonance imaging studies [4].

The increasing demand for MR neurography reflects the potential of this technique in terms of better patient management and care. For example, Baumer et al recently reported that in patients with unclear sensory symptoms, magnetic resonance neurography could confirm the diagnosis of thoracic outlet syndrome and significantly change patient management [5]. In this study, magnetic resonance neurography could depict fine fibrous bands which caused neural compression of brachial plexus structures [5].

Regardless what imaging technique is used, ultrasound or magnetic resonance imaging, the mainstay of imaging diagnosis is detailed knowledge about nerve anatomy. This syllabus and the 2017 Davos Workshops aim to guide the learner towards understanding of the nerve anatomy, appreciation of technical aspects, and knowledge of normal and abnormal nerve appearances. The focus will be magnetic resonance neurography, particularly on methods that use fairly basic MR pulse sequences for high resolution cross-sectional imaging of nerves. Often mentioned imaging techniques such as diffusion weighted, diffusion tensor imaging and tractography will not be described in the syllabus because to date, those techniques only play a limited role in the clinical routine. Even in the abovementioned centers where nerve imaging is an established part of the daily clinical business, they are only used as complementary to standard imaging techniques [6].

J. Hodler et al. (eds.), *Musculoskeletal Diseases 2017-2020*, DOI 10.1007/978-3-319-54018-4_14

Peripheral Neuromuscular Anatomy

The axon, the basic anatomic unit of a peripheral nerve, is surrounded by a connective tissue layer which is referred to as endoneurium. It consists of Schwann cells and connective tissue stroma. Axons can be myelinated or unmyelinated depending on the presence of Schwann cells. Bundles of axons are grouped together and organized into a fascicle, which is covered by a tissue layer referred to as perineurium. Multiple fascicles, which are sheathed by the epineurium, a layer that is the most outer cover, finally form the peripheral nerve trunk. The connective tissue layers, i.e. the perineurium, form the blood nerve barrier. Within a peripheral nerve, there is normal axonal flow of endoneurium fluid like the cerebral spinal fluid flow in the central nervous system [2].

The fascicular structure of peripheral nerves is well visible on nerve ultrasound as well as magnetic resonance neurography images. To date, the fascicular level represents the highest level of spatial resolution that both US and MRI can resolve. It is not possible to directly visualize the axonal level of a nerve. Indirectly, the anatomic integrity at the axonal level can be assessed by functional imaging techniques such as diffusion tensor imaging [7].

Anatomic variations of peripheral nerves occur with aging. In children and young adults, the peripheral nerve usually appears tight and compact with thick fascicles, whereas in senior adults, increasing intraneural fat can be found. In addition, prominent vessels mimicking bright fascicles can be identified with increasing age within the nerve. Skeletal muscles usually do not show signs of aging over many years. However, with increasing age fatty streaks within skeletal muscles should be considered normal, as compared to young adults or children where muscles usually appear compact and homogenous on all imaging techniques.

Pathophysiology, Classification Systems and Nerve Regeneration

Various didactic approaches exist to describe and categorize the pathophysiology of peripheral neuropathies. Pathologic conditions of peripheral nerves include traumatic injuries (crush, compression or penetration), compression or entrapment neuropathies, as well as hereditary, inflammatory and infectious conditions. Tumors are not very frequent, but represent another group of pathology. Beginners in peripheral nerve evaluation should focus on common etiologies such as trauma and entrapment, as the other diseases are usually rare and should always get a second opinion from an expert in nerve imaging [6].

Traumatic Injuries

Traumatic injuries are most commonly described according to the Seddon classification system. In this system, three different types of nerve injury are described: neuropraxia, axonotmesis and neurotmesis [8]. Neuropraxia is the lowest level of injury, meaning that the nerve, i.e. the axons, remains intact but the signaling ability is hampered. Axonotmesis is the second degree. It's meaning is easy to remember as in axonotmesis the axons are damaged. The surrounding soft tissue remains intact and preserves the nerve trunk from discontinuity. The latter is present in the third and highest degree, neurotmesis, which is characterized by disrupted nerve fibers and full loss of nerve function.

Another popular system is the Sunderland classification [8]. Class I and II injuries are the same as Seddon's neuropraxia and axonotmesis, respectively (Table 1). Class III-V lesions are included in Seddon's neurotmesis. Class III

Table 1 The Seddon and Sunderland classification systems [8]

						Electrophysiology			MRN findings
Class of nerve injury	Myelin	Axon	Endoneurium	Perineurium	Epineurium	Sensory nerve action potential	Compound motor action potential	Electromyography	
I- *Neurapraxia*	Abnormal	Normal	Normal	Normal	Normal	Normal	Normal or conduction block	Normal but interference pattern decreased	Hyperintense nerve
II- *Axonotmesis*	Abnormal	Abnormal	Normal	Normal	Normal	Amplitude decreased	Amplitude decreased	interference pattern and spontaneous activity decreased	Hyperintense and thickened nerve with/ without prominent fascicles
III	Abnormal	Abnormal	Abnormal	Normal	Normal				
IV	Abnormal	Abnormal	Abnormal	Abnormal	Normal				Heterogeneous nerve signal with lateral or fusiform neuroma in continuity
V-*Neurotmesis*	Abnormal	Abnormal	Abnormal	Abnormal	Abnormal	Absent	Absent	No motor unit potentials	Complete nerve gap

lesions have lesions of the endoneurium but the perineurium and epineurium must remain intact. Class IV lesions have a damage to the perineurium in addition to Class III lesions. Class V lesions are the most severe lesions with complete nerve transection. Class IV and V lesions typically lead to significant nerve dysfunction and usually require immediate surgical treatment. Class I-III lesions can be treated conservatively, however, detailed diagnosis and lesion characterization is needed for any management decision.

Nerve Compression and Entrapment Neuropathies

Nerve compression typically occurs at specific anatomic sites leading to what is termed an entrapment neuropathy [9]. Typically, these are chronic conditions. Classic examples for nerve compression or entrapment syndromes are carpal tunnel syndrome and cubital tunnel syndrome. However, compression neuropathies may occur at many more sites or tunnels in the body including the pelvic floor region, the popliteal space, the tarsal tunnel, the dorsal foot, the thoracic outlet, the infraclavicular region, quadrilateral space, the elbow, the forearm, the canal of Guyon, etc. It is beyond the scope of this syllabus to explain these lesions in detail, but the most important upper extremity entrapment syndromes e.g. have been described in the 2013 IDKD syllabus book as well as other good review articles [10–13].

External nerve compression blocks the normal flow of endoneurium fluid. In addition, compression of the venous flow occurs which typically leads to vascular congestion and local hyperemia at the compression side and proximal to it. This is important to understand as abnormalities on magnetic resonance neurography images will show correspondingly signal changes of the nerve at the side of compression and proximal to it. The pathophysiology of entrapment syndromes is different from acute nerve pathologies, as the development of compressive neuropathy depends mostly on long-term or repetitive pressure within these tunnels and the fact that nerves typically can withstand only little external pressure. At more than 15 mmHg, the venous drainage of the nerves is increasingly hampered, and at over 40 mmHg the arterial blood supply is affected. Irreversible structural nerve damage begins at pressures of around 80 mmHg [3]. In patients where the external compression continues for a longer period, there is a loss of myelin with associated risk of permanent axonal damage, Wallerian degeneration, nerve infarction and nerve fibrosis [14].

Spontaneous nerve healing in chronic nerve compression or entrapment syndromes is very unlikely. However, with surgery, good results and nerve recovery can be achieved, i.e. when the diagnosis is made prior to chronic and often irreversible nerve changes [15]. The latter is characterized by fat and/or fibrous tissue proliferation around the affected axons.

Nerve Regeneration

Nerve regeneration usually proceeds slowly from the anterior horn cells of the spinal cord (the location of the main cell body of a peripheral nerve) to the neuromuscular endplate a rate of 1 mm per day or approximately 1 in. per month. Therefore, depending on the length of the nerve fibers, it is easy to calculate the likely recovery time. For "spontaneous" recovery of long extremity nerves, it may take up to 1–1½ years. As a practical example, it may take up to 2 years to return full motor function to the distal forearm after a brachial plexus injury [16].

It must be also noted that functional nerve recovery does not occur in all pathologies. There can be a persistent lack of full sensory and/or motor function; there is typically no guarantee that even with primarily successful surgical therapy that normal function will be restored. The latter can be seen especially in chronic pathologies or hereditary neuropathies such as Charcot-Marie-Tooth disease (CMT) where either formation of "axon-deficient myelin ovoid" in axonal degeneration (CMT II) or "repeated myelination-related onion-bulb formation" (CMT I) is observed.

Technical Considerations and Normal Appearance of Nerves

For successful magnetic resonance neurography, the most practical advice may be the following: "simply use the best equipment which you have available". This includes the magnet, the radiofrequency coils, the pulse sequences and the software [17].

Scanner

Magnetic resonance neurography can be performed on 1.5 and 3.0 Tesla clinical scanners. When available, 3.0 Tesla is preferred due to the increased signal-to-noise ratio and superior contrast-to-noise ratio at higher spatial resolution. Especially 3-dimensional (3D) isotropic imaging benefits from higher field strength and shorter acquisition times. With high-end field strength, some drawbacks may arise such as increased B0 inhomogeneities that might cause poor fat suppression when spectral saturation pulses are used. Therefore, the use of STIR (short tau inversion recovery) or Dixon type fat suppression may be beneficial at 3.0 Tesla [17]. Another concern at 3.0 Tesla is the increased specific absorption rate, which might cause longer examination times. Of course, technical tricks exist to address these latter limitations such as reducing the refocusing flip angle to shortened acquisition time (e.g. 130° instead of 150°). However, despite some drawbacks, most experts favor the use of 3.0 Tesla scanners.

Coils

Whenever possible, the use dedicated multichannel surface coils is advised. These should be—as always in magnetic resonance imaging—be placed as close as possible to the anatomy of interest. While seemingly simple, this can be quite challenging when imaging several anatomic regions needing different coils or if a larger field-of-view needs to be covered. Some scanners allow combined use of multiple coils, whereas with other scanners, coils need to be changed during the study.. Dedicated joint coils can also be used in combination with flex or surface coils in some scanners which, for example, allows the use of high-resolution wrist coils to examine the median nerve in the wrist in combination with a flex coil that covers the forearm. This combination allows seamless examination of the median nerve in the forearm, wrist and hand at the same time. If a specific field-of-view is still too large to be covered even with the use of coil combination, then a stepwise-approach, first using nerve ultrasound to narrow down the possible site of injury and with subsequent dedicated magnetic resonance imaging of that remaining nerve section may be helpful. Along these lines, it is important that referring physicians understand the tradeoffs between spatial resolution and anatomic coverage in magnetic resonance neurography. It is almost always preferable to scan a small region in high detail than to try to survey a large amount of anatomy for possible nerve pathology.

Training of the technician/technologist is an often forgotten but nevertheless extremely important issue. Technicians should also be taught to identify target anatomic structures (they should be able to identify the nerve-of-interest); to correctly position patients (e.g. the region-of-interest should be placed in the scanners isocenter whenever possible); and to correctly plan pulse sequences (e.g. to avoid wraparound artifacts).

Sequences

Much has been written about pulse sequence developments for magnetic resonance neurography and several new techniques have been published including variations of 3D FSE (fast spin echo) acquisitions. The latter are based on technical advancements and are available as product sequences (e.g. Siemens; SPACE; Philips: VISTA, Views; and GE: Cube) [4]. The basic principle of the sequences when used and optimized for magnetic resonance neurography is to reduce the refocusing flip angles to decrease the sensitivity to flow. When assessing images, it is obvious that these sequences adequately suppress the arterial signal, however, venous signal contamination remains a frequent problem due to slow flow. Hence, these 3D FSE sequences are often combined with either a weak gradient pulse to reduce venous signal or with motion sensitizing driven equilibrium (MSDE) for further reduction of the venous flow signal. For example, SHINKEI (nerve-SHeath signal increased with INKed rest-tissue RARE Imaging) is a 3D FSE sequence variant with SPAIR for fat suppression and MSDE for blood suppression [18]. These 3D sequences are especially helpful for brachial and/or lumbosacral plexus imaging [19].

While advanced 3D sequences are helpful (Fig. 1), the mainstay for peripheral nerve imaging, especially in the extremities, is the use of conventional pulse sequences including T1, T2, T2 with fat saturation, STIR, and post contrast T1 fat suppression FSE type imaging. Most routine neurography protocols are based on these sequences and extended by some of the new techniques including the abovementioned 3D techniques and diffusion weighted imaging or diffusion tensor imaging techniques. In the author's opinions, proton density (PD) weighting is not advised for magnetic resonance neurography because normal nerves display intrinsically brighter signal on PD sequences, making it difficult to assess for pathological nerve hyperintensity.

The morphological sequences should be of the highest possible in plane resolution, while typically a lower through plane resolution (= thicker slice thickness) is accepted e.g.

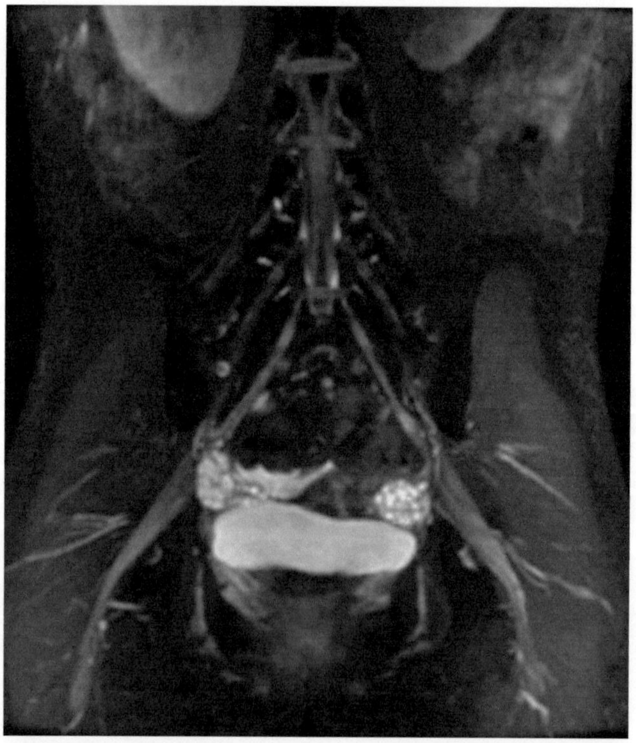

Fig. 1 20 year old woman with diffuse lumbosacral neuritis. Coronal maximum intensity projection (MIP) created from a 3D, T2 weighted fat suppressed acquisition of the lumbosacral plexus at 3.0T. While MIP images can nicely display nerve abnormalities, the primary interpretation is made on source images

for better field-of-view coverage in extremities. Whether axial planes, sagittal or coronal planes are preferred depends on the anatomy of interest as well as the personal choice of the radiologists. In our personal experience, axial planes provide the most accurate information and allow true cross-section imaging of the peripheral nerve, especially in the extremities. Coronal and sagittal planes can be helpful for illustration purposes, but it is often difficult to evaluate small nerves on longitudinal planes due to their course that brings them in or out of plane.

A final note needs to be made on fat suppression as it is of utmost importance in peripheral nerve imaging to achieve a robust and spatially homogeneous fat suppression. Global variations in signal intensity across an image from inhomogeneous fat suppression or other coil effects can make a nerve appear relatively more hyperintense than its contralateral counterpart (e.g. right versus left sciatic nerve), creating an opportunity for incorrect diagnosis. As mentioned above, the selective use of STIR sequences and Dixon type fat suppression can be helpful, especially in the 3.0 Tesla environment [20].

Normal and Abnormal Imaging Appearances

Typically, eight different criteria are used in the assessment of peripheral nerves [2, 6]:

Size

A normal peripheral nerve shows a similar size compared to the adjacent arteries. This is best viewed on axial slices. Normal peripheral nerves gradually decrease in size from proximal to distal. This is a basic rule which can often help to identify the site of pathology, especially in compressive or entrapment syndromes, where the nerve diameter may increase proximal to the site of compression (see above). Focal or diffuse nerve enlargements are a sign of a possible pathology as well. In cases where the nerve is consistently larger than the adjacent artery over a long distance, a reader may be fooled into interpreting the nerve as normal but "well seen", however the consistent enlargement of a nerve relative to the adjacent artery is indeed the pathology; such diffusely thickened nerves should raise the suspicion for an inflammatory or infectious etiology.

Signal Intensity

The second most important criteria to assess is signal intensity. The normal nerve on T1-weighted and T2-weighted images appears isointense to skeletal muscle. On T2-weighted fat suppressed images, the normal nerve signal is isointense to minimally hyperintense. On the 3D FSE sequences, a normal peripheral nerve appears uniform and symmetrically hyperintense. Pathology is indicated by an even higher hyperintensity on T2-weighted sequences, approaching the T2 signal of adjacent veins. Any elevation in signal intensity of peripheral nerve might be considered suspicious.

Fascicular Pattern

As mentioned above, the fascicular pattern of peripheral nerves can be appreciated on high-resolution MR images (Fig. 2). This is especially true for axial T1 -weighted and T2-weighted sequences. The fascicular pattern should always be present and should never be effaced. In case of single or multiple fascicle enlargement or even disruption, nerve pathology must be considered (Fig. 3). Also, any diffuse loss of the fascicular pattern should raise the suspicion for pathology. Experienced readers have a very good feeling for the fascicular pattern of different peripheral nerves at different anatomic locations. Beginners are advised to train themselves to interpret peripheral nerve anatomy and signal intensities on every scan they read, even if it is not a magnetic resonance neurography examination. For example, train yourself while reading standard knee examinations and look for look for the size, signal intensity, and fascicular pattern of the peroneal and tibial nerves. Doing the same in other body regions as well will soon help beginners to develop to an expert.

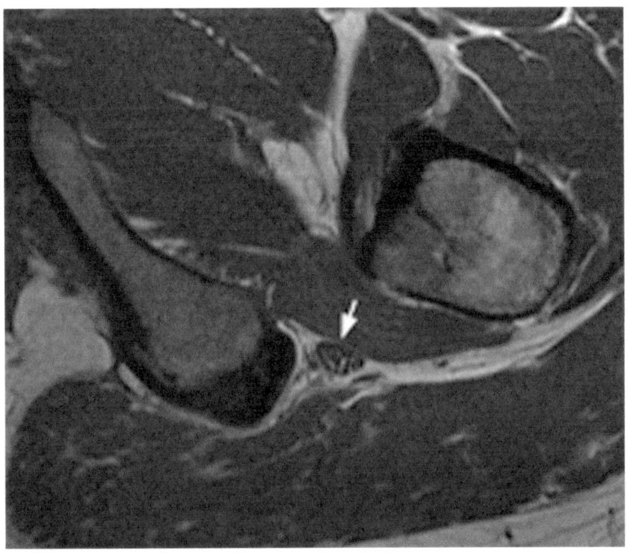

Fig. 2 Normal fascicular pattern of the sciatic nerve (*arrow*) at the level of the ischial tuberosity. Axial T1 weighted image obtained at 3.0T

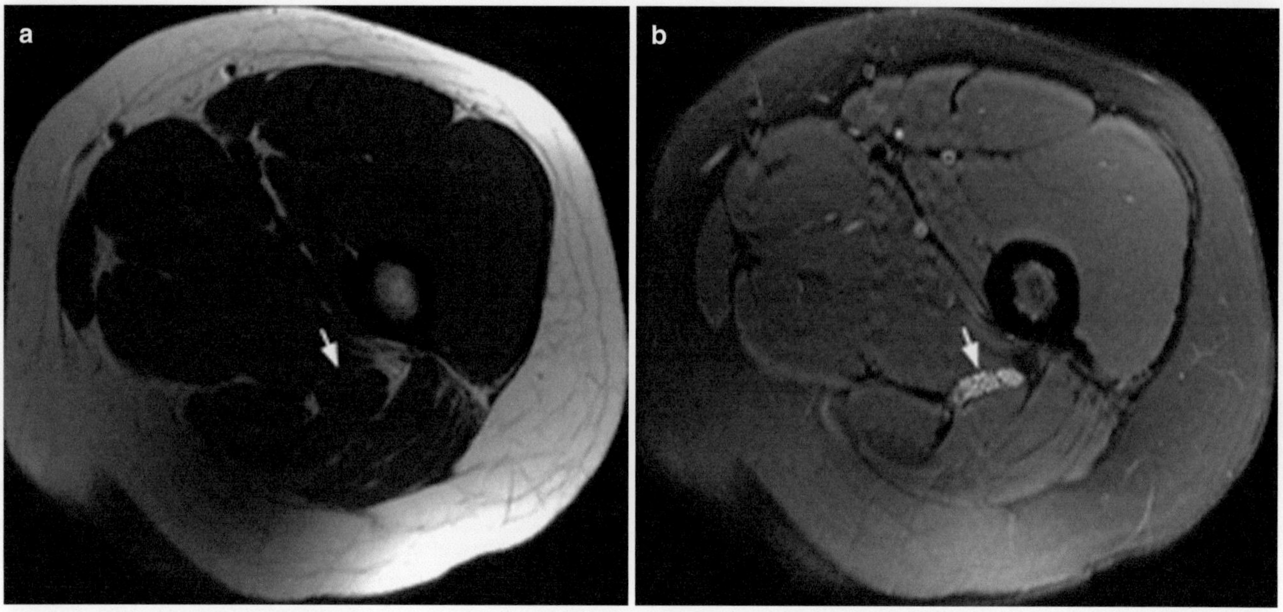

Fig. 3 21 year old woman with hereditary neuropathy liable to pressure palsies (HNPP). (**a**) Axial T1 weighted image of the mid thigh shows enlarged sciatic nerve (*arrow*) consisting of its tibial and common peroneal components. (**b**) Axial T2 fat suppressed image at the same level demonstrated markedly enlarged nerve (*arrow*) with hyperintense fascicles. In this patient, the entirety of both sciatic nerves were involved

Course

Normal peripheral nerves show a smooth course without deviations. Normal peripheral nerves also have few branches, and most branches are well known, especially the larger branches of large nerves. Those branches always course towards the innervated muscles. Normal peripheral nerves do not exhibit wavy courses, sharp angles, or diffuse branching. Bifid nerves can occur, such as in the pelvis where the sciatic nerve might be divided into two portions as a normal variant [21]. Any focal or diffuse deviation or sharp angulation should raise the suspicion of pathology.

Continuity

Normal peripheral nerves follow an uninterrupted, continuous course. Any discontinuity represents an abnormality. It is important to be aware that artifacts, especially nearby metal implants can lead to apparent zones of discontinuity and this should not be misinterpreted.

Perineural Fat

Peripheral nerves are usually surrounded by a clean fat plane. Depending on the actual anatomic site, this fat plane can be thick or thin. Sometimes it is hardly visible, i.e. in slim patients as well as when the peripheral nerve runs parallel to skeletal muscle (such as in the forearm). However, perineural stranding on T1- or T2-weighted images and encasement along a peripheral nerve must be considered abnormal, especially after surgery or penetrating injuries. Chronic nerve compression from external sources can also lead to perineural fibrosis/scarring which must be detected as it hampers "spontaneous" recovery. Axial slices might be the best to detect perineural fat effacement.

Contrast Enhancement

Normal peripheral nerves do not take up gadolinium based contrast agents after intravenous injection. Exceptions include areas of deficient blood-nerve barrier such as the dorsal nerve root ganglion. In tumors and infections there is also typically disruption of the blood-nerve barrier, which can be seen as focal or diffuse contrast enhancement. There are different philosophies on the use of gadolinium based contrast agents in standard magnetic resonance neurography examinations. Some experts use them in dedicated cases only such as in postoperative conditions or where inflammatory or infectious diseases are suspected. Other experts routinely use contrast agents as they want to improve the sensitivity for nerve pathology overall. For one of the authors of this syllabus, the use of contrast agents is routine and seen to have advantages, particularly when patients referred for magnetic resonance neurography examinations come with an unclear clinical history. For the other author, almost all neurography studies are performed as non-contrast examinations, with contrast used selectively in cases where the tumor or a diffuse neuritis is suspected, or if the patient is post-operative for a nerve condition.

Muscles

Muscle denervation is a sequela of a neurogenic pathology. Identification of the muscles involved and knowledge about the innervation pattern of the motor nerves in that body part can assist in the identification of the exact site of nerve lesion. In the acute or subacute setting, denervation may result in muscle edema manifest as increased T2 signal, without necessarily showing decreased muscle bulk. In more chronic denervation, muscles may show fatty infiltration and atrophy. Muscle abnormalities only occur in neuropathies where motor branches of nerves are affected. Pure sensory neuropathies are not expected to cause muscle denervation

Conclusions

A number of pathological conditions can affect peripheral nerves, and it is important for the radiologist to be vigilant in examining nerves in any magnetic resonance study. This syllabus has provided a short overview of neuromuscular anatomy and relevant pathophysiology. Moreover, it has discussed technical requirements and described the normal and abnormal appearance of nerves. A structured approach for nerve assessment has been provided by describing eight criteria that often prove useful in the clinical routine. For further reading, the list of references should be helpful.

References

1. Pham M, Baumer T, Bendszus M (2014) Peripheral nerves and plexus: imaging by MR-neurography and high-resolution ultrasound. Curr Opin Neurol 27(4):370–379
2. Chhabra A, Andreisek G (2012) Magnetic resonance neurography. Jaypee, London
3. Filler AG, Howe FA, Hayes CE et al (1993) Magnetic resonance neurography. Lancet 341(8846):659–661
4. Chhabra A, Zhao L, Carrino JA et al (2013) MR neurography: advances. Radiol Res Pract 2013:809568
5. Baumer P, Kele H, Kretschmer T et al (2014) Thoracic outlet syndrome in 3T MR neurography-fibrous bands causing discernible lesions of the lower brachial plexus. Eur Radiol 24(3):756–761
6. Chhabra A (2014) Peripheral MR neurography: approach to interpretation. Neuroimaging Clin N Am 24(1):79–89
7. Eppenberger P, Andreisek G, Chhabra A (2014) Magnetic resonance neurography: diffusion tensor imaging and future directions. Neuroimaging Clin N Am 24(1):245–256
8. Chhabra A, Ahlawat S, Belzberg A, Andreseik G (2014) Peripheral nerve injury grading simplified on MR neurography: as referenced to Seddon and Sunderland classifications. Indian J Radiol Imaging 24(3):217–224
9. Andreisek G, Burg D, Studer A, Weishaupt D (2008) Upper extremity peripheral neuropathies: role and impact of MR imaging on patient management. Eur Radiol 18(9):1953–1961
10. Andreisek G, Bencarino J (2013) Neuropathies of the upper extremity. In: Hodler J (ed) Musculoskeletal diseases. Springer, Milan
11. Deniel A, Causeret A, Moser T, Rolland Y, Dreano T, Guillin R (2015) Entrapment and traumatic neuropathies of the elbow and hand: an imaging approach. Diagn Interv Imaging 96(12): 1261–1278
12. Donovan A, Rosenberg ZS, Cavalcanti CF (2010) MR imaging of entrapment neuropathies of the lower extremity. Part 2. The knee, leg, ankle, and foot. Radiographics 30(4):1001–1019
13. Petchprapa CN, Rosenberg ZS, Sconfienza LM, Cavalcanti CF, Vieira RL, Zember JS (2010) MR imaging of entrapment neuropathies of the lower extremity. Part 1. The pelvis and hip. Radiographics 30(4):983–1000
14. Beaulieu C, Does MD, Snyder RE, Allen PS (1996) Changes in water diffusion due to Wallerian degeneration in peripheral nerve. Magn Reson Med 36(4):627–631
15. Thawait SK, Wang K, Subhawong TK et al (2012) Peripheral nerve surgery: the role of high-resolution MR neurography. AJNR Am J Neuroradiol 33(2):203–210
16. Chhabra A, Lee PP, Bizzell C, Soldatos T (2011) 3 Tesla MR neurography—technique, interpretation, and pitfalls. Skelet Radiol 40(10):1249–1260
17. Chhabra A, Flammang A, Padua A Jr, Carrino JA, Andreisek G (2014) Magnetic resonance neurography: technical considerations. Neuroimaging Clin N Am 24(1):67–78
18. Kasper JM, Wadhwa V, Scott KM, Rozen S, Xi Y, Chhabra A (2015) SHINKEI—a novel 3D isotropic MR neurography technique: technical advantages over 3DIRTSE-based imaging. Eur Radiol 25(6):1672–1677
19. Soldatos T, Andreisek G, Thawait GK et al (2013) High-resolution 3-T MR neurography of the lumbosacral plexus. Radiographics 33(4):967–987
20. Reeder SB, Yu H, Johnson JW et al (2006) T1- and T2-weighted fast spin-echo imaging of the brachial plexus and cervical spine with IDEAL water-fat separation. J Magn Reson Imaging 24(4):825–832
21. Kraus E, Tenforde AS, Beaulieu CF, Ratliff J, Fredericson M (2016) Piriformis syndrome with variant sciatic nerve anatomy: a case report. PM R 8(2):176–179

Postoperative Knee

Hassan Douis and Mark E. Schweitzer

Introduction

Reconstruction of the anterior cruciate ligament and meniscal surgery are the two most common indications when surgery for internal derangement of the knee is performed. In contrast, repairs of the medial collateral ligament and the medial patellofemoral ligament are less commonly performed whilst posterior cruciate ligament reconstructions remain relatively rare. In case of continued or recurrent pain or instability after surgery, MRI is frequently performed. Therefore, knowledge of common surgical techniques, familiarity with normal MRI-findings of the postoperative knee and the potential complications after knee surgery is crucial to derive to an accurate diagnosis.

MRI-Protocol of the Postoperative Knee

When considering an appropriate MRI-protocol for the evaluation of the postoperative knee, it is crucial to take into consideration that susceptibility artefacts due to metal implants or metal fragments may significantly hamper interpretation of the MRI-study. It is therefore vital to adjust and optimize the MR-imaging protocol in order to minimize metal artefacts.

At our institution, conventional MRI is used as the first imaging investigation in the assessment of the postoperative knee with the acquisition of fat-suppressed proton-density-weighted sequences in the axial, sagittal and coronal plane, a sagittal T2W SE and a coronal T1W SE sequence. In contrast, direct MR-arthrography at our institution is primarily used for assessment of the integrity of the postoperative meniscus. There remains controversy if patients after meniscus surgery should undergo conventional MRI first followed by MR-arthrography in cases of diagnostic uncertainty or whether to perform direct MR-arthrography as the first MR-investigation [1]. For direct MR-arthrography, our protocol is to perform T1W SE sequences with fat-suppression in the axial, sagittal and coronal plane and a fat-suppressed fluid-sensitive sequence in the sagittal plane after intra-articular injection of 30–40 ml of dilute gadolinium (2 mmol/l gadopentate dimeglumine).

Anterior Cruciate Ligament (ACL)

ACL-Reconstruction

The most widely used surgical techniques for reconstruction of the anterior cruciate ligament utilize bone-patellar tendon-bone autograft or a hamstring tendon autograft where usually the semitendinosus tendon and gracilis tendon are harvested although occasionally only the semitendinosus tendon is used [2–5]. The ACL can be reconstructed using a single-bundle technique or a double-bundle technique. The single-bundle technique remains by far the most widely used ACL-reconstruction technique [6]. This technique reconstructs the stronger anteromedial bundle and is performed by creating one femoral tunnel and one tibial tunnel. In contrast, the technically more challenging double-bundle reconstruction aims to reproduce the native anatomy of the ACL by reconstructing both the anteromedial and posterolateral bundle of the ACL separately. This technique requires the creation of two femoral tunnels and two tibial tunnels and placement of two grafts [2–4, 7]. A recent Cochrane database meta-analysis demonstrated that the double-bundle technique achieved better anteroposterior and rotational knee stability. Functional outcomes were similar to the single-bundle technique [8].

H. Douis (✉)
Department of Radiology, University Hospital Birmingham, Mindelsohn Way, Birmingham, West Midlands B15 2GW, UK
e-mail: hassan.douis@uhb.nhs.uk

M.E. Schweitzer
Department of Radiology, Stony Brook University, HSC level 4, Room 120, Stony Brook, NY 11794-8460, USA
e-mail: Mark.schweitzer@stonybrookmedicine.edu

J. Hodler et al. (eds.), *Musculoskeletal Diseases 2017-2020*, DOI 10.1007/978-3-319-54018-4_15

Normal Postoperative MRI-Findings After ACL-Reconstruction

The normal signal characteristics of ACL-graft reconstruction are dependent on the age and type of the graft. Within the first 3–4 months after ACL-graft reconstruction, the graft is avascular and is therefore typically of low signal intensity on all pulse sequences. Four to eight months after surgery, the graft gradually undergoes revascularization and resynovialisation resulting in mild increased signal intensity of the graft on both T1-weighted and T2-weighted images. 12–18 months after surgery, the ACL-graft will start to resemble histologically a ligament and therefore on MR, the signal will return to a low signal intensity on all pulse sequences (Fig. 1). This process is also termed "ligamentization" of the tendon graft. It is crucial not to misinterpret the increased signal intensity of the tendon graft which is observed during some of the stages of the ligamentization process as a sign of impingement [5, 9, 10].

Hamstring tendon grafts demonstrate distinct imaging features due to the nature of the graft reconstruction. The two tendons are sutured together, folded onto one another, and subsequently sutured together again, resulting in a graft composed of four separate bundles folded twice (so-called M-technique). This unique configuration of the hamstring tendon graft therefore results in linear areas of mild to moderate increased signal intensity on fluid-sensitive sequences between the double-folded graft which is due to entrapped foci of fluid and granulation tissue between the graft bundles. With this particular graft reconstruction, fluid may also be observed within the femoral and tibial tunnel [5, 10].

Correct position of the femoral and tibial tunnels is crucial. Figure 2 demonstrates the accurate position of the tunnels and the graft. The graft typically demonstrates a straight, taut configuration and should lie dorsal to Blumensaat's line. In order to assess accurate tunnel position, it is useful to divide the AP-diameter of the intercondylar notch and the tibial plateau each in four equal-length segments (see Fig. 2). On sagittal images, the femoral tunnel should lie at the intersection of the posterior femoral cortex and the posterior intercondylar roof (at or dorsal to segment 4 of the femur; see Fig. 2). In contrast, the tibial tunnel should be posterior to Blumensaat's line with the centre of the tunnel situated in

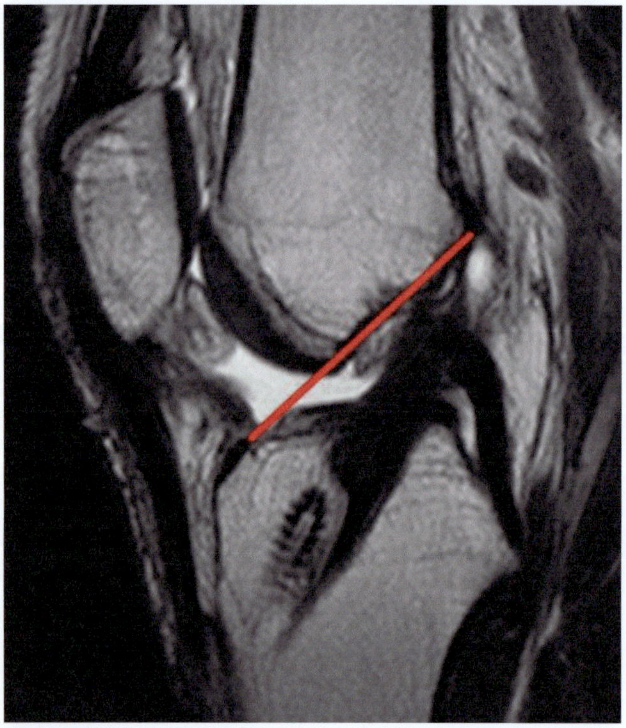

Fig. 1 Sagittal T2-weighted image of a normal ACL reconstruction. The graft is of homogenous low signal intensity 18 months after surgery. Also note the graft and the tibial tunnel are located posterior to Blumensaat's line (*red line*)

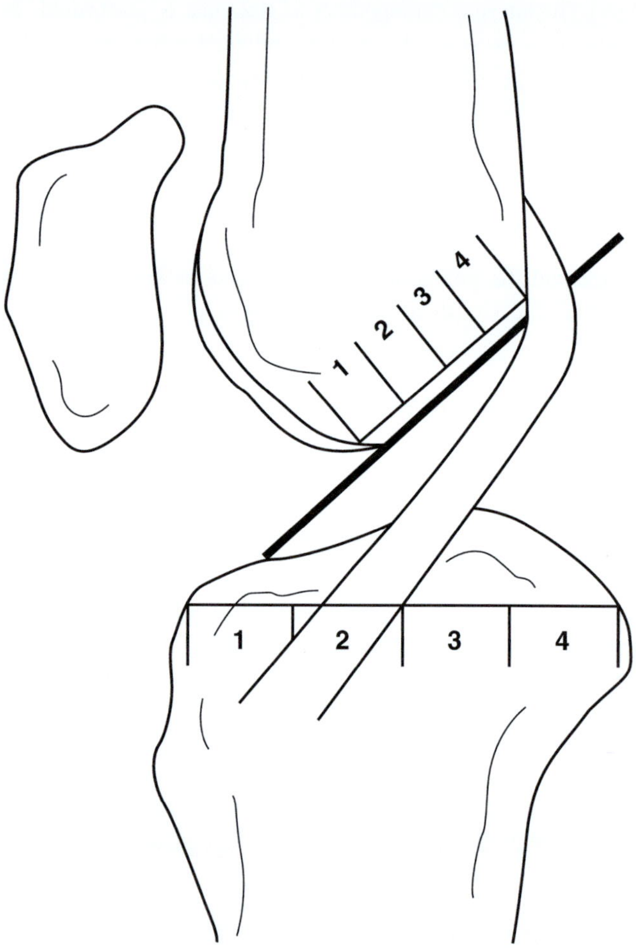

Fig. 2 The drawing shows the correct position of the femoral and tibial tunnels as well as the graft in relation to Blumensaat's line after single-bundle reconstruction. Note that the graft is located posteror to Blumensaat's line. (drawing adapted from: Woertler K (2014) Anterior cruciate ligament reconstruction. In: Woertler K, Waldt S (eds) Measurements and classifications in musculoskeletal radiology. Thieme, Stuttgart, New York, p 58

segment 2 of the tibia as demonstrated in Figs. 1 and 2 [2–4, 10]. On coronal images, the femoral tunnel should be at the posterosuperior corner of the intercondylar notch at 10–11 o'clock for the right knee and at 1–2 o'clock for the left knee. Similarly, the tibial tunnel on coronal images should be centred on the intercondylar eminence [2–4]. A far anterior femoral tunnel or a far posterior tibial tunnel position may cause instability of the graft. In contrast, a tibial tunnel position that is too anteriorly located may result in a more horizontal alignment of the graft and in possible graft impingement.

Complications of ACL Reconstruction

Complications after ACL-reconstruction include: graft rupture, graft stretching, graft impingement, arthrofibrosis, cyst formation and tunnel widening, mucoid degeneration of the graft, hardware failure and impingement due to metalwork, intra-articular loose bodies, infection and donor site pathology.

Graft Rupture

The ACL-graft is most susceptible to injury during the revascularisation process of the graft which occurs 4–8 months after surgery. However, graft ruptures typically occur after trauma and are clinically characterized by instability. Similar to the MRI-diagnosis of complete preoperative ACL-tears, MRI-findings of complete postoperative ACL-graft ruptures can be divided into direct and indirect signs. Direct signs of ACL-graft rupture are complete discontinuity or deficiency of the graft fibres and fluid-like increased signal intensity completely traversing the graft. Indirect signs of ACL-graft rupture are anterior tibial translation, buckling of the PCL, posterior displacement of the posterior horn of the lateral meniscus and new bone marrow oedema-like signal affecting the posterolateral tibial plateau and the lateral femoral condyle. The accuracy of conventional MRI in the diagnosis of ACL-rupture after graft reconstruction is however slightly lower than the diagnostic accuracy for ACL-tears in the preoperative knee. Furthermore, indirect signs of ACL-graft rupture are not specific for ACL-graft rupture and may also be present in cases of malposition of the ACL-graft. In contrast, MR-arthrography has been reported to have a sensitivity of 100% and a specificity of 89–100% in the diagnosis of postoperative ACL-graft tears [3–5, 10].

Graft Impingement

Graft impingement can result in restriction of knee joint extension and increases the risk of graft rupture. Graft impingement may be due to tunnel positioning or less

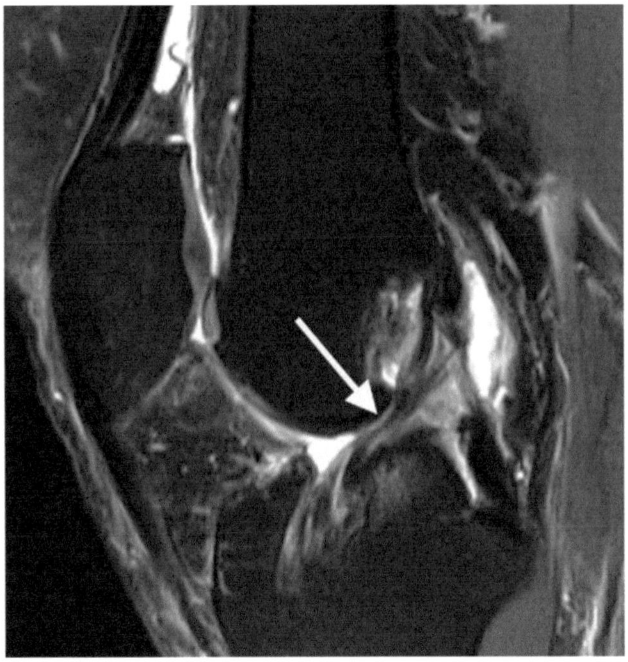

Fig. 3 Sagittal intermediate-weighted fat-saturated image of ACL-reconstruction demonstrating graft impingement. The graft is frayed, shows increased signal intensity within the distal 2/3 of the fibres and demonstrates kinking at the anterior margin of the intercondylar notch (*arrow*)

commonly due to osteophyte formation or the result of protrusion of tunnel screws. The most common cause for graft impingement is a far anterior position of the tibial tunnel whilst a far lateral placement of the tibial tunnel is less common. In these cases, the ACL-graft abuts the roof or the side wall of the intercondylar notch during knee extension therefore resulting in graft shearing and fraying which ultimately may cause graft rupture [11]. On MRI, in addition to malposition of the graft, graft impingement demonstrates increased signal intensity within the fibres at the site of impingement on T1-and T2-weighted images and kinking of the graft at the anterior margin of the intercondylar notch (Fig. 3). Within the first 12 months after graft reconstruction, it can be difficult to differentiate if signal changes within the graft are due to impingement or due to revascularisation. Signal change limited to the distal 2/3 of the graft, kinking of the graft as well as persistence of the signal changes beyond 12 months after surgery favour the diagnosis of graft impingement [5, 10].

Arthrofibrosis

Patients suffering from arthrofibrosis clinically present with restricted movement and pain. The incidence of arthrofibrosis after ACL-graft reconstruction is 5–10% [12]. Two distinct forms of arthrofibrosis are described: localised anterior arthrofibrosis and diffuse arthrofibrosis [7, 10].

Localized Anterior Arthrofibrosis

Localised anterior arthrofibrosis (also called "cyclops lesion") is characterised by a well-defined nodule immediately anterior to the ACL-graft at the level of the tibial plateau. On arthroscopy, it bears resemblance to the single eye of the giant "cyclops" in Greek mythology. Histologically, cyclops lesions largely consist of fibrous granulation tissue with some cases containing bony fragments and synovium [13]. Whilst cyclops lesions are observed in 1–10% of all patients after ACL-graft reconstruction, only a minority of patients are symptomatic (up to 2% of all patients after ACL-graft reconstruction) [13, 14]. Symptoms are thought to be due to impingement of the cyclops lesion between the femur and tibia which may result in an audible clunk. Whilst the aetiology of cyclops lesions remains uncertain, it has been postulated that they may originate from a residual tibial ACL stump, infrapatellar fat pad metaplasia, or the graft itself. On MRI, cyclops lesions appear as nodular lesions located immediately anterior to the distal aspect of the ACL-graft and are of low to intermediate signal intensity on all pulse sequences (Fig. 4) [13, 14]. The diagnostic accuracy of MRI in the detection of cyclops lesions is 85% and increases to more than 90% in lesions larger than 1 cm [13].

Diffuse Arthrofibrosis

Diffuse arthrofibrosis is associated with significant restriction of movement which is due to extensive fibrosis located anterior to the ACL-graft extending into Hoffa's fat pad, the suprapatellar recess and sometimes into the posterior aspect of the knee joint. On MRI, diffuse arthrofibrosis manifests as diffuse areas of low signal intensity on all pulse sequences which is more pronounced than the scar tissue observed after knee surgery [3, 4, 7, 15].

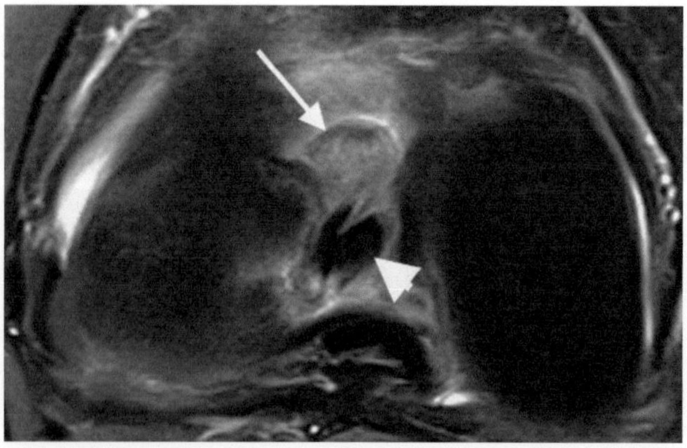

Fig. 4 Axial intermediate-weighted fat-saturated image after ACL-reconstruction demonstrating a cyclops lesion. A well-defined nodular lesion which is of intermediate signal intensity (*long thin arrow*) located immediately anterior to the ACL-graft (*thick, small arrow*) is in keeping with a cyclops lesion

Tunnel Widening and Cyst Formation

In the early postoperative period, it is common to observe a small amount of fluid in the fixation tunnels which may moderately enlarge. However, cyst formation within the tunnel with subsequent tunnel widening exceeding 20 mm may be due to incomplete graft incorporation. The tibial tunnel is most commonly affected. Occasionally, cysts may extend into the pretibial region resulting in a clinically palpable swelling. Cyst formation is more common with hamstring grafts. Its association with graft failure remains uncertain. However, extensive tunnel expansion may complicate ACL graft revision surgery. On MRI, cyst formation results in increased tunnel diameter. Within the tunnel there is low signal intensity on T1-weighted images and increased signal intensity on T2-weighted images in keeping with fluid and/or granulation tissue [3, 16]. Furthermore, granulation tissue will demonstrate avid enhancement after gadolinium administration. Osteolysis is particularly well identified adjacent to bioabsorbable grafts due to minimal susceptibility artefacts [10].

Donor-Site Morbidity

Occasionally, complications may arise at the donor site. This particularly affects bone-patellar tendon-bone grafts where patellar tendinosis, patellar tendon rupture or patellar fracture may occur [4]. However increased signal intensity and thickening of the patellar tendon as well as a central gap at the site of tendon harvesting are normal postoperative findings within the first 2 years after surgery [3, 17]. It is therefore crucial to correlate the clinical and imaging findings.

Posterior Cruciate Ligament (PCL)

Posterior cruciate ligament injury is rare, and are mainly partial-thickness tears which may be treated conservatively. There has been increased interest in PCL-reconstructions in order to treat PCL instability and prevent premature osteoarthritis. Therefore, current indications for PCL-reconstruction are: acute or chronic PCL injuries with significant instability, associated avulsion fracture, and the presence of multiple ligamentous injuries [18].

PCL-Reconstruction

PCL-reconstruction largely utilize the same grafts as those used for ACL-reconstruction. The fixation of the graft may be directly onto the tibia (so-called "inlay technique") or through the tibial tunnel (also called "transtibial tunnel technique"), the latter being associated with impingement of the graft at

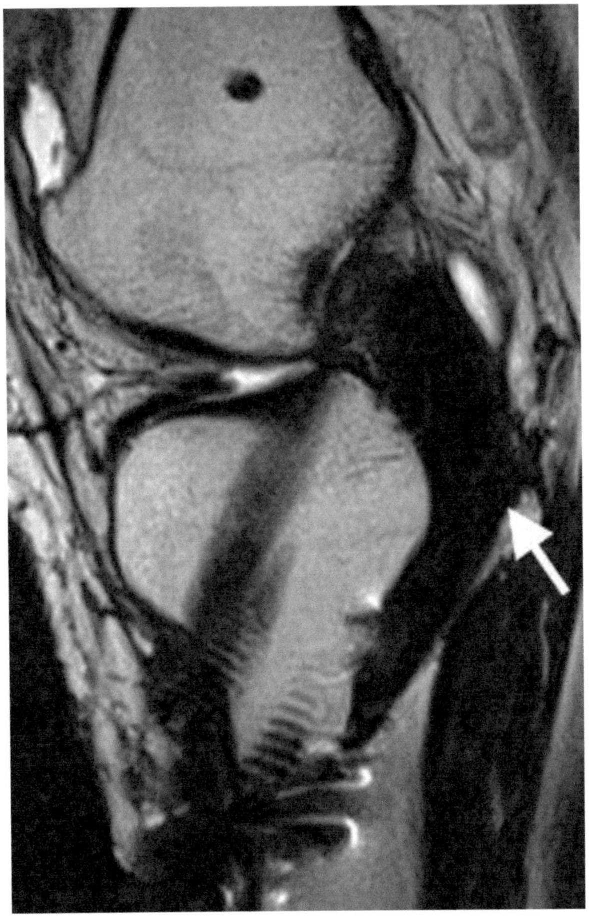

Fig. 5 Sagittal T2-weighted image of a normal PCL reconstruction using the transtibial tunnel technique. The PCL graft is thickened however it is of homogenous low signal intensity. Note the "killer turn" in the opening of the tibial tunnel (*arrow*), which is associated with impingement

the so-called "killer turn" point which occurs at the opening of the tibial tunnel (Fig. 5). Both single-bundle and double-bundle techniques are utilized. The single-bundle technique reconstructs the anterolateral bundle of the PCL and requires the creation of one femoral and one tibial tunnel. The double-bundle technique reconstructs both the anterolateral and the posteromedial bundle of the PCL and requires the drilling of two femoral tunnels and one single tibial tunnel. The double-bundle technique is technically more challenging and has not been proven to be superior [18, 19].

Normal Postoperative MRI-Findings After PCL-Reconstruction

The reconstructed PCL-graft undergoes the same signal changes as the ACL-graft. Thickening of the PCL-graft is frequently observed (Fig. 5) [20]. The position of the femoral tunnel in the single-bundle technique should be in the anterior half of the insertion site of the native PCL at 11 o'clock in the right knee or at 1 o'clock in the left knee on coronal images and it should be 8–10 mm away from the articular margin. The tibial fixation site on the sagittal images should be located in the middle of the posterior half of the retrospinal surface, 8–15 mm distal to the articular surface. On axial images, it should be immediately medial to the articular midline. A too anterior location of the tibial tunnel, a too posteriorly located or excessively high located femoral tunnel may result in instability. Bone marrow adjacent to the tunnels and the fixation sites may be present within the first 12 months after surgery [18].

Complications of PCL Reconstruction

Complications of PCL and ACL graft reconstruction are similar and include: graft rupture, graft laxity and impingement, arthrofibrosis, cyst formation and tunnel widening. Graft impingement is a noteworthy complication as it may occur due to the "killer turn" position in the transtibial technique or due to erroneous location of the tunnels [18, 20, 21]. On MRI, thickening and increased signal intensity on T1- and T2WI may be seen within the graft, which persists or worsens over time [18].

Medial Collateral Ligament (MCL)

Although isolated MCL injuries are usually treated conservatively, a complete tear of the MCL in combination with other ligamentous injuries or an isolated full-thickness tear which has failed conservative treatment may require surgery [22]. The MCL may be repaired using staples or sutures. On MRI after surgery, the MCL is typically thickened and of increased signal intensity on T2WI, occasionally demonstrating new bone formation. Later, the repair site may diminish in thickness and shows a decrease in signal intensity within the ligament in keeping with scar tissue formation [3].

Disruption of the MCL repair will appear as discontinuity of the ligament with fluid at the site.

Medial Patellofemoral Ligament (MPFL)

MPFL Surgery

Lateral patellar dislocation may result in medial patellofemoral ligament laxity or tear which in turn may lead to recurrent patellar dislocation. In these patients, MPFL repair or reconstruction is indicated if conservative treatment has failed. The concept of MPFL reconstruction is relatively new. However, the technique has gained popularity recently. The goal is to restore patellofemoral stability.

Various techniques have been described, including primary repair with or without augmentation, reconstruction using autologous tendon, allografts, and synthetic grafts. In MPFL reconstruction, a single- or double-bundle technique is used to fix the graft to the medial distal femur and the medial patella. Patellar fixation may be achieved by placement of bone anchors, creation of a patellar tunnel or by using a quadriceps autograft tendon. Femoral fixation can be performed by placement of a bone anchor, tunnel formation and screw placement, post and washer fixation and suturing [23, 24].

Normal Postoperative MRI-Findings of MPFL Reconstruction

On MRI, the normal graft is low signal intensity on T1- and T2-weighted images and appear continuous, taut and orientated along the anatomical course of the native MPFL. The patella and femoral anchor sites should be near the point of the expected native MPFL insertion [23, 25].

Complications of MPFL Reconstruction

Postoperative complications include patellar fracture, quadriceps avulsion fracture, protrusion of bone anchors or screws, graft laxity, persistent patellar instability and recurrent patellar dislocation which may lead to graft failure. On MRI, graft failure demonstrates fluid-like increased signal intensity within the graft, with partial or complete disruption of graft fibres [23, 25].

Meniscus

Meniscal Surgery

The aim of meniscal surgery is to improve patient symptoms and to maintain meniscal tissue. Loss of meniscal tissue is associated with an increased risk of osteoarthritis. The three forms of meniscal surgery are: meniscal repair, partial (or rarely total) meniscectomy and meniscal transplantation. Possible causes for persistent or recurrent postoperative pain are residual meniscal tears after partial meniscectomy, nonhealing meniscal sutures, dislocated meniscal fragments, meniscal re-tear after new trauma, cartilage defects and the development of osteoarthritis.

Indications for meniscal repair are post-traumatic vertical tears located in the peripheral ("red zone") meniscus, greater than 1 cm in length. The fragments can be fixed using a variety of sutures, bio absorbable arrows, tacks or darts. Partial meniscectomy is indicated if a tear is not amenable to repair. It may be performed as circumferential or segmental. A circumferential meniscectomy involves resection of the inner aspect of the meniscus whilst a segmental resection involves focal resection of almost the complete width of part of the meniscus. Meniscal transplantation is reserved for young patients who have symptomatic, irreparable meniscus tears or who have undergone previous meniscectomy with continued pain. It can be performed using allografts or synthetic scaffold implants (which are either polyurethane or collagen-based meniscal implants). In the procedure, anterior and posterior meniscal anchors are fixed using bone plugs and sutures with the margin of the meniscus sutured to the capsule.

Normal MRI-Findings After Meniscal Surgery

After successful meniscal repair, the meniscus may demonstrate a normal appearance and normal low signal intensity on all MR-sequences. However, within the first 12 months after successful repair, meniscal suture material may show linear increased signal intensity on T2WI which may simulate a re-tear.

In contrast, partial meniscectomy may show diminution of meniscal size and change in meniscal shape which include blunting of the meniscal margins or truncation of the meniscal horns. Furthermore, pre-existing increased signal intensity within the substance of the meniscus due to mucoid degeneration may extend into the resection surface margin of the meniscus after partial meniscectomy and mimic a re-tear.

On serial MRI, meniscal allograft transplantation show progressive increased signal intensity within the meniscus for at least a year, decreased width and increased thickness of the body segment as well as mild to moderate meniscus extrusion. Similarly, synthetic scaffold implants are initially of diffuse increased signal intensity on short and long TE pulse sequences due to the high water content within the scaffold which tends to diminish as the scaffold matures. Meniscus extrusion can be a normal postoperative finding [1, 26].

MRI of Recurrent Meniscal Tears

Taking into account the above mentioned mimickers of meniscal tears on conventional MRI of the postoperative meniscus, it is not surprising that the diagnostic accuracy of conventional MRI in the diagnosis of meniscal tears after meniscal surgery is lower when compared to MRI of the preoperative knee. This is predominantly the case for partial meniscectomies where more than 25% of the

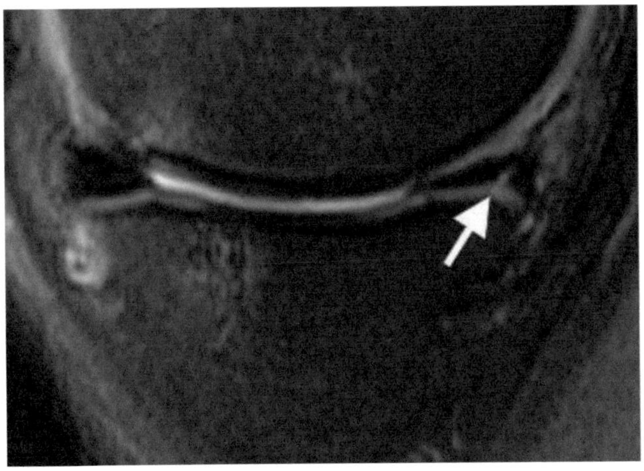

Fig. 6 Sagittal intermediate-weighted fat-saturated image of a recurrent meniscal tear after partial meniscectomy. The posterior horn of the medial meniscus demonstrates linear fluid-like increased signal intensity which extends into the articular surface (*arrow*). Arthroscopy confirmed a recurrent meniscal tear

meniscus was resected and for meniscal repairs. This diagnostic dilemma in the diagnosis of meniscal re-tears is also highlighted by the fact that the sensitivity and specificity of meniscal re-tears varies considerably dependent on the diagnostic criteria used. Whilst "fluid-like" increased signal intensity which extends from the meniscal substance into the meniscal surface on T2WI shows a high specificity in the diagnosis of recurrent meniscal tears (Fig. 6), its sensitivity remains low. In contrast, the mere presence of linear increased signal intensity within the meniscal substance which extends into the meniscal surface on T2WI demonstrates a high sensitivity but low specificity in the diagnosis of recurrent meniscal tears. However, the presence of meniscal fragmentation or displaced meniscal tissue is in keeping with a recurrent meniscal tear [1, 26, 27].

In view of these significant limitations of conventional MRI in the diagnosis of recurrent meniscal tears in the postoperative knee, direct MR-arthrography has been advocated. On direct MR-arthrography, extension of contrast into the meniscal substance is in keeping with a recurrent meniscal tear. The increased diagnostic accuracy of direct MR-arthrography when compared to conventional MRI particularly holds true in cases of partial meniscectomy where more than 25% of meniscal tissue has been excised and after meniscal repair. In these patients, direct MR-arthrography demonstrates a diagnostic accuracy of 85–92% whilst the diagnostic accuracy of conventional MRI is only 66–80%. In contrast, in cases where less than 25% of the meniscal volume has been resected, direct MR-arthrography and conventional MRI show similar diagnostic accuracy [28, 29].

CT arthrography is a useful alternative in the diagnosis of recurrent meniscal tears demonstrating a sensitivity of 79–100% and specificity of 78–89% [30].

Conclusion

MR imaging is crucial in the diagnosis of postoperative complications of the knee. Knowledge of common surgical techniques, the expected normal postoperative MRI-findings and typical pathological findings affecting the ligaments and menisci is essential in the interpretation of the postoperative knee.

Postoperative Shoulder

Introduction

Since most modern shoulder surgery is done arthroscopically, usually with non metallic devices, and with devises geographically distinct from the are of clinical interest, in general no modifications of pulse sequences are needed when imaging the postoperative shoulder. We also believe arthrography is similarly unnecessary. The most we would suggest in terms of sequences is a doubling of the bandwidth.

When looking at a postoperative shoulder, the first decision is the general family of surgery that was performed. These families of surgeries fall into three categories. Category 1 is most common and that is patients who have cuff and impingement related issues. Category 2 is the second most common and related to instability procedures. Category 3 is more protean and includes things such as arthoplasties and fractures. Category 3 since it is the most diverse and least commonly goes to advanced imaging will not be covered in the remainder of this chapter.

Cuff Surgery

In Category 1, there are two types of rotator cuff repairs [31]. Most commonly it is tendon-to- bone, where one will see some type of artifact within the subchondral surface of a lateral humeral head [32]. This artifact rarely degrades the image and usually no special sequence modifications are necessary. Much less common is tendon-to-tendon reconstructions [33]. In these reconstructions, one sees a suture line within the tendon. Both of these procedures are evaluated similar to a virgin cuffs with the exception that the grayish signal can be seen in a postoperative cuff fairly commonly. Rarely does this signal look like fluid unless the tendon is abnormal. Hence, to call a retear fluid must be seen [34]. In either type of reconstruction if the tendon appears retracted it is also involved in a retear In these postoperative cuff reconstructions, careful attention should made to the muscle mass. Patients who had atrophy of varying degrees pre-operatively tend to have a poorer operative result. The classifications of muscle atrophy are based upon the robustness of the size of the muscle and or the degree of the fatty infiltration of the muscle [35, 36]. The reference standard for fatty infiltration is the deltoid. If the fat in the supraspinatus muscle exceeds the deltoid atrophy can be called confidently. Be careful to use the sagittal images to assess for early atrophy, but the coronal images only for more severe atrophy. With retraction the tendon will look artifactually smaller on the sagittal images perhaps leading one to overcall atrophy on this plane alone.

Non Cuff Impingement Surgery

Rotator cuff surgeries are commonly associated with acromioplasties. Acromioplasties can be done arthroscopically where the MR signs are relatively subtle, or they can be done open, this is much less common. Open acromioplasties, however, have a more overt appearance postoperatively. The best plane to evaluate for changes on the undersurface of the acromion is the sagittal plane, usually just lateral to the acromioclavicular joint.

Acromioclavicular Joint Procedures

Notably osteoarthritis of the acromioclavicular joint is infrequently symptomatic. Hence be careful in the virgin shoulder to be conservative in your description of the extent of articular disease. In a small percentage of cases, the acromioclavicular joint is addressed at shoulder surgery [37]. Sometimes mere shaving of the osteophyte is done. This can be called a cheilectomy. Usually it is the undersurface and acromial sided osteophytes, which are shaved. Occasionally, resection of the distal clavicle is performed. This is a remarkably effective procedure for acromioclaviular pain.

It should be noted that the acromioclavicular joint is a relatively common cause of symptoms in the recalcitrant postoperative patient. Hence, it is our preference to overcall arthritic disease of the acromioclavicular joint in the postoperative patient. In terms of symptoms the presence of marrow edema and effusions as these are a more common symptom generated in a postoperative patient.

Bursectomy

The subacromial subdeltoid bursa is often resected at surgery, but tends to regrow and a virgin criteria can be used for subacromial bursal collections [38, 39]. Often when this bursa regrows the fat stripe may be interrupted or less visible. However, it has been our experience that imaging interpretation for the presence of surgery in this region is somewhat inaccurate.

Postoperative Instability

Instability procedures fall into three general categories [40]. The first addresses the labrum and the second are capsular, and the third are mechanical reconstructions. The labrum is most often reattached, rarely shaved or resected. Hence, relatively virgin signs can be used in a postoperative labrum, with the exception of that it might be slightly rounded postoperatively [41]. Internal signal is rarely seen postoperatively. It is our opinion that intra articular contrast is not necessary in these groups of patients. This is especially true if a 3T unit is available but even true for 1.5T scanners with more powerful gradients.

The second group is often termed a capsulorrhaphy . The capsule can be tightened closer to the glenoid or the labrum. This is more often performed arthroscopically then open currently. These suture lines are better seen with gradient echo techniques with longer TE's. Historically heat was used to tighten the capsule with rather poor results. Rather than assessing for the capsule directly, the best way to assess for the capiciousness of the capsule is by the visible joint volume.

Reconstruction procedures for instability often involve osseous and tendon transfer. Most often currently this is provided by coracoid positioning. These are best evaluated by conventional radiography and CT and rarely come to MR imaging. Rarely is recurrent instability seen in these patients.

Hill-Sachs deformities can be engaging if they are large and less lateral. This is a quite rare phenomenon. These engaging Hill-Sachs are reconstructed and will demonstrate residual marrow edema for a relatively long period of time. Otherwise edema under a Hill-Sachs is a sign of a recurrent dislocation.

Slap Repairs

SLAP repairs usually involve an anchor placed in the superior glenoid. As stated above this anchor rarely leads to artifact that degrades the images. These reattachments are usually water tight, and often there is residual signal at the site of the reattachment. Hence, this is a situation where direct arthrography should be utilized in order to determine if contrast imbibes into the reattachment site. It should be noted that recurrent SLAP tears are quite uncommon [42].

Adhesive Capsulitis

Frozen shoulder is not an infrequent complication of an shoulder operation. The MR signs of this are

1. obliteration of fat within the anterior cuff interval
2. thickening of the corico-humeral ligament
3. thickened synovium in the axillary recess
4. fluid in the biceps tendon sheath but not in the superior glenoid recess [43]

References

1. Boutin RD, Fritz RC, Marder RA (2014) Magnetic resonance imaging of the postoperative meniscus: resection, repair, and replacement. Magn Reson Imaging Clin N Am 22:517–555
2. Meyers AB, Haims AH, Menn K, Moukaddam H (2010) Imaging of anterior cruciate ligament repair and its complications. AJR Am J Roentgenol 194:476–484
3. Tsifountoudis I, Karantanas AH (2016) Current concepts on MRI evaluation of postoperative knee ligaments. Semin Musculoskelet Radiol 20:74–90
4. Walz DM (2016) Postoperative imaging of the knee: meniscus, cartilage, and ligaments. Radiol Clin N Am 54:931–950
5. White LM, Kramer J, Recht MP (2005) MR imaging evaluation of the postoperative knee: ligaments, menisci, and articular cartilage. Skelet Radiol 34:431–452
6. Ahlden M, Samuelsson K, Sernert N, Forssblad M, Karlsson J, Kartus J (2012) The Swedish national anterior cruciate ligament register: a report on baseline variables and outcomes of surgery for almost 18,000 patients. Am J Sports Med 40:2230–2235
7. Sanders TG (2011) Imaging of the postoperative knee. Semin Musculoskelet Radiol 15:383–407
8. Mundi R, Bhandari M (2016) Cochrane in CORR ((R)): double-bundle versus single-bundle reconstruction for anterior cruciate ligament rupture in adults (review). Clin Orthop Relat Res 474:1099–1101
9. Frick MA, Collins MS, Adkins MC (2006) Postoperative imaging of the knee. Radiol Clin N Am 44:367–389
10. Woertler K (2009) MRT des Kniegelenks nach Kreuzband- und Meniskusoperationen. Radiologieup2date 9:67–81
11. Howell SM, Clark JA (1992) Tibial tunnel placement in anterior cruciate ligament reconstructions and graft impingement. Clin Orthop Relat Res:187–195
12. Cosgarea AJ, DeHaven KE, Lovelock JE (1994) The surgical treatment of arthrofibrosis of the knee. Am J Sports Med 22:184–191
13. Bradley DM, Bergman AG, Dillingham MF (2000) MR imaging of cyclops lesions. AJR Am J Roentgenol 174:719–726
14. Recht MP, Piraino DW, Cohen MA, Parker RD, Bergfeld JA (1995) Localized anterior arthrofibrosis (cyclops lesion) after reconstruction of the anterior cruciate ligament: MR imaging findings. AJR Am J Roentgenol 165:383–385
15. Casagranda BU, Maxwell NJ, Kavanagh EC, Towers JD, Shen W, Fu FH (2009) Normal appearance and complications of double-bundle and selective-bundle anterior cruciate ligament reconstructions using optimal MRI techniques. AJR Am J Roentgenol 192:1407–1415
16. Kulczycka P, Larbi A, Malghem J, Thienpont E, Vande Berg B, Lecouvet F (2015) Imaging ACL reconstructions and their complications. Diagn Interv Imaging 96:11–19
17. Kartus J, Lindahl S, Kohler K, Sernert N, Eriksson BI, Karlsson J (1999) Serial magnetic resonance imaging of the donor site after harvesting the central third of the patellar tendon. A prospective study of 37 patients after arthroscopic anterior cruciate ligament reconstruction. Knee Surg Sports Traumatol Arthrosc 7:20–24
18. Alcala-Galiano A, Baeva M, Ismael M, Argueso MJ (2014) Imaging of posterior cruciate ligament (PCL) reconstruction: normal postsurgical appearance and complications. Skelet Radiol 43:1659–1668
19. Qi YS, Wang HJ, Wang SJ, Zhang ZZ, Huang AB, Yu JK (2016) A systematic review of double-bundle versus single-bundle posterior cruciate ligament reconstruction. BMC Musculoskelet Disord 17:45
20. Sherman PM, Sanders TG, Morrison WB, Schweitzer ME, Leis HT, Nusser CA (2001) MR imaging of the posterior cruciate ligament graft: initial experience in 15 patients with clinical correlation. Radiology 221:191–198
21. Noyes FR, Barber-Westin SD (2005) Posterior cruciate ligament revision reconstruction, part 1: causes of surgical failure in 52 consecutive operations. Am J Sports Med 33:646–654
22. DeLong JM, Waterman BR (2015) Surgical repair of medial collateral ligament and posteromedial corner injuries of the knee: a systematic review. Arthroscopy 31:2249–2255. e2245
23. Torabi M, Wo S, Vyas D, Costello J (2015) MRI evaluation and complications of medial patellofemoral ligament reconstruction. Clin Imaging 39:116–127
24. Panagopoulos A, van Niekerk L, Triantafillopoulos IK (2008) MPFL reconstruction for recurrent patella dislocation: a new surgical technique and review of the literature. Int J Sports Med 29:359–365
25. Meyers AB, Laor T, Sharafinski M, Zbojniewicz AM (2016) Imaging assessment of patellar instability and its treatment in children and adolescents. Pediatr Radiol 46:618–636
26. Barber BR, McNally EG (2013) Meniscal injuries and imaging the postoperative meniscus. Radiol Clin N Am 51:371–391
27. Lim PS, Schweitzer ME, Bhatia M et al (1999) Repeat tear of postoperative meniscus: potential MR imaging signs. Radiology 210:183–188
28. Applegate GR, Flannigan BD, Tolin BS, Fox JM, Del Pizzo W (1993) MR diagnosis of recurrent tears in the knee: value of intraarticular contrast material. AJR Am J Roentgenol 161:821–825
29. Magee T, Shapiro M, Rodriguez J, Williams D (2003) MR arthrography of postoperative knee: for which patients is it useful? Radiology 229:159–163
30. Mutschler C, Vande Berg BC, Lecouvet FE et al (2003) Postoperative meniscus: assessment at dual-detector row spiral CT arthrography of the knee. Radiology 228:635–641
31. Adler RS (2013) Postoperative rotator cuff. Semin Musculoskelet Radiol 17:12–19. doi:10.1055/s-0033-1333909
32. Owen RS, Iannotti JP, Kneeland JB, Dalinka MK, Deren JA, Oleaga L (1993) Shoulder after surgery: MR imaging with surgical validation. Radiology 186:443–447. doi:10.1148/radiology.186.2.8421748
33. Zanetti M, Hodler J (2004) MR imaging of the shoulder after surgery. Magn Reson Imaging Clin N Am 12:169–183. doi:10.1016/j.mric.2004.01.003
34. Zanetti M, Jost B, Hodler J, Gerber C (2000) MR imaging after rotator cuff repair: full-thickness defects and bursitis-like subacromial abnormalities in asymptomatic subjects. Skelet Radiol 29:314–319
35. Gladstone JN, Bishop JY, Lo IKY, Flotow EL (2007) Fatty infiltration and atrophy of the rotator cuff do not improve after rotator cuff repair and correlate with poor functioning outcome. Am J Sports Med 35:719–728. doi:10.1177/0363546506297539
36. Randelli P, Spennacchio P, Ragone V, Arrigoni P, Casella A, Cabitza P (2012) Complications associated with arthroscopic rotator cuff

repair: a literature review. Musculoskelet Surg 96:9–16. doi:10.1007/s12306-011-0175-y

37. Shubin Stein BE, Ahmad CS, Pfaff CH, Bigliani LU, Levine WN (2006) A comparison of magnetic resonance imaging findings of the acromioclavcular join in symptomatic versus asymptomatic patients. J Shoulder Elb Surg 15:56–59. doi:10.1016/j.jse.2005.05.013
38. McMenamin D, Koulouris G, Morrison WB (2008) Imaging of the shoulder after surgery. Eur J Radiol 68:106–119. doi:10.1016/j.ejrad.2008.02.050
39. Henkus HE, de Witte PB, Neilssen RGHH, Brand R, van Arkel ERA (2009) Bursectomy compared with acromioplasty in the management of subacromial impingement syndrome: a prospective randomised study. J Bone Joint Surg Br 91:504–510
40. Bancroft LW, Wasyliw C, Pettis C, Farley T (2012) Postoperative shoulder magnetic resonance imaging. Magn Reson Imaging Clin N Am 20:313–325. doi:10.1016/j.mric.2012.01.010
41. Wagner SC, Schweitzer ME, Morrison WB, Fenlin JM Jr, Bartolozzi AR (2002) Shoulder instability: accuracy of MR imaging performed after surgery in depicting recurrent injury—initial findings. Radiology 222(1):196–203. doi:10.1148/radiol.222101553
42. Probyn LJ, White LM, Salonen DC, Tomlinson G, Boynton EL (2007) Recurrent symptoms after shoulder instability repair: direct MR arthrographic assessment-correlation with second-look surgical evaluation. Radiology 245(3):814–823
43. Emig EW, Schweitzer ME, Karasick D, Lubowitz J (1995) Adhesive capsulitis of the shoulder: MR diagnosis. AJR 164(6):1457–1459

Soft Tissue Tumors in Children

Diego Jaramillo

The approach to soft tissue tumors is very different in the child than in the adult. The majority of soft tissue tumors in children are benign, their origin usually being vascular, fibrous or neurogenic [1]. The incidence of malignancy is much lower: STS occur with an incidence of 11 per million [2] whereas the incidence in adults is approximately three times greater [3]. Particularly in children over six years of age, malignant soft tissue tumors in the absence of a predisposing condition such as NF are very rare. On the other hand, the most common soft tissue tumors are vascular malformations. Many soft tissue tumors occur in association with telltale findings in the skin (birthmarks in vascular malformation, café-au-lait spots) or with known syndromes. This review will focus on those aspects of soft tissue tumors that are unique to the pediatric population.

Vascular Lesions

There are two main types of vascular lesions in children: vascular malformations, that are present at birth and grow at the same rate as the body, and vascular tumors that generally arise in infancy, grow and regress. The International Society for the Study of Vascular Anomalies has developed a classification [4] (ISSVA.org) that is currently accepted. It divides the tumors into benign, locally aggressive and malignant.

Hemangiomas and Related Tumors

The most common benign tumors are the hemangiomas of infancy and the congenital hemangiomas, the most important locally aggressive lesion is the Kaposiform hemangioendothelioma, and the two malignant lesions, although extremely rare in children, are angiosarcoma and epithelioid hemangiothelioma. Vascular malformations are classified based on the vessel of origin (lymphatic malformations (LM), venous malformations (VM), arterial malformations (AM), or capillary malformations (CM); whether they are simple or combined; and whether they are associated with other abnormalities. The most important of these include limb overgrowth with CM + VM ± LM in Klippel-Trenaunay syndrome; limb overgrowth with CM + arteriovenous fistuals in Parkes Weber syndrome; VM ± spindle-cell hemangioma with enchondroma in Maffucci syndrome; and CM, VM and/or LM + asymmetrical somatic overgrowth in Proteus syndrome.

This discussion will be limited to infantile hemangioma and venous and lymphatic malformation which are the most common.

Hemangiomas of infancy are the most common vascular tumors in infants [5]. Other hemangiomas include congenital hemangiomas that are fully grown at birth and may decrease in size over the first few months of life (rapidly involuting congenital hemangiomas or RICH) or not involute at all (non-involuting congenital hemangiomas or NICH).

Infantile hemangiomas are positive for glucose transporter 1 (GLUT1); this marker helps in the differentiation with congenital hemangiomas which are GLUT1 negative [5]. Girls are affected 3 times more than boys, the lesions are multiple in 20% [1] and 60% affect the head and neck. The lesions appear in the first few months of life, proliferate rapidly for a few months and by one year age they begin a slow phase of involution which lasts years. Hemangiomas contain tissue and arterial vessels (Fig. 1), and during involution become fatty.

Kaposiform hemangioendothelioma is the other important tumor, often presenting clinically with Kassabach-Merritt phenomenon, and characterized by a large soft tissue mass which is infiltrative, has fast-flowing vessels, although less than infantile hemangiomas, and shows no involution. It can be congenital and on imaging show poorly defined margins. Suggestive findings include subcutaneous stranding and hemosiderin deposition, but the diagnosis requires biopsy.

D. Jaramillo
Department of Radiology, Miami Children's Hospital, 3100 S.W. 62nd Ave, Miami, FL 33155, USA
e-mail: Diegjar1@gmail.com

J. Hodler et al. (eds.), *Musculoskeletal Diseases 2017-2020*, DOI 10.1007/978-3-319-54018-4_16

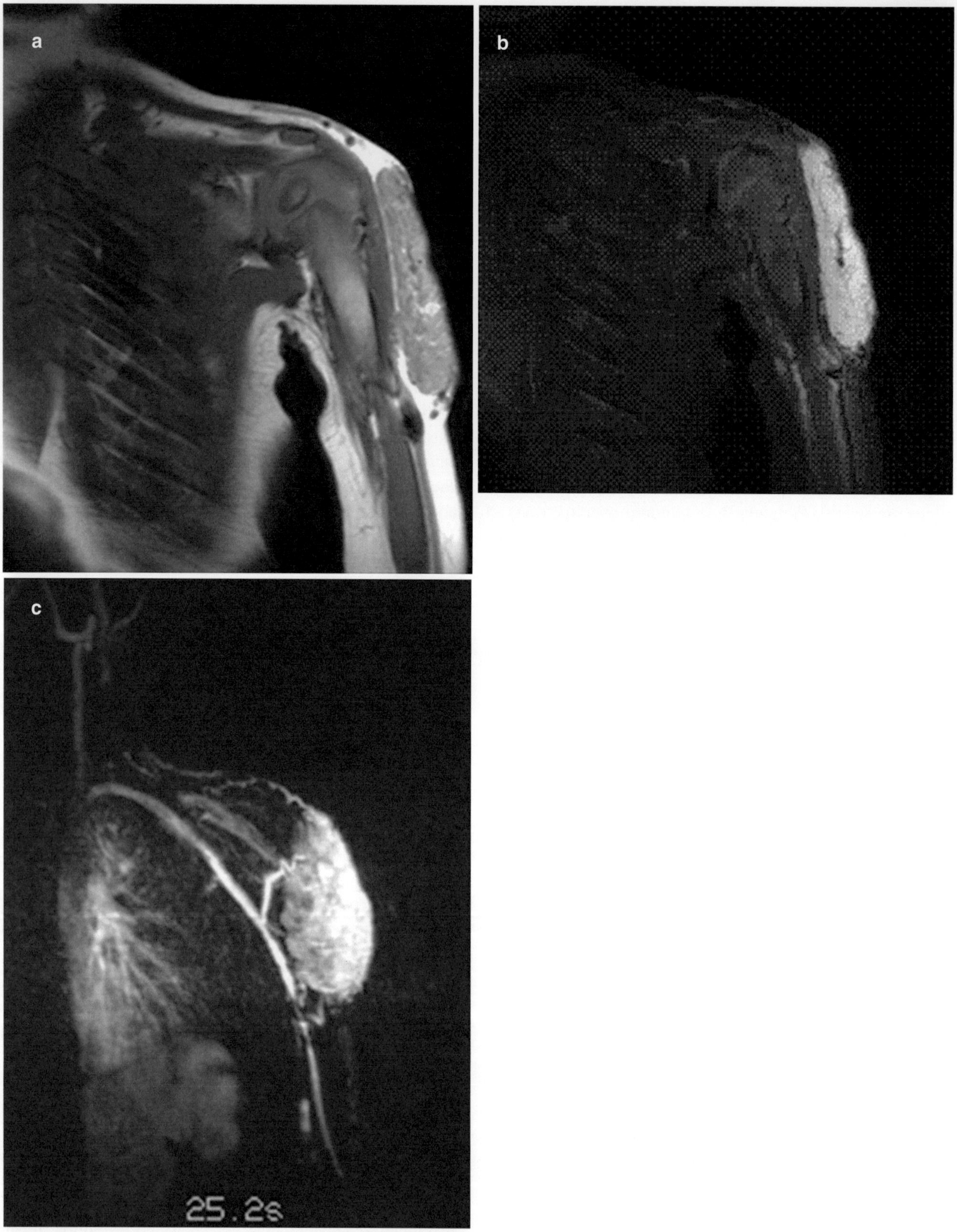

Fig. 1 Infantile hemangioma. 10-month old boy with an enlarging mass on the proximal left arm. (**a**) Coronal T1-weighted image shows a lobulated, relatively well-defined mass in the superficial soft tissues of the proximal arm. There is a vessel with a flow void inferior to the mass indicating a fast-flowing vessel. (**b**) Gadolinium-enhanced T1-weighted image shows diffuse enhancement of the mass. There is a vessel with flow void seen within the substance of the lesion. (**c**) Image from a time-resolved MR angiogram shows that there is a major feeding arterial vessel and that there is very early enhancement of the mass

Vascular Malformations

Vascular malformations are disorders of endothelial morphogenesis. They are congenital lesions and do not proliferate or have a soft tissue mass. The most common, venous and lymphatic, do not have fast flowing vessels.

Venous malformations are present at birth but may not become apparent until childhood. They contain endothelial-lined large vascular spaces or varicosities, containing thrombi. Unlike hemangiomas, they are as frequent in the limbs as in the head and neck [6] (Fig. 2). They do not contain fast flowing vessels, but often the vascular spaces are interspersed with fat.

Lymphatic malformations may contain large cystic spaces or be microcystic. Seventy to 80% occur in the head and neck [7] and usually are detected in the first years of life. The macrocystic variety is most commonly imaged and shows multiple fluid filled spaces. The contents vary in echogenicity and signal characteristics, and can often be highly proteinaceous and hemorrhagic, thus showing increased echogenicity and high SI on T1-weighted images and large fluid-levels. The lesions can involve multiple anatomic spaces, and, in particular, cervical lesions can have a significant mediastinal extension.

Imaging Approach to Vascular Lesions

The first step is to evaluate for fast-flowing vessels, seen as spaces with arterial waveforms on US and flow voids on MRI. If there are fast flowing vessels, is there are soft tissue mass? If the answer is yes, this constitutes a tumor, likely a congenital hemangioma. The tumoral component is typically echogenic and enhancing. If there is no mass, it is likely to be a malformation with an arterial component such as an arteriovenous malformation or fistula. If there are no fast-flowing vessels, it is paramount to determine whether the vascular spaces contain blood, indicated by a venous waveform on sonography and enhancement on contrast-enhanced MRI. Enhancing lesions are usually venous malformations; non-enhancing lesions are typically lymphatic malformations. Other characteristics suggesting venous malformation include thrombi or phleboliths within the vascular spaces, seen as low SI on water sensitive sequences, and multiple fluid levels.

Myofibroblastic Tumors

Fibroblastic and myofibroblastic tumors account for slightly more than 10% of soft tissue tumors in children [8]. Although they represent a wide variety of lesions, they all share a

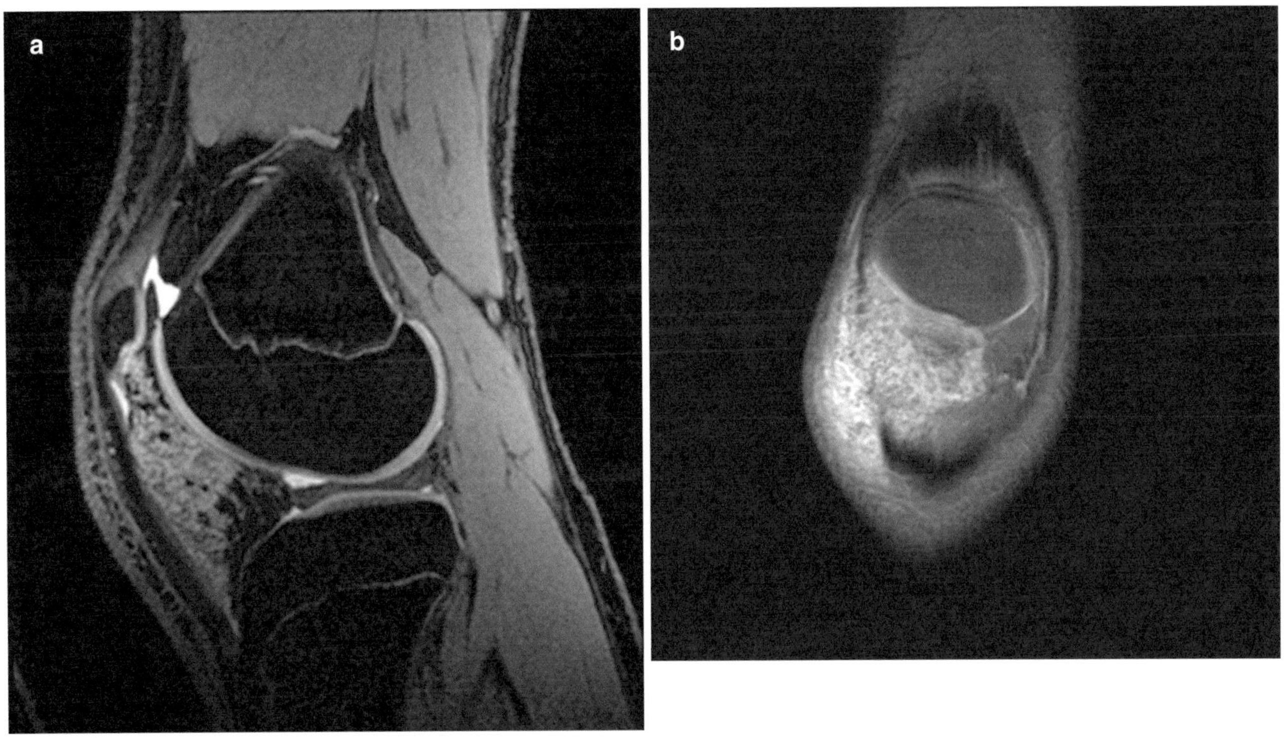

Fig. 2 Synovial venous malformation in a 13-year old girl with episodes of joint swelling. (**a**) Sagittal 3D gradient echo (DESS) image shows a multilobular mass high SI mass occupying a significant portion of Hoffa's fat pad and abutting the articular cartilage. Small round low SI structures correspond to phleboliths or small thrombi. (**b**) Coronal gadolinium-enhanced T1-weighted image shows diffuse enhancement of the mass indicating that it is a venous malformation

proliferation of fibrous tissue with extension along the fascial planes. They are usually echogenic, of low or intermediate SI on T2-weighted images. They present in different anatomic locations and age groups and can have peculiar characteristics such as a large mass with deformity of the adjacent bone (infantile fibrosarcoma), multiple subcutaneous or intramuscular lesions (infantile myofibromatosis), plaquelike pattern of growth pattern (Gardner fibroma), or presence of fat (lipofibromatosis). I will focus on those types that are unique to children.

Cranial Fasciitis

Although nodular fasciitis is the most common fibroblastic tumor, it is more often seen in adults than children. In newborns and young infants, cranial fasciitis, a form of nodular fasciitis, presents as low SI proliferations of fibrous tissue in the scalp. In cranial fasciitis, imaging shows lesions of 1–2 cm in diameter with well-defined margins and a fascial tail.

Infantile Myofibromatosis

Infantile myofibromatosis is the most common benign fibrous tumor in infancy. It often presents in the neonatal period and almost always in the first two years of life. It can be unifocal, more often in the head and neck, or multicentric, involving the skin, subcutaneous tissues, muscle and bone. One distinguishing characteristic is central necrosis, which results in a hypoechoic center which has high SI on water sensitive images and peripheral enhancement after contrast administration. When there is associated bony involvement, the lesions are metaphyseal or metadiaphyseal, lytic, well-circumscribed.

Fibromatosis Colli

Fibromatosis colli is a selective fibrous proliferation of the sternocleidomastoid muscle presenting in the first two months of life. It is more common in the right side, may be associated with birth trauma, and results in torticollis and a palpable neck mass. The US appearance is characteristic, with the sternocleidomastoid being replaced by a fusiform echogenic mass.

Desmoid Fibromatosis

Desmoid Fibromatosis is the most common pediatric fibrous tumor [8]. There are two peaks, one in childhood around 5 years of age, and the other in early adulthood. Lesions are locally aggressive and often recurrent, but not metastasizing [8, 9]. Localized forms are more common than multifocal, and the lesions occur most often in the extremities and trunk. Although there is abundant fibrous tissue, the signal characteristics are complex, with areas of low SI intermixed with high SI on T2-weighted images. Desmoid can present in isolation or be part of Gardner's syndrome.

Myositis Ossificans

Myositis ossificans, a post-traumatic lesion occurring often in the second decade of life, has three phases: an early proliferative phase, a phase of early calcification (seen 4–6 weeks after trauma) and a phase of late calcification after. Unlike soft tissue sarcomas, the calcification in myositis ossificans is always better defined in the outside. Imaging, particularly MRI during the early phase can be confusing as the lesion is very heterogeneous [8, 9].

Congenital Infantile Fibrosarcoma

Congenital fibrosarcoma (Fig. 3) presents as a large mass in the extremity or trunk either at birth or during the first months of life. Radiographs show elongation, bowing or attenuation of the bone adjacent to the tumor without focal destruction. The masses are heterogeneous and very vascular and are often confused with a hemangioma or vascular malformation [10]. Congenital fibrosarcoma has a more favorable prognosis that its adult counterpart.

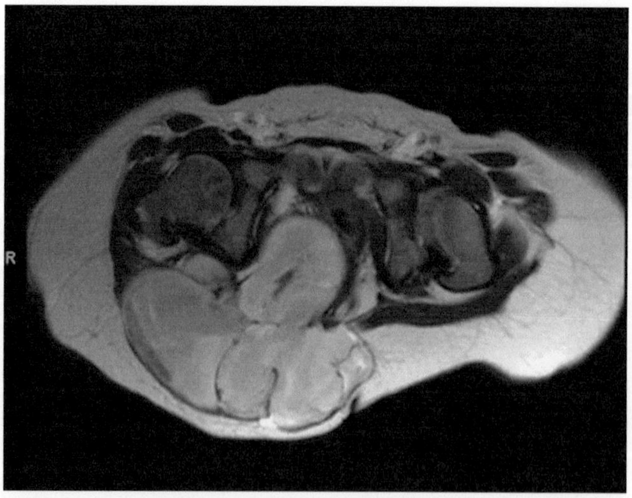

Fig. 3 Infantile fibrosarcoma in a 2-week old girl with a buttock mass. Axial T2-weighted image shows a heterogeneous soft tissue mass extending from the ischiorectal fossa into the gluteal region

Granuloma Annulare

Granuloma annulare is a subcutaneous lesion that is seen most commonly in younger children 2–5 years old, and most frequently in the pretibial region and in the occipital scalp. It is an inflammatory condition that manifests as a rapidly enlarging mass. It is benign and self-limited. On US it is echogenic and ill-defined and on MRI it is of low SI on T1, high SI on T2 and showing avid contrast enhancement.

Neurofibromatosis

Neurofibromas can be single or plexiform. Plexiform neurofibromas are the hallmark of NF1 and can be superficial or deep, each with very different imaging characteristics [11]. Deep plexiform NF are composed by cords of nervous and fibrous tissue surrounded by glycoproteinaceous matrix. These cords follow the course of major nerves, as they contain the nerve fibers. Optimal imaging involves whole body STIR. When plexiform neurofibromas are imaged transversely, the appearance of each cord is that of a target (Fig. 4), with a center that has low SI on STIR and enhances, surrounded by a high SI on STIR periphery which is non-enhancing. A typical neurofibroma contains many targets. When imaged longitudinally, the length of the cord can be appreciated, so that a lesion appears as a tangle of cords.

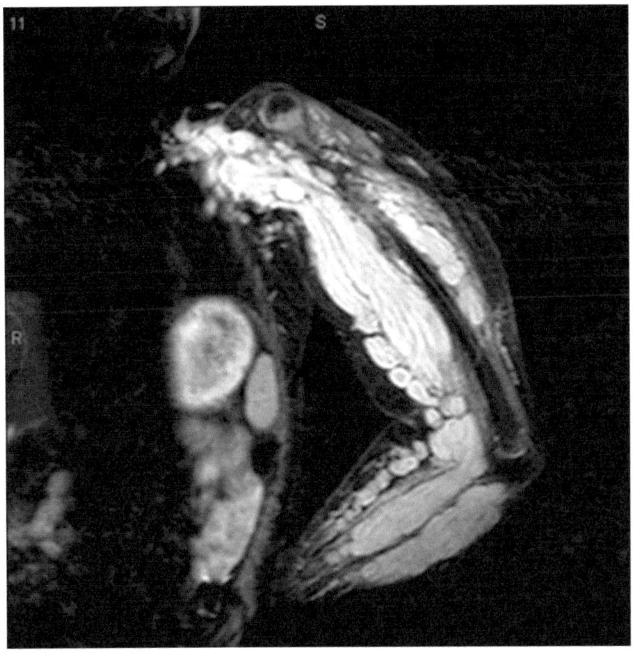

Fig. 4 Plexiform neurofibroma in a 12-year old boy with NF1. Coronal STIR image shows a large plexiform neurofibroma extending throughout the entire left upper extremity. The portions sectioned longitudinally have a cord-like appearance, whereas those sectioned transversely have a target appearance with a low SI center surrounded by a high SI periphery

A second form of neurofibromatosis is superficial. These lesions are primarily dermal and subdermal, plaquelike, and their borders are ill-defined [12]. They can have abundant vessels and therefore be confused with a vascular lesion.

Malignant degeneration of a neurofibroma into a malignant peripheral nerve sheath tumor is rare, occurring in less than 5% of cases, and the tumors usually present after the third decade [3]. These tumors can have some of the findings of other neural tumors such as splitting the fat or having a tail, but they may simply be a complex heterogenous mass which is non-specific.

Patients with NF1 require imaging to evaluate the specific involvement of certain structures like joints, abdominal or mediastinal structures (best done with MRI) [13, 14]; to evaluate for growth or response to therapy (best done with whole body MRI); and to exclude MPNST (best done with PET/CT [11] or PET/MRI).

Diffuse Malformations

There are lesions that may extend into various anatomic compartments and contain a proliferation of various mesenchymal elements. Macrodystrophia lipomatosa consists of a proliferation of fat associated with bone overgrowth. Typically it involves tissues in the course of the median nerve or the medial plantar nerve. Proteus syndrome has a combination of somatic overgrowth, vascular lesions, hamartomas and fat proliferation.

Soft Tissue Sarcomas

Soft tissue sarcomas constitute approximately 7% of malignancies in the pediatric age group [2].

Rhabdomyosarcoma is the most common sarcoma in children, constituting 50–60% of all STS [10]. Two thirds of these arise in children under 6 years of age. Other soft tissue sarcomas include synovial sarcoma, infantile fibrosarcoma, malignant peripheral nerve sheath tumors, and malignant fibrous histiocytoma [15]. STS are sometimes seen in association with cancer predisposition syndromes, such as Li-Fraumeni syndrome and Beckwith-Wiedeman syndrome or with chromosomal translocations, most notably the 11/22 translocation of Ewing Sarcoma/PNET [10].

Rhabdomyosarcomas

In children, rhabdomyosarcomas are more frequently of the embryonal type (Fig. 5), affecting younger children, primarily in the head and neck and genito-urinary (GU) tract (20%);

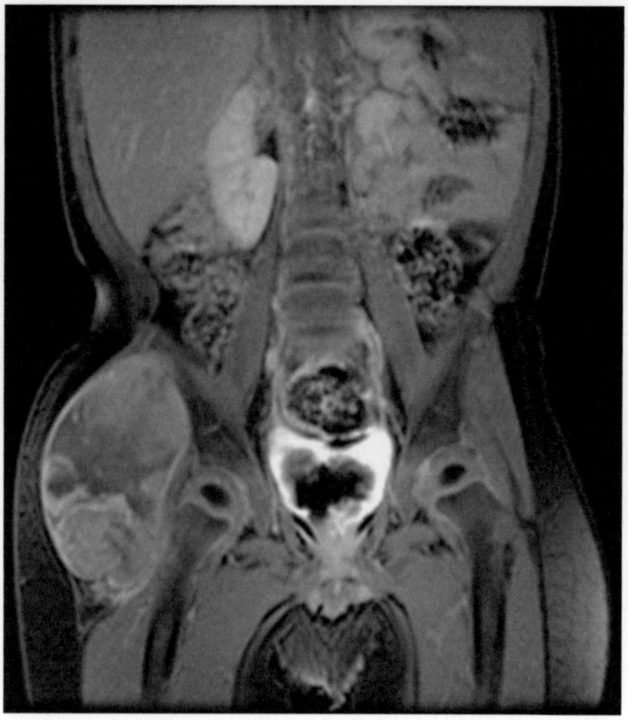

Fig. 5 Rhabdomyosarcoma in a 4-year-old boy. Coronal gadolinium-enhanced T1-weighted image shows a large, partially necrotic mass just lateral to the right hip joint. Biopsy revealed that the tumor was of the embryonal type

or the alveolar type, affecting the extremities of older children. Head and neck tumors constitute 40% of all rhabdomyosrcomas, and tumors of the GU tract and extremities constitute 20% each [10], Alveolar rhabdomyosarcomas of the extremities are heterogenous masses, usually highly vascularized on US and MRI. At times they can contain cystic components [16]. Alveolar tumors have a worse prognosis, particularly if they have the PAX3 mutation [2].

Sinovial Sarcoma

Synovial sarcoma is the second most common soft tissue sarcoma in children [2]. Synovial sarcomas, do not arise in the synovium of joints. They are often periarticular. Synovial sarcomas are often well-defined and on T2-weighted images can have a deceiving cyst-like appearance.

Conclusion

Soft tissue tumors have very different etiologies in children than adults. It is important to become familiar with those pathologies, and specifically with the fact that most lesions are vascular in origin and most often benign, to formulate an imaging approach.

References

1. Laor T (2004) MR imaging of soft tissue tumors and tumor-like lesions. Pediatr Radiol 34:24–37
2. Thacker MM (2013) Malignant soft tissue tumors in children. Orthop Clin North Am 44:657–667
3. Jagannathan JP, Tirumani SH, Ramaiya NH (2016) Imaging in soft tissue sarcomas: current updates. Surg Oncol Clin N Am 25:645–675
4. Dasgupta R, Fishman SJ (2014) ISSVA classification. Semin Pediatr Surg 23:158–161
5. Navarro OM (2016) Magnetic resonance imaging of pediatric soft-tissue vascular anomalies. Pediatr Radiol 46:891–901
6. Olivieri B, White CL, Restrepo R et al (2016) Low-flow vascular malformation pitfalls: from clinical examination to practical imaging evaluation—part 2, venous malformation mimickers. AJR Am J Roentgenol 206:952–962
7. White CL, Olivieri B, Restrepo R et al (2016) Low-flow vascular malformation pitfalls: from clinical examination to practical imaging evaluation—part 1, lymphatic malformation mimickers. AJR Am J Roentgenol 206:940–951
8. Sargar KM, Sheybani EF, Shenoy A et al (2016) Pediatric fibroblastic and myofibroblastic tumors: a pictorial review. Radiographics 36:1195–1214
9. Laffan EE, Ngan BY, Navarro OM (2009) Pediatric soft-tissue tumors and pseudotumors: MR imaging features with pathologic correlation: part 2. Tumors of fibroblastic/myofibroblastic, so-called fibrohistiocytic, muscular, lymphomatous, neurogenic, hair matrix, and uncertain origin. Radiographics 29:e36
10. Sangkhathat S (2015) Current management of pediatric soft tissue sarcomas. World J Clin Pediatr 4:94–105
11. Salamon J, Mautner VF, Adam G et al (2015) Multimodal imaging in neurofibromatosis type 1-associated nerve sheath tumors. Rofo 187:1084–1092
12. Lim R, Jaramillo D, Poussaint TY et al (2005) Superficial neurofibroma: a lesion with unique MRI characteristics in patients with neurofibromatosis type 1. AJR Am J Roentgenol 184:962–968
13. Delgado J, Jaramillo D, Ho-Fung V et al (2014) MRI features of plexiform neurofibromas involving the liver and pancreas in children with neurofibromatosis type 1. Clin Radiol 69:e280–e284
14. Zacharia TT, Jaramillo D, Poussaint TY et al (2005) MR imaging of abdominopelvic involvement in neurofibromatosis type 1: a review of 43 patients. Pediatr Radiol 35:317–322
15. Ahlawat S, Fayad LM (2015) De novo assessment of pediatric musculoskeletal soft tissue tumors: beyond anatomic imaging. Pediatrics 136:e194–e202
16. Navarro OM (2009) Imaging of benign pediatric soft tissue tumors. Semin Musculoskelet Radiol 13:196–209

Primary Bone Tumors in Children

Peter J. Strouse

Imaging of pediatric bone tumors begins with radiography. Radiographs serve to confirm the presence of a tumor, to identify the site (bone, location within bone), to characterize (aggressive vs. non-aggressive), to formulate a differential diagnosis and to guide further imaging work up. Clinical presentation and radiographic characteristics will determine the need for further imaging. The differential diagnosis of a bone tumor can be narrowed, often to a single diagnosis, by answering a few simple questions [1, 2]:

How old is the child? Childhood bone tumors have a proclivity to occur within characteristic age ranges (Table 1).

What bone is involved? What part of the bone is involved? Tumors have a proclivity to occur in certain bones and at characteristic locations within those bones (Table 2). Distribution of tumor location may change with patient age.

Is the tumor unifocal or multifocal? Multifocality narrows the differential to a shorter list (Table 3).

Is the tumor aggressive or non-aggressive (Table 4)? In general, non-aggressive appearing lesions tend to be benign and aggressive appearing lesions tend to be malignant, but this does not hold uniformly. Non-aggressive lesion have well-defined margins often with sclerosis, expand bone contour via slow growth, have single-layered, smooth periosteal new bone, if any, and do not have an associated soft tissue mass (Fig. 1). Aggressive lesions have poorly defined margins, an ill-defined zone of transition to normal bone, permeative or frank bone destruction without remodeling, aggressive periosteal new bone (sunburst [hair on end], layered [onion-skin], interrupted [Codman triangle]), and may have an associated soft tissue mass (Fig. 2).

Table 1 Pediatric bone tumors—Peak age of occurrence

Age group	Tumors
Infant and toddler ≤5 years old	Infantile myofibromatosis Leukemia Langerhans cell histiocytosis (multifocal) Metastatic neuroblastoma Osteofibrous dysplasia
Child 5–10 years old	Ewing sarcoma of long bone Langerhans cell histiocytosis (unifocal)
Adolescent 10–20 years old	Aneurysmal bone cyst Chondroblastoma Chondromyxoid fibroma Ewing sarcoma of axial skeleton Fibrous dysplasia Osteochondroma Leukemia (second peak) Nonossifying fibroma/fibrous cortical defect Osteoblastoma Osteoid osteoma Osteosarcoma Periosteal chondroma Primary lymphoma of bone Simple bone cyst
Adult ≥20 years old	Adamantinoma Enchondroma Giant cell rumor (rare until physes fuse) Parasteal osteosarcoma Periosteal osteosarcoma

Note: Reproduced with permission from Kaste SC, Strouse PJ, Fletcher BD, Neel MD (2008) Benign and malignant bone tumors. In: Slovis TL (ed) Caffey's pediatric diagnostic imaging, 11th edn, Mosby, p 2912–2969 (copyright Elsevier)

P.J. Strouse
Section of Pediatric Radiology, C. S. Mott Children's Hospital, Department of Radiology, University of Michigan Health System, 1540 E. Hospital Drive, Ann Arbor, MI 48109-4252, USA
e-mail: pstrouse@umich.edu

J. Hodler et al. (eds.), *Musculoskeletal Diseases 2017-2020*, DOI 10.1007/978-3-319-54018-4_17

Table 2 Pediatric bone tumors—Location in long bones

Epiphysis	Chondroblastoma Giant cell tumor (after physeal fusion) Langerhans cell histiocytosis
Metaphysis	Aneurysmal bone cyst Chondromyxoid fibroma Enchondroma Leukemia Metastases Nonossifying fibroma/fibrous cortical defect[a] Osteochondroma[a] Osteoid osteoma Osteosarcoma Parosteal osteosarcoma Simple bone cyst[a]
Diaphysis	Adamantinoma Ewing sarcoma/primitive neuroectodermal tumor Fibrous dysplasia Nonossifying fibroma/fibrous cortical defect (in older patients)[a] Osteofibrous dysplasia Osteoid osteoma Periosteal osteosarcoma Simple bone cyst (in older patients)[a]

Note: Reproduced with permission from Kaste SC, Strouse PJ, Fletcher BD, Neel MD (2008) Benign and malignant bone tumors. In: Slovis TL (ed) Caffey's pediatric diagnostic imaging, 11th edn, Mosby, p 2912–2969 (copyright Elsevier)

[a]Osteochondromas, nonossifying fibromas/fibrous cortical defects and simple bone cysts begin in the metaphyses. With maturation, the lesions may "migrate" into the metaphysis and diaphysis as the physis grows away from the lesion

Table 3 Pediatric bone tumors—Multifocal lesions

Brown tumors (hyperparathyroidism)
Cystic angiomatosis/lymphangiomatosis
Enchondroma (Ollier disease, Maffucci syndrome)
Fibrous dysplasia (McCune-Albright syndrome)
Infantile myofibromatosis
Langerhans cell histiocytosis
Leukemia
Metastases (i.e., from neuroblastoma)
Multifocal osteosarcoma
Nonossifying fibroma/fibrous cortical defects
Osteochondroma (oteochondromatosis)

Note: Reproduced with permission from Kaste SC, Strouse PJ, Fletcher BD, Neel MD (2008) Benign and malignant bone tumors. In: Slovis TL (ed) Caffey's pediatric diagnostic imaging, 11th edn, Mosby, p 2912–2969 (copyright Elsevier)

Table 4 Pediatric bone tumors—Aggressive vs. nonaggressive radiographic appearance[a]

Nonaggressive	Aneurysmal bone cyst Chondroblastoma Chondromyxoid fibroma Enchondroma Fibrous dysplasia Nonossifying fibroma/fibrous cortical defect Osteoblastoma Osteoid osteoma Osteochondroma Simple bone cyst
Indeterminate	Adamantinoma Desmoplastic fibroma Giant cell tumor Langerhans cell histiocytosis Osteofibrous dysplasia
Aggressive	Ewing sarcoma/primitive neuroectodermal tumor Leukemia Lymphoma Metastases Osteoblastoma (aggressive form) Osteosarcoma

Note: Reproduced with permission from Kaste SC, Strouse PJ, Fletcher BD, Neel MD (2008) Benign and malignant bone tumors. In: Slovis TL (ed) Caffey's pediatric diagnostic imaging, 11th edn, Mosby, p 2912–2969 (copyright Elsevier)

[a]Lesions are listed based on their most common radiologic presentation. With some lesions, variation from the norm is common

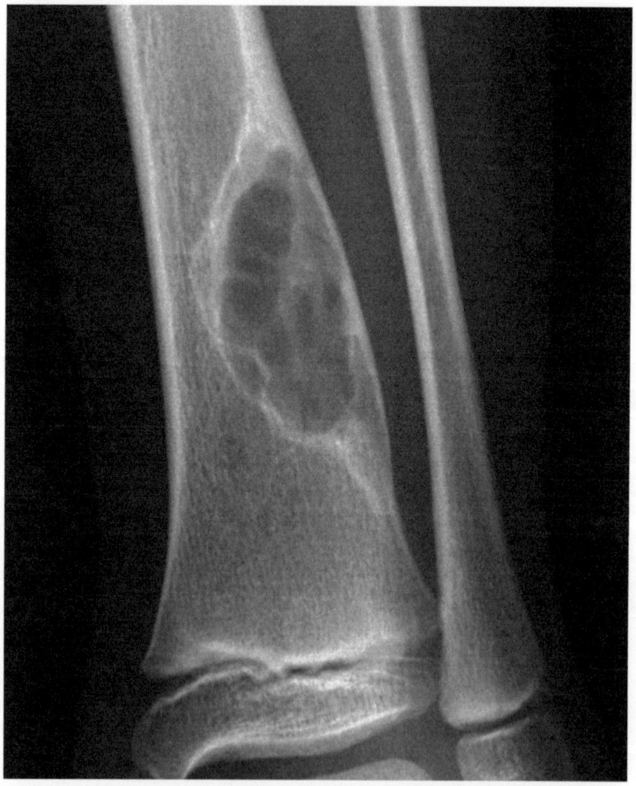

Fig. 1 7-year-old boy with non-ossifying fibroma (NOF) of the distal tibia. The lesion has characteristics of a non-aggressive process—well-defined sclerotic margins, absence of periosteal new bone, thinned but intact overlying cortex consistent with slow growth. The eccentric location and lobulated, multilocular appearance are consistent with an NOF

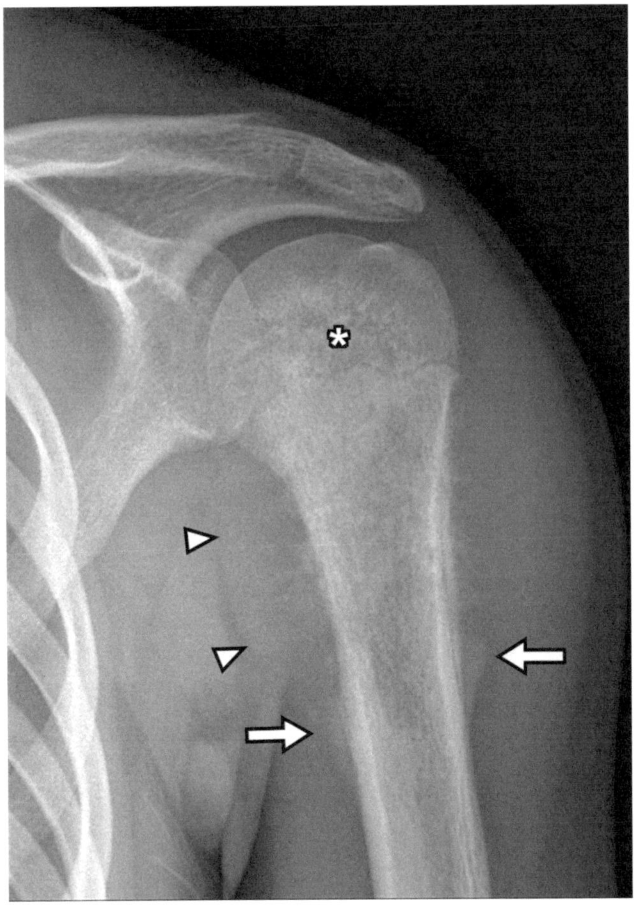

Fig. 2 12-year-old girl with osteosarcoma. The lesion has characteristics of an aggressive process—permeative bone destruction, poorly defined margins, layered and interrupted periosteal new bone (Codman's triangle, *arrows*), soft tissue mass. Some spiculated osteoid production is seen within the soft mass around the bone. Ill-defined lucency and sclerosis within the humeral head suggests epiphyseal extension (*asterisk*), confirmed by subsequent MRI

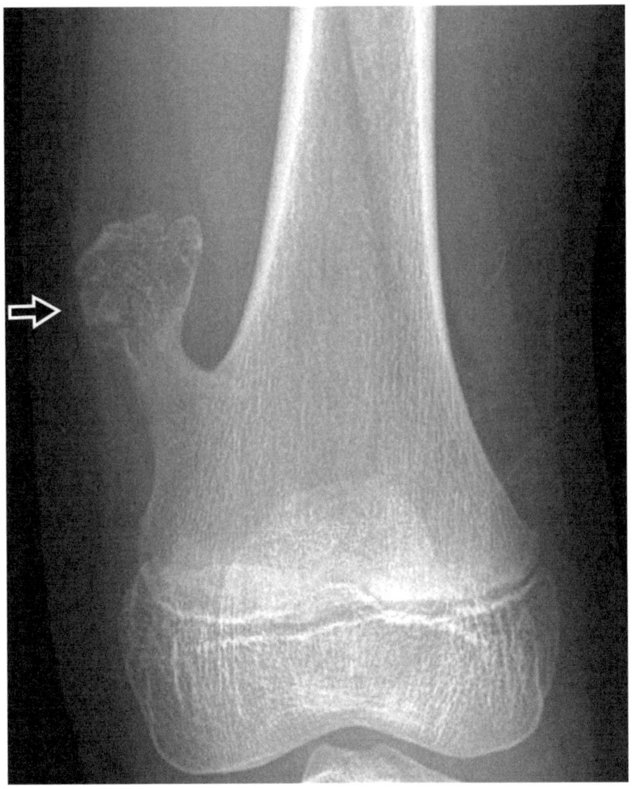

Fig. 3 11-year-old boy with a pedunculated osteochondroma of the distal femoral metaphysis. The lesion (*arrow*) has cortex and medullary space contiguous with that of the underlying femur and is oriented away from the growth plate as is characteristic

Benign Bone Tumors

The majority of pediatric bone tumors are benign. Many benign bone tumors have characteristic presentations, locations and appearances [1, 2]. Radiographs may suffice for diagnosis. Knowledge of the typical appearance of common benign lesions aids in limiting concern for a more ominous diagnosis, unnecessary imaging and some biopsies. CT or MR may be useful for characterization and anatomical delineation [3].

Cartilaginous Tumors

Osteochondroma

Osteochondromas have a cartilaginous cap with a growth plate at its interface with the underlying bone [4, 5]. Lesions are well-defined and occur in metaphyses and metaphyseal equivalents. Cortex and medullary space are in contiguity with the underlying bone (Fig. 3). Lesions vary from pedunculated to sessile. Growth ceases with skeletal maturity.

Most osteochondromas are asymptomatic. Some may produce symptoms due to encroachment of adjacent structures including vasculature, nerves, muscles and tendons or other bones [6]. Malignant degeneration is extraordinarily rare in childhood. Malignant transformation to chondrosarcoma is suggested with growth after skeletal maturity, new pain, bone destruction or a cartilaginous cap of greater than 1.5–2 cm thickness.

Multiple hereditary osteochondromatosis (MHE) is an autosomal dominant disorder usually presenting before age 10 years. MHE patients may have secondary osseous deformities which limit function and are more prone to axial lesions which may encroach on visceral structures or the spinal canal.

Enchondroma

Enchondromas are most common in the small tubular bones of the hands and feet and with the metaphyses/metadiphyses of long bones [4]. It is the most common pediatric bone tumor in the hand. The incidence of enchondroma increases with age, peaking in the third decade.

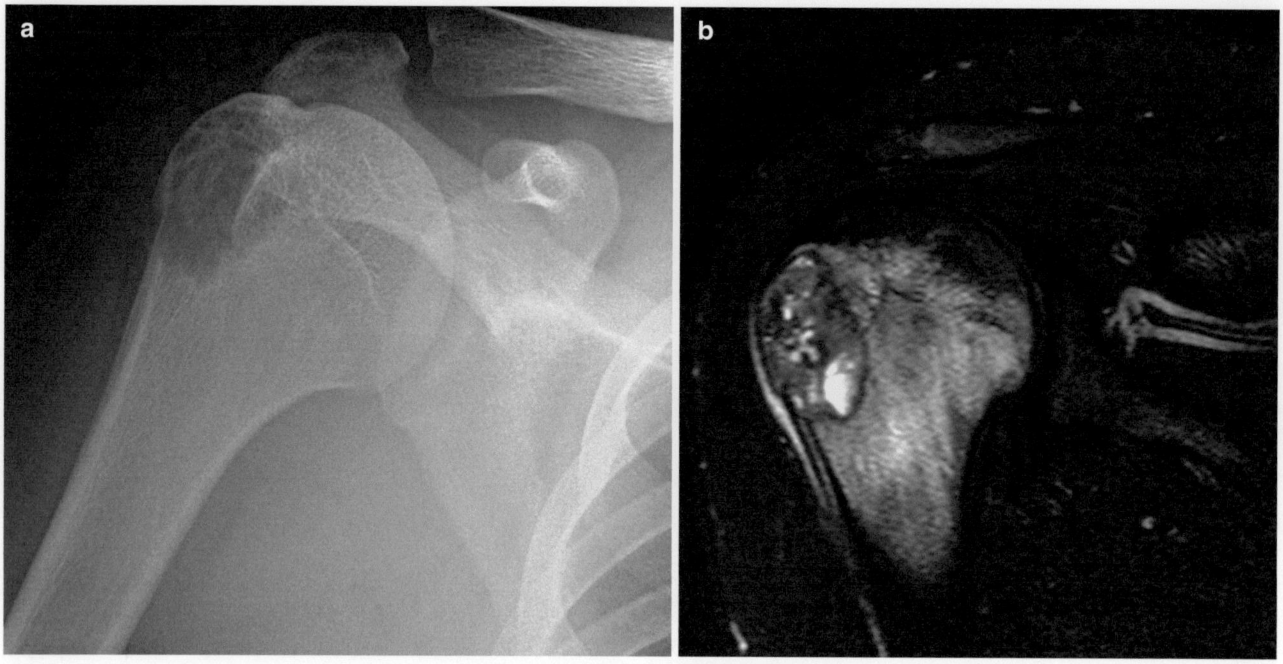

Fig. 4 15-year-old boy with chondroblastoma. The patient presented with increasing shoulder pain over four months. (**a**) External rotation anteroposterior radiograph of the right shoulder shows a well-defined lucent lesion centered in the greater tuberosity of the proximal humeral epiphysis extending into adjacent metaphysis. (**b**) Fat-saturated coronal T2-weighted MR image (TR 4947, TE 60 ms) show a predominantly solid, well-defined lesion with scattered areas of high and low signal. The solid portions of the lesion paralleled articular cartilage on all sequences. Abundant bone marrow edema is seen adjacent to the lesion.

Enchondromas are well-defined, lucent lesions Overlying cortex may be thinned. Focal, punctate cartilage matrix may be seen, but is better defined by CT. On MRI, lesions follow cartilage in signal appearing isotense to muscle on T1-weighted images and high signal on T2-weighted images. Adjacent bone marrow edema is absent. Lesions enhance with contrast, varying in enhancement pattern from homogeneous to peripheral.

Enchondromatosis (Ollier disease) is non-hereditary mesodermal dysplasia. The hands are most often affected and may be substantially deformed and functionally limited. Lesions in long bones and the pelvis tend to be larger, expansile and striated. Maffucci syndrome is enchondromatosis in conjunction with soft tissue vascular malformations, typically venous malformations. Metachondromatosis is a rare disorder combining osteochondromatosis and enchondromatosis.

Chondroblastoma

Chondroblastomas are most common in the second decade and occur in epiphyses, apophyses, carpal and tarsal bones and the patella [4, 7]. Larger lesions may extend into the adjacent metaphysis. Chondroblastomas are inflammatory and produce pain leading to presentation.

On radiography, lesions are well-defined and lucent, with a mildly sclerotic border. Non-aggressive periosteal new bone is seen on the adjacent metaphysis (Fig. 4). Lesion anatomy, borders and cartilage matrix are better seen with CT. On MRI, lesion signal intensity parallels cartilage; however, a cystic component is common. Adjacent bone marrow and soft tissue edema and joint effusion are best seen on MRI [8].

Cysts

Simple (Unicameral) Bone Cyst

Simple bone cysts are of uncertain etiology. Lesions are substantially more common in boys than girls. Bone cysts are seen in the metaphysis and metadiaphysis of long bones [9]. The proximal humerus is the most common site followed by the proximal femur. Axial sites are rare, the most common being the calcaneus. With growth, the growth plate moves away from a bone cyst. Lesions are centered within the medullary space, well-defined and have a mildly sclerotic cyst wall. Overlying cortex may be thinned and mildly expanded. Septations may be seen. Bone cysts are the most common cause for pathologic fracture in children. The fallen fragment sign is diagnostic of a simple bone cyst (Fig. 5). On MRI, the cyst wall

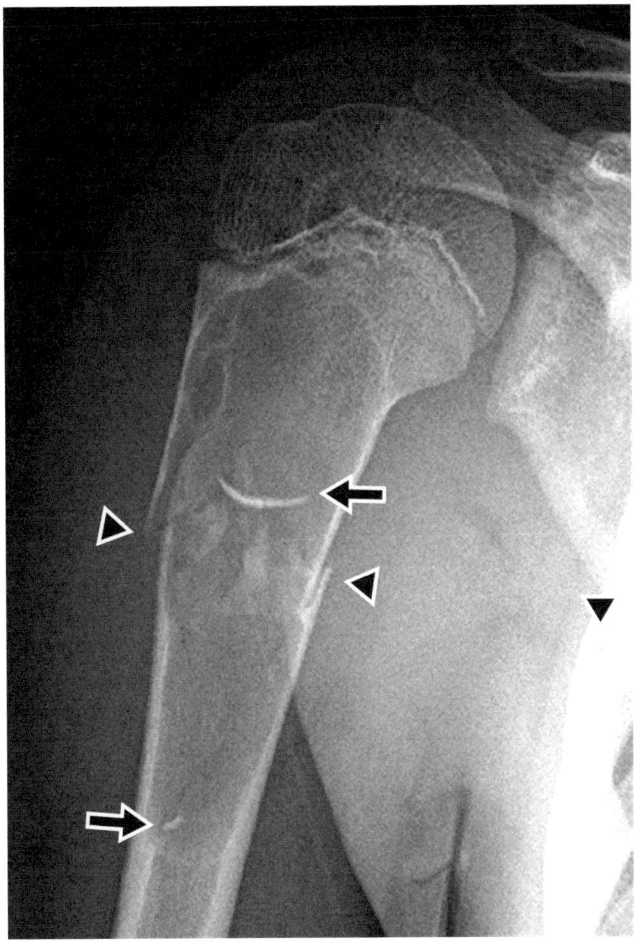

Fig. 5 11-year-old boy with a pathologic fracture through a simple bone cyst of the proximal humerus. The lesion is well-defined and slightly expansile with thinning of the overlying cortex. A fracture (*arrowheads*) is seen through the midpoint of the lesion with small fallen fragments (*arrows*)

enhances mildly with uniform thickness. Adjacent bone marrow edema is absent in the absence of fracture or stress related to the cyst.

Aneurysmal Bone Cyst (ABC)

Aneurysmal bone cysts (ABCs) are composed of communicating loculations contain blood and lined by fibrous walls containing spicules of bone, fibrous tissue, red blood cells and hemosiderin [9]. An underlying lesion may be found in up to one third of cases.

ABC most commonly occurs in children and young adults. It is rare under 5 years of age. The lesion is most common in long bone metaphyses, but can occur in flat bones. Most ABCs are intramedullary but eccentric, with cortical and subperiosteal (surface) lesions being much less common.

ABCs appear as well-defined, multiloculated, expansile, lucent lesions, classically described as a "soap bubble" [9]. Overlying cortex is remodeled and thinned. With CT or MR, fluid-fluid levels due to blood products within locules of the lesion are characteristic. Septations enhance; however, any solid component may signal the presence of an underlying lesion.

Fibrous Tumors

Fibrous Cortical Defect (FCD)/Non-ossifying Fibroma (NOF)

Fibrous cortical defect and non-ossifying fibromas are histologically identical fibroxanthomatous lesions differentiated by size alone [10]. FCDs are defined as less than 2 cm and NOFs as greater than 2 cm. Most FCDs and NOFs are found incidentally on radiographs performed for trauma or for other reasons. FCDs and NOFs are most common in the metaphases of the legs. Lesions are well defined with a sclerotic border and eccentric, located in the cortex (Fig. 1) [10]. Lesions may be multiple. Most FCDs are unilocular whereas NOFs are frequently multilocular and lobulated. Overlying cortex is thinned and may be expanded. With maturation lesions become sclerotic. Lesions are well-defined by CT. On MR, lesions are well defined without adjacent bone marrow edema [11]. Younger lesions may show some high signal on T2-weighting and some enhancement [11]. Older lesions are low signal on all sequences.

Fibrous Dysplasia

Fibrous dysplasia is a focal dysplastic process of unknown etiology. It is usually solitary with approximately 25% having polyostotic disease. Characteristic locations include the proximal femurs, craniofacial bones and ribs. On radiography, lesions expand the medullary space, centrally or eccentrically. Overlying cortex may be thinned with endosteal scalloping and expansion. The appearance of the lesion varies with the proportions of fibrous tissue and dysplastic bone contained [10, 12]. Lesions may appear lucent or have a classic "ground glass" appearance (Fig. 6). Margins are well-defined and usually sclerotic. Bowing of the proximal femur is a characteristic finding. Lesions are well characterized by CT or MR [10, 12]. On MR, T2-weighted signal varies with the composition of the lesion ranging from hyperintense to hypointense.

McCune-Albright syndrome occurs in females and is characterized by unilateral polyostotic fibrous dysplasia in association with precocious puberty and dermal café-au-lait spots.

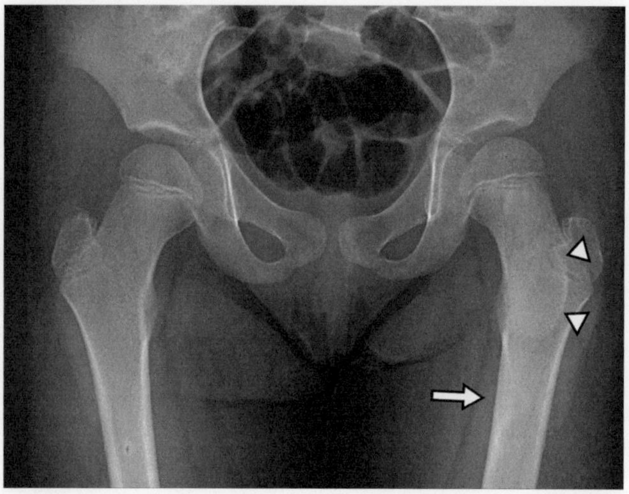

Fig. 6 6-year-old girl with McCune-Albright syndrome and polyostotic fibrous dysplasia. A well-defined, mild sclerotic, ground-glass lesion (*arrowheads*) is seen within the intertrochanteric proximal left femur. A less well-defined, mildly sclerotic lesion is seen further distal (*arrow*). A prominent vascular groove is seen end-on in the proximal right femur

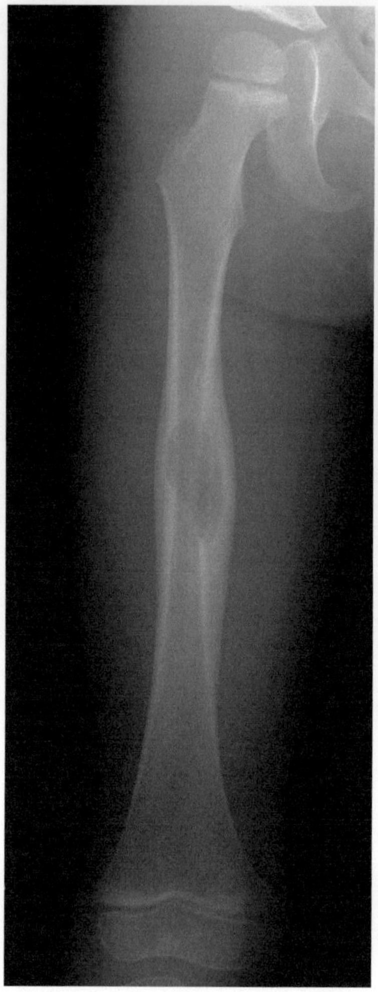

Fig. 7 4-year-old boy with Langerhans cell histiocytosis. The patient presented with thigh pain after minor trauma. A well-defined "punched-out" lucent lesion is seen in the mid femoral diaphysis. There is destruction of the medial cortex; however, the lesion is enveloped in a homogenous, thick layer of non-aggressive appearing periosteal new bone. Imaging work-up demonstrated several lesions in the skull

Langerhans Cell Histiocytosis

Langerhans cell histiocytosis (LCH) is a proliferative lesion of uncertain etiology Lesions occur in a continuum ranging from a single osseous lesion to an aggressive multiorgan, systemic process [13, 14]. LCH occurs throughout childhood into young adulthood. It is most common before 15 years of age, peaking in the toddler years. Patients with a solitary lesion present with pain, tenderness to palpation and, occasionally, a soft tissue mass originating from bone. The most common site of LCH is the skull but common sites of involvement include the pelvis, ribs, spine and long bones, especially the femur. Lesions are metaphyseal or diaphyseal, intramedullary and expanding through cortex with associated remodeling and non-aggressive periosteal reaction (Fig. 7) [13, 14]. Lesions are characterized by well-defined, minimally sclerotic borders. Occasionally, lesions may occur be permeative or have more aggressive appearing layered periosteal new bone. Lesions often have mixed aggressive and non-aggressive characteristics.

In the skull, lesions appear "punched-out" or with a beveled edge due to differential involvement of the inner and outer tables. "Floating teeth (maxilla) and vertebra plana (vertebra) are classic LCH appearances [13, 14]. Multifocality is suggestive of LCH, particularly when individual lesions are characteristic in appearance and location.

On CT or MRI, lesions are well-defined. Associated soft tissue masses are common. On MR, extensive adjacent bone marrow and soft tissue edema may be seen. Lesions are high signal on T2-weighting and enhance relatively homogeneously and densely.

Osteoid Tumors

Osteoid Osteoma

Osteoid osteoma is a small, inflammatory neoplasm with characteristic presentation and imaging [15, 16]. Patients present with pain which is classically worse at night and relived by aspirin. The lesion may present throughout childhood and young adulthood, peaking in the second decade and rarely presenting after 35 years of age.

Osteoid osteoma is composed of a nidus with or without a sequestrum at it center, surrounded by sclerotic bone [15, 16]. By definition, the nidus is 1.5 cm in diameter or less. Lesions are usually cortical, less commonly intramedullary and least commonly subperiosteal. Lesions can occur in any

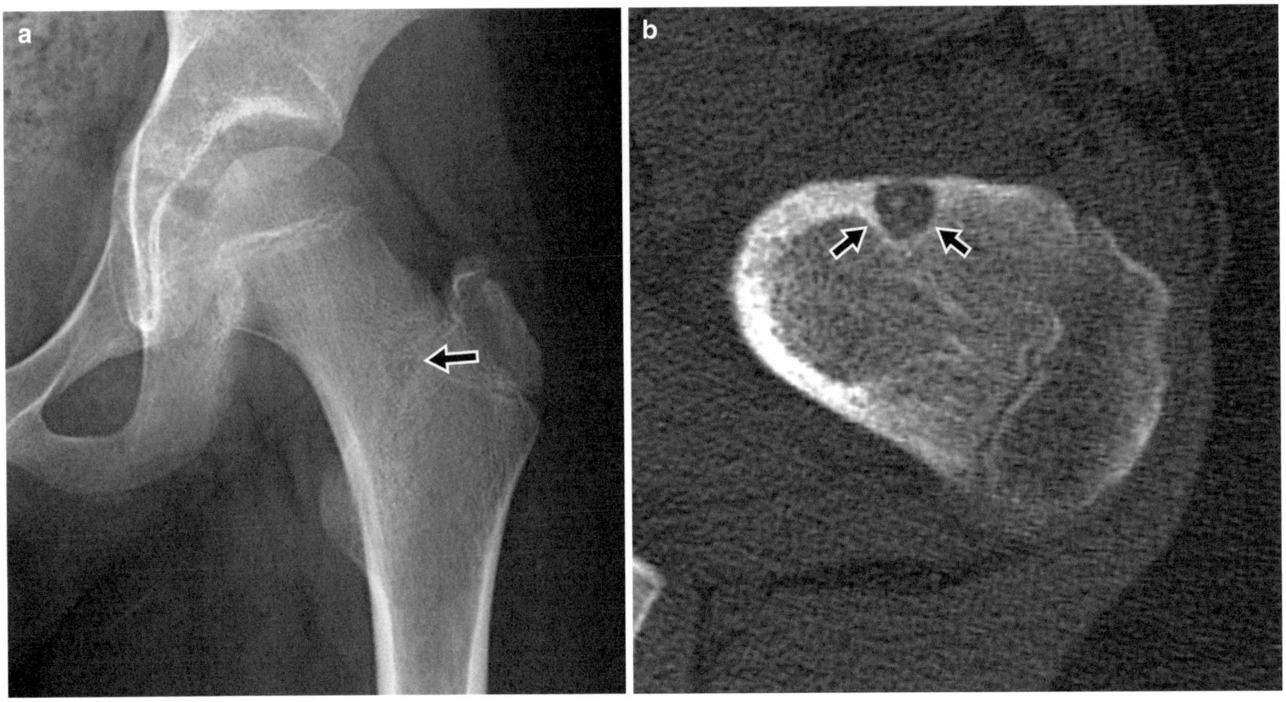

Fig. 8 9-year-old girl with osteoid osteoma of the femoral neck. The girl presented with hip pain and decreased range of movement. (**a**) Anteroposterior radiograph shows a faint, round lucent lesion at the base of the femoral neck (*arrow*). (**b**) Axial CT image shows a well-dined lucent lesion centered in the anterior cortex (*arrows*). A small opacity is seen centrally within the lesion. There is mild cortical thickening

bone; however, the femur is most common followed by the tibia. Interarticular lesions mimic arthritis. There is associated cortical thickening and non-aggressive periosteal new bone. CT is preferred for delineation of osteoid osteomas as it shows the bony changes best (Fig. 8). Associated bone and soft tissue edema is better shown on MR but may also mask the lesion itself.

Ostoblastoma

Osteoblastoma is related to osteoid osteoma but larger [15]. By definition, lesions larger than 1.5 cm are labeled as osteoblastoma. Common locations are the posterior elements of the spine, the proximal metaphysis and diaphysis of the femur, the tibia and the neck of the talus. Lesions may be cortical or intramedullary. Radiologic appearance varies between three patterns: osteoid osteoma-like, but larger; ABC-like, particularly in the spine; and, aggressive malignant appearing.

Malignant Bone Tumors

The majority of malignant pediatric bone tumors are either osteosarcoma (approximately two thirds) or Ewing sarcoma (approximately one third) [17]. Other sarcomas are extremely rare in children. Sarcomatous degeneration of an osteochondroma or enchondroma is distinctly rare in the pediatric age group, even in patients with underlying conditions (i.e. multiple hereditary osteochondromatosis or enchondromatosis). Primary lymphoma of bone does occur in children and is in the differential for an aggressive appearing osseous tumor, but is less common than osteosarcoma or Ewing sarcoma.

Children with malignant bone tumors commonly present with pain and swelling. Symptoms are usually gradual in onset; however, not infrequently patients present after an episode of relatively minor trauma. As malignant tumors are most common in adolescents, athletic activity is also sometimes related to symptoms and lesions must be differentiated from a stress injury [18].

Osteosarcoma

Osteosarcoma is the most common pediatric primary bone tumor. Incidence increases later in the first decade with a peak in adolescence at approximately 12-years-old in girls and 16-years-old in boys [17]. Five-year survival is now approximately 60%. Factors include age, race, anatomic site (axial worse than appendicular), pathologic subtype, stage and response to chemotherapy [17]. Tumors are usually treated with neo-adjuvant, multidrug chemotherapy followed by surgery focused at limb salvage and further chemotherapy.

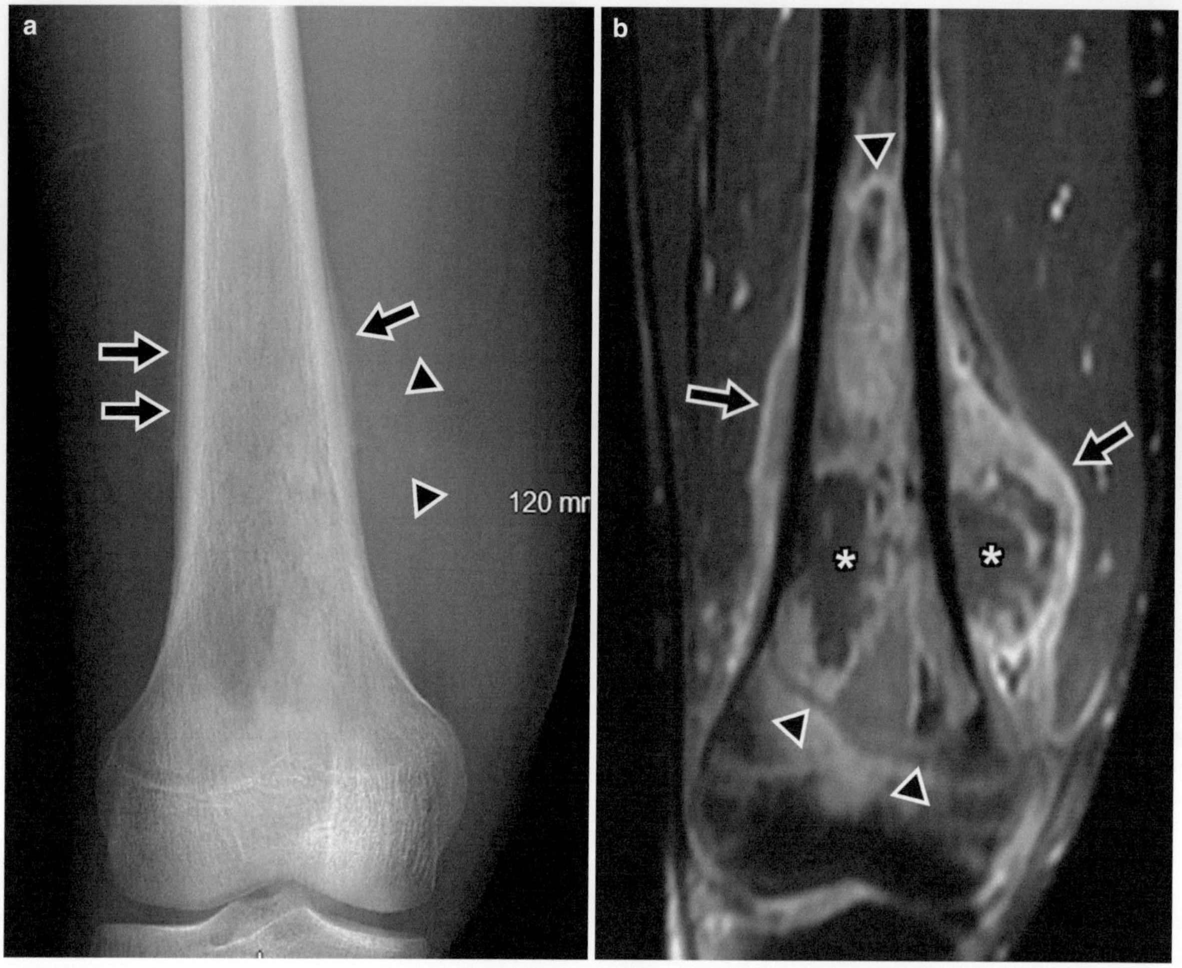

Fig. 9 15-year-old boy with osteosarcoma of the distal femur. (**a**) Anteroposterior radiograph shows an ill-defined mixed lucent and sclerotic lesion in the distal femoral metaphysis and diaphysis. Periosteal new bone (*arrows*) is mildly irregular. Faint opacities project in soft tissues medially (*arrowheads*). (**b**) Coronal fat-saturated T1-weighted image after gadolinium-based contrast (TR 467, TE 8 ms) shows the intramedullary extent of the tumor (*arrowheads*) and extraosseous soft tissue extension (*arrows*). Areas of necrosis do not enhance (*asterisks*)

Most osteosarcomas are conventional high-grade intramedullary tumors [17]. Teliangiectactic osteosarcomas are expansile lesions which may mimic benign tumors. Surface osteosarcomas include parosteal (low grade), periosteal and high-grade surface types [19].

Osteosarcoma is most common in the metaphyses of growing bones. The most common site is the distal femur at the knee. Osteosarcoma can theoretically occur within any bone, but is less common in flat bones of the axial skeleton.

On radiography, osteosarcoma appears as an aggressive lesion with poorly defined margins, permeative bone destruction, aggressive periosteal new bone (layered, spiculated, interrupted) and an associated soft tissue mass (Figs. 2 and 9) [20, 21]. The diagnosis can be specifically suggested when there is abundant osteoid production within the lesion within bone or within the associated soft tissue mass (Fig. 10).

Telangiectatic osteosarcoma often appears similar to a simple or aneurysmal bone cyst on radiography. Any aggressive features on radiography and any solid component (even very small) on MRI, suggests a more ominous

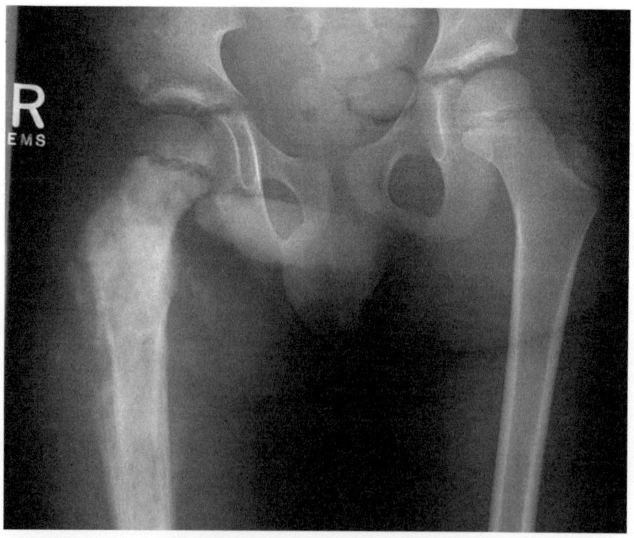

Fig. 10 6-year-old boy with osteosarcoma of the proximal femur. The lesion is ill-defined, with permeative change, cortical destruction, aggressive periosteal new bone (layered, speculated, interrupted) and associated soft tissue mass. The degree of opacity is in keeping with abundant osteoid production of an osteosarcoma rather than just reactive sclerosis

lesion requiring histological sampling. Parosteal and periosteal osteosarcomas are relatively uncommon, but have characteristic appearances. Parosteal osteosarcoma usually appears as a lobular, juxtacortical, ossified mass (differential diagnosis includes osteochondoma and myositis ossificancs) [17, 19]. Periosoteal osteosarcoma usually appears as fusiform mass with or without scalloping of the underlying cortex, spiculated periosteal new bone and Codman triangles [17, 19].

Ewing Sarcoma

Ewing sarcoma is the second most common pediatric bone tumor. It occurs throughout childhood into early adulthood [17, 22]. Ewing sarcoma is slightly more common in the first decade of life than osteosarcoma. It is a small round blue cell tumor probably of neural crest origin. Ewing sarcoma usually arises in bone but may arise in soft tissues (extraosseous Ewing sarcoma). In general, prognosis is worse than for osteosarcoma and depends on age, location, tumor size and staging (metastatic disease). Treatment involves multi-agent chemotherapy, radiation and surgery. Axial lesions are more challenging to treat and resect.

Ewing sarcoma most commonly occurs in the diaphyses and metadiaphyses of the long bones and within flat bones of the axial skeleton [17, 22]. On radiography, the lesions appear aggressive with poorly-defined margins, permeative bone bone destruction, aggressive periosteal new bone (layered [onion skin], interrupted) and associated soft tissue mass (Figs. 11 and 12). There may be reactive sclerosis with the interosseous portion of the mass, but there is no frank osteoid production, unlike osteosarcoma. Occasionally, Ewing sarcoma is eccentric or surface in location, producing an aggressive-appearing scalloping of the underlying bone (Fig. 11).

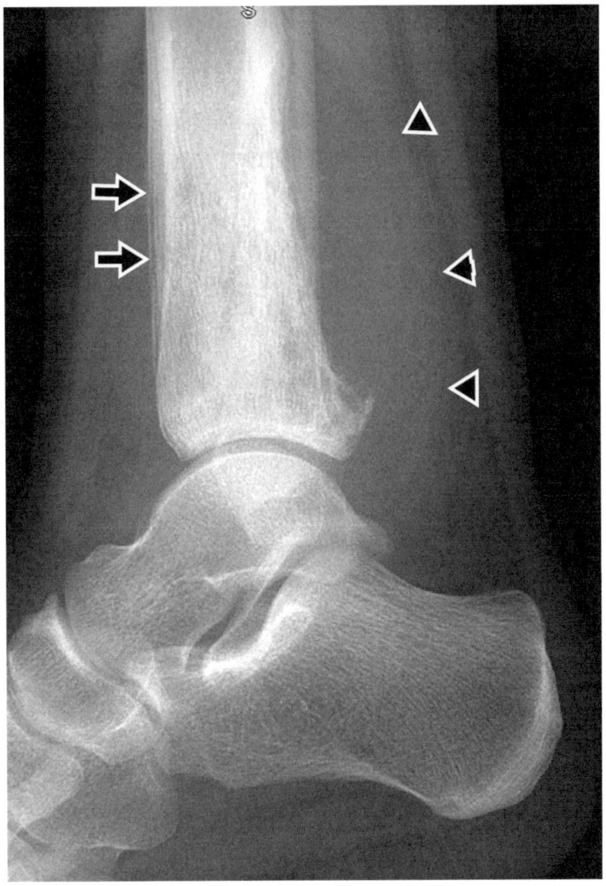

Fig. 11 13-year-old girl with Ewing sarcoma of the distal tibia. The posterior aspect of the tibia shows scalloped bone destruction with a soft tissue mass (*arrowheads*). Faint spiculations of bone are seen within the scalloping. Aggressive layers periosteal new bone is seen anteriorly (*arrows*). Reactive sclerosis is noted. In this case, imaging findings are indistinguishable from osteosarcoma although scalloping of the cortex is more frequently seen with Ewing sarcoma. On staging work-up, diffuse skeletal metastases and pulmonary metastases were found

Imaging Work-Up of Malignant Tumors

As noted, imaging of malignant tumors begins with radiography. Radiography serves to identify a lesion as aggressive or non-aggressive in appearance and guide further imaging and clinical work-up.

MRI is used for characterization of the tumor and delineation of extent (Fig. 9) [17, 21–23]. MR defines the intramedullary extent of tumor and involvement of physes/epiphyses. MR shows soft tissue extension and involvement of adjacent neurovascular structures. Although multiplanar, multisequence MRI without gadolinium-based contrast media suffices for delineation of most malignant bone tumors, contrast aids in characterization and by defining areas of necrosis (Fig. 9). Dynamic gadolinium enhancement has been used in some centers for prediction and monitoring of response to chemotherapy [17, 24].

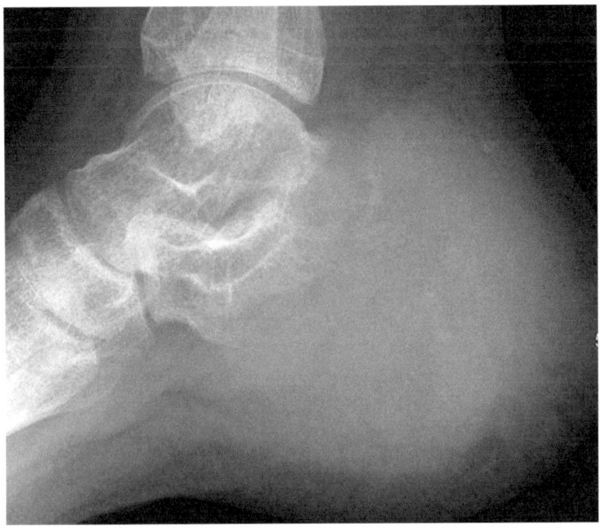

Fig. 12 13-year-old boy with Ewing sarcoma of the calcaneus. The body and posterior calcaneus are destroyed and replaced by a large soft tissue mass. Margins with the remaining bone of the anterior calcaneus are poorly defined

Skip lesions are not infrequent in pediatric musculoskeletal tumors, particularly with a primary osteosarcoma in the distal end of a long bone. Initial MRI studies should thus include images of the entire bone to evaluate for skip lesions. Conventional T1-weighted images without fat saturation and STIR (short tau inversion recovery) images are performed in the sagittal and/or coronal planes. With monitored cases, if these image are negative for tumor, the field of view can be narrowed for better evaluation of the primary tumor on subsequent sequences.

Definitive diagnosis of bone tumors requires biopsy and histological access. Traditionally, biopsies are performed as an incisional surgical biopsy to assure adequate tissue is obtained for analysis. Increasingly, image guided biopsy is utilized. It is imperative that the track of biopsy (surgical or needle) is carefully considered with reference to eventual surgical management of the tumor as the track is considered contaminated and requires resection.

Staging of malignant bone tumors is completed by performing CT of the chest for pulmonary metastases and imaging for distant bone metastatic disease. Traditionally, Tc99m-methylenediphophonate bone scans have been done to assess for other sites of bone disease. More recently, 18F-fluorodeoxyglucose PET, whole-body MRI and now PET-MRI scans have been increasing used [25–27].

Imaging of osteosarcoma and Ewing sarcoma in children is largely therapy protocol driven, both at presentation and in follow-up. Follow-up studies are performed at set intervals unless interval symptoms or concerns for recurrence develop. MRI is performed to monitor response to therapy and for surveillance to exclude recurrence. In assessing response to therapy, MRI can assess change in tumor size, tumor necrosis, tumor vascularity (enhancement pattern and dynamics), change in relationship to other structures (vasculature, nerves), response of metastatic foci, net metastatic disease and complications of therapy [17, 22]. CT of the chest is also regularly performed in follow-up of treated patients. MRI is usually involved monitoring of the primary site; however, after limb-salvage surgery, images are limited my metal artifact. Serial PET imaging is also valuable in assessing for recurrence or new metastatic disease. Post-surgical changes and altered weight bearing may produce areas of increased activity on PET scans which must be differentiated from recurrent tumor.

Primary Osseous Lymphoma

Although rare, primary osseous non-Hodgkin lymphoma is within the differential diagnosis for an aggressive appearing bone lesion in a pediatric patient [28]. The appearance overlaps with osteosarcoma and Ewing sarcoma. Lesions vary from predominantly lytic to sclerotic. Associated regional lymph node enlargement may suggest the diagnosis as this is less common with osseous sarcomas. Diagnosis is made by biopsy and histological examination.

Differential Diagnosis of an Aggressive Bone Lesion in a Child

Aggressive (i.e. methicillin-resistant *Staphylococcus aureus*) or indolent infection (i.e. *Mycobacterium tuberculosis*) may have imaging features mimicking an aggressive tumor, particularly on radiography. Traumatic stress injuries may mimic an aggressive tumor both in presentation and imaging appearance. Some Langerhans cell histiocytosis lesions may have aggressive features including layered periosteal new bone and associated soft tissue mass. Osseous metastatic disease and leukemia may produce osseous lesions but are usually multifocal. In an infant or toddler, the most likely diagnosis for an aggressive-appearing metaphyseal lesion is metastatic neuroblastoma.

Conclusion

Imaging plays an integral part to the diagnosis, management and follow-up of pediatric bone tumors, benign and malignant. At presentation, distinction of non-aggressive from aggressive lesions by radiography guides further imaging. CT (for some non-aggressive lesions) and MRI (for all aggressive lesions) are valuable for further characterization and delineation of extent.

References

1. Kaste SC, Strouse PJ, Fletcher BD, Neel MD (2008) Benign and malignant bone tumors. In: Slovis TL (ed) Caffey's pediatric diagnostic imaging, 11th edn, Mosby, p 2912–2969
2. Nichols RE, Dixon LB (2011) Radiographic analysis of solitary bone lesions. Radiol Clin N Am 49:1095–1114
3. Khanna G, Bennett DL (2012) Pediatric bone lesions: beyond the plain radiographic evaluation. Semin Roentgenol 47:90–99
4. Douis H, Saifuddin A (2012) The imaging of cartilaginous bone tumours. I. Benign lesions. Skelet Radiol 41:1195–1212
5. Murphy MD, Choi JJ, Kransdorf MJ et al (2000) Imaging of osteochondroma: variants and complications with radiologic-pathologic correlation. Radiographics 20:1407–1434
6. Woertler K, Linder N, Gosheger G et al (2000) Osteochondroma: MR imaging of tumor-related complications. Eur Radiol 10:832–840
7. Sailhan F, Chotel F, Parot R (2009) Chondroblastoma of bone in a pediatric population. J Bone Joint Surg Am 91:2159–2168
8. Weatherall PT, Maale GE, Mendelsohn DB et al (1994) Chondroblastoma: classic and confusing appearance at MR imaging. Radiology 190:467–474
9. Mascard E, Gomez-Brouchet A, Lambot K (2015) Bone cysts: unicameral and aneurysmal bone cyst. Orthop Traumatol Surg Res 101:S119–S127
10. Fitzpatrick KA, Taljanovic MS, Speer DP et al (2004) Imaging findings of fibrous dysplasia with histopathologic and intraoperative correlation. AJR Am J Roentgenol 182:1389–1398

11. Jee WH, Choe BY, Kang HS et al (1998) Nonossifying fibroma: characteristics by MR imaging with pathologic correlation. Radiology 209:197–202
12. Smith SE, Kransdorf MJ (2000) Primary musculoskeletal tumors of fibrous origin. Semin Musculoskelet Radiol 4:73–88
13. Azouz EM, Saigal G, Rodriguez MM et al (2005) Langerhans' cell histiocytosis: pathology, imaging and treatment of skeletal involvement. Pediatr Radiol 2005:103–115
14. Stull MA, Kransdorf MJ, Dvaney KO (1992) Langerhans cell histiocytosis of bone. Radiographics 12:801–823
15. Yalcinkaya U, Doganavsargil B, Sezak M et al (2014) Clinical and morphological characteristics of osteoid osteoma and osteoblastoma: a retrospective single-center analysis of 204 patients. Ann Diagn Pathol 18:319–325
16. Laurence N, Epelman M, Markowitz RI et al (2012) Osteoid osteomas: a pain in the night diagnosis. Pediatr Radiol 42:1490–1501
17. Kaste SC (2011) Imaging pediatric bone sarcomas. Radiol Clin N Am 49:749–765
18. Krych A, Odland A, Roase P et al (2014) Oncologic conditions that simulate common sports injuries. J Am Acad Orthop Surg 22:223–234
19. Kaste SC, Fuller CE, Saharia A et al (2006) Pediatric surface osteosarcoma: clinical, pathologic, and radiologic features. Pediatr Blood Cancer 47(2):152–162
20. Clayer M (2015) Many faces of osteosarcoma on plain radiographs. ANZ J Surg 85:22–26
21. Suresh S, Saifuddin A (2007) Radiological appearance of appendicular osteosarcoma: a compreshensive pictorial review. Clin Radiol 62:314–323
22. Murphey MD, Senchak LT, Mambalam PK et al (2013) From the radiologic pathology archives: ewing sarcoma family of tumors: radiologic-pathologic correlation. Radiographics 33: 803–831
23. Rana KA, Meyer J, Ibrahim S et al (2013) The role of imaging of malignant bone tumors in children and young adults. Curr Probl Cancer 37:181–191
24. Guo J, Reddick WE, Glass JO et al (2012) Dynamic contrast-enhanced magnetic resonance imaging as a prognostic factor in predicting event-free and overall survival in pediatric patients with osteosarcoma. Cancer 118:3776–3785
25. Dalrup-Link HE, Franzius C, Link TM et al (2001) Whole-body MR imaging for detection of bone metastases in children and young adults: comparison with skeletal scintigraphy and FDG PET. AJR Am J Roentgenol 177:229–236
26. Eftekhari F (2009) Imaging assessment of osteosarcoma in childhood and adolescence: diagnosis, staging, and evaluating response to chemotherapy. Cancer Treat Res 152:33–62
27. Choudhry AA, Gul M, Could E et al (2016) Utility of positron emission tomography-magnetic resonance imaging in musculoskeletal imaging. World J Radiol 28:268–274
28. Milks KS, McLean TW, Anthony EY (2016) Imaging of primary pediatric lymphoma of bone. Pediatr Radiol 46:1150–1157

Shoulder: Glenohumeral Instability

Monica Tafur, Sarah Koles, Ara Kassarjian,
and Lawrence M. White

Glenohumeral Instability

The glenohumeral joint is a classic ball and socket type joint which allows a broad range of movement but whose shallow glenoid component compromises the inherent stability of the joint. Only 25–30% of the humeral head contacts the glenoid surface [1]. The joint is fortified by both intrinsic and extrinsic components. Internally, the glenoid fibrocartilaginous labrum is a strong cuff around the bony glenoid which serves to deepen the socket and cradle the humeral head. The labrum and synovial fluid create an intrinsic vacuum within the joint believed to further stabilize the joint [2]. Strong anterior glenohumeral ligaments (superior, middle and inferior) act as static stabilizers and provide support along the anterior and inferior joint, and blend with the thinner glenohumeral joint capsule [3]. The labroligamentous complex (anterior band of the inferior glenohumeral ligament (IGHL) and labrum) is the strongest stabilizer of the joint [4]. The labrum is a fibrocartilaginous dense tissue circumferentially deepening the glenoid articular surface. This is attached to the glenoid bone, glenoid cartilage and glenohumeral ligaments and superiorly with the tendon of the long head of the biceps. The strength of the labrum and its glenoid attachment increases with age so labral injuries are more common in younger patients [5, 6].

Bony morphology such as glenoid version, typically a slight anteversion relative to the scapular spine, prevents posterior displacement of the humeral head. Extrinsically, the rotator cuff tendons, long head of biceps tendon and deltoid muscle lend added stability to the joint by acting as dynamic stabilizers. The rigid scapula and the acromioclavicular articulation are adjacent bony struts that further protect the shoulder girdle. Compromise of any of the intrinsic or extrinsic stabilizers of the joint can lead to joint laxity and result in either unidirectional or multidirectional glenohumeral instability.

Clinical apprehension testing of anterior shoulder instability is a reliable test although other clinical tests to diagnose instability, or specifically evaluate individual structural contributors of instability, are less reliable. Likewise, arthroscopic visualization of some glenohumeral pathologies associated with instability can be challenging [7]. Imaging, specifically MR arthrography, can bridge this medical gap by identifying structural components causing glenohumeral instability, associated pathology and sequelae of chronic instability. Imaging findings can thereby augment clinical findings and allow clinicians to further stratify patients who would be best managed surgically.

Imaging Techniques

MR arthrography has long been considered the imaging "gold standard" for assessing glenohumeral instability.

MR arthrography is indicated in patients with glenohumeral instability and may be of benefit in athletes with unclear shoulder pain and a negative conventional non-arthrographic MRI [6]. Direct MR arthrography involves injection of a dilute gadolinium chelate into the glenohumeral joint using either fluoroscopic or sonographic guidance. Intra-articular positioning can be confirmed with a small volume injection of iodinated contrast media with fluoroscopy, or by visualization of joint distension with injection under ultrasound. In some centres, the arthrogram injectant includes a small volume of anaesthetic, adding a further diagnostic component to the study. Pre- and post- injection

M. Tafur • L.M. White (✉)
Joint Department of Medical Imaging, University of Toronto,
585 University Avenue, Toronto, ON M5G 2N2, Canada
e-mail: monica.tafur@uhn.ca; lawrence.white@uhn.ca

S. Koles
Mayfair Diagnostics, 132 Mayfair Place, 6707 Elbow Dr SW,
Calgary, AB T2V 0E3, Canada
e-mail: skoles@radiology.ca

A. Kassarjian
Corades S. L., Calle Galeon 2, Majadahonda, Madrid 28220, Spain
e-mail: akassarjian@gmail.com

J. Hodler et al. (eds.), *Musculoskeletal Diseases 2017-2020*, DOI 10.1007/978-3-319-54018-4_18

pain scores can add valuable diagnostic information when attempting to differentiate intra- or extra-articular causes of pain [8]. In recent years, there have been studies which have shown anesthetics have varying degrees of cartilage toxicity [9]. A recent controlled in vivo study however showed no histologic cartilage damage after five consecutive weekly intra articular injections of bupivacaine [10].

Indirect MR arthrography, with delayed joint opacification through intravenous injection, is of limited utility in assessing shoulder stability. The capsular distension and extension of contrast into subtle or effaced labral tears afforded by direct MR arthrography provides an advantage over an indirect MR arthrography or unenhanced MRI [8, 11]. Direct MR arthrography has a sensitivity of 88–98% and a specificity of 91–100% for the diagnosis of labral tears [6]. ABER positioning further increases the conspicuity of anteroinferior or other labral pathology [12]. MR arthrography is also more sensitive and specific for partial thickness articular sided rotator cuff tears [6].

Although there is great variability in local preferences, MR arthrographic imaging with a dedicated shoulder coil typically includes a coronal oblique T1 TSE (or FSE) and intermediate (i.e., TE 30–60 ms) TSE sequence with fat suppression, and a sagittal oblique T1 TSE with or without fat suppression. In the transverse plane, an axial T1 TSE with or without fat suppression, and sometimes an intermediate TSE sequence in ABER (abducted and externally rotated) position is obtained. A *maximal* slice thickness of 3.5 mms, a *maximum* field of view of 16 cms, and a *minimum* matrix of 256 × 256 is suggested in the recent guidelines of the European Society of Musculoskeletal Radiology for Imaging of Sports Injuries [13]. Depending on local hardware and software capabilities, higher resolution imaging can be obtained [14].

Non-enhanced MRI may be adequate if performed after a recent shoulder dislocation as the joint will be distended physiologically by the post-traumatic joint effusion. As the quality of imaging and access to 3T imaging has increased, non-arthrographic 3T MRI has also been suggested as a sufficient diagnostic tool for shoulder instability. However, subtle findings associated with instability are not always seen at unenhanced 3T MR imaging and recent studies continue to support MR arthrography, either with 1.5T or 3T imaging, as the most comprehensive imaging test for the assessment of shoulder instability [15].

As most of the key contributing structures to shoulder instability are intra-articular, ultrasound has been of limited benefit, although ultrasound can diagnose associated rotator cuff tendon pathology and some forms of extra-articular impingement.

Radiography is an excellent and accessible method to assess glenohumeral joint integrity and alignment. Anteroposterior images depict a curvilinear glenohumeral overlap, reflecting the glenoid socket articulating with the convex humeral head. Congruity of the joint on this view is confirmed by a smooth, not angled, inferior glenohumeral line. Loss of this congruity is seen in anterior or posterior subluxation, or dislocation (Fig. 1a, b). In addition, fractures or intra-articular dependent ossific bodies can be visualized. An anteroposterior (AP) radiograph with internal rotation is more sensitive in the detection of Hill Sachs lesions of the humeral head. Oblique AP views (e.g., Grashey views) allow

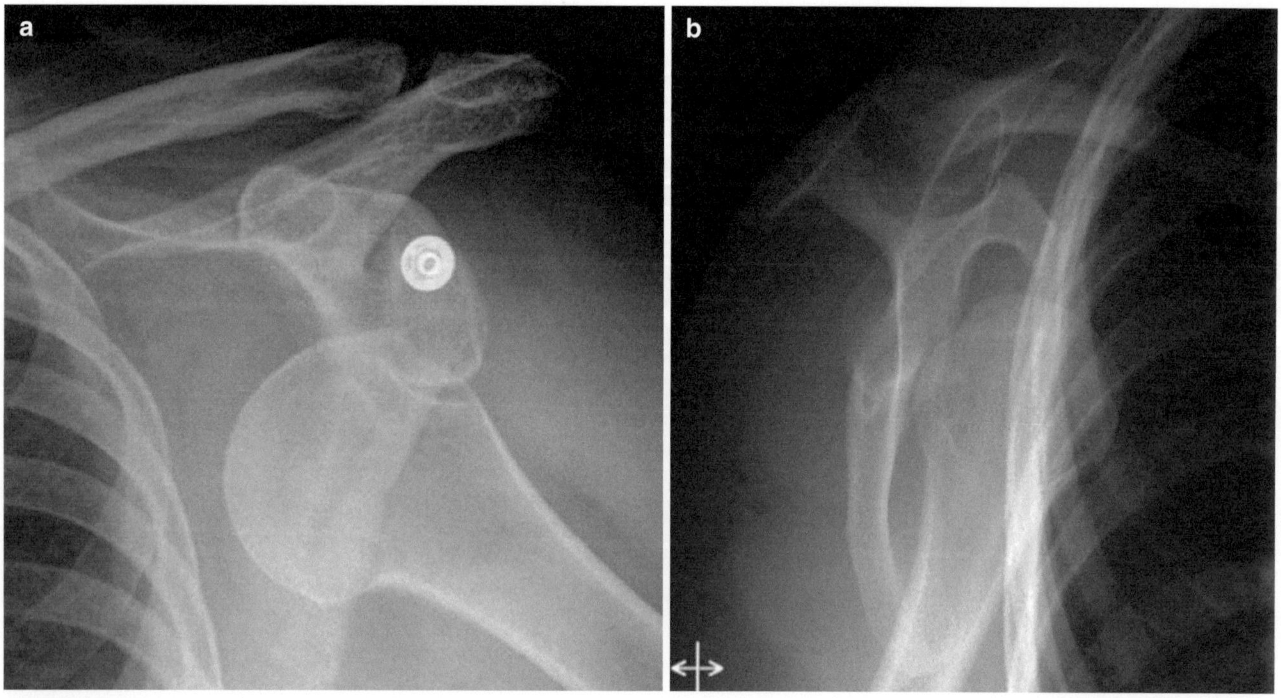

Fig. 1 Anterior shoulder dislocation. AP (**a**) and scapular Y-view (**b**) radiographs demonstrate anteroinferior glenohumeral dislocation

an en face assessment of the joint space. Glenoid rim abnormalities related to prior dislocations, such as bony Bankart lesions, may be subtly seen. Similarly, this view permits assessment of the posterolateral humeral head contour which may be depressed or indented after prior dislocations (Hill Sachs deformity). Lateral radiographs can be obtained by two different techniques. A trans-scapular view is aligned with the axis of the scapular body. Glenohumeral dislocation can be assessed, as can inferior or superior subluxation. Alternatively, if the patient can be comfortably positioned, a trans-axillary view provides the most reliable assessment of the glenohumeral joint alignment, including subtle subluxations, and can assess the glenoid margin for the presence of bony Bankart lesions.

Computed tomography (CT) is valuable for confirmation of subtle bone lesions associated with instability and for orthopedic surgical planning. A tailored thin cut CT with direct axial, coronal, sagittal and 3D reformats oriented relative to the scapular spine provides a thorough assessment of the glenoid bony morphology and version. Furthermore, evaluation of associated Bankart or Hill Sachs lesions, specifically whether they are "engaging" or apt to lock with repeat dislocation, is of value for orthopaedic triage. CT arthrography is performed in a manner similar to MR arthrography but using nonionic contrast instead of MRI contrast and a viable option for patients who cannot undergo MR imaging. Capsular and cartilage integrity, bone morphology and alignment are well assessed with CT arthrography, as are the glenohumeral ligaments. Positioning with external rotation and active supination increases detection of SLAP tears [15]. With improved CT imaging, MR and CT arthrography are more recently considered equivalent in diagnosing SLAP tears and full thickness rotator cuff tears. Although MR arthrography remains better at predicting engaging Hill Sachs deformities, CT arthrography is better at identifying humeral avulsion of the GHL (HAGL) and glenoid rim fractures [7].

Anterior Glenohumeral Instability

Glenohumeral instability is a spectrum of pathology including dislocation, subluxation and hyperlaxity of the joint [6]. Stability of the glenohumeral joint has historically been subdivided into two main categories based on mechanism of injury. A post-traumatic mechanism typically results in unidirectional instability, is associated with a Bankart injury and often requires surgery; acronym of TUBS (traumatic, unidirectional, Bankart, surgery). The most common instability condition of the glenohumeral joint is secondary to an anterior shoulder dislocation which is traumatic 95% of the time and has a peak occurrence in males 22–33 years old. The estimated incidence of shoulder dislocation in the USA is 23.9 per 100,000 person-years [16]. The most common cause of traumatic anterior instability is due to glenohumeral dislocation, typically anteroinferior dislocation of the humerus after forced abduction and external rotation [7]. This can result in capsular stripping or laxity, labroligamentous tearing, and cartilage or bone defects.

The incidence of recurrent dislocations depends on the cacophony of soft tissue and bony injuries, and patient age. Recurrent dislocations are more frequent in younger patients. For example, young males suffered from recurrent injuries 87% of the time during a 5-year follow-up [17]. The possibility of recurrent shoulder instability in all age populations after non-operative management is 55–67% [18]. In those with recurrent dislocation and injury, surgical stabilization of the glenohumeral joint is more effective than immobilization and rehabilitation alone [19].

Regardless of the etiology, shoulder instability is a very common pathology. Beyond pain, or activity limited by apprehension of recurrent dislocation, chronic glenohumeral instability can initiate a cycle of premature joint degeneration, rotator cuff tearing and impingement [6]. These pathologies can secondarily result in progressive glenohumeral instability and further degeneration of the joint and associated stabilizers.

Anatomical and Biomechanical Considerations

The fibrocartilaginous labrum circumferentially deepens the glenoid articular surface. This is attached to the glenoid bone, glenoid cartilage and glenohumeral ligaments (GHLs) and superiorly with the long head of biceps tendon. The inferior glenohumeral ligament (IGHL) and labrum are intimate and often considered one entity, the "labroligamentous complex". The IGHL is the largest of the glenohumeral ligaments and the most consistent stabilizer of the glenohumeral joint. It is composed of a thick anterior band and a smaller posterior band with an intervening axillary pouch. In abduction, there is increased tension on the IGHL with the anterior band limiting anterior translation of the humerus in external rotation and the posterior band limiting humeral translation in internal rotation. The anterior band of the IGHL arises from the glenoid between 2–5 o'clock, and the posterior band between 7–9 o'clock. Both bands have a broad lateral insertion on the humeral anatomic neck [20].

The superior glenohumeral ligament (SGHL) may originate from the anterosuperior labrum, the long head of the biceps tendon, or directly off the middle glenohumeral ligament. It extends anteriorly parallel to the base of the coracoid process. The middle glenohumeral ligament (MGHL) is the most variable in its appearance. Just over 50% of the time, the MGHL arises directly from the labrum. Otherwise, it arises at the origin of the superior glenohumeral ligament. A cordlike MGHL is present in 17% and a true Buford complex (absent anterosuperior labrum and cord-like MGHL) is present in less than 2% of people [21].

Imaging Findings in Anterior Glenohumeral Dislocation

Injuries to the stabilizing tissues of the shoulder joint observed in the setting of traumatic anterior glenohumeral dislocation are described according to a spectrum of labroligamentous, cartilaginous, periosteal and osseous pathology associated with anterior glenohumeral instability.

A Bankart lesion is a detachment of the labroligamentous complex off the anteroinferior glenoid, typically seen after a traumatic dislocation. On MR imaging, the labrum is separated from the bony glenoid but remains attached to the anterior band of the IGHL (Fig. 2). On non-contrast MRI, the tear may be seen although without a joint effusion, the actual separation of a non-displaced labral tear may be difficult to discern. MR arthrograms have higher sensitivity as intra-articular contrast will track beneath the torn labrum and affected structures such as the periosteum. Bankart lesions are the most common post-traumatic lesions associated with anterior instability. As these lesions are unstable, they are unlikely to heal by primary intention and are often surgically managed.

A fragment of the anterior inferior glenoid bone avulsed with the labroligamentous complex during dislocation is referred to as a bony Bankart lesion (Fig. 3). The larger the glenoid bony fragment, the greater the risk of instability, even after stabilization of soft tissue defects [22]. The size

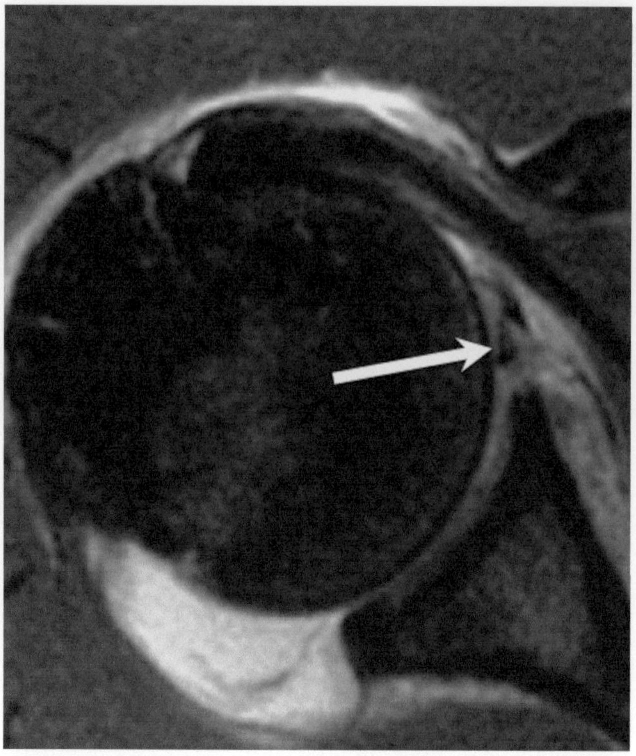

Fig. 2 Bankart lesion. Axial fat-suppressed PD image shortly after dislocation demonstrates a classic Bankart lesion with the anteroinferior labroligamentous complex (*arrow*) separated from the glenoid rim. Due to the acute setting, the joint effusion acts as positive intra-articular contrast

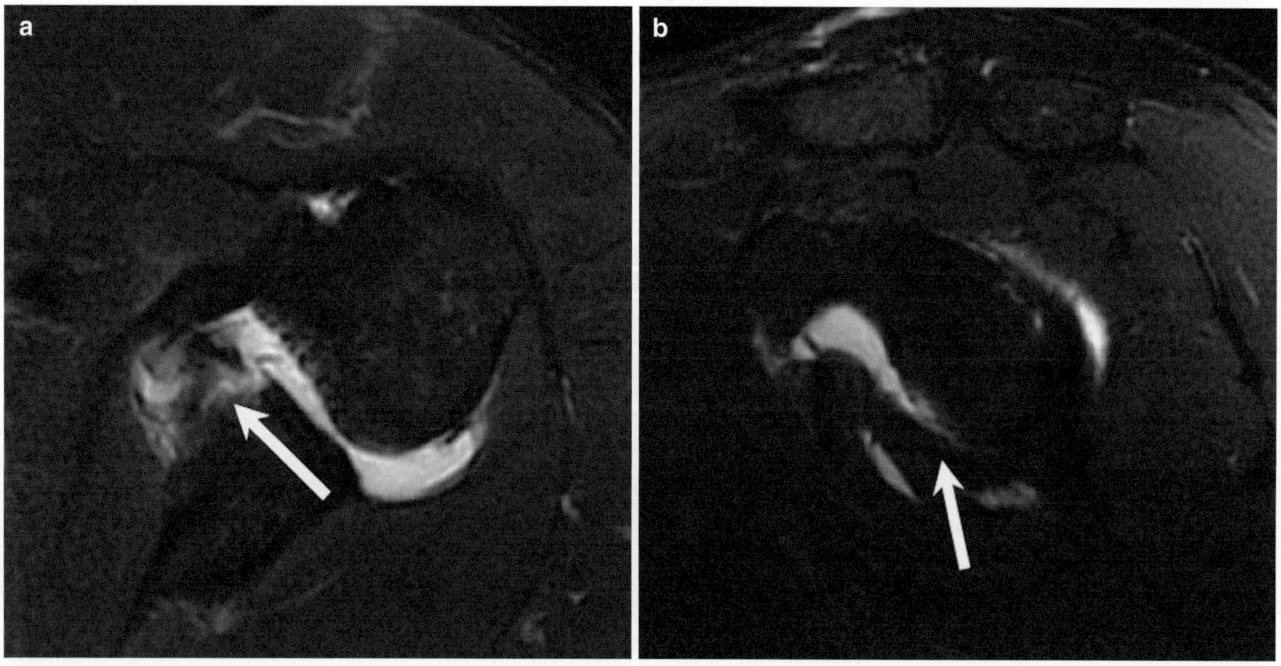

Fig. 3 Bony Bankart lesion. Axial and sagittal fat-suppressed T1-weighted images demonstrate a bony Bankart lesion (*arrow*) with a fracture along the anteroinferior glenoid rim

and configuration of the bone lesion will determine if bone grafting is required. This is best assessed by CT. Most osseous Bankart lesions may be repaired arthroscopically, although an open procedure may be needed if bone grafting is required.

There are many injuries associated with Bankart lesions. Anterior labroligamentous periosteum sleeve avulsion (ALPSA) is the most frequent, seen in 22% of all anteroinferior labroligamentous lesions arthroscopically. They are correctly diagnosed on MR arthrography 77% of the time and seen as a fluid- or contrast-filled cleft beneath the anteroinferior glenoid periosteum which itself may be medially displaced (Fig. 4) [23]. The second most common associated injury is the Perthes lesion where the torn anteroinferior labrum remains non-displaced and attached to periosteum stripped off the anterior scapula (Fig. 5). This occurs in up to 11% of shoulders at arthroscopy for anterior instability, but can be difficult to visualize arthroscopically without probing. Compared to arthroscopy, these lesions are correctly identified on MR arthrography only 50% of the time [23], although they can be better visualized with ABER positioning [5]. A glenolabral articular disruption (GLAD) is infrequent, accounting for less than 3% of anteroinferior labral tears. In one study, all GLAD lesions were correctly diagnosed on MR arthrography pre-arthroscopy with contrast undercutting a fragment of cartilage attached to the torn anteroinferior labrum (Fig. 6) [23].

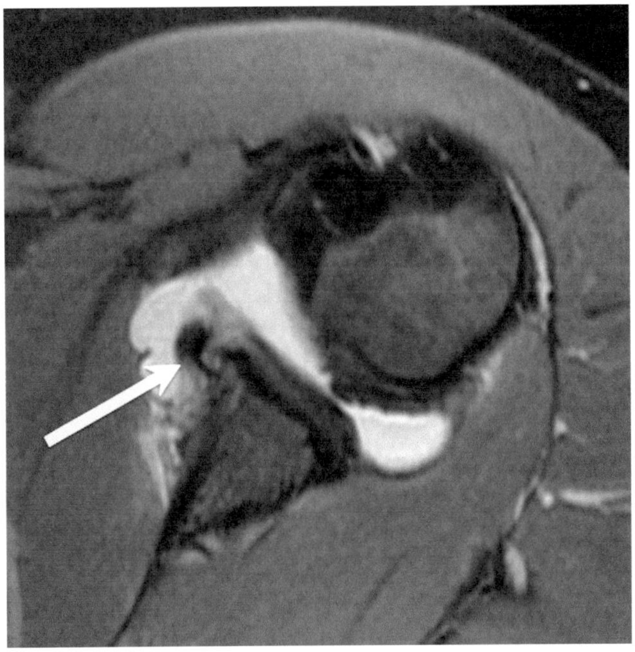

Fig. 4 ALPSA lesion. Axial fat-suppressed PD-weighted image shortly after dislocation demonstrates an ALPSA lesion with medialization of the labrum and periosteum (*arrow*) nicely outlined by the joint effusion

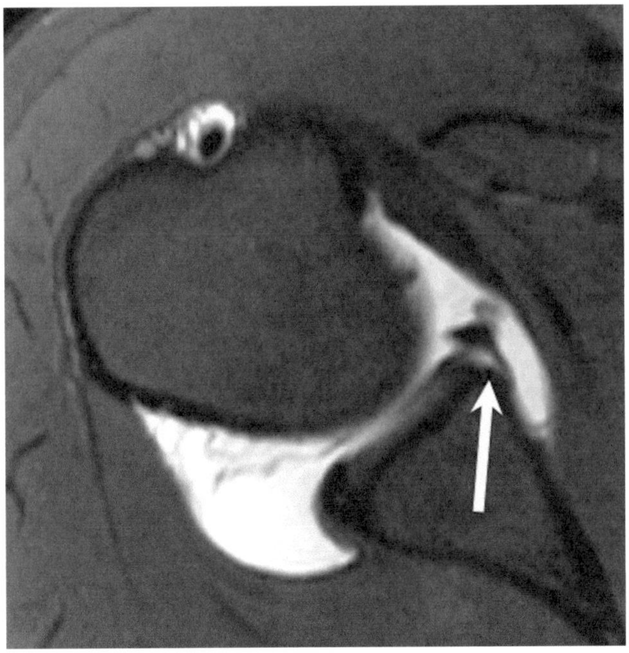

Fig. 5 Perthes lesion. Axial fat-suppressed T1-weighted image demonstrates a Perthes lesions (*arrow*) with periosteal stripping but without medicalization of the labrum or periosteum

Humeral avulsion of the inferior GHL (HAGL) is documented arthroscopically in 1.5–9.3% of cases but the incidence is higher (up to 26.9%) in patients with anterior glenohumeral instability without a Bankart lesion [24]. HAGL can be a difficult diagnosis on imaging. In one review, only 50% of the HAGL lesions were diagnosed on imaging compared to arthroscopy [25]. On MR, a J-shaped axillary pouch, or focal extravasation of intra-articular contrast or joint effusion is seen passing through the torn humeral attachment (Fig. 7). Rarely a bony humeral avulsion of the glenohumeral ligament (BHAGL) can occur and may occasionally be seen on radiographs [25]. Glenoid avulsion of the GHL (GAGL) is an uncommon associated injury also diagnosed with contrast or joint fluid extravasating through the torn attachment of the glenohumeral ligament on the glenoid [20].

Hill Sachs deformity occurs when the superolateral humeral head impacts against the inferior glenoid during dislocation or relocation (Fig. 8). The size of a Hill Sachs lesion is an important factor in glenohumeral instability: larger defects (greater than one third of the focal humeral head circumference) or those with a long axis paralleling the glenoid, are considered "engaging" and associated with repeated subluxations or dislocations [22]. These deformities are often more shallow in patients with underlying hyperlaxity. On MR arthrography, these are accurately seen only 40% of the time compared to arthroscopy.

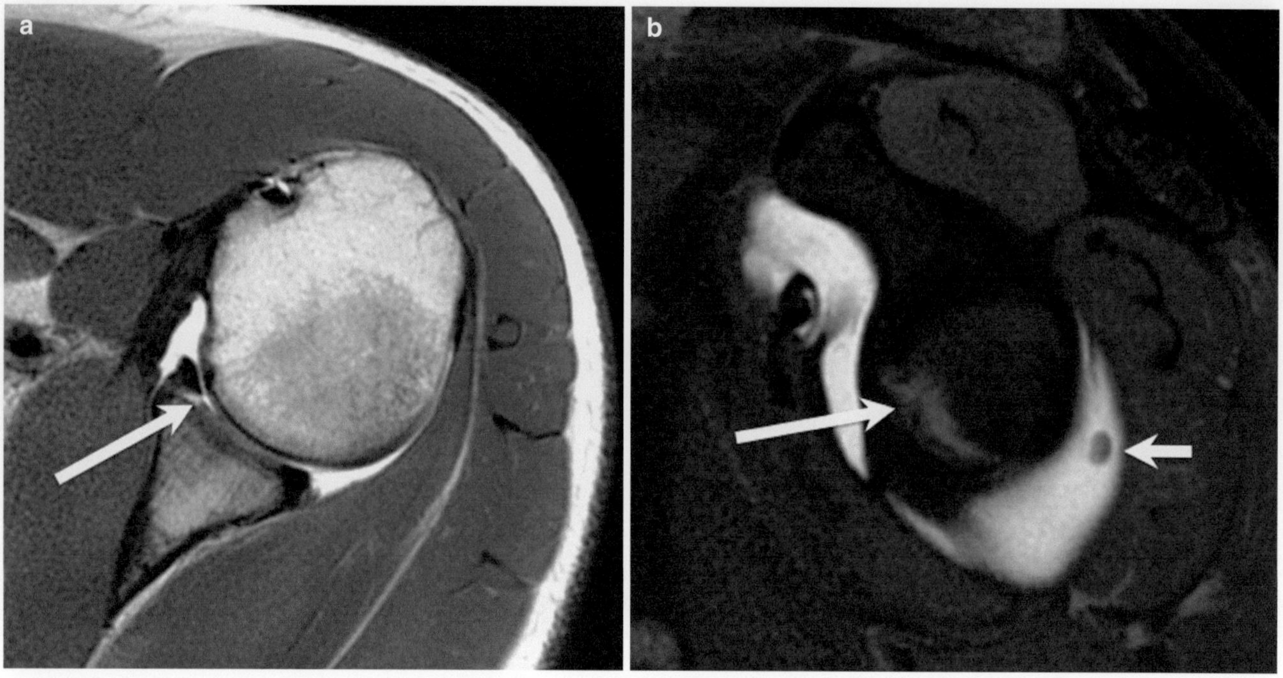

Fig. 6 GLAD lesion. Axial T1-weighted (**a**) and sagittal oblique fat-suppressed T1-weighted (**b**) images demonstrate a GLAD lesion with an anteroinferior glenoid cartilage defect (*arrow* in **a**) and anteroinferior labral tear (*long arrow* in **b**) and loose cartilage fragment (*short arrow* in **b**)

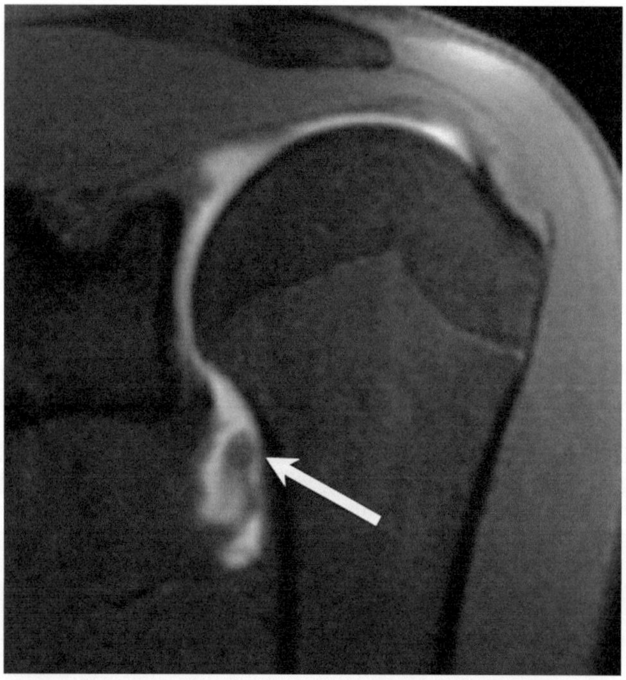

Fig. 7 HAGL lesion. Coronal oblique fat suppressed T1-weighted image demonstrates a HAGL lesion with the distal fibers of the inferior glenohumeral ligament avulsed from the humerus (*arrow*) and adjacent contrast extravasation

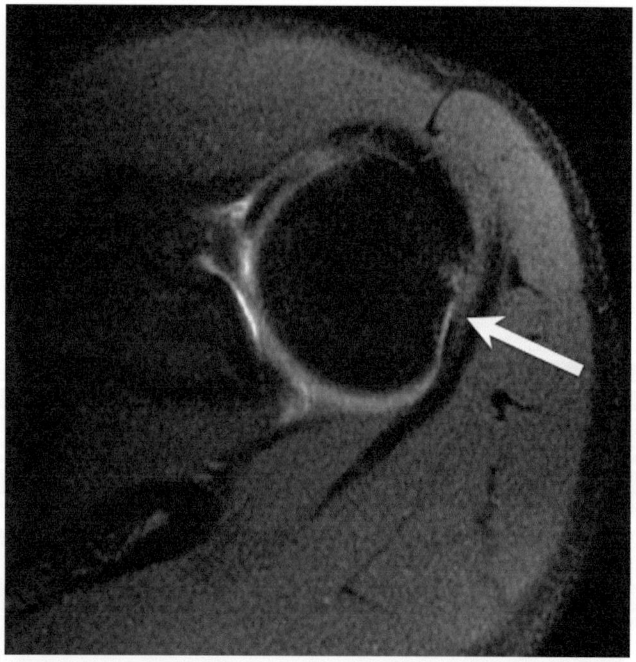

Fig. 8 Hill-Sachs lesion. Axial fat-suppressed T1-weighted image demonstrates a Hill-Sachs lesion (*arrow*) with flattening of the posterolateral aspect of the humeral head due to an impaction fracture

Occasionally, a cyst arises from fluid imbibing through a labral tear and may be paralabral or extend further by dissecting into adjacent tissues. Some cysts communicate with intra-articular contrast extending through the labrum. Cysts extending into the suprascapular notch can cause mass effect on the suprascapular nerve which innervates the supraspinatus and infraspinatus muscle. This can result in atrophy of these muscles. If such a cyst extends into the spinoglenoid notch, it may selectively compress the descending suprascapular nerve and cause denervation of the infraspinatus muscle only. A cyst extending into the quadrilateral space in the axilla may cause denervation of axillary nerve and atrophy of trees minor in isolation [5].

Posterior Glenohumeral Instability

Posterior glenohumeral instability refers to the symptoms and signs resulting from excessive posterior translation of the humeral head relative to the glenoid, and constitutes approximately 5–10% of all cases of shoulder instability. Posterior glenohumeral instability includes a continuum of pathologic changes ranging from chronic posterior dislocation to the more common recurrent posterior subluxation [26]. Common features of posterior glenohumeral instability include traumatic posterior dislocations, a redundant posterior capsule, posterior labroligamentous tears and osteochondral lesions [27].

Recurrent posterior subluxation has become an increasingly recognized cause of shoulder instability. Affected patients are most commonly 20–30 year-old males, who are involved in overhead sports (e.g., baseball pitcher, volleyball, baseball, swimming) or contact sports (e.g., football, wrestling, hockey, or rugby) [28]. Symptoms can also develop insidiously, aggravated by repetitive minor injury when the shoulder is in flexion, adduction and internal rotation [27].

Anatomical and Biomechanical Considerations

Posterior shoulder instability results from several not entirely understood pathological processes, in which several predisposing factors may coexist in the same patient. A variety of osseous or soft tissues abnormalities are associated with the development of posterior instability, or may be seen as secondary complications of posterior instability itself [29].

Any loss in posterior glenoid bone stock or structural irregularities such as glenoid erosion, glenoid hypoplasia/dysplasia, posterior glenoid rim deficiency, excessive glenoid retroversion, or excessive humeral retroversion, may predispose to posterior instability. Non-united prior reverse osseous Bankart lesions may also be a predisposing cause of recurrent posttraumatic posterior shoulder instability [29].

Injury of the primary posterior labrocapsular soft tissue stabilizers of the shoulder may impair their function resulting in an increased posterior translation of the humeral head relative to the glenoid. The inferior glenohumeral ligament (IGHL) and the posteroinferior capsule represent the primary soft tissue restraints of the posterior shoulder in 90° of abduction [30]. The posterior capsule, defined as the area between the intraarticular portion of the biceps tendon and the posterior band of the IGHL, is the thinnest portion of the entire joint capsule and therefore, vulnerable to injury [31]. Other structures that are important in maintaining posterior stability of the glenohumeral joint include the rotator interval and the rotator cuff. The rotator interval functions as a "check-rein" against excessive motion and limits posteroinferior glenohumeral translation [32]. The subscapularis tendon has been proven to be the most significant rotator cuff tendon in preventing posterior translation of the humeral head [31].

Posterior Glenohumeral Dislocation

Posterior glenohumeral dislocation is considered to be a rare injury accounting for 2–5% of all shoulder dislocations. It was first described in 1839 by Sir Astley Cooper in a patient who had sustained an epileptic seizure [29]. The true incidence of posterior glenohumeral dislocation is difficult to estimate because of the high frequency of missed diagnosis on clinical examination and radiographs. The even less frequent posterior fracture-dislocation accounts for 0.9% of all shoulder dislocations [33].

Posterior glenohumeral dislocation is an acute entity associated with direct or indirect trauma. While the term "dislocation" is commonly used, this condition more accurately presents as a "subluxation" as there is commonly some remaining contact between the humeral head and the glenoid [34]. Patients who experience a posterior dislocation may develop a fixed, or locked, posteriorly dislocated shoulder that often requires reduction with additional treatment typically determined by the size of associated osseous defects and the duration of the dislocation [33].

Similar to anterior shoulder dislocations, posterior dislocations are classified according to the anatomic position of the humeral head relative to the glenoid and surrounding osseous structures, with subacromial posterior dislocation being more frequent than subglenoid and subspinous dislocation patterns [35].

Anatomic and Biomechanical Considerations

Multiple mechanisms have been implicated in the etiology of posterior glenohumeral dislocation, most commonly resulting from indirect trauma during violent muscle contraction as seen in the setting of epileptic seizures, electric shock or electroconvulsive therapy. Posterior glenohumeral dislocation may also result from major trauma such as motor vehicle accidents or sports injuries when an axial load is applied on an adducted, flexed and internally rotated arm as seen with a FOOSH (fall on outstretched hand) type injury [35].

Posterior glenohumeral dislocation is associated with a variety of lesions of the posterior labrocapsular complex caused by tensile stress on the posterior band of the IGHL, or by direct compressive and shearing stress applied by the humeral head on the posterior labrum, during posteroinferior dislocation [5].

Imaging Findings in Posterior Glenohumeral Dislocation

The reverse Hill-Sachs lesion is the most frequent anatomic lesion seen following an acute traumatic posterior shoulder dislocation. The prevalence of reverse Hill-Sachs lesions varies in the literature and has been described in up to 86% of patients who have experienced an acute posterior shoulder dislocation [27, 36]. A reverse Hill-Sachs lesion occurs as a result of impaction of the posteroinferiorly displaced humeral head onto the glenoid rim, and is diagnosed when any loss of the normal convexity in the anteromedial aspect of the humeral head is seen (Fig. 9). On radiographs, this lesion may be suspected when a vertical line is identified parallel to the glenoid and has been called the "trough sign" [34]. Reverse Hill-Sachs lesions usually involve less that 25% of the circumference of the articular surface of the humeral head and are infrequently associated with fractures of the tuberosities or the subcapital humerus [36].

The reverse osseous Bankart lesion is typically seen in patients with posterior shoulder instability who had experienced a significant traumatic posterior shoulder dislocation.

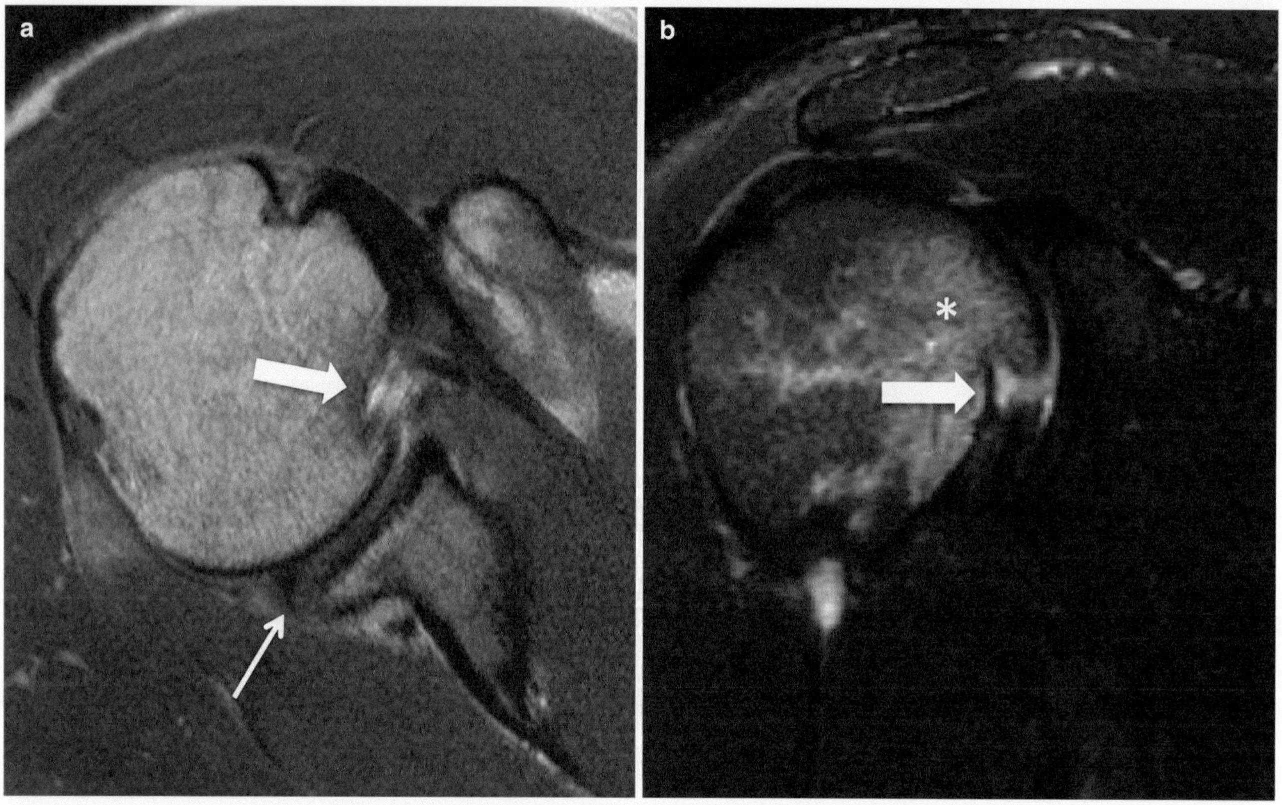

Fig. 9 Posterior glenohumeral dislocation. Axial intermediate-weighted (**a**), coronal fat suppressed T2-weighted (**b**) and axial intermediate-weighted (**c**) MR images demonstrate a large reverse Hill-Sachs lesion in the anteromedial aspect of the humeral head (*thick arrows*). Note the prominent adjacent bone marrow edema (*asterisk*) on the fluid-sensitive MR sequence (**b**). Tears of the posteroinferior labrum (*thin arrows*) and scapular periosteum (*arrowhead*) are seen in keeping with a reverse Bankart lesion

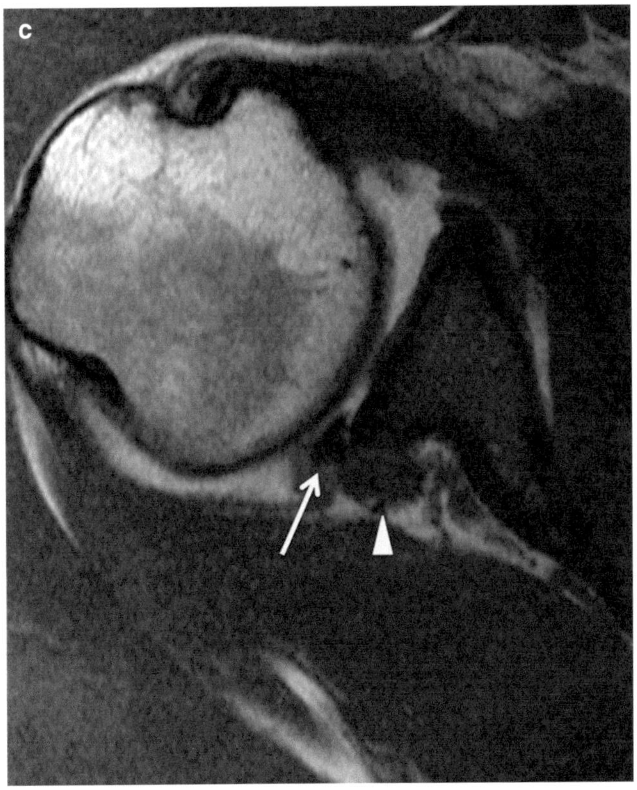

Fig. 9 (continued)

Reverse osseous Bankart lesions occur in 31% of patients after an acute traumatic posterior glenohumeral dislocation and are defined as traumatic fractures of the posterior osseous glenoid rim [36].

Lesions of the posterior labrocapsular complex include reverse soft tissue Bankart lesions, posterior labrocapsular periosteal sleeve avulsion (POLPSA) lesions, and Kim's lesions [5, 28]. Reverse soft tissue Bankart and POLPSA lesions were the most frequent lesions observed in a prior imaging study of acute posterior dislocation patients, with a prevalence of 11% and 10% respectively [36].

Posterior labral tears are less frequent than anterior labral tears and occur in approximately 2–5% of all cases of shoulder instability [37]. On Magnetic Resonance Arthrography (MRA), a posterior labral tear can be manifest by extension of intra-articular contrast material into the substance of the posterior labrum, contrast undercutting the normal labral interface with the posterior glenoid rim, or disruption of posterior labral continuity with possible displacement of labral tissue from its expected normal anatomic position [36]. Isolated posterior tears are uncommon (5%) and are usually associated with other osseous or rotator cuff abnormalities [5].

The reverse Bankart lesion is defined as a posteroinferior labral tear associated with disruption of the posterior scapular periosteal or capsular attachment [38]. MRA demonstrates a displaced and detached posteroinferior labrum between the 6 o'clock and 10 o'clock positions, and a defect in the adjacent scapular periosteum (Figs. 9 and 10). On occasions, gadolinium may be seen outlining the medial aspect of the posterior glenoid neck secondary to the scapular periosteal tear [27].

The POLPSA lesion is defined as an avulsion of the posterior labrum by the posterior inferior glenohumeral ligament/capsule with the posterior labral periosteal attachment to the posterior glenoid neck remaining intact. Unlike the reverse soft tissue Bankart lesion, the scapular periosteal attachment of the posterior labrum is not torn in the POLPSA lesion. The term POLPSA was coined in 1998 for this type of injury, due to the similarity in appearance with the ALPSA lesion seen in cases of anterior-inferior glenohumeral instability and dislocation [38, 39].

Kim's lesion is a deep/intrasubstance detachment of the posteroinferior labrum from the glenoid rim with injury at the adjacent chondrolabral junction or "marginal crack". This type of lesion usually results from a posteroinferiorly directed force on the labrum. Recognition of the presence of a Kim's lesion is crucial at arthroscopy, as it constitutes an apparently concealed lesion at surgery. On MRA, Kim's lesion is seen as a combination of incomplete labral avulsion, loss of labral height and seemingly intact chondrolabral junction [5, 27].

Injury to the rotator cuff can be seen after an acute posterior shoulder dislocation and has been described in 2–19% of acute posterior shoulder dislocation patients [40]. Tears of the teres minor and inferior fibers of the infraspinatus can accompany posterior labrocapsular injury and can be seen as edema or as gadolinium-filled tendon defects on MRA [41]. Contusion or tears can also involve the subscapularis after an acute traumatic dislocation or in the setting of recurrent posterior dislocation [27]. Massive tears of the rotator cuff tears associated with posterior glenohumeral dislocation are rare and only few cases have been reported in the literature [40]. Injuries to the rotator interval and long head of the biceps tendon (LHBT) have also been described in the spectrum of soft tissue injuries seen with posterior glenohumeral dislocation [27, 36].

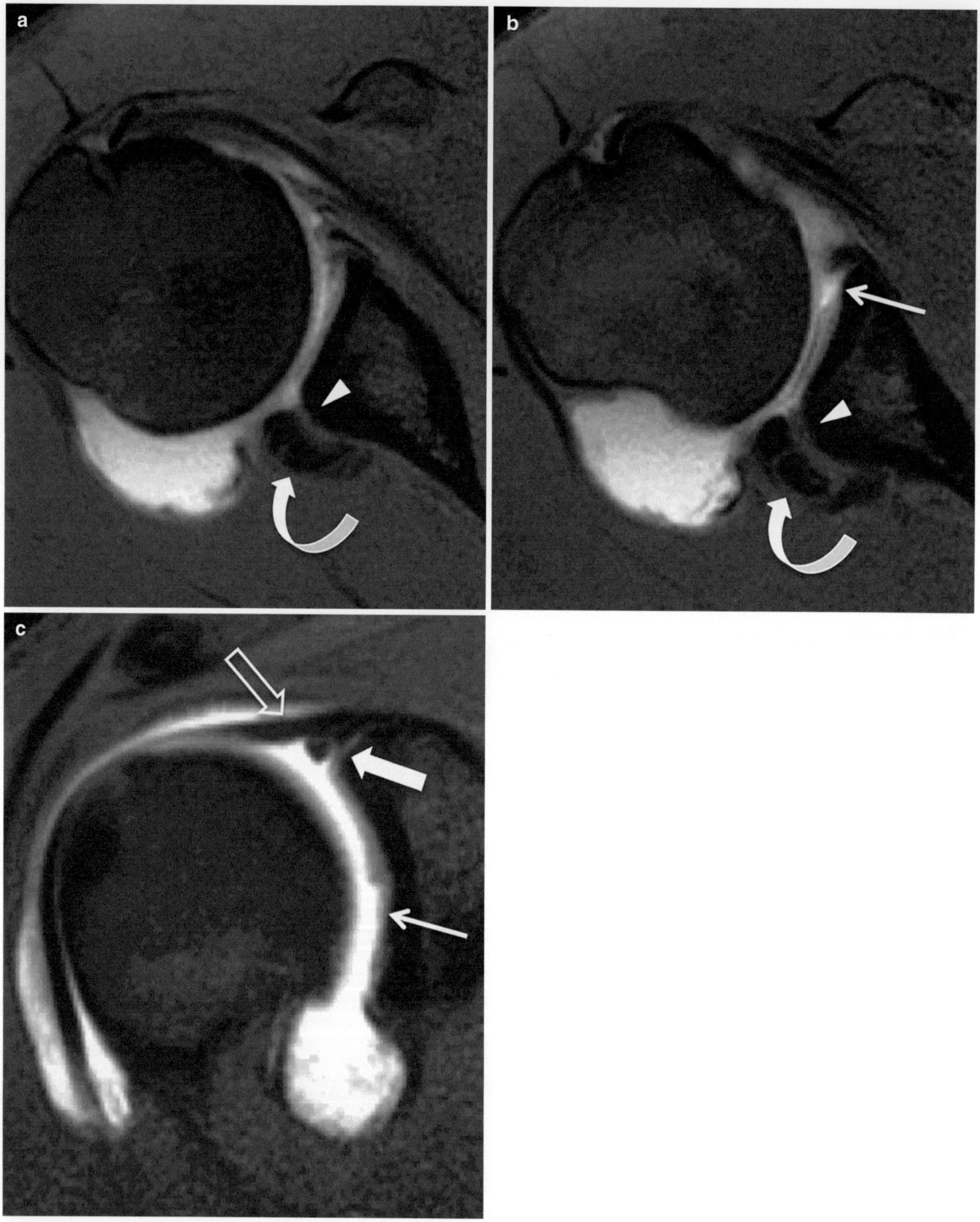

Fig. 10 Acquired multidirectional microinstability in a hockey player with history of symptomatic subluxation. Axial (**a** and **b**) and coronal (**c**) fat suppressed T1-weighted MR arthrographic images show a displaced fracture of the posteroinferior glenoid involving the adjacent labrum (*curved arrow*) consistent with a reverse osseous Bankart lesion. Note the blunted posteroinferior margin of the glenoid (*arrowhead*). A small type II SLAP lesion (*thick arrow*) and a focal full-thickness chondral defect (*thin arrow*) are also seen on the same patient. LHBT = open arrow

Multidirectional Glenohumeral Instability

Shoulder instability includes a spectrum of conditions, ranging from unidirectional posttraumatic dislocation or TUBS (traumatic, unilateral, Bankart lesion, surgery) to atraumatic multidirectional microinstability or AMBRI (atraumatic, multidirectional, bilateral, rehabilitation, inferior capsular shift) [42]. Several classification systems for shoulder instability have been proposed, however, the contribution of multiple factors to this condition makes such a classification difficult [43].

Multidirectional shoulder instability may develop as a consequence of a traumatic injury of the anterior and/or posterior capsulolabral structures, or develop as a consequence of existing predisposing developmental anatomic factors such as glenoid dysplasia/retroversion or capsule hyperlaxity. Atraumatic multidirectional instability of the shoulder was first described by Neer and Foster, and was defined as dislocation of the glenohumeral joint in more than one direction without a previous history of major trauma [44]. More recently revised diagnostic criteria for this condition includes the presence of instability in the inferior direction and at least one other direction (anterior or posterior) [42, 45].

Multidirectional instability usually occurs in young patients, and presents with subtle non-specific symptoms, usually occurring during activities that require repetitive overhead movements. In sedentary patients, this condition affects young women with poor muscular development [46].

Anatomic and Biomechanical Considerations

Multidirectional instability can be complicated by an acute traumatic event and result in unidirectional macroinstability; conversely, a shoulder with unidirectional macroinstability can sustain repetitive microtrauma resulting in symptomatic instability in more than one direction [42].

Ligamentous hyperlaxity is an important predisposing factor for multidirectional shoulder instability, and results from an excess of elastin in the capsular tissue. Capsular hyperlaxity can be congenital or acquired after repetitive microtrauma or a single major traumatic episode [45]. Scapular position has also been implicated as a contributing etiologic factor to multidirectional instability with a reduced scapular inclination contributing to inferior shoulder instability [47].

Imaging Findings in Multidirectional Instability

Although considered a clinical diagnosis, radiographs or CT imaging may be of use in evaluation of patients with atraumatic multidirectional instability, delineating possible glenoid dysplasia or hypoplasia, glenoid bone loss or humeral head defects. However, osseous defects in patients with multidirectional instability are not common [42].

Magnetic Resonance Imaging (MRI), particularly MRA, is considered crucial in the evaluation of the capsuloligamentous structures of the shoulder. Subjective assessment of capsular widening and distention have been show to have high interobserver variability. On MRA, cross-sectional dimensions of glenohumeral joint capsular distension with contrast material, measured on axial and sagittal images, have been shown to be increased in patients with posterior or multidirectional instability but not in patients with anterior instability [47]. The width and presence of herniation of the joint capsule of the rotator interval have been evaluated as indirect signs of a capacious capsule on MRA with variable results. Lee and colleagues found an increased width of the rotator interval in a group of patients with atraumatic multidirectional instability [30]. The crescent and triangle signs on abduction external rotation (ABER) position on MRA have been proposed as useful diagnostic features of patients with multidirectional instability with good sensitivity (48–62%) and excellent specificity (94–100%). The crescent sign is defined as the presence of a crescent-shaped layer of intra-articular contrast material between the humeral head and the anterior band of the IGHL. The triangle sign refers to the presence of a triangular accumulation on intra-articular contrast material between the humeral head, the articular surface of the glenoid and the anterior band of the IGHL [48].

Findings on MR imaging can reflect the dominant direction of instability in patients with atraumatic multidirectional instability, with Bankart lesions described in 53% of cases of anteroinferior dominant instability, and with increased chondrolabral and osseous retroversion identified in cases of posteroinferior multidirectional instability [30].

Microinstability of the Glenohumeral Joint

The concept and definition of microinstability varies in the literature. The term microinstability may be used at the most basic level when referring to any pathologic laxity that results in altered glenohumeral joint mechanics without a frank dislocation. More selectively, microinstability may be defined as the pathology involving the superior and superior-posterior aspects of the glenohumeral joint, associated with decentering of rotation of the humeral head relative to the glenoid [43].

Acquired Multidirectional Microinstability—Throwing Shoulder

In the throwing athlete, repetitive overhead throwing motions place high forces on the shoulder predisposing this group of patients to a variety of injuries in the glenohumeral joint. These injuries have been classically described in baseball pitchers, but they can occur in any sport or vocation that involves repetitive overhead movements of the upper extremity [49].

Anatomic and Biomechanical Considerations

Knowledge of the phases of the throwing motion is important to understand the spectrum of injury that may be found in the throwing athlete. The overhead throwing motion occurs in six phases, sequentially described as; wind-up, early-cocking, late-cocking, acceleration, deceleration, and follow-through (Fig. 11). Of these six phases, the late-cocking phase with abduction and maximal external rotational positioning of the arm, and deceleration requiring violent muscle contraction to slow down arm rotation during throwing are the phases most implicated in the patho-etiology of micro-instability of the shoulder [50].

The microtraumatic stress placed upon the shoulder associated with repetitive shoulder throwing activities are theorized to result in osseous and soft tissue adaptations that affect the stability and mobility of the glenohumeral joint. Throwing athletes have been shown to demonstrate 9–16° increased external rotation of their throwing arm compared to non-throwing athletes with a corresponding decrease in internal rotation of the arm in 90° of abduction. It has been accepted that maximal external rotation and associated capsular structural adaptations are required for throwing athletes to be able to develop the high arm speeds required in competitive throwing sports. However these same capsular adaptations in their extreme may result in shoulder micro- or macro-instability [49, 50].

Two theories have been proposed to explain the pathoetiology of microinstability in the throwing shoulder. The first theory proposes that pathologic laxity, secondary to repetitive stretching of the anterior capsule at the extremes of shoulder abduction and external rotation (experienced during the late-cocking phase of throwing), leads to anterior translation of the humeral head on the glenoid. Eccentric muscular contraction and soft tissue capsular micro-tearing may further increase anterior capsular laxity with resultant posterior decentering of humeral head position relative to the glenoid when the upper extremity is place in an abducted and externally rotated position, which contribute to posterosuperior glenohumeral impingement. The second theory proposes that progressive scarring of the posterior glenohumeral capsule, due to tensile stresses experienced during the deceleration-phase of throwing, leads to decreased internal rotation of the shoulder, starting a pathologic cascade process that results in posterosuperior shift of the glenohumeral rotation point during abduction and external rotation, maximal during the late cocking phase [39].

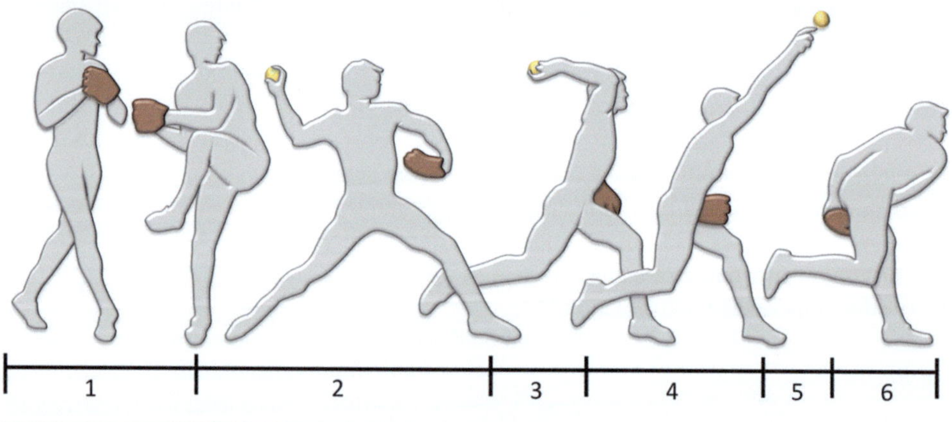

1. Wind-up	Readying phase with minimal shoulder stress.
2. Early cocking	Minimal load, moves the shoulder into 90º abduction and 15° horizontal abduction.
3. Late cocking	Begins with the planting of the striding leg and ends with the shoulder in maximum external rotation of 170° to 180° and 90° to 100° of abduction. This results in posterior translation of the humeral head on the glenoid and an increased risk of developing microinstability-related injuries.
4. Acceleration	Rotates the shoulder to the ball release point of 90° rotation.
5. Deceleration	Begins at ball release and ends with cessation of humeral rotation to 0°. Horizontal adduction increases to 35°. This phase is recognized as the most violent phase of the throwing cycle with joint loads at their greatest. The shoulder is more prone to injury during this phase.
6. Follow-through	The rebalancing phase. The body moves forward with the arm until motion stops.

Fig. 11 Diagram showing the phases of the throwing cycle

Imaging Findings in Acquired Multidirectional Microinstability—Throwing Shoulder

Injuries associated with acquired microinstability of the throwing shoulder observed at imaging classically include, rotator cuff tears, anterior labral fraying, SLAP lesions and posterior-superior glenohumeral impingement (Fig. 10) [50].

Posterosuperior glenohumeral impingement, first described by Walch and colleagues, refers to contact of the undersurface of the posterior supraspinatus tendon and anterior infraspinatus tendon, with the posterosuperior labrum. During maximal abduction and external rotation of the shoulder, decentering of the humeral head relative to the glenoid may result in the posterosuperior rotator cuff becoming pinched between the superior labrum and greater tuberosity of the humerus. In the throwing athlete, posterosuperior glenohumeral impingement usually occurs during the late-cocking phase [51]. Findings on conventional MR imaging and MR arthrography of posterosuperior glenohumeral impingement include: (1) articular-sided partial thickness tears of the posterior supraspinatus and anterior infraspinatus tendons; (2) SLAP lesions; (3) subcortical humeral head cysts; and in some cases evidence of frank anterior capsule micro-tearing and/or posterior capsular thickening and contracture [39, 52].

Other pathologic lesions which may be seen as a result of acquired microinstability in throwing athletes include tendinosis of the long head of the biceps tendon (LHBT) and Bennett's lesions. Biceps tendinosis is a common cause of shoulder pain in the throwing athlete. In such patients, the LHBT may be exposed to attritional repetitive microtraumatic injury during abduction and external rotation where the tendon may be overriding the lesser tuberosity. The Bennett's lesion, described in throwing athletes is reflective of reactive mineralization of the posteroinferior capsule at its insertion on the glenoid due to repetitive posterior capsular stress [53].

SLAP Lesions

Superior labral anterior to posterior (SLAP) lesions are frequent labral abnormalities centered at the biceps labral complex, which may extend anteriorly or posteriorly and involve adjacent capsuloligamentous structures [54].

SLAP lesions often occur with overhead repetitive motions but also may be seen after an acute traumatic event. Reported prevalence of SLAP lesions at arthroscopy range from 3.9% to 11.8% [55, 56]. The clinical diagnosis of a SLAP lesion is challenging with non-specific shoulder pain as the most common presentation. Additional symptoms include popping, clicking, catching, weakness, stiffness and instability [57].

Anatomic and Biomechanical Considerations

Normal anatomic variants are frequently seen in the antero-superior labrum and should not be confused with SLAP lesions. These anatomic variants include the sublabral recess or sulcus (Fig. 12a), the pseudo-SLAP lesion and cartilage undercutting [5].

The sublabral sulcus or recess represents the most frequent labral variant, with a reported prevalence of up to 73% on cadaveric studies. It is a recess between the inner apical margin of the labrum and the glenoid cartilage and is usually located from the 11-o'clock to the 1-o'clock positions. MRA has demonstrated sensitivities of 81–92% and a specificity of 100% for detection of sublabral recesses [58]. Recognizing the presence of a sublabral sulcus is important as it may mimic a type II SLAP lesion. A sulcus should demonstrate smooth margins and should parallel the underlying glenoid cartilage (Fig. 12).

The pseudo-SLAP lesion refers to a swallow recess between the LHBT and the superior labrum. On MRA, it is seen as a small contrast-filled cleft, which is better appreciated on oblique coronal images [5, 59].

The "magic angle effect" can contribute to increased signal intensity in the posterosuperior labrum particularly on MR sequences with short echo times, and may mimic pathology. The circumferential collagen fibers of the posterosuperior labrum are oriented at approximately 55° in relation with the static magnetic field (B_0) where the magic angle effect is maximal [57]. Intermediate signal intensity may also be seen at the chondrolabral junction, which corresponds to the transitional zone of fibrocartilage and should not be mistaken for a labral tear [5].

SLAP lesions have been theorized to occur secondary to a number of possible biomechanical mechanisms in which excess stress is applied to the superior labrum and biceps anchor. Peel back stresses upon the biceps anchor are seen in the setting of the abducted and externally rotated shoulder, where the LHBT acquires a more vertical and posterior orientation transmitting tensile forces to the superior labrum, which promote tensile upward peeling away of the superior labrum and biceps anchor from the superior glenoid rim and supraglenoid tubercle. Repetitive traction of the LHBT upon the superior labrum is also common during overhead movements, particularly the late cocking phase and deceleration phase of throwing. Compressive shearing stress upon the superior labrum between the glenoid rim and greater tuberosity of the humerus may be seen in the setting of superior-posterior impingement or in the setting of a FOOSH type injury in which the subluxating humeral head impacts the superior labrum [54].

SLAP Classification and MR Imaging Findings

The term SLAP was first coined by Snyder and colleagues in 1990, who described four lesion types [60]. Subsequently

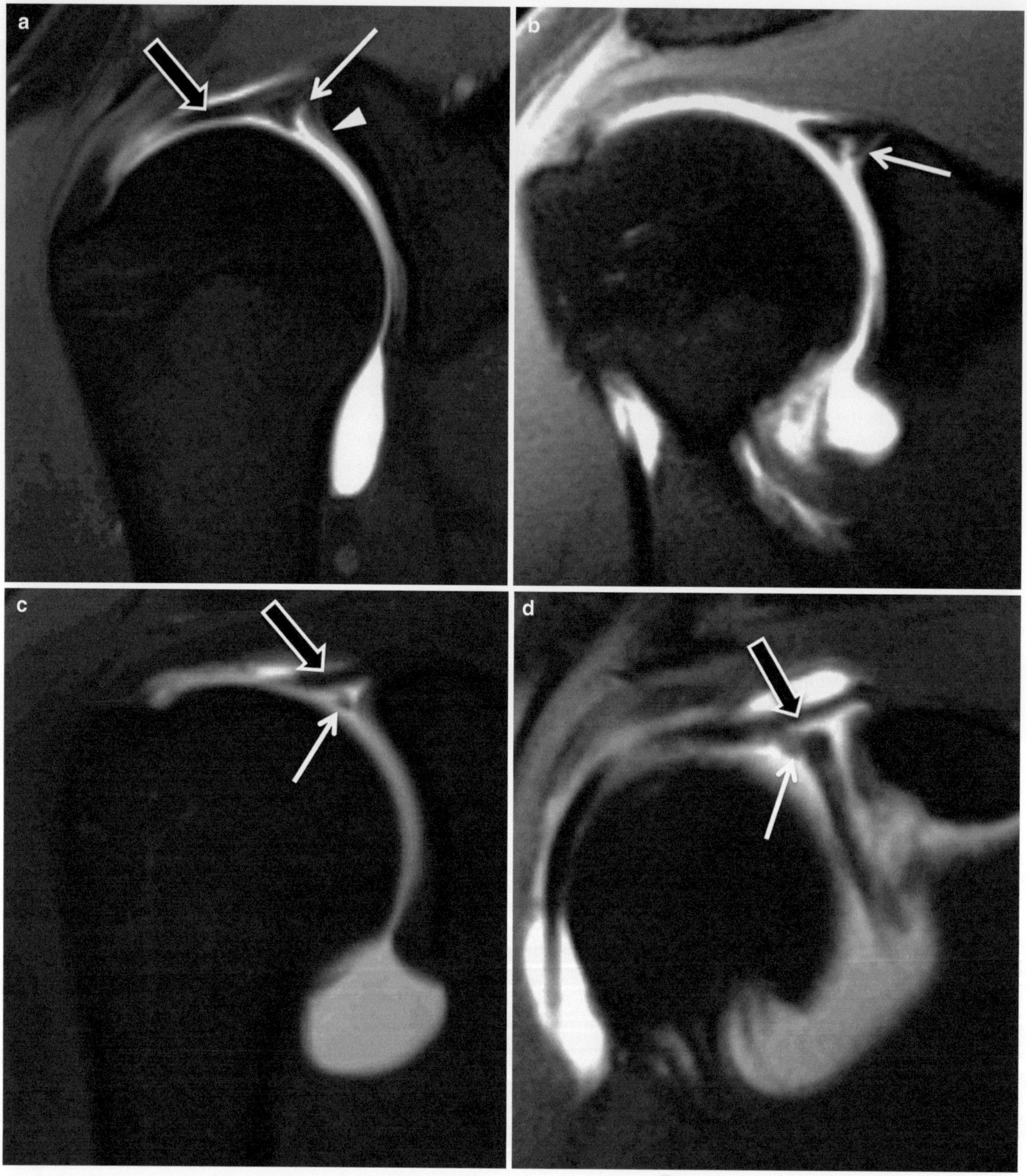

Fig. 12 Coronal fat suppressed T1-weighted MR arthrographic images showing a sublabral recess (**a**), SLAP type II lesion (**b**), SLAP type III lesion (**c**) and SLAP type lesion IV (**d**). **a**. Note the smooth margins and the parallel orientation to the underlying glenoid cartilage (*arrowhead*) of the sublabral sulcus (*thin arrow*). **b**. The SLAP type II lesion involves the superior labrum/biceps anchor, has irregular margins and a more oblique orientation (*thin arrow*). **c**. A small and displaced hypointense labral fragment (*thin arrow*), which represents a bucket-handle tear, is noted on the SLAP type III lesion. **d**. A bucket-handle tear of the superior labrum with extension into the LHBT is demonstrated on the SLAP type IV lesion (*thin arrow*). LHBT = thick arrows

Table 1 Classification of SLAP lesions

Type	Description
Type I	Fraying of the superior labrum
Type II	Tear of the superior labrum extending into the biceps anchor
Type IIa	Mainly involving the anterior labrum
Type IIb	Mainly involving the posterior labrum
Type IIc	Involving the anterior and posterior labrum
Type III	Bucket-handle tear
Type IV	Bucket-handle tear extending into the long head of the biceps tendon (LHBT)
Type V	Bankart lesion with superior extension
Type VI	Unstable flap tear
Type VII	Extension into the middle glenohumeral ligament (MGHL)
Type VIII	Extension into the posterior labrum, more extensive than type IIb
Type IX	Circumferential tear of the labrum
Type X	Extension into the rotator interval

SLAP II lesions were further subdivided into SLAP types IIa, IIb and IIc lesions [61]. Since 1991 several additional types of SLAP lesions have been included with 10 different types of SLAP reported in the literature (Table 1) [5, 54, 56], although the original I–IV classification system by Snyder and colleagues remains the most frequently used.

Studies have shown MRA has been shown to have higher sensitivity (82–100%), specificity (69–98%), and accuracy (74–94%) for the detection of SLAP lesions as compared to results seen with conventional MRI (sensitivity 66–98%, specificity 71–90% and accuracy 77–96%) [43, 62].

On MRA, SLAP lesions may be manifest by: detachment and displacement of the superior labrum from the glenoid rim, contrast material extending superiorly into the glenoid attachment of the LHBT origin on coronal images, irregular delineation of the LHBT origin or substance of the superior labrum on coronal and sagittal images, or the visualization of contrast material between the labrum and the glenoid rim on axial images [5, 62].

SLAP type I lesions are defined as degenerative type lesions and typically demonstrate irregular labral margins with or without heterogeneous increased signal intensity within the substance of the labrum. Type 1 lesions are common findings especially with advancing patient age and are considered by many to be within the spectrum of potentially asymptomatic findings in overhead throwing athletes. Type II lesions are the most frequent SLAP lesions with a discrete tear, with a reported frequency of 47% [62]. SLAP type II lesions are characterized by a discrete tear of the anterosuperior labrum (between the 10 o'clock to the 2 o'clock position) with partial or full detachment of the superior labrum and LHBT from the glenoid resulting in an unstable labral-biceps anchor [60]. An irregularly marginated contrast-filled cleft, or any lateral orientation of contrast extension within the substance of the superior labrum are helpful differentiation features from a superior labral recess or sulcus (Fig. 12), as is the presence of possible associated paralabral cysts. SLAP type III lesions represent displacible longitudinal tears of the anterosuperior labrum, similar to a bucket-handle tear of the knee meniscus, and SLAP type IV lesions are bucket-handle tears of the anterosuperior labrum extending into the LHBT.

References

1. Feldman F (2006) Radiology of shoulder prostheses. Semin Musculoskelet Radiol 10(1):5–21
2. Pagnani MJ, Warren RF (1994) Stabilizers of the glenohumeral joint. J Shoulder Elb Surg 3(3):173–190
3. Massengill AD, Seeger LL, Yao L, Gentili A, Shnier RC, Shapiro MS, Gold RH (1994) Labrocapsular ligamentous complex of the shoulder: normal anatomy, anatomic variation, and pitfalls of MR imaging and MR arthrography. Radiographics 14(6): 1211–1223
4. Edwards SL, Lee JA, Bell JE, Packer JD, Ahmad CS, Levine WN, Lu B, Blaine TA (2010) Nonoperative treatment of superior labrum anterior posterior tears: improvements in pain, function and quality of life. Am J Sports Med 38(7):1456–1466
5. De Coninck T, Ngai SS, Tafur M, Chung CB (2016) Imaging the glenoid labrum and labral tears. Radiographics 36(6):1628–1647
6. Waldt S, Metz S, Burkart A, Mueller D, Bruegel M, Rummeny EJ, Woertler K (2006) Variants of the superior labrum and labrobicipital complex: a comparative study of shoulder specimens using MR arthrography, multi-slice CT arthrography and anatomical dissection. Eur Radiol 16(2):451–458
7. Jarraya M, Roemer FW, Gale HI, Landreau P, D'Hooghe P, Guermazi A (2016) MR-arthrography and CT-arthrography in sports related glenolabral injuries: a matched descriptive illustration. Insights Imaging 7(2):167–177
8. Fox MG, Petrey WB, Alford B, Huynh BH, Patrie JT, Anderson MW (2012) Shoulder MR arthrography: intraarticular anesthetic reduces periprocedural pain and major motion artifacts but does not decrease imaging time. Radiology 262(2):576–583
9. Piper SL, Kramer JD, Kim HT, Feeley BT (2011) Effects of local anesthetics on articular cartilage. Am J Sports Med 39(10):2245–2253
10. Iwasaki K, Sudo H, Kasahara Y, Yamada K, Ohnishi T, Tsujimoto T, Iwasaki N (2016) Effects of Multiple intra-articular injections of 0.5% bupivacaine on normal and osteoarthritic joints in rats. Arthroscopy 32(10):2026–2036
11. Mohana-Borges AV, Chung CB, Resnick D (2003) Superior labral anteroposterior tear: classification and diagnosis on MRI and MR arthrography. AJR Am J Roentgenol 181(6):1449–1462
12. Tian CY, Cui GQ, Zheng ZZ, Ren AH (2013) The added value of ABER position for the detection and classification of anteroinferior labroligamentous lesions in MR arthrography of the shoulder. Eur J Radiol 82(4):651–657
13. "ESSR guidelines for MR imaging of sports injuries 2016" (2016). http://www.essr.org/html/img/pool/ESSR%20MRI%20Protocols%20Shoulder.pdf. Accessed 30 Oct
14. Woertler K, Waldt S (2006) MR Imaging in sports-related glenohumeral instability. Eur Radiol 16(12):2622–2636
15. Major NM, Browne J, Domzaiski T, Cothran RL, Helms CA (2011) Evaluation of the glenoid labrum with 3-T MRI: is intraarticular contrast necessary? AJR Am J Roentgenol 196(5):1139–1144

16. Zacchilli MA, Owens BD (2010) Epidemiology of shoulder dislocations presenting to emergency departments in the United States. J Bone Joint Surg Am 92(3):542–549
17. Chandnani VP, Gagliardi JA, Murnane TG, Bradley YC, DeBerardino TA, Spaeth J, Hansen MF (1995) Glenohumeral ligaments and shoulder capsular mechanism: evaluation with MR arthrography. Radiology 196(1):27–32
18. Owens BD, Duffey ML, Nelson BJ, DeBerardino TM, Taylor DC, Mountcastle SB (2007) The incidence and characteristics of shoulder instability at the United States Military Academy. Am J Sports Med 35(7):1168–1173
19. Jakobsen BW, Johannsen HV, Suder P, Søjbjerg JO (2007) Primary repair versus conservative treatment of first-time traumatic anterior dislocation of the shoulder: a randomized study with 10-year follow-up. Arthroscopy 23(2):118–123
20. Mannem R, DuBois M, Koeberl M, Kosempa D, Erickson S (2016) Glenoid avulsion of the glenohumeral ligament (GAGL): a case report and review of the anatomy. Skelet Radiol 45(10):1443–1448
21. De Maeseneer M, Van Roy F, Lenchik L, Shahabpour M, Jacobson J, Ryu KN, Handelberg F, Osteaux M (2000) CT and MR arthrography of the normal and pathologic anterosuperior labrum and labral-bicipital complex. Radiographics 20:S67–S81
22. Burkhart SS, De Beer JF (2000) Traumatic glenohumeral bone defects and their relationship to failure of arthroscopic Bankart repairs: significance of the inverted-pear glenoid and the humeral engaging Hill-Sachs lesion. Arthroscopy 16(7):677–694
23. Waldt S, Burkart A, Imhoff AB, Bruegel M, Rummeny EJ, Woertler K (2005) Anterior shoulder instability: accuracy of MR arthrography in the classification of anteroinferior labroligamentous injuries. Radiology 237(2):578–583
24. Bokor DJ, Conboy VB, Olson C (1999) Anterior instability of the glenohumeral joint with humeral avulsion of the glenohumeral ligament. A review of 41 cases. J Bone Joint Surg Br 81(1):93–96
25. Bui-Mansfield LT, Taylor DC, Uhorchak JM, Tenuta JJ (2002) Humeral avulsions of the glenohumeral ligament: imaging features and a review of the literature. AJR Am J Roentgenol 179(3):649–655
26. Bradley JP, Baker CL III, Kline AJ, Armfield DR, Chhabra A (2006) Arthroscopic capsulolabral reconstruction for posterior instability of the shoulder: a prospective study of 100 shoulders. Am J Sports Med 34(7):1061–1071
27. Harish S, Nagar A, Moro J, Pugh D, Rebello R, O'Neill J (2008) Imaging findings in posterior instability of the shoulder. Skelet Radiol 37(8):693–707
28. Shah N, Tung GA (2009) Imaging signs of posterior glenohumeral instability. AJR Am J Roentgenol 192(3):730–735
29. Van Tongel A, Karelse A, Berghs B, Verdonk R, De Wilde L (2011) Posterior shoulder instability: current concepts review. Knee Surg Sports Traumatol Arthrosc 19(9):1547–1553
30. Lee HJ, Kim NR, Moon SG, Ko SM, Park JY (2013) Multidirectional instability of the shoulder: rotator interval dimension and capsular laxity evaluation using MR arthrography. Skelet Radiol 42(2):231–238
31. Tannenbaum EP, Sekiya JK (2013) Posterior shoulder instability in the contact athlete. Clin Sports Med 32(4):781–796
32. Gaskill TR, Braun S, Millett PJ (2011) Multimedia article. The rotator interval: pathology and management. Arthroscopy 27(4):556–567
33. Kokkalis ZT, Iliopoulos ID, Antoniou G, Antoniadou T, Mavrogenis AF, Panagiotopoulos E (2016) Posterior shoulder fracture-dislocation: an update with treatment algorithm. Eur J Orthop Surg Traumatol. doi:10.1007/s00590-016-1840-5. [Epub ahead of print]
34. Cicak N (2004) Posterior dislocation of the shoulder. J Bone Joint Surg Br 86(3):324–332
35. Sheehan SE, Gaviola G, Gordon R, Sacks A, Shi LL, Smith SE (2013) Traumatic shoulder injuries: a force mechanism analysis-glenohumeral dislocation and instability. AJR Am J Roentgenol 201(2):378–393
36. Saupe N, White LM, Bleakney R, Schweitzer ME, Recht MP, Jost B et al (2008) Acute traumatic posterior shoulder dislocation: MR findings. Radiology 248(1):185–193
37. Badge R, Tambe A, Funk L (2009) Arthroscopic isolated posterior labral repair in rugby players. Int J Shoulder Surg 3(1):4–7
38. Yu JS, Ashman CJ, Jones G (2002) The POLPSA lesion: MR imaging findings with arthroscopic correlation in patients with posterior instability. Skelet Radiol 31(7):396–399
39. Beltran LS, Nikac V, Beltran J (2012) Internal impingement syndromes. Magn Reson Imaging Clin N Am 20(2):201–211. ix–x
40. Luenam S, Kosiyatrakul A (2013) Massive rotator cuff tear associated with acute traumatic posterior shoulder dislocation: report of two cases and literature review. Musculoskelet Surg 97(3):273–278
41. Hottya GA, Tirman PF, Bost FW, Montgomery WH, Wolf EM, Genant HK (1998) Tear of the posterior shoulder stabilizers after posterior dislocation: MR imaging and MR arthrographic findings with arthroscopic correlation. AJR Am J Roentgenol 171(3):763–768
42. Merolla G, Cerciello S, Chillemi C, Paladini P, De Santis E, Porcellini G (2015) Multidirectional instability of the shoulder: biomechanics, clinical presentation, and treatment strategies. Eur J Orthop Surg Traumatol 25(6):975–985
43. Chang EY, Fliszar E, Chung CB (2012) Superior labrum anterior and posterior lesions and microinstability. Magn Reson Imaging Clin N Am 20(2):277–294. x–xi
44. Neer CS II, Foster CR (1980) Inferior capsular shift for involuntary inferior and multidirectional instability of the shoulder. A preliminary report. J Bone Joint Surg Am 62:897–908
45. Macmahon PJ, Palmer WE (2012) Magnetic resonance imaging in glenohumeral instability. Magn Reson Imaging Clin N Am 20(2):295–312. xi
46. Longo UG, Rizzello G, Loppini M, Locher J, Buchmann S, Maffulli N et al (2015) Multidirectional instability of the shoulder: a systematic review. Arthroscopy 31(12):2431–2443
47. Dewing CB, McCormick F, Bell SJ, Solomon DJ, Stanley M, Rooney TB et al (2008) An analysis of capsular area in patients with anterior, posterior and multidirectional shoulder instability. Am J Sports Med 36(3):515–522
48. Schaeffeler C, Waldt S, Bauer JS, Kirchhoff C, Haller B, Schroder M et al (2014) MR arthrography including abduction and external rotation images in the assessment of atraumatic multidirectional instability of the shoulder. Eur Radiol 24(6):1376–1385
49. Cohn RM, Jazrawi LM (2012) The throwing shoulder: the orthopedist perspective. Magn Reson Imaging Clin N Am 20(2):261–275
50. Meister K (2000) Injuries to the shoulder in the throwing athlete. Part one: biomechanics/pathophysiology/classification of injury. Am J Sports Med 28(2):265–275
51. Heyworth BE, Williams RJ III (2009) Internal impingement of the shoulder. Am J Sports Med 37(5):1024–1037
52. Giaroli EL, Major NM, Higgins LD (2005) MRI of internal impingement of the shoulder. AJR Am J Roentgenol 185(4):925–929
53. Wright RW (2004) Prevalence of the Bennett lesion of the shoulder in major league pitchers. Am J Sports Med 32(1):121–124
54. Chang D, Mohana-Borges A, Borso M, Chung CB (2008) SLAP lesions: anatomy, clinical presentation, MR imaging diagnosis and characterization. Eur J Radiol 68(1):72–87
55. Snyder SJ, Banas MP, Karzel RP (1995) An analysis of 140 injuries to the superior glenoid labrum. J Shoulder Elb Surg 4(4):243–248
56. Maffet MW, Gartsman GM, Moseley B (1995) Superior labrum-biceps tendon complex lesions of the shoulder. Am J Sports Med 23(1):93–98

57. Bydder M, Rahal A, Fullerton GD, Bydder GM (2007) The magic angle effect: a source of artifact, determinant of image contrast, and technique for imaging. J Magn Reson Imaging 25(2):290–300
58. Smith DK, Chopp TM, Aufdemorte TB, Witkowski EG, Jones RC (1996) Sublabral recess of the superior glenoid labrum- study of cadavers with conventional nonenhanced MR imaging, MR arthrography, anatomic dissection, and limited histologic examination. Radiology 201(1):251–256
59. Dunham KS, Bencardino JT, Rokito AS (2012) Anatomic variants and pitfalls of the labrum, glenoid cartilage, and glenohumeral ligaments. Magn Reson Imaging Clin N Am 20(2):213–228. x
60. Ahsan ZS, Hsu JE, Gee AO (2016) The Snyder classification of superior labrum anterior and posterior (SLAP) lesions. Clin Orthop Relat Res 474(9):2075–2078
61. Morgan CD, Burkhart SS, Palmeri M, Gillespie M (1998) Type II SLAP lesions: three subtypes and their relationships to superior instability and rotator cuff tears. Arthroscopy 14(6): 553–565
62. Bencardino JT, Beltran J, Rosenberg ZS, Rokito A, Schmahmann S, Mota J et al (2000) Superior labrum anterior-posterior lesions: diagnosis with MR arthrography of the shoulder. Radiology 214(1):267–271

MR Imaging of the Rotator Cuff and Rotator Interval

Marcelo R Abreu and Michael Recht

Anatomy of the Rotator Cuff

The rotator cuff is comprised of the supraspinatus, infraspinatus, subscapularis, and teres minor muscles and tendons. The four muscles of the rotator cuff act as stabilizers of the glenohumeral joint. The supraspinatus is primarily a shoulder abductor. The supraspinatus muscle originates along the dorsal surface of the scapula. The muscle fibers course in a lateral orientation and converge to form an anterior tendon although there is also a second smaller posterior tendon of the supraspinatus. The supraspinatus tendon is bordered superiorly by the subacromial-subdeltoid bursa and inferiorly by the joint capsule. Anteriorly, the more distal supraspinatus tendon converges with the coracohumeral ligament, and posteriorly it merges with the anterior fibers of the infraspinatus tendon. At the distal aspect of the rotator cuff, the supraspinatus and infraspinatus tendons splay out and interdigitate, forming a common continuous insertion on the middle facet of the humeral greater tuberosity. The supraspinatus tendon is best evaluated in the coronal oblique plane and the sagittal oblique plane, with the latter being helpful in evaluating the most anterior fibers of the supraspinatus. The region just medial to the convergence of the posterior fibers of the supraspinatus and the anterior fibers of the infraspinatus has been referred to as the posterior rotator interval [1].

The infraspinatus muscle externally rotates the shoulder, originating in the infraspinous fossa. The infraspinatus has a multipennate configuration, usually with three tendons, with the myotendinous junction having a somewhat fanlike configuration. The infraspinatus is best evaluated in the coronal oblique and sagittal oblique planes [1, 2].

M.R. Abreu (✉)
Hospital Mae de Deus, Costa 40, Porto Alegre, RS 90110-270, Brazil
e-mail: marcelorad@gmail.com

M. Recht
NYU Langone Medical Center, 660 First Ave., New York, NY 10016, USA
e-mail: Michael.Recht@nyumc.org

The teres minor muscle originates along the upper two thirds of the lateral border of the scapula and blends into the posterior glenohumeral joint capsule more distally. The infraspinatus and teres minor externally rotate the shoulder, with the former also being an abductor and the latter being a weak adductor.

The subscapularis muscle is a strong adductor and internal rotator. The subscapularis muscle originates from the subscapular fossa along the anterior aspect of the scapula. It inserts primarily on the lesser tuberosity, with superficial fibers extending to the greater tuberosity. Similar to the infraspinatus, the subscapularis has a multipennate configuration. The deep fibers of the subscapularis tendon blend with and reinforce the anterior capsule of the glenohumeral joint. The mid and distal portions of the middle glenohumeral ligament blend with the capsule and deep fibers of the subscapularis before inserting into the lesser tuberosity. The subscapularis is best evaluated in the axial and sagittal oblique planes.

MR Imaging

On MR imaging, a normal, healthy tendon should appear with low signal intensity on all sequences. There are however, some exceptions/pitfalls to this statement. One exception is that on short TE imaging the magic angle phenomenon may result in increased signal in regions where the tendon courses at a 55-degree angle in relation to the main magnetic field. Magic angle artifact should resolve on T2-weighted (long TE) sequences, thus differentiating it from true tendon pathology. Additionally, volume averaging between the tendon and adjacent tissues such as muscle, fascia, fat, and cartilage may result in increased tendon signal on short TE imaging. Again, use of T2-weighted imaging and assessing tendons in at least two planes can increase confidence in differentiating volume averaging from true intratendinous signal abnormalities. The tendon microanatomy itself can lead to false pathologic diagnosis especially when using high resolution imaging, when visualization of tendon fascicles can simulate tears and tendinopathy. Better understanding of

J. Hodler et al. (eds.), *Musculoskeletal Diseases 2017-2020*, DOI 10.1007/978-3-319-54018-4_19

tendon microanatomy, such as tendon fusions (example: distal fusion of supraspinatus and infraspinatus tendons near the footprint) and normal multipennate configuration of some tendons of the cuff, can minimize false positive diagnosis.

Impingement Syndromes

In 1972 Neer stated that the vast majority of rotator cuff pathology was secondary to impingement but it is now felt that the etiology is multifactorial with contributions from impingement, vascular insufficiency, aging and/or metabolic conditions.

There are two types of impingement, external and internal impingement syndromes. External impingement syndromes include subacromial and subcoracoid impingement. Subacromial impingement, which is the most common impingement syndrome, occurs with overhead activities. It occurs secondary to impingement of the cuff, primarily the supraspinatus tendon, within the coracoacromial arch (Drawing 1). The impingement can be caused by primary structural abnormalities of the arch such as acromioclavicular osteophytes, an abnormally shaped acromion such as a "hooked" acromion, subacromial enthesophytes, or an *os acromiale* (Fig. 1). MR findings of subacromial impingement include tendon changes, structural abnormalities of the coracromial arch and subacromial-subdeltoid bursitis. In subcoracoid impingement the subscapularis tendon is impinged between the coracoid and the lesser tuberosity. Findings in subcoracoid impingement include narrowing of the coracohumeral interval, partial articular sided tears of the subscapularis tendon and subcoracoid bursitis.

Internal impingement syndromes include both posterosuperior and anterosuperior impingement. In posterosuperior impingement the undersurface of the posterior cuff becomes entrapped between the humeral head and the posterior glenoid when the arm is abducted and externally rotated. Although contact may be physiologic in this position, with constant repetition, such as in overhead athletes, it can lead to attrition and partial tears of the undersurface of the cuff as well as tears of the posterior superior labrum and osteochondral changes in the greater tuberosity.

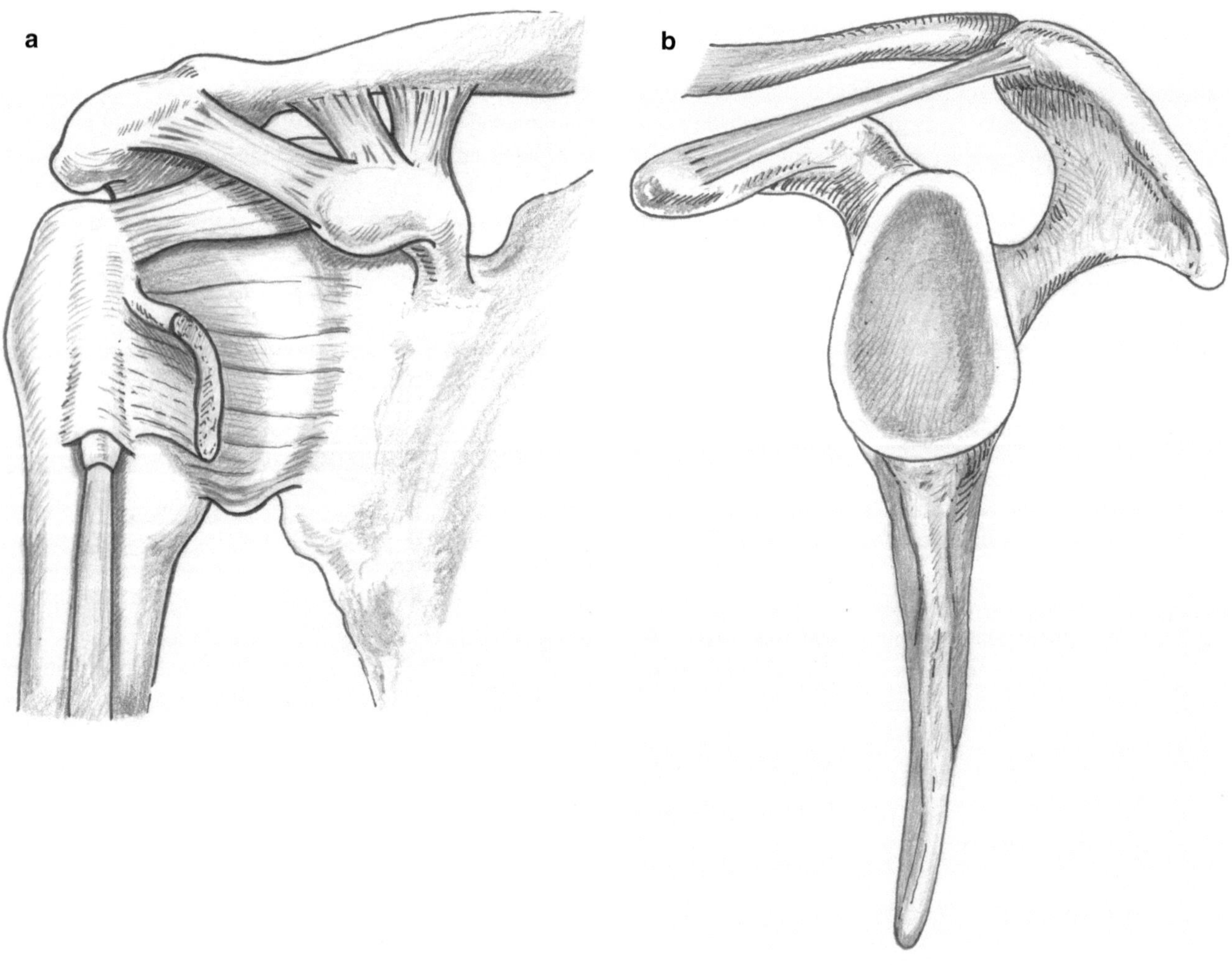

Drawing 1 Hand drawing of shoulder anatomy. (**a**) Coronal view of the osseous and ligamentous components of the subacromial tunnel formed by the acromium, the coracoid, the coracoacromial ligament and the coraracoclavicular ligament, with the supraspinatus tendon passing inside the tunnel. (**b**) Sagittal view of osseous and ligamentous arch

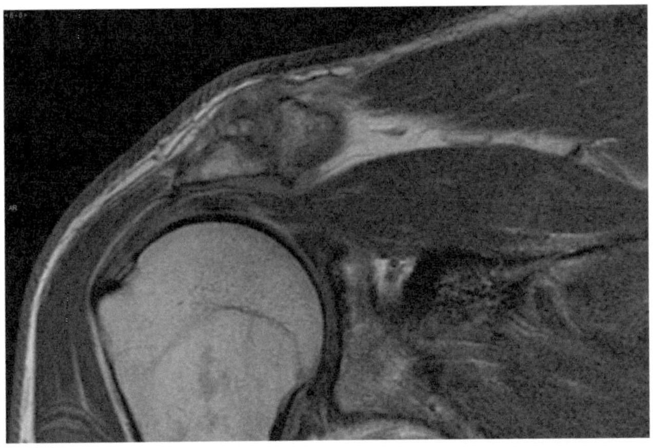

Fig. 1 Coronal oblique T1-weighted image showing acromioclavicular joint degenerative changes with inferior osteophytes causing supraspinatus impingement

Anterosuperior impingement is much less common than posterosuperior impingement and occurs when the subscapularis tendon is trapped between the anterior humeral head and the anterosuperior glenoid and labrum during forward flexion of the arm.

Tendinosis (Tendinopathy)

Tendinosis histopathologically refers to tendon degeneration with collagen fiber disorientation, increased intrasubstance deposition of mucoid, and absence of inflammatory cells (thus the term tendinitis is inappropriate). The typical MR appearance of tendinosis is abnormal signal intensity associated with morphology changes (Figs. 2 and 3). The signal changes of tendinopathy typically are of intermediate

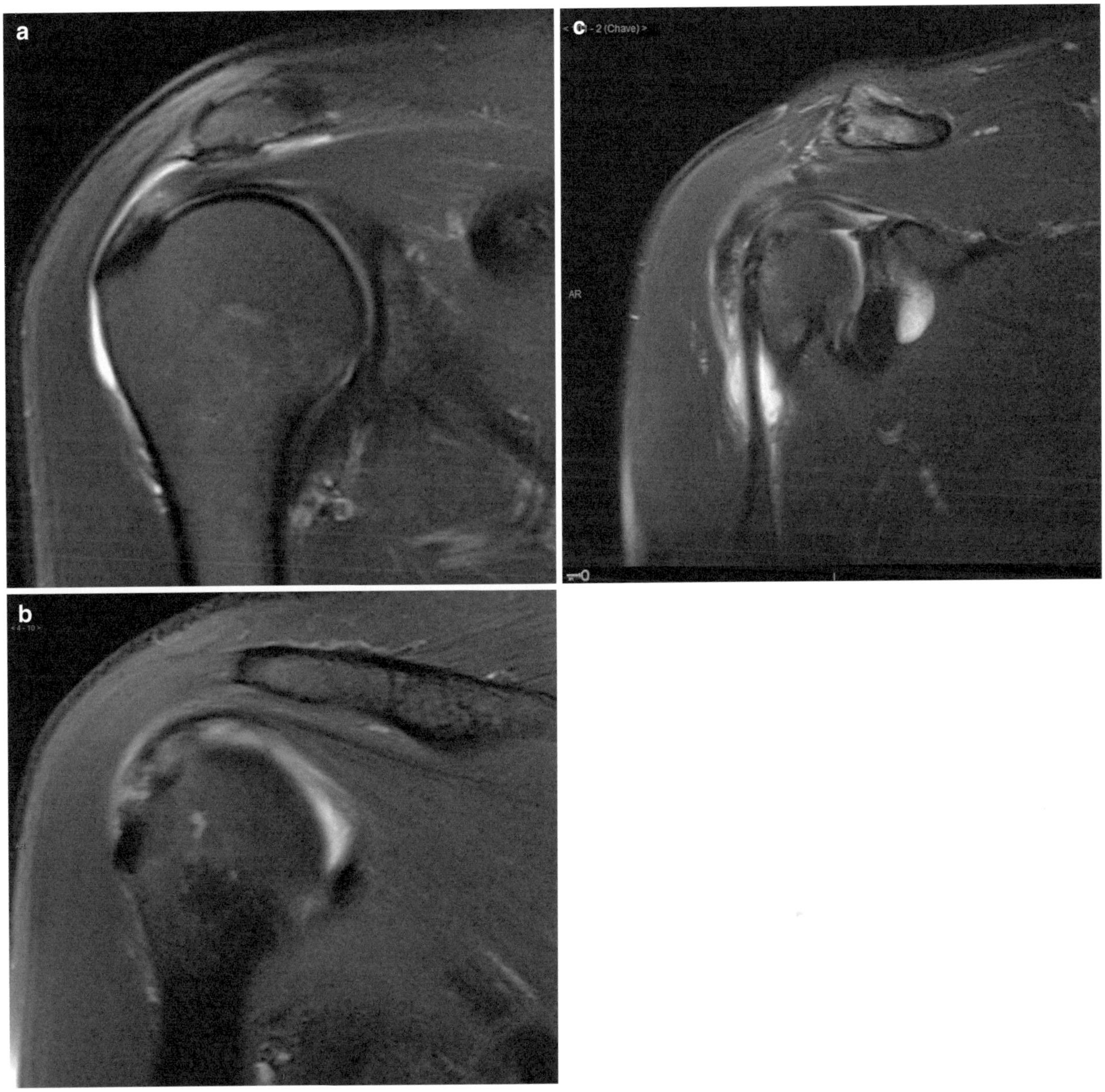

Fig. 2 Coronal oblique T2-weighted fat suppressed images showing subacromial bursitis and tendinosis of supraspinatus (**a**), infraspinatus (**b**) and intra-articular portion of long head of biceps tendon (**c**)

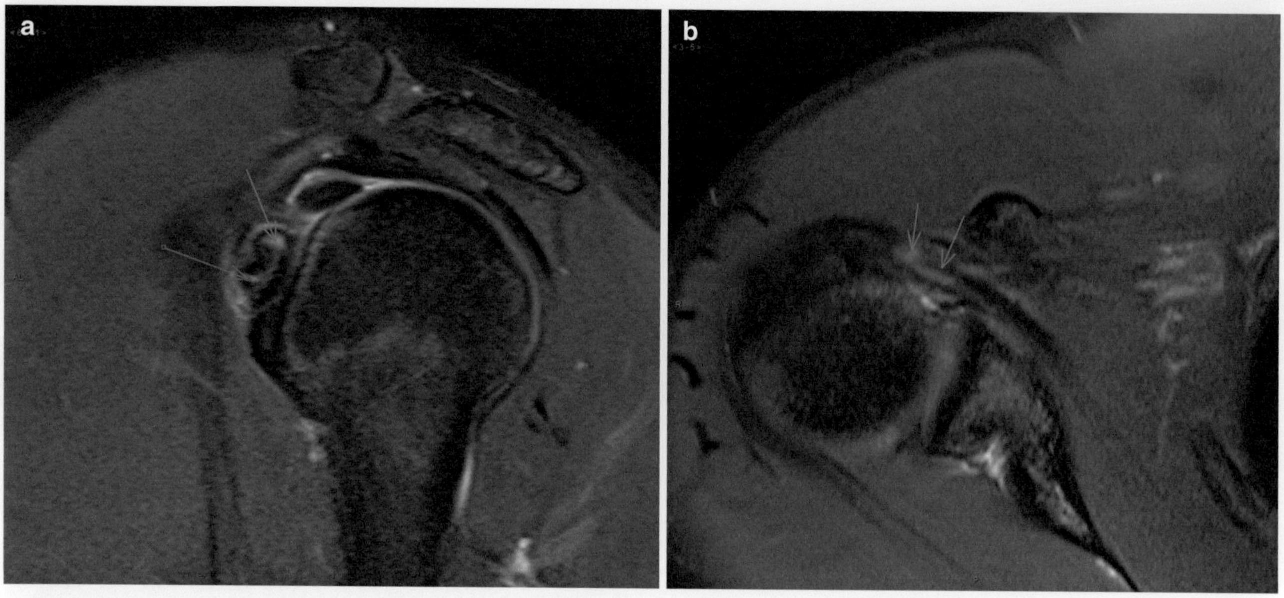

Fig. 3 (**a**) Sagittal T2-weighted fat suppressed image showing tendinosis of the superior fibers of subscapularis (*arrows*), note the intra-articular thick long head of the biceps tendon superiorly with mild signal abnormality consistent with mild tendinosis (**b**) axial T2-weighted fat suppressed image demonstration high signal of the superior fibers of the subscapularis tendon, not as intense as fluid, characterizing focal tendinosis

signal on both short and long TE imaging. In particular with tendinosis there is no fluid-like signal intensity on long TE images. This allows one to differentiate tendinosis from frank tendon tearing. Because of the pitfalls described above that can lead to intermediate signal on short TE images in normal tendons, we believe that one should be very hesitant to call tendinopathy in tendons with normal morphology. The associated morphology changes typically consist of abnormal thickening of the involved tendon. Classically, rotator cuff tears occur in the insertional fibers of the cuff tendons in regions of preexisting tendinopathy [3].

MR Imaging of Tendon Tears

Tendon tears are classified into full thickness or partial thickness tears. Full thickness tears are subclassified as complete or incomplete depending on if all or only some of the tendons of a muscle are involved. Partial thickness tears are subdivided by the location of the tear into articular-sided, intratendinous, and bursal-sided tears. Although rotator cuff tears typically appear as areas of fluid signal intensity on T2-weighted images, in about 10% of tears, the region of tendon discontinuity is low in signal on T2-weighted images, possibly because of chronic scarring and fibrosis. These tears may be visualized at MR arthrography because intraarticular contrast fills the tear. On conventional MR imaging, secondary signs of cuff tear, such as tendon retraction (measured in the medial-lateral dimension), may be the only indication of a full-thickness tear.

Partial Tears

Partial-thickness rotator cuff tears can be described according to the surface of the tendon involved as well as the percentage of tendon involved (Drawing 2).

Partial-thickness articular surface tears are characterized by a focal region of fiber discontinuity that is filled with fluid-like signal intensity on T2-weighted imaging. Fat-suppressed T2-weighted imaging can increase lesion conspicuity by better demonstrating the high T2 signal tendon defect). Articular surface tears are the most common type and are easily diagnosed with standard MR imaging when a joint effusion is present (Fig. 4). In the absence of a joint effusion, articular surface partial-thickness tears may be difficult to identify, particularly in the setting of granulation tissue or scarring. Delamination of the involved portion of the tendon may occur, most often involving the articular surface of the supraspinatus tendon (Drawing 3). Delaminated tears can lead to cyst formation within the associated or adjacent muscle, the so called sentinel cyst. Those cysts usually are restricted to the muscle belly and typically do not cause symptoms, in contrast to the paralabral ganglion cysts that may cause nerve compression.

Intrasubstance or concealed tears are characterized by intratendinous T2 fluid-like signal without extension to either the bursal or articular surface (Fig. 5). These lesions will not fill with gadolinium on MR arthrography because of lack of communication between the tear and the articular surface of the tendon. Intrasubstance tears will not be seen by the arthroscopist as they do not communicate with the tendon surface.

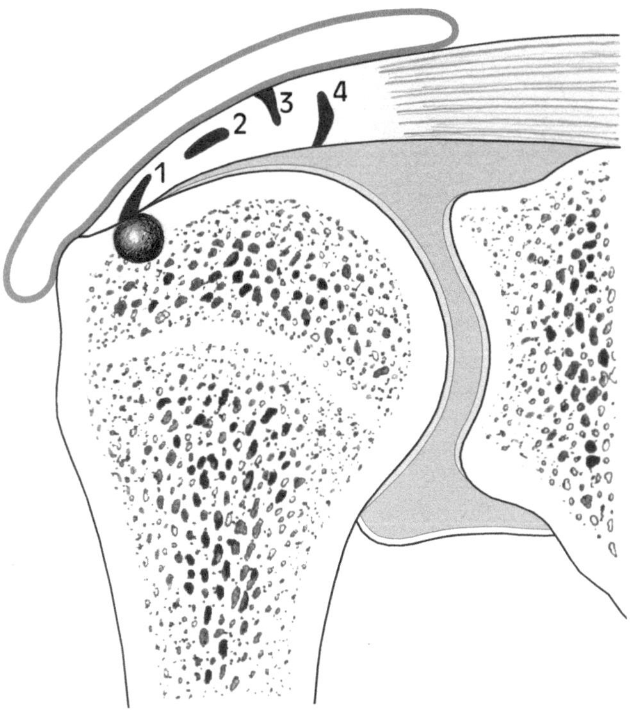

Drawing 2 Hand drawing of partial thickness tear types (coronal view of the supraspinatus tendon). 1. Intrasubstance footprint tear with adjacent bone cyst. 2. Intrasubstance tear. 3. Bursal side tear. 4. Undersurface tear

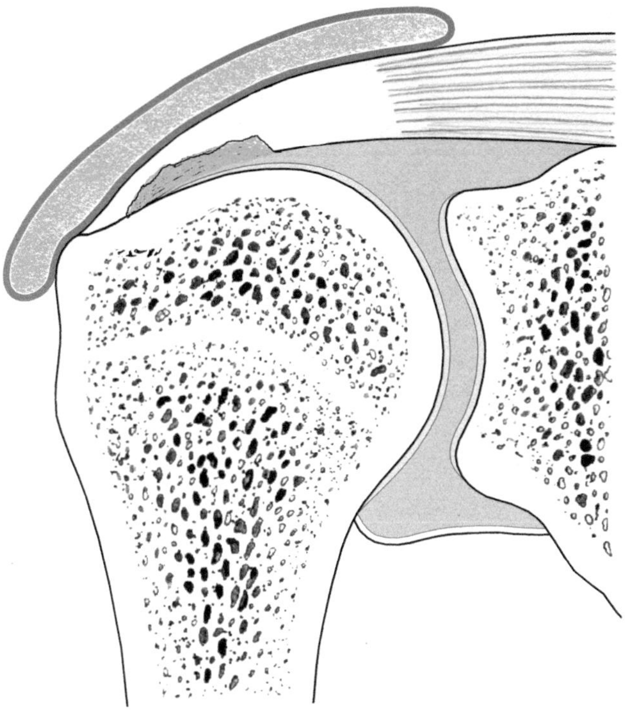

Drawing 3 Partial thickness undersurface delaminated tear

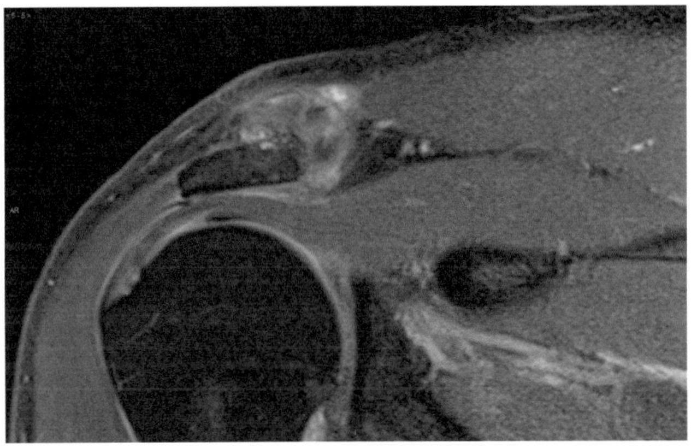

Fig. 4 Coronal oblique T2-weighted fat suppressed image showing supraspinatus partial thickness undersurface tear, and acromioclavicular joint degenerative changes with inferior osteophytes

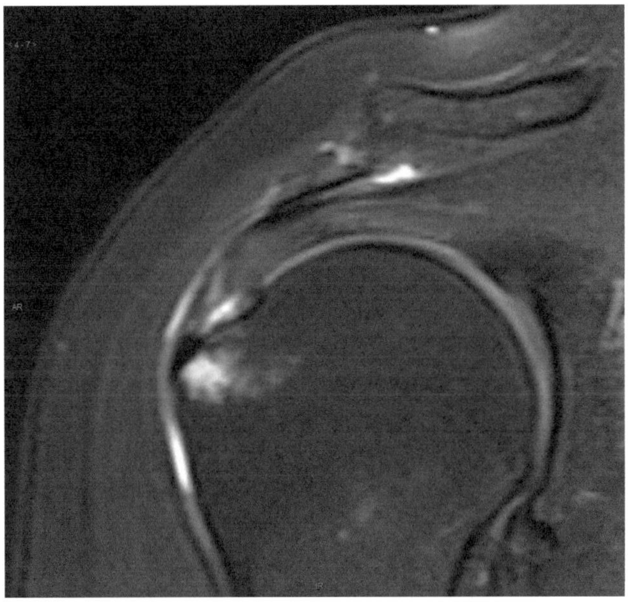

Fig. 5 Coronal oblique T2-weighted fat suppressed image showing partial thickness intrasubstance tear at the footprint, with adjacent bone marrow edema, tendinosis and bursitis

Partial-thickness bursal surface tears demonstrate abnormal increased T2 signal along the superior (bursal) surface of the tendon (Fig. 6). The articular surface remains intact. When there is fluid in the subacromial bursa, the tears are well visualized, particularly on T2-weighted images. However, these tears may not be visible on T1-weighted MR arthrographic images as the intra-articular gadolinium will not enter the gap in the tendon because of intact articular surface fibers. In addition, the presence of bursal fluid may not be appreciated on T1-weighted imaging. For these reasons, it is crucial to include at least one T2-weighted sequence on all MR arthrographic exams to assess for fluid-filled bursal surface tears. The extent of the partial tear can further be

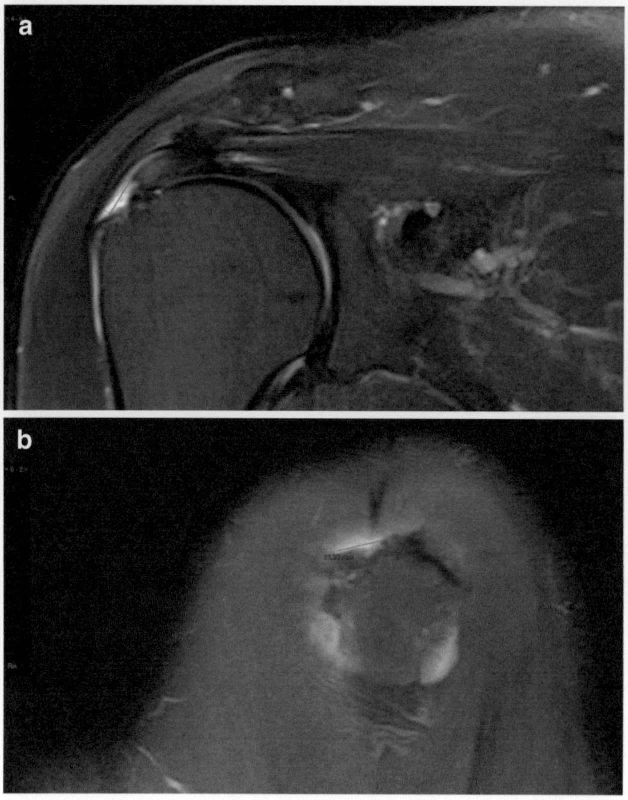

Fig. 6 (**a**) Coronal oblique T2-weighted fat suppressed image showing partial thickness bursal side tear of the supraspinatus tendon, tendinosis and subacromial bursitis. (**b**) Sagittal T2-weighted image demonstrating the partial thickness bursal side tear, transverse length

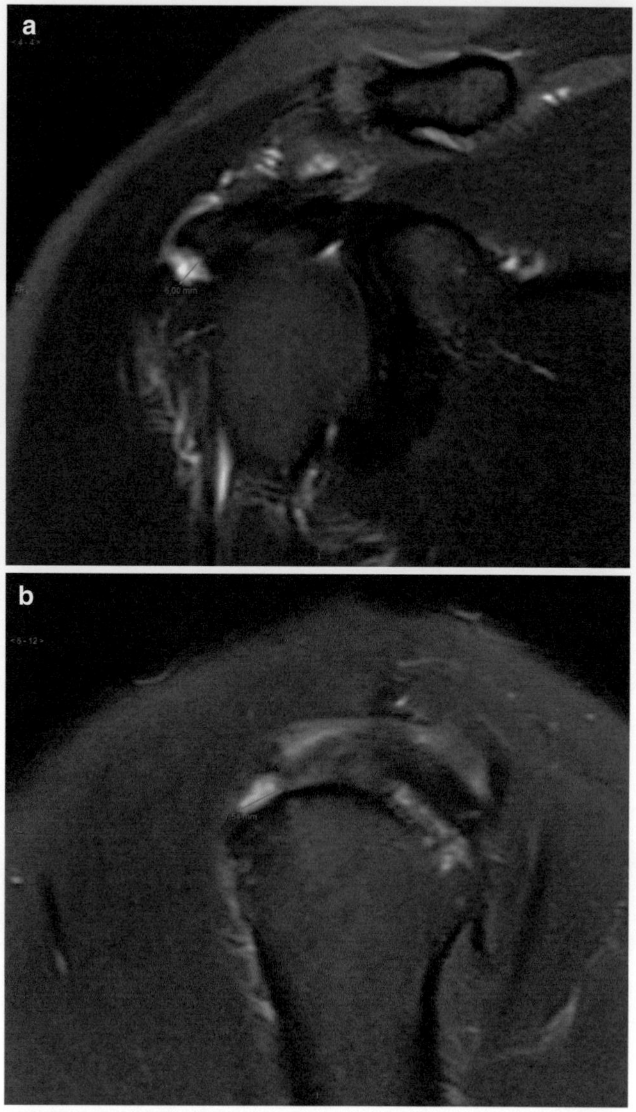

Fig. 7 (**a**) Coronal oblique T2-weighted fat suppressed image showing full thickness tear of the anterior fibers of the supraspinatus tendon. (**b**) Sagittal T2-weighted image demonstrating the supraspinatus full thickness tear transverse length

Table 1 Extent of partial tear of the rotator cuff tendons

Grade I for tears < 3 mm
Grade II for extension 3–6 mm
Grade III if > 6 mm

declared according to the depth; a commonly used grading system is shown in (Table 1) [4, 5].

Full Thickness Tears

Tears of the supraspinatus tendon most commonly arise at the anterior aspect of the tendon immediately adjacent to its attachment onto the greater tuberosity (Fig. 7). Supraspinatus tears can extend posteriorly into the infraspinatus tendon or anteroinferiorly through the rotator interval to involve the medial aspect of the coracohumeral ligament and superior subscapularis tendon fibers, a situation that is associated with more severe supraspinatus atrophy and poor prognosis [6]. A full-thickness supraspinatus tear allows communication between the articular and the bursal compartments.

Infraspinatus tendon tears are often associated with supraspinatus tendon tears and may be observed in younger athletes with overhead activities and posterosuperior

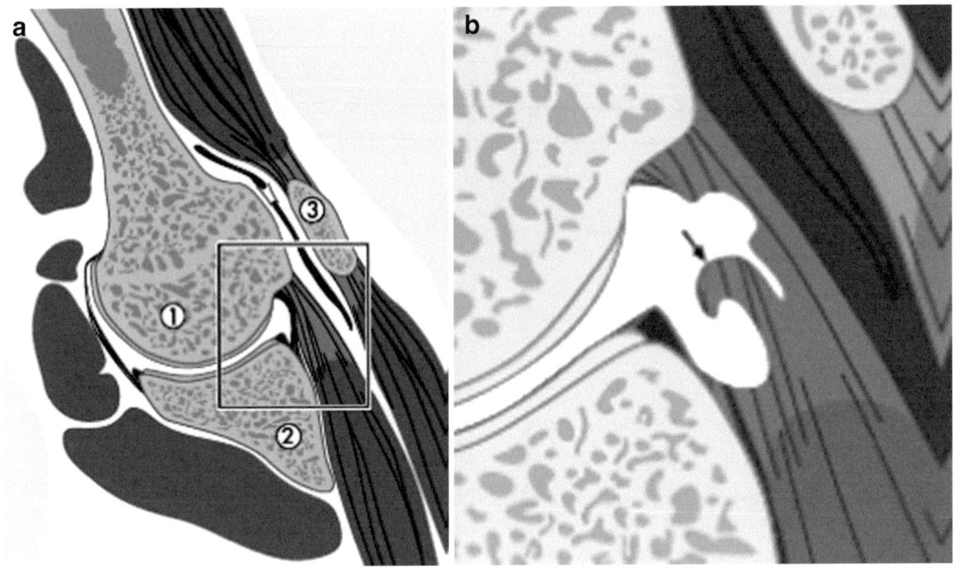

Drawing 4 (**a**) Schematic illustration of the anatomy of the glenohumeral joint in ABER position. 1 Humeral head, 2 Glenoid, 3 Acromion. (**b**) Detail illustrations demonstrate: tear with torn edge of the articular surface. (Modified from Schreinemachers SA, et al (2009) Detection of partial-thickness supraspinatus tendon tears: is a single direct MR arthrography series in ABER position as accurate as conventional MR arthrography? Skeletal Radiol 38:967–975)

impingement, in which there is often an articular side delamination of the cuff. The so-called ABER view (abduction and external rotation arm position) in conventional MRI or MR arthrography has been proposed to increase the sensitivity for detection of these tears. For younger patients and patients suspected of having posterior superior impingement and partial-thickness undersurface tears, the ABER position is valuable in demonstrating lesions of posterior superior impingement and undersurface tears of the rotator cuff as well as non-displaced tears of the anterior inferior labrum in patients with glenohumeral instability [7, 8] (Drawing 4). Teres Minor tendon tears are rare and present most commonly as partial tears accompanied by infraspinatus tears.

When describing rotator cuff tears there are a number of features that need to be described: the size, retraction, tear shape, and status of the muscle

Size

The size (AP dimension) of a full thickness tear has important implications on both the decision to perform surgery as well as the surgical approach, the postoperative prognosis, and the possibility of tear recurrence. DeOrio and Cofield classified rotator cuff tears on the basis of greatest dimension [9] as show on Table 2.

Table 2 Rotator cuff full thickness tears DeOrio and Cofield classification

small	<1 cm
medium	1–3 cm
large	3–5 cm
massive	>5 cm

Retraction

Retraction is defined as the medial-lateral extent of the tear. We can measure the retraction assuming its origin at the footprint or give information about its location regarding the acromioclavicular (AC) joint. The tendon can be lateral to the AC joint, at the AC joint or medially to the AC joint. It has been suggested that a tear is suspected to be irreparable if MR imaging depicts retraction medial to the AC joint, although this is controversial.

Shape

The shape of a rotator cuff tear is important in the selection of a surgical technique. Tears can be classified arthroscopically into three basic shapes according to the tear geometry as viewed from the tendon surface: crescentic, U shaped

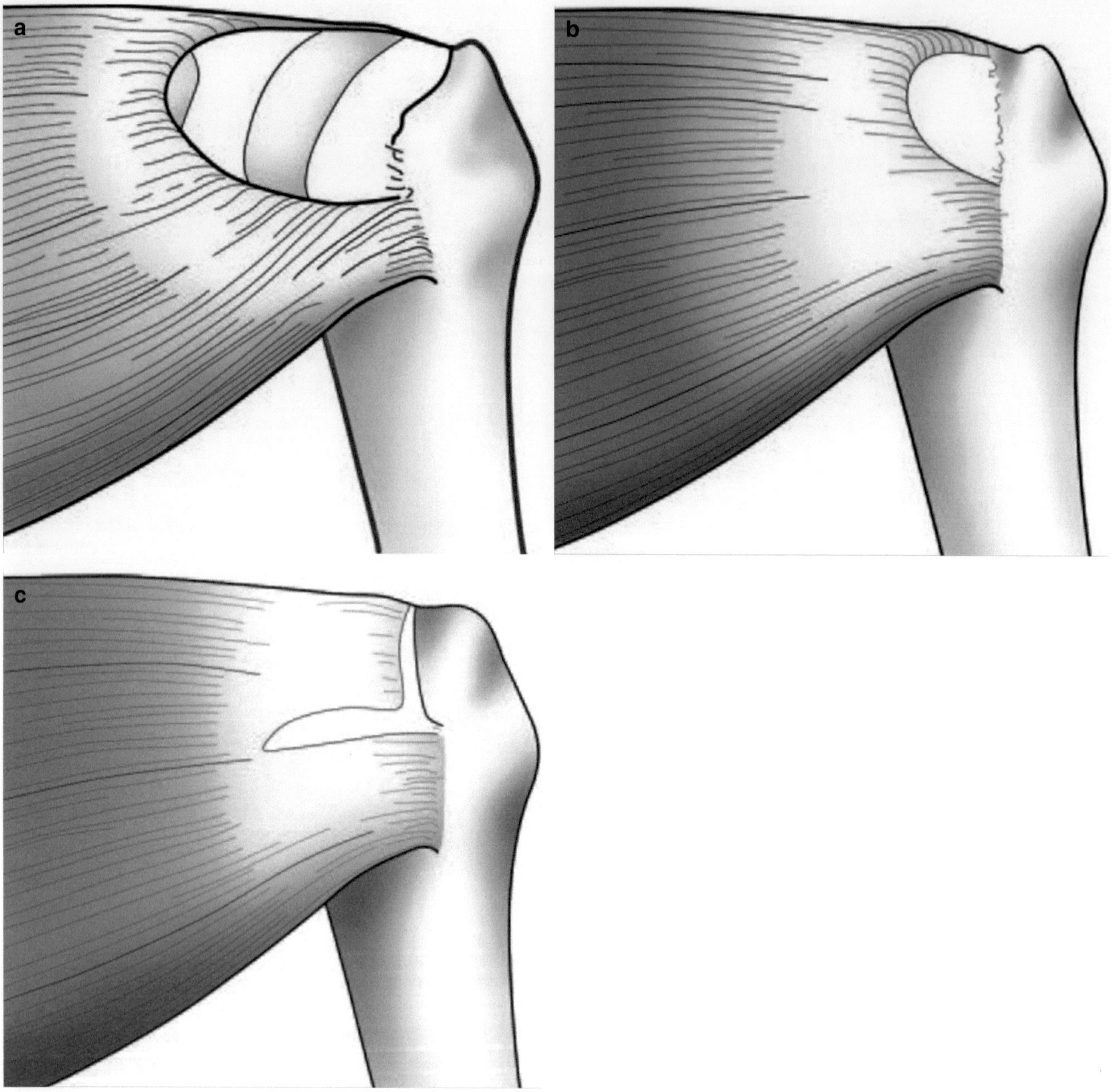

Drawing 5 Full thickness tear shape. Drawings illustrate a U-shaped tear (**a**) a crescentic tear (**b**) and an L-shaped tear (**c**). (Modified from Morag Y, et al (2006) MR imaging of rotator cuff injury: what the clinician needs to know. Radiographics 26:1045–1065)

and L shaped (Drawing 5). In crescentic tears, the tendon pulls away from the greater tuberosity but typically does not retract far medially and therefore can be reattached to bone with minimal tension. In crescenteric tears the antero-posterior diameter of the tear is greater than its medial-lateral diameter. In L and U shaped tears the medial-lateral dimension of the tear is greater than the antero-posterior dimension. The difference between the L and U tears is whether or not the anterior or posterior attachments of the tendon are intact (U shaped) or disrupted (L shaped) (Drawing 5).

Muscle Status

When rotator cuff tendons are torn it is important to evaluate the associated muscle belly for its status, particularly the presence of any fatty atrophy (Fig. 8). The presence of

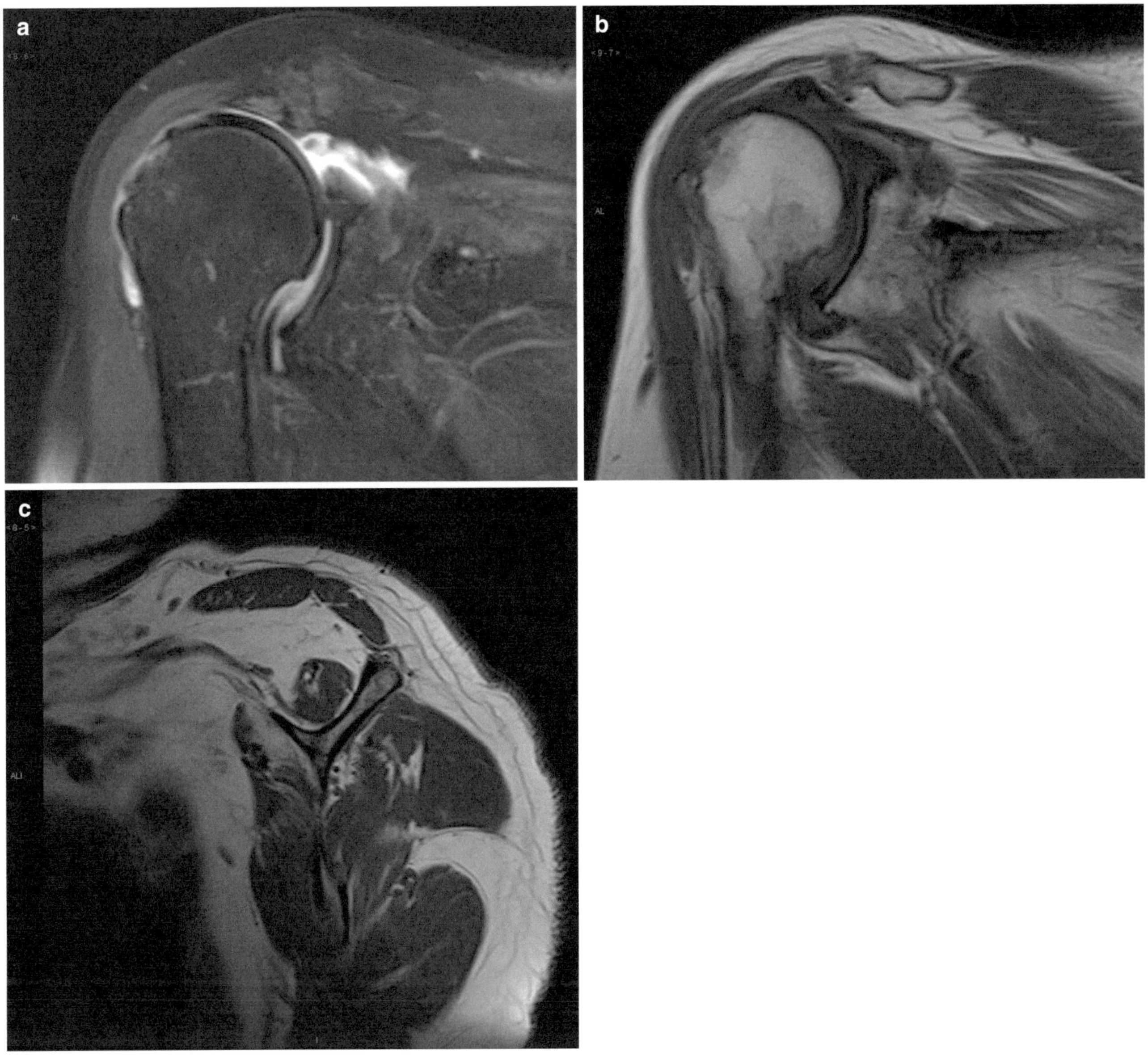

Fig. 8 (**a**) Coronal oblique T2-weighted fat suppressed image showing full thickness total surface tear of the supraspinatus tendon with retraction, cranial migration the humeral head, and impingement with the superior labrum. (**b** and **c**) Coronal oblique and sagittal T1-weighted images showing atrophy of the supraspinatus muscle with fatty infiltration

fatty atrophy is considered a poor prognostic sign and a contraindication for surgery. Qualitative assessment of the fatty degeneration of the rotator cuff muscles can be made using the Goutallier classification [10], initially described for computed tomography and later adapted for MR (Table 3).

Table 3 Goutallier classification of muscle fatty degeneration

Stage 0 Normal muscle without fat
Stage I Few fatty streaks within the muscle
Stage II Less fat than muscle within the muscle
Stage III Same amount of fat and muscle within the muscle
Stage IV More fat than muscle within the muscle

Miscellaneous Conditions

Calcific Tendinitis

Hydroxyapatite deposition disease (HADD) typically affects middle-aged persons and represents a common cause of joint pain, related primarily to periarticular deposition of calcific material within tendons. Asymptomatic hydroxyapatite deposits are common, and may be found in the periarticular soft tissues of virtually every joint. Clinical symptoms range from chronic or recurrent joint pain associated with a limited range of motion to acute severe pain and tenderness. It is estimated that HADD afflicts 3% of the asymptomatic adult population and 7% of those with shoulder pain. The shoulder is the most commonly affected region, where symptomatic HADD is usually referred to as "calcific tendinitis", or "calcific bursitis", or "calcific tendinobursitis". The critical zone of the supraspinatus tendon (approximately 1 cm from its insertion in the greater tuberosity) is, by far, the most frequently affected site. It is common for hydroxyapatite deposits of the rotator cuff to migrate to adjacent tissues such as subacromial bursa, along the course of the tendon toward the myotendinous junction, or less commonly intra-osseously. The calcific deposits have a globular appearance and low-signal intensity at all MR imaging sequences (Fig. 9)

When the calcification deposits migrate to bones, muscle or bursae, there is associated increased signal intensity with T2 weighted MR imaging sequences because of the inflammatory process that develops with the migration (most symptomatic stage of the disease). After and during the migration we can observe increased bursal fluid or tenosynovial fluid (when adjacent to long head of the biceps tendon). After that very symptomatic stage the calcification deposits can reabsorb and evenly disappear. It can be difficult to appreciate small amounts of calcification of MR and the use of radiographs or ultrasound may be helpful to confirm the presence of calcifications [11–13].

Muscle Denervation

Etiologies for denervation include both inflammatory conditions such as acute brachial neuritis and compressive neuropathies. Fluid-sensitive MR sequences such as T2 fat saturated and short tau inversion recovery, or STIR, are useful for detecting the increased T2 weighted signal associated with acute denervation. T1-weighted imaging is ideal for depicting fatty infiltration and muscle atrophy secondary to chronic denervation.

Acute brachial neuritis, also known as Parsonage-Turner syndrome, may result in atraumatic shoulder pain and weakness, thereby mimicking a rotator cuff tear. Although the pain may resolve in weeks or months, weakness of the affected muscles may persist and result in fatty atrophy. Although the supraspinatus and infraspinatus are typically affected, the deltoid and rhomboid muscles may also be affected.

The most common cause of nerve compression around the shoulder is compression of the suprascapular nerve by

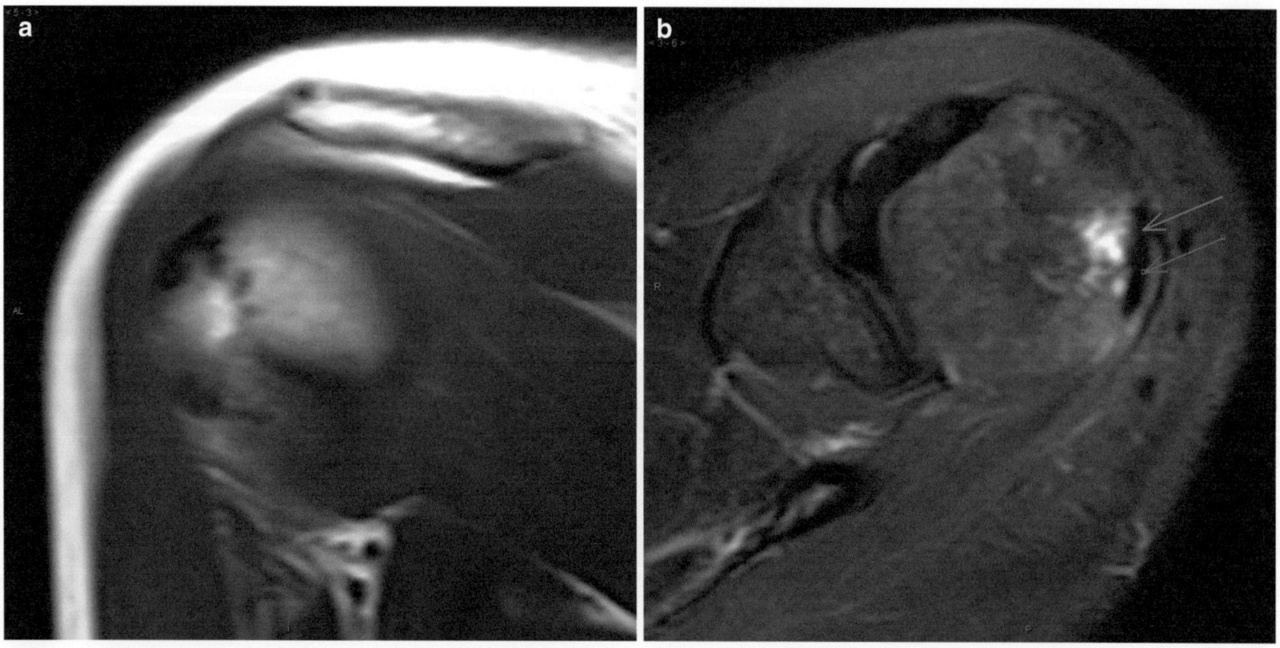

Fig. 9 (**a**) Coronal oblique T1-weighted image showing calcific tendinitis of the infraspinatus tendon visualized as focal low signal intensity hidroxiapatite deposits at the footprint. (**b**) Axial T2-weighted fat suppressed image showing infraspinatus calcification as low signal intensity and inflammatory reactive bone marrow as high signal intensity

paralabral cysts secondary to labral tears. The suprascapular nerve courses through the suprascapular notch to enter the supraspinatus fossa where it gives off branches to the supraspinatus muscle and then courses through the spinoglenoid notch to enter the infraspinatus fossa and gives off branches to the infraspinatus muscle. The level of nerve compression can be inferred by identifying the involved muscles. Involvement of both the supraspinatus and infraspinatus implies a more proximal compression at the level of the suprascapular notch, while isolated infraspinatus involvement is consistent with disease affecting the nerve at the level of the spinoglenoid notch.

The axillary nerve courses in the quadrilateral space and can suffer entrapment in this location, leading to the quadrilateral space syndrome. MR imaging can be useful for detection the etiology of the nerve compression. which can be secondary to paralabral cysts or by fibrous bands, which may be difficult to identify on MR imaging. Isolated edema/fatty atrophy of the teres minor muscle may be detected, sometimes accompanied by edema/fatty atrophy of the deltoid. If no structural abnormality is demonstrated, secondary signs of denervation become important in aiding the diagnosis of quadrilateral space syndrome [14–16].

Rotator Interval

The rotator interval, the triangular shaped region demarcated by the coracoid process medially and the converging margins of the supraspinatus and subscapularis tendons laterally, contains several structures important for the stability and proper biomechanical functioning of the shoulder. These include the coracohumeral ligament (CHL), the superior glenohumeral ligament (SGHL), and the intra-articular portion of the long head of the biceps tendon (LHB).

The CHL arises from the lateral aspect of the coracoid process and inserts on both the lesser tuberosity (the medial band of the CHL) and on the greater tuberosity (the lateral band of the CHL). The medial band of the CHL blends with the fibers of the SGHL to form the biceps pulley (sling) that surrounds the medial and inferior aspect of the intra-articular portion of the LHB.

The lateral band of the CHL surrounds the superior and lateral aspect of the intra-articular LHBT before inserting on the greater tuberosity of the humerus. The SGHL is a fold of the glenohumeral joint capsule that has a variable origin and inserts on the humerus just above the lesser tuberosity. The LHB arises from the posterosuperior labrum, the supraglenoid tubercle or a combination of both. The tendon courses obliquely through the rotator interval before it exits the joint in the intertubercular groove.

The biceps pulley plays an important role in the stability of the intra-articular biceps tendon. It limits medial subluxation of the tendon when the arm is abducted and externally rotated. The superior insertion of the intra-articular subscapularis tendon also provides medial support of the biceps tendon by contributing to the medial wall of the bicipital groove. Disruption of the pulley can lead to instability of the tendon with either subluxation or dislocation. Disruption can occur secondary to trauma [17] or overuse, such as repetitive overhead activity [18]. In addition, the pulley can be injured in associated with tears of the far anterior supraspinatus and far superior subscapularis tendons that extend to involve the coracohumeral and/or superior glenohumeral ligaments [18, 19].

The clinical diagnosis of biceps pulley lesions can be difficult and it is also frequently difficult to identify abnormalities of the pulley on MR imaging, because of the small size of the anatomic structures involved, unless there is associated biceps subluxation/dislocation. There are two main classification systems of biceps pulley injuries, the Bennett [20] and Habermeyer [21] classifications, which are based on the anatomic structures injured.

References

1. Minagawa H, Itoi E, Konno N et al (1998) Humeral attachment of the supraspinatus and infraspinatus tendons: an anatomic study. Arthroscopy 14(3):302–306
2. Soslowsky LJ, Carpenter JE, Bucchieri JS, Flatow EL (1997) Biomechanics of the rotator cuff. Orthop Clin North Am 28(1): 17–30
3. Khan KM, Cook JL, Bonar F, Harcourt P, Astrom M (1999) Histopathology of common tendinopathies. Update and implications for clinical management. Sports Med 27(6):393–408
4. Ellman H, Kay SP (1991) Arthroscopic subacromial decompression for chronic impingement: two to five-year results. J Bone Joint Surg Br 73(3):395–398
5. Snyder SJ, Pachelli AF, Del Pizzo W, Friedman MJ, Ferkel RD, Pattee G (1991) Partial thickness rotator cuff tears: results of arthroscopic treatment. Arthroscopy 7(1):1–7
6. Essman JA, Bell RH, Askew M (1991) Full-thickness rotator-cuff tear: an analysis of results. Clin Orthop Relat Res 265:170–177
7. Lee SY, Lee JK (2002) Horizontal component of partial-thickness tears of rotator cuff: imaging characteristics and comparison of ABER view with oblique coronal view at MR arthrography initial results. Radiology 224(2):470–476
8. Jung J-Y, Jee W-H, Chun HJ, Ahn MI, Kim Y-S (2010) Magnetic resonance arthrography including ABER view in diagnosing partial-thickness tears of the rotator cuff: accuracy, and inter- and intra-observer agreements. Acta Radiol 51(2):194–201
9. DeOrio JK, Cofield RH (1984) Results of a second attempt at surgical repair of a failed initial rotator cuff repair. J Bone Joint Surg Am 66(4):563–567
10. Fuchs B, Weishaupt D, Zanetti M, Hodler J, Gerber C (1999) Fatty degeneration of the muscles of the rotator cuff: assessment by computed tomography versus magnetic resonance imaging. J Shoulder Elb Surg 8(6):599–605
11. Kachewar SG, Kulkarni DS (2013) Calcific tendinitis of the rotator cuff: a review. J Clin Diagn Res 7:1482–1485
12. Uhthoff HK, Loehr JW (1997) Calcific tendinopathy of the rotator cuff: pathogenesis, diagnosis, and management. J Am Acad Orthop Surg 5:183–191

13. Pereira B, Chang E, Resnick D, Patria M (2016) Intramuscular migration of calcium hydroxyapatite crystal deposits involving the rotator cuff tendons of the shoulder: report of 11 patients. Skelet Radiol 45:97–103
14. Steinmann SP, Moran EA (2001) Axillary nerve injury: diagnosis and treatment. J Am Acad Orthop Surg 9(5):328–335
15. Yanny S, Toms AP (2010) MR patterns of denervation around the shoulder. AJR Am J Roentgenol 195(2):W157–W163
16. Cothran RL Jr, Helms C (2005) Quadrilateral space syndrome: incidence of imaging findings in a population referred for MRI of the shoulder. AJR Am J Roentgenol 184(3):989–992
17. Walch G, Nove-Josserand L, Boileau P, Levigne C (1998) Subluxations and dislocations of the tendon of the long head of the biceps. J Shoulder Elb Surg 7:100–108
18. Gerber C, Sebesta A (2000) Impingement of the deep surface of the subscapularis tendon and the reflection pulley on the anterosuperior glenoid rim: a preliminary report. J Shoulder Elb Surg 9:483–490
19. Habermeyer P, Krieter C, Tang KL, Lichtenberg S, Magosch P (2008) A new arthroscopic classification of articular-sided supraspinatus footprint lesions: a prospective comparison with Snyder's and Ellman's classification. J Shoulder Elb Surg 17:909–913
20. Bennett WF (2001) Subscapularis, medial, and lateral head coracohumeral ligament insertion anatomy. Arthroscopic appearance and incidence of "hidden" rotator interval lesions. Arthroscopy 17:173–180
21. Habermeyer P, Magosch P, Pritsch M, Scheibel MT, Lichtenberg S (2004) Anterosuperior impingement of the shoulder as a result of pulley lesions: a prospective arthroscopic study. J Shoulder Elb Surg 13:5–12

Spine Degeneration and Inflammation

David J. Wilson and Victor Cassar-Pullicino

Introduction

At some point in our lives almost all of us will suffer from back pain. The clear majority will be suffering from degenerative disease of the discs or facet joints. A small minority will have tumours, insufficiency fractures, inflammatory joint disease or infection. Differentiation of these conditions is clearly critical for management. In this syllabus, we will cover degeneration and inflammatory joint disease and describe how imaging and image guided intervention are important in precise diagnosis and planning therapy. Brief mention will be made of the alternative diagnoses.

Anatomy

The spine comprises of segments comprising of a vertebral body, articulations with adjacent vertebrae and in the thoracic region with ribs. The sacrum is a specialised segment where vertebrae are embryological fused and the whole structure acts as a part of the pelvic ring. These articulations are at risk from degenerative and inflammatory disorders.

Ligaments and muscles bridge vertebral segments and allow flexion, extension, tilt and rotation. It is useful to think of a mechanical segment as comprising of the vertebra and its attachments.

The intervertebral disc's function is to allow the above movements at the same time as maintaining transverse stability. The disc sits at the division of a mechanical segment and is subject to considerable physical load. The joints between vertebrae must slide and rotate to allow movement. The annulus fibrosis is bound to the edge of the vertebral body and comprises 15–25 concentric layers. Within the disc the nucleus pulposus is soft and very hydrated. It transmits hydrostatic pressure and acts as a buffer between the end plates.

The spine will experience compression, tensile force, shear force, bending movement and torsional movement. Normal function of joints, ligaments and muscle spreads these loads across many segments. However, when disease intervenes focal load will increase at adjacent segments which must move more dramatically to compensate for less movement at disease levels. It is therefore common that symptoms in one part of the spine precipitate pain and dysfunction throughout the vertebral column.

We should not consider the vertebral body to be a simple building block. It has a trabecular internal structure which responds to load applied in different ways. The discs distribute load across the vertebral body and when they become degenerate point pressures may become very much higher than in the young person's spine. In older patients, the bone mineral quantity is reduced often considerably and these two processes combine to cause catastrophic collapse presenting as insufficiency fracture. The combination of osteoporosis and degenerative disease with mechanical dysfunction are major factors in this very common disorder.

Ligamentous attachments in the spine are extensive and complex. Some ligaments restrain the spinal segment from

D.J. Wilson (✉)
St Luke's Radiology, Latimer Road, Oxford OX3 7PF, UK
e-mail: davidwilson.stlukes@btconnect.com

V. Cassar-Pullicino
Department of Radiology, The Robert Jones and Agnes Hunt Orthopaedic Hospital, Oswestry, Shropshire SY10 7AG, UK
e-mail: Victor.Pullicino@rjah.nhs.uk

J. Hodler et al. (eds.), *Musculoskeletal Diseases 2017-2020*, DOI 10.1007/978-3-319-54018-4_20

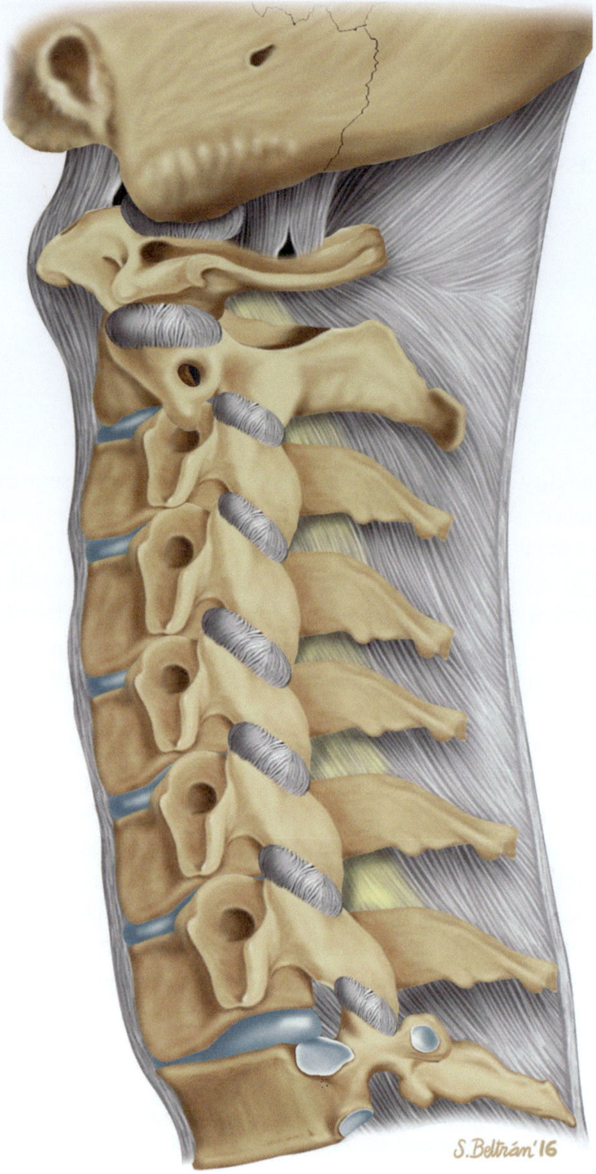

Fig. 1 Diagram of ligamentous and joint capsule attachments in the cervical spine

excessive motion but others provide integral stability binding vertebra to disc, most particularly the posterior and anterior longitudinal ligaments. It is easy to underestimate the complexity of the ligamentous structures around the sacroiliac region, there are anterior and posterior complexes with deep and superficial layers posteriorly. These envelop the articulation of the sacrum to the pelvis. The sacroiliac joint has both fibrous and synovial components and is therefore at risk in patients with systemic inflammatory disease of joints.

This concept of mechanical activity is very important when considering disease; it is easy to view the spine as a solid static structure but observation and the above descriptions should make it clear that movement is a primary function and the one that is most frequently lost in patients who present with pain and dysfunction. Imaging is currently based on static description of morphology and abnormalities of function are more difficult to determine [1] (Figs. 1 and 2).

Degenerative Disease

The degenerative process seems to be an inevitable consequence of ageing. The changes may be observed in the third decade and progress throughout life. The mechanisms are:

1. relatively poor blood supply to the intervertebral discs
2. multiple micro injuries to discs
3. cartilage wear in the joints
4. reduction in the number of chondrocytes
5. vascular ingrowth into the disc
6. marginal osteophytes on vertebral bodies and joints
7. herniation of discs
8. osteopenia and osteoporosis
9. biomechanical overload due to disease at other segments

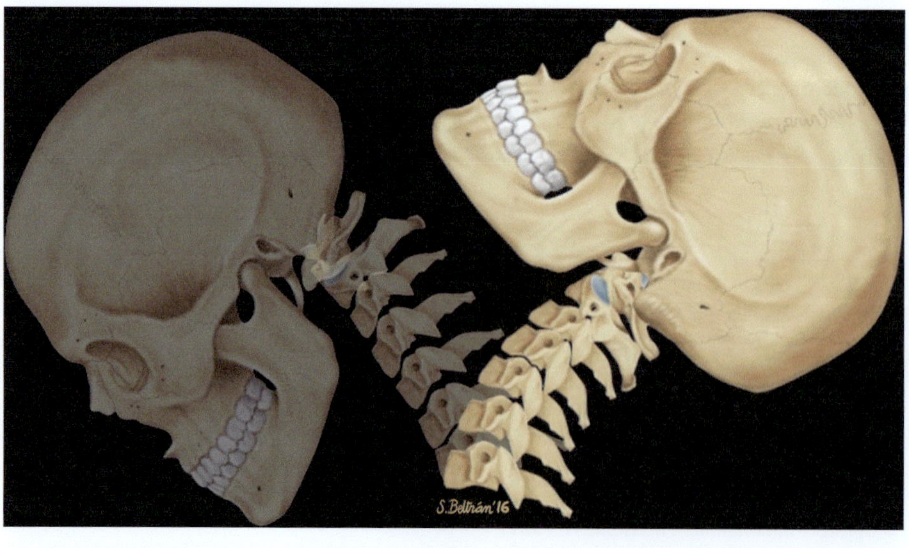

Fig. 2 Diagram to demonstrate spine movement of up to 130° in the sagittal plane

There is a genetic element to the speed of progress of degeneration probably related to the proteoglycan binding of collagen fibres. More linkages mean stiffer collagen which is more brittle, fewer linkages mean softer collagen more likely to tear and displace.

The micro trauma element of degeneration is accelerated by impact and multiple minor traumatic incidents and therefore has an occupational and sporting association.

Manifestations of Degenerative Disease

Discs

Small tears within the disc lead to annular tears. A tear may be seen as a defect in the annulus, containing soft tissue material which may take on an increased water content. There is considerable debate as to whether these tears with high signal material are a cause of localised back pain [2–4]. Tears with scar tissue and repair produce low MRI signal. There is considerable debate over alterations in water content in the annulus, some regard this as the main cause of reduced MRI signal on all sequences but others believe that scar tissue from micro trauma is a major element. The consequence of all these changes is reduction in pliability and tension within the annulus and a tendency for disc height reduction. This in turn leads to buckling of the longitudinal ligaments. Less commonly described in imaging interpretation but probably a much more important factor in morbidity is mechanical instability due to loss of tension within the annulus and laxity of the margins of the disc. Frank herniation of disc material through tears in the annulus fibrosis (Fig. 3) may not only compress adjacent nerve roots but also releases several chemical irritants including prostaglandin, tumour necrosis factor alpha (TNFα) and interleukins [5]. These chemicals may be part of the localised pain response and are potentially toxic to the adjacent nerves.

The loss of height in an intervertebral disc will in turn create mechanical instability and this will lead to osteophytes that may impinge on adjacent nerves [6].

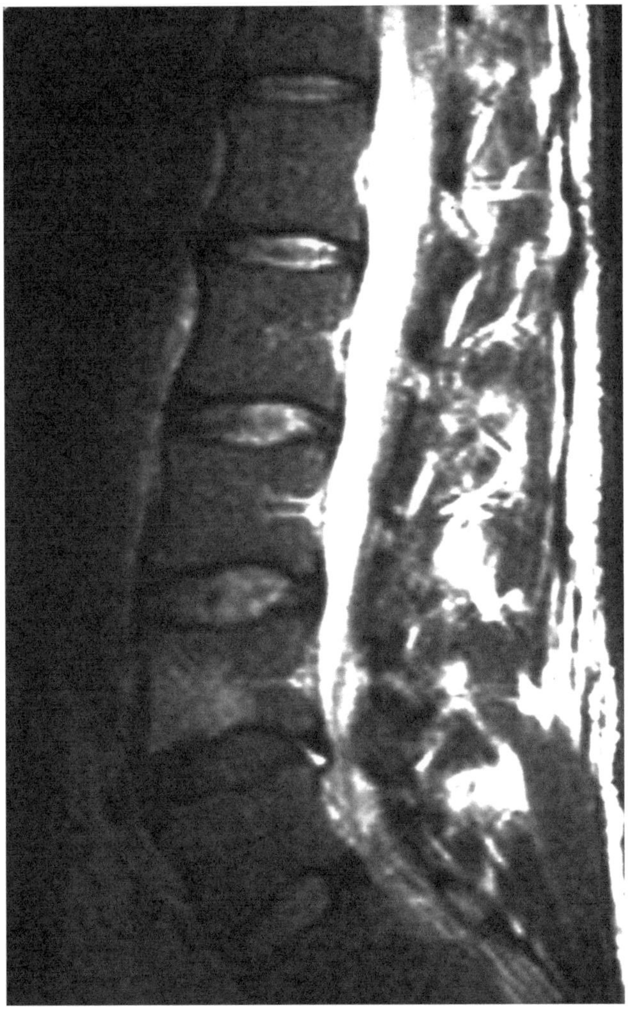

Fig. 3 MRI of annular tear

Facet Joints

As for all synovial joints, articular cartilage wear and mechanical instability lead to osteoarthritis with localised pain and osteophytes. New bone formation around the joint may considerably limit movement which in turn places additional load on adjacent segments. As degeneration is inevitably widespread and extremely common it may be very

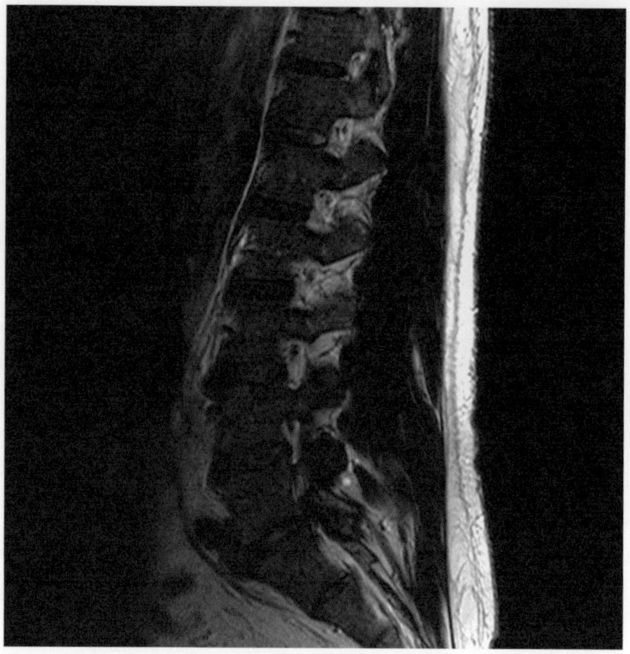

Fig. 4 Facet joint arthritis with a synovial cyst

difficult to determine the origin of pain as the presence of facet joint arthropathy does not predict that pain arises from this area. Synovial cysts may arise from the joint and may compress nerve roots. Haemorrhage into the cysts may increase the pressure. The fundamental problem is that facet joint disease is very common and we have no imaging technique that scans for the origin of pain. The presence of facet joint changes does not necessarily indicate an origin of pain, similarly, joints that look relatively normal may be the source of symptoms. Systems are closely interrelated and there is association between muscle atrophy and facet joint disease, it may be that spine instability is exacerbated by this connection [7] (Fig. 4).

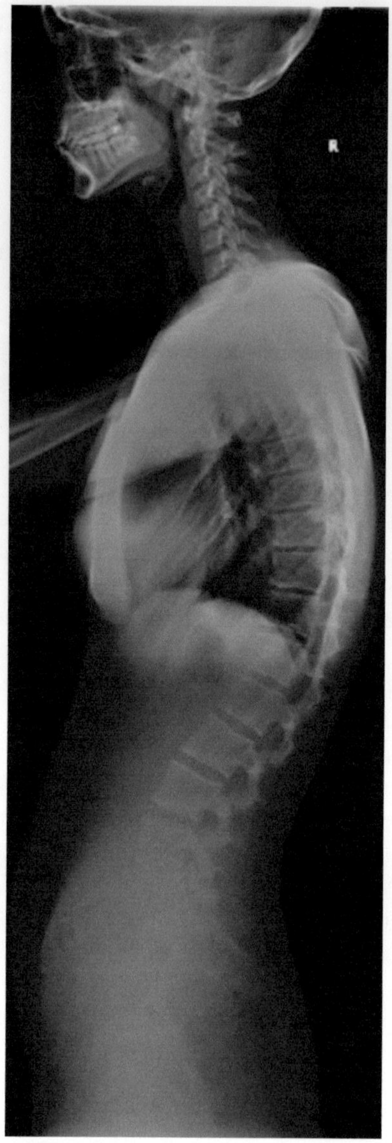

Fig. 5 Scheuermann's disease

End Plates

MRI is often used to assess the end plates. The changes include Schmorl's nodes which are indentations in the end plate surface (Fig. 5) and probably represent adolescent disc protrusion through bone that is too soft to accept the loads applied. There is a genetic predisposition and severe cases affecting multiple levels may lead to progressive kyphosis probably? due to damage to growth in the anterior part of the vertebral body; this condition is termed Scheuermann's disease or idiopathic adolescent kyphosis. This may be a factor in later facet joint arthritis and segmental instability.

Stress of the end plate may lead to the changes described by Modic et al. which may be characterised by their MRI signal as, bone oedema, fatty infiltration and sclerosis. There is some evidence that end plate stress changes particularly those with oedema are linked to back pain [8, 9] but there is poor evidence to show that lumbar surgery results are related to the stage of end plate change

Spinal Stenosis

Individuals are born with spinal canals of differing dimension. Those with narrow canals need very little disc protrusion or osteophytes formation to cause pressure on the cord or cauda equina. Spinal stenosis is when the spinal canal is rendered too narrow due to disc or joint disease for normal blood supply to reach the neural structures. Patients will typically complain of back and leg pain which comes on after walking (spinal claudication), this eases after several minutes' rest.

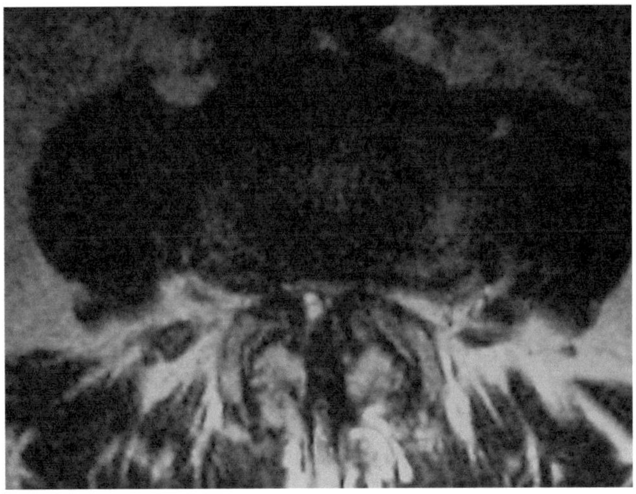

Fig. 6 MRI spinal stenosis

The disease is progressive and rarely undergoes spontaneous resolution. Therefore, surgery is an important treatment method and imaging is essential in plotting the extent and severity. There is considerable literature on the efficacy of surgery but a recent Cochrane review suggested that fusion plus decompression was no better than conventional decompression alone [10] (Fig. 6).

Inflammatory Disorders

The underlying pathology of target organs in spinal inflammatory disorders dictates the imaging appearances throughout the natural history of the disease processes. Although overlap exists, inflammatory disorders can predominantly affect the synovial articulations of the spine (rheumatoid disease) or primarily the enthesis of ligaments and intervertebral discs (seronegative spondyloarthropathies). The various disease states are not static but rather need to be viewed as dynamic and progressive usually resulting in complications. In rheumatoid disease it is primarily the cervical spine that is involved but it is very rare that the rheumatoid arthritis patient presents with cervical spine manifestations as the first mode of presentation. On the other hand seronegative spondyloarthropathies usually present with axial manifestations of enthesitis as the first mode of presentation which are easily overlooked.

Spondyloarthropathy may result from a wide range of inflammatory disorders. They include rheumatoid arthritis, ankylosing spondylitis, psoriatic arthropathy, reactive arthritis, Bechet's disease, Reiter's syndrome and SAPHO syndrome. Synovial involvement of the cervical spine in seropositive inflammatory states have a predilection for the facet joints, and in particular the C1–C2 articulations. In the seronegative spondyloarthropathy the inflammatory site is the enthesis where the collagen of the ligaments or intervertebral disc annulus enters bone directly. The cause of the inflammatory process is the generation of cytokines which results in oedema, bone erosion, disorganisation of bone and ligament structure which promotes a reactive osteitis and eventually ossification of the ligaments commencing at the enthesis interface. The seronegative spondyloarthropathies can be further categorised based on the imaging findings equated to the clinical features and laboratory findings. Although multiple modalities such as radiography, CT and scintigraphy can be employed to assess the inflammatory sites within both the axial and appendicular skeleton, it is primarily MRI which is the optimal imaging modality to assess inflammatory disorders of the spine due to its high sensitivity and specificity. Although contrast enhanced MR studies are not usually required for diagnosis, they can distinguish between active and inactive disease and also help in assessing the response to anti-inflammatory therapy.

Clinical Features

Rheumatoid arthritis very commonly affects the spine especially the cervical region and the odontoid peg [11]. Erosion of the peg may lead to severe subluxation and may be life-threatening. Imaging is important when patients are being considered for intubation anaesthesia whether they have symptoms or not. Disease modifying drugs are having a profound effect in the degree of spinal involvement by the rheumatoid process if treated early.

Ankylosing spondylitis is the prototype of the seronegative arthropathies. Associated with HLA-B27 this is a disease more common in men with an onset mean of 25 years. It usually presents with back pain and morning stiffness. Untreated the disease will progress to bony ankylosis of joints which renders the spine at risk of transverse fractures (banana fracture) with relatively minor injury. In the acute phase the pain arises from inflamed entheses (the insertion of ligaments) at the corner of the vertebral bodies (Romanus lesion or shiny corner). The disease commonly affects the sacroiliac joints and the costovertebral joints. Using MR imaging bone oedema is the hallmark but care must be taken to observe even small numbers of lesions as they may be fairly subtle and only visible on water sensitive fat suppressed sequences. Early diagnosis is key as disease modifying drugs and physical therapy should be commenced as early as possible.

Sacroiliitis

Sacroiliitis is the hallmark of all spondyloarthropathies. It is a fundamental component required in establishing the diagnosis of ankylosing spondylitis but it is also relevant to the other spondyloarthropathies. In ankylosing spondylitis it is bilateral and symmetrical, while in psoriatic spondyloarthropathy and reactive arthritis it may be bilateral or unilateral. Involvement of the axial skeleton is unusual and indeed rare in the absence of sacroiliitis.

Conventional radiography remains the initial diagnostic imaging modality recommended despite its low sensitivity and relatively high false negative rate in early disease. There are inherent limitations to the proper radiographic assessment of the sacroiliac joints which arise because the joints themselves are divergent in the AP projection which is why a PA projection is usually a better option of assessing the sacroiliac joints. It is also well known that conventional radiography can miss advanced sacroiliitis. Early inflammatory sacroiliitis can result in a loss of the sharpness of the subchondral bone outline of the joint which then progresses to becoming irregular due to the presence of erosions which in turn produces an appearance of localised joint widening. Sclerosis of the subchondral bone on either side of the joint is fairly diagnostic in established disease, especially when it involves the inferior and middle portion of the joint and is more pronounced on the iliac side. However, in established disease the sacroiliac joint may also exhibit loss of sharpness due to ossification across the joint leading to ankylosis. In practice however, radiological detection of sacroiliiac joint changes is challenging with poor inter-observer and intra-observer reliability for the changes in early disease.

The relatively late development of radiographic changes in ankylosing spondylitis undeniably is one of the factors which can delay the diagnosis. MR imaging however, has revolutionised the early diagnosis of sacroiliitis. This is primarily dependent on the pericartilage osteitis which is an important feature of ankylosing spondylitis which produces bone marrow oedema which is well picked up on the oedema sensitive sequences such as T2 weighted sequences with fat suppression or the STIR sequence. The T1 weighted spin-echo sequences are however better at depicting articular erosions. The degree of the oedema may vary ranging from florid, fairly extensive areas of periarticular oedema to more focal and localised zones of oedema paralleling the joint line. It is usually the inferior iliac portion of the joint that is involved in the early stages of sacroiliac inflammatory change. Some studies have positively related the degree of marrow oedema on MR to BMD status. Gadolinium enhanced MR studies have been advocated in active disease as there is a rise in the MR signal at the point of enhancement in the joint space and periarticular tissues in the first two minutes. However, contrast enhancement is particularly useful if the oedema sensitive sequence (STIR) is equivocal. Using contrast enhancement MRI can not only distinguish active from inactive disease, but it can also monitor the treatment response where a decrease in the enhancement even in the persistent presence of bone marrow oedema has been shown to be strongly correlated with a good clinical response to treatment. There are various ways of utilising post contrast MR imaging in the assessment of sacroiliac disease. They are particular helpful in determining whether the instituted drug regime is working, identify a need to alter the drug regime, and stop drug regimes if they are not working in view of the significant side effects and high cost.

Although the oedema sensitive sequences in particular the T2 sequences with fat suppression are very sensitive and specific in visualisation of bone marrow oedema, joint widening and joint fluid, they are not as good in identifying subtle erosions due to the relatively low spatial resolution compared with CT. The high spatial resolution inherent in CT identifies subtle erosions and subchondral sclerosis in sacroiliac joint involvement. CT indeed is the preferred modality for the detection of very early erosions of the sacroiliac joints and their early ankylosis. However, one needs to bear in mind that sclerosis on its own can have a similar appearance in both active disease and in burnt out inflammation.

Axial Skeleton

Ankylosing spondylitis is the seronegative spondyloarthropathy prototype. It is primarily a disease of the axial skeleton involving the sacroiliac joints and the spine. The primary target organ is the enthesis where the spinal longitudinal ligaments and annulus fibrosus merge directly with the bone. In the early manifestations of inflammation an osteitis is produced by the inflammatory response which leads to bone marrow oedema and then subsequently this is followed by reactive sclerosis and eventually ossification of the involved ligaments. There is usually an orderly progression of involvement of the spine commencing firstly in the thoracolumbar and lumbosacral regions and then advancing to the midlumbar, midthoracic and eventually the cervical spine.

Spondylitis

Spondylitis occurs in about 50% of ankylosing spondylitis patients although females are relatively less affected. The earliest changes are due to enthesitis at the insertion of the outer fibres of the annulus fibrosus on the ring apophysis of the vertebral end plate. Although this occurs circumferentially, it is predominantly the anterior attachment that usually produces the more florid manifestations. Subtle erosions with reactive sclerosis in the vertebral corners are seen which radiographically have been referred to as Romanus lesions when viewed as erosions, and "shiny corners" when the erosion is associated with sclerosis due to

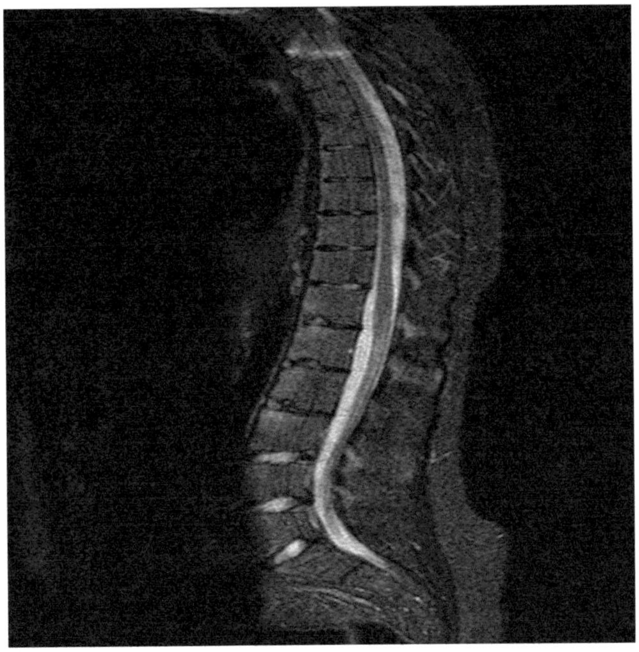

Fig. 7 Romanus lesion

the reactive osteitis. The Romanus erosive disease (Fig. 7) may also produce an apparent squaring of the anterior outline of the vertebral body. The Romanus lesions are, however, short lived and resolve by producing resultant syndesmophyte formation. The syndesmophytes represent the ossification of the outer fibres of the annulus fibrosus in ankylosing spondylitis. They are seen radiographically as very fine and symmetric in appearance bridging the intervertebral space. This may initially appear at a single disc level but usually progresses to involve multiple segments producing the so-called characteristic "bamboo spine". The same inflammatory process results in ossification of the longitudinal ligaments which insert onto the vertebral bodies producing squaring of the vertebral body appearance as the fusion progresses.

MR imaging is the most sensitive diagnostic tool for the identification of discovertebral inflammatory disease. The Romanus lesions are identified on the sagittal sequences and characterised by a triangular pattern of bone marrow oedema at the corners of the vertebral end plates highlighted by low T1 signal and high T2 fat sat and STIR sequence appearance. The small erosion may be overlooked when compared with the areas of oedema. After the acute Romanus lesion phase subsides, the chronic lesions are identified by a fatty marrow replacement at the sites of enthesis inflammation within the vertebral bodies, highlighted by a high T1 signal and a low signal on STIR and T2 fat sat sequences. Multiple contiguous areas of high T1 signal can be seen in vertebral bodies and in particular at their corners in segments of the spine which have undergone extensive fusion. The intervertebral disc in cases of long term spinal fusion can also undergo changes producing a high T1 inherent MR signal. This has been related to the presence of calcification or alternatively the presence of marrow within mature transdiscal ankylosis.

Contrast enhanced MR studies and diffusion weighted MR sequences have also been employed in the detection of inflammatory disease of the spine. They can be useful in the acute phase of inflammatory change, particularly in the early manifestations of the disease. In acute Romanus lesions contrast medium injection usually renders the erosions more clearly defined. Comparative studies, however, with STIR sequences have concluded that there is very little advantage as both have high intra- and inter-observer reliability and more active lesions are seen on the STIR sequences. In cases where the STIR sequence is equivocal dynamic Gadolinium DTPA studies have been found useful.

Although there is no doubt that MR imaging has revolutionised the role of imaging in the early and active phases of inflammatory disorders of the spine, one also needs to bear in mind that it does have a particular drawback in identifying the syndesmophytes which are the hallmark of established disease. Syndesmophytes are not well seen by MRI and easily overlooked because the low signal of the syndesmophyte is similar to the low signal of the normal anterior longitudinal ligament and annulus fibrosus. Similarly MRI can overlook ossification and fusion of other spinal elements namely the apophyseal joints, paraspinal ligaments and interspinous ligaments. It is still the case that radiographic diagnosis is very easy when compared to MRI in the chronic case where there is established soft tissue ossification.

Spondylodiscitis

There are two types of spondylodiscitis that can be detected within the discovertebral junction. *Primary spondylodiscitis*, or as it is sometimes known Anderson Type A lesions, resemble Schmorl's nodes exhibiting a rim of oedema within the vertebral body, a focal endplate defect, and enhancement of the marrow oedema as well. The primary spondylodiscitis usually is a sign of early discovertebral involvement with a stable spinal status. In the *secondary spondylodiscitis*, or as they are sometimes known the Anderson Type B lesions, there is more extensive and florid discovertebral disease and destruction. These are particularly well demonstrated on CT and MRI. The degree of vertebral destruction is usually mild but there is often extensive bony oedema and bony sclerosis, and in long established cases the endplates can be completely destroyed on both sides of the intervertebral disc. In Anderson Type B lesions the spine is unstable at the site of involvement due to increased mobility. This increased mobility could be at a level between fused segments or be associated with deficiency of the posterior elements where there is a pseudoarthrosis due to a fracture. It is therefore imperative that the posterior elements are assessed assiduously to differentiate Type A from Type B Anderson lesions as the latter are associated with pain and instability and can give rise to neurological dysfunction.

Costo-Vertebritis

This is the hallmark of spondyloarthropathy usually starting in the lower thoracic spine.

Complications of Inflammatory Joint Disease

The most important spinal complications in ankylosing spondylitis include *osteoporosis, fracture, instability, cauda equine syndrome*, and *spinal stenosis*.

Osteoporosis increases in prevalence directly with increased patient age, increased severity of spinal involvement, increased disease duration and peripheral arthritis. The vertebral marrow signal is usually increased on the T1 sequences as a result of the osteoporosis. The osteoporosis obviously increases the chances of vertebral compression fractures, posterior element fractures, pseudoarthrosis, and unstable fractures from relatively minor trauma.

Fractures of the cervical spine may occur after a minor fall or injury to the head and neck. Typically the conventional radiographs show a chalk-stick type of break either through the disc or the vertebral body anteriorly and horizontally through the posterior fused elements. A common spinal location for fracture is the thoracolumbar and cervicothoracic and lastly the lumbosacral junction. By definition all three columns of the spine are involved in this type of fracture. There is a high risk of missing the fracture at the time of initial evaluation particularly if radiographic techniques are not optimal. A delayed diagnosis can lead to the development of a true pseudoarthrosis resulting in instability and cord injury. Increasingly it has been shown that conventional radiography is not sufficient in excluding a fracture complicating a fused spine in ankylosing spondylitis. Any ankylosing spondylitis patient suffering minor trauma who complains of pain should have advanced imaging preferably by CT, as this will show the full extent of the fracture in both the axial and the reconstructive sagittal and coronal images. If the patient has neurological deficit MR is essential in assessing the status of the cord and in particular whether there is an epidural haematoma or disc/bone fragment compressing the cord.

Cauda Equina Syndrome is a rare but specific complication following longstanding ankylosing spondylitis. It invariably occurs in a fused spine and is most common in the lumbar region. Dural ectasia producing leptomeningeal succulations are common resulting in erosions of primarily the posterior neural arch. This is best evaluated with CT or MR imaging. MR will show enlargement of the spinal canal with arachnoid diverticulae, erosion of the laminae and adherent nerve roots.

Spinal Stenosis

It is important that one remembers that the ligamentous ossification that takes place as a result of the chronic inflammatory reactive process can also involve the ligaments within the spinal canal, namely the longitudinal ligament and the ligamentum flavum. As a result of this ossification there can be encroachment onto the contents, namely the cord and nerve roots. Neurological deficit in patients with ankylosing spondylitis could have a number of causes but C1–C2 subluxation, fracture, pseudoarthrosis, ligamentous ossification and cauda equine syndrome would tend to be the most common list that one needs to remember in directing imaging to the spine to assess the underlying reason for the neurological deficit.

Other Spondyloarthropathies

Reiter's disease, psoriatic arthropathy, Bechet's disease and reactive arthropathy may all cause changes like those seen in acute ankylosing spondylitis. Advanced fusion of the spine is much less common. Reiter's disease typically produces asymmetric inflammatory arthropathy in the sacroiliac joints with relative preservation of one side of the joint, it is associated with urethritis and uveitis and is sexually transmitted. Bechet's disease is associated with mouth ulcers and multisystem disease. Psoriatic arthropathy is associated with peripheral arthropathy, skin and nail disorders. Note that the skin disease may be relatively minor in advanced cases of spondyloarthropathy [12] (Fig. 8).

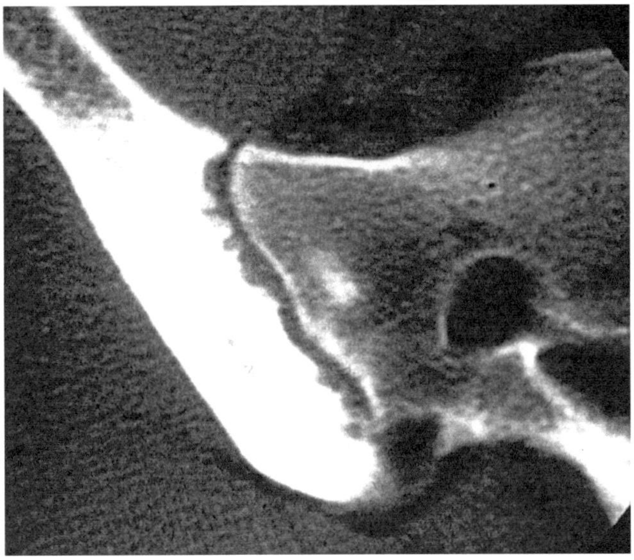

Fig. 8 Reiter's syndrome sacroiliitis

Imaging

Conventional Radiographs

Conventional radiographs of the spine have a principal role in assessing patients with trauma. This includes patients suspected of insufficiency fracture. However, it is now well recognised that they have limited if any value in the assessment of patients with back pain and are of minimal value in judging whether degenerative changes are affecting the patient in a way that might require interventional techniques. The appearances of advanced ankylosing spondylitis are typical but it might be argued that if you are trying to assess the disease at this stage you are far too late. National guidance of the United Kingdom now states that conventional radiographs are not indicated for the investigation of back pain.

Computed Tomography

CT is the ideal method of assessing complex fractures and detecting destructive tumours. It will not demonstrate inflammatory changes at the early stage when they would be best treated and it was felt not to show bone oedema. It is much less effective at judging nerve root compression.

MRI

MRI is the workhorse for the assessment and diagnosis of spinal disease. It is the preferred imaging for patients with back pain that fails to respond to conservative measures and those patients who have adverse clinical features or signs that might suggest infection, tumour or insufficiency fracture. It is without doubt the best technique for assessing nerve root compression. Perhaps the only weakness is when there is metal implanted surgically and despite newer metal artefact suppression techniques the image will be distorted at the level of the metal. MRI has particular strength in assessing for bone oedema and haemorrhage in acute subtle fractures.

Isotope Bone Scintigraphy and White Cell Scintigraphy

These techniques have a particular use in patients where pain is unexplained by MRI or when there are so many abnormalities found using MRI that it is uncertain which is the origin. Increased metabolic activity or white cell accumulation at a particular site may point to this as the most likely origin of symptoms. The radiation dose and the non-specificity of the techniques are sufficient to make this a second line test rather than a primary investigation.

Interventional Techniques

In the assessment of patients with degenerative arthropathy, disc degeneration and nerve root irritation, local anaesthetic blocks optionally with the use of steroids may allow the examiner to determine the exact origin of pain. 12 h of complete relief after a 1 mL injection of bupivacaine clinches the origin of the symptoms. Therapeutic interventions include anaesthetic and steroid blocks to joints or nerve roots, radiofrequency Rhysolysis to denervate facet joints, laser and radiofrequency disc ablation for disc generated pain and percutaneous annuloplasty for symptomatic disc protrusion and are all potential techniques in the spine. Sacroiliac joint injections and sacroiliac ligament injections may help to determine whether the joint or the surrounding tissues are the origin of pain. Radiofrequency denervation of the sacroiliac joint may be useful [13] (Fig. 9).

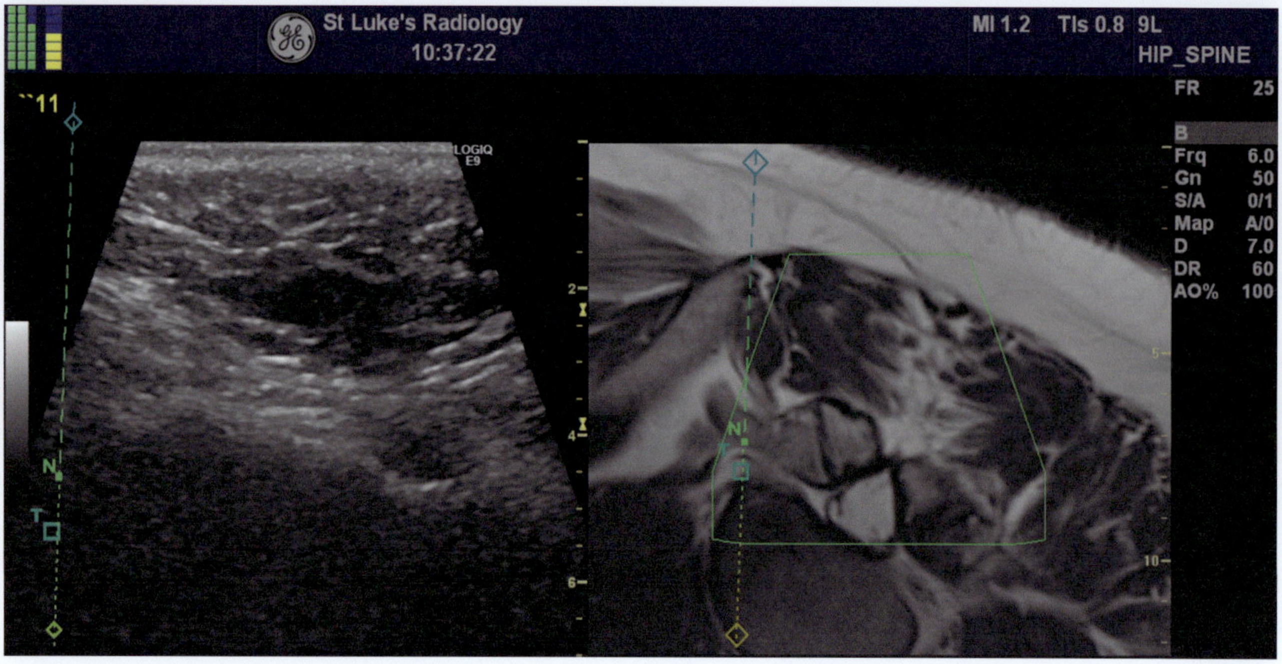

Fig. 9 Fusion imaging guided nerve root block

References

1. Adams MA, Bogduk N, Burton K, Dolan P (2013) The biomechanics of back pain, 3rd edn. Churchill Livingstone, Elsevier
2. Bogduk N, Aprill C (1993) On the nature of neck pain, discography and cervical zygapophysial joint blocks. Pain 54:213–217
3. Aprill C, Bogduk N (1992) High-intensity zone: a diagnostic sign of painful lumbar disc on magnetic resonance imaging. Br J Radiol 65:361–369
4. Jha SC, Higashino K, Sakai T et al (2016) Clinical significance of high-intensity zone for discogenic low back pain: a review. J Med Investig 63:1–7
5. Goupille P, Mulleman D, Valat JP (2006) Radiculopathy associated with disc herniation. Ann Rheum Dis 65:141–143
6. An HS, Masuda K, Inoue N (2006) Intervertebral disc degeneration: biological and biomechanical factors. J Orthop Sci 11:541–552
7. Sebro R, O'Brien L, Torriani M, Bredella MA (2016) Assessment of trunk muscle density using CT and its association with degenerative disc and facet joint disease of the lumbar spine. Skelet Radiol 45: 1221–1226
8. Maatta JH, MacGregor A, Karppinen J, Williams FM (2016) The relationship between Modic changes and intervertebral disc degeneration. BMC Musculoskelet Disord 17:371
9. Xu L, Chu B, Feng Y, Xu F, Zou YF (2016) Modic changes in lumbar spine: prevalence and distribution patterns of end plate oedema and end plate sclerosis. Br J Radiol 89:20150650
10. Machado GC, Ferreira PH, Yoo RI et al (2016) Surgical options for lumbar spinal stenosis. Cochrane Database Syst Rev 11: CD012421
11. Macovei LA, Rezus E (2016) Cervical spine lesions in rheumatoid arthritis patients. Rev Med Chir Soc Med Nat Iasi 120:70–76
12. Leone A, Marino M, Dell'Atti C, Zecchi V, Magarelli N, Colosimo C (2016) Spinal fractures in patients with ankylosing spondylitis. Rheumatol Int 36:1335–1346
13. Pope TL, Bloem HL, Beltran J, Morrison WB, Wilson DJ (2015) Musculoskeletal imaging, 2nd edn. Saunders, Elsevier

Imaging of Spine Trauma

Mark W. Anderson and Suzanne E. Anderson

Introduction

An estimated 2–10% of blunt trauma patients will be found to have a fracture of the cervical, thoracic or lumbar spine with up to 20% of these having a one or more additional non-contiguous fractures [1].

A pre-eminent goal when assessing these patients is to detect any bone or soft tissue injury that compromises the stability of the spinal column or results in actual or potential damage to the spinal cord or nerve roots. Poor management, due to either a delay in diagnosis or improper immobilization, may lead to neurologic deterioration and potentially devastating consequences [2].

"Clearing" the Spine

In order to minimize the chance of mismanagement, a patient presenting after blunt trauma should be considered to have a significant spinal injury until proven otherwise. The process of clearing the spine is typically accomplished through a combination of clinical examination and imaging studies, with the patient immobilized until that is accomplished.

Clinical Clearance

The National Emergency X-Radiography Utilization Study Group (NEXUS) and the Canadian C-spine Rule, both proposed various clinical criteria for determining which patients should undergo radiography after blunt trauma [3, 4]. While both of these tools have been advocated for use with mildly injured patients, subsequent studies, using CT rather than radiography as a gold standard, have reported that significant injuries may be missed when they are used with severely injured blunt trauma patients [5].

Criteria that have been advocated as indications for obtaining a CT examination of the cervical spine include:

- Midline pain or tenderness
- Neurologic deficit
- Altered mental status
- Distracting injuries (e.g., pelvic/extremity fractures)
- Features which typically trigger a trauma team activation (e.g., Glasgow Coma Scale score < 14; severe anatomic injuries; a high risk mechanism such as a high speed MVA > 35 mph; fall from >20 ft; etc) [5, 6].

Imaging Clearance

Numerous studies have demonstrated that radiography is woefully insensitive for detecting cervical spine fractures when compared to CT with one meta-analysis reporting a pooled sensitivity of 52% for radiography versus 98% for CT [7]. As a result, CT has become that primary screening modality of the spine in these patients and has virtually replaced radiographic evaluation in most centers.

MR imaging should only be obtained *after* a CT scan given its relatively poor sensitivity for fracture detection

M.W. Anderson (✉)
University of Virginia Health Sciences Center, 1218 Lee Street, Charlottesville, VA 22901, USA
e-mail: mwa3a@virginia.edu

S.E. Anderson
Kantonsspital Baden, Im Ergel 1, 5404 Baden, Baden, Kanton Aarau 5404, Switzerland
e-mail: andersonsembach@bluewin.ch

J. Hodler et al. (eds.), *Musculoskeletal Diseases 2017-2020*, DOI 10.1007/978-3-319-54018-4_21

(55% compared with CT in one study) [8]. Because of its superb ability to demonstrate soft tissue pathology (cord, nerve root, ligament, disc, hematoma), it is complementary to CT in this clinical setting. Indications for MRI include neurologic deficit, persistent pain after a negative CT, assessing for ligamentous or other soft tissue injury in the obtunded patient, and subsequent neurologic deterioration [9].

Despite these strengths of MR imaging many authors now suggest that if a high quality CT is negative for injury, even in the obtunded patient, further evaluation with MR imaging is not needed [10]. At this point, however, this remains controversial and a recently published practice guideline suggests that the use of MRI in conjunction with CT should be individualized to each institution [11].

Classifcation Schemes

Numerous classification systems for categorizing spine injuries have been proposed in an attempt to develop a common language for communication, as well as for providing information regarding prognosis and the need for treatment.

The Denis classifcation [12] divided the spine into three columns: (1) anterior—anterior longitudinal ligament (ALL) and anterior 2/3 of vertebra and disc; (2) middle—posterior 1/3 of vertebra and disc and posterior longitudinal ligament (PLL); and (3) posterior—all elements posterior to the PLL (Fig. 1). The importance of the middle column for spine stability was stressed and major injuries were divided into four categories: compression, burst, "seat belt" (distraction), and fracture dislocation.

In 1994, Magerl described a new system based on the AO fracture classification used in the extremities [13]. Injuries were divided into three categories: A = compression, B = distraction, C = translation (Fig. 2). These three categories were further subdivided into three groups, each of which contained three subgroups. The higher the grade in all of these categories, the more severe the injury. This extremely comprehensive system is commonly used by surgeons, but its high degree of complexity limits its usefulness in daily practice and has contributed to poor reproducibility in several studies.

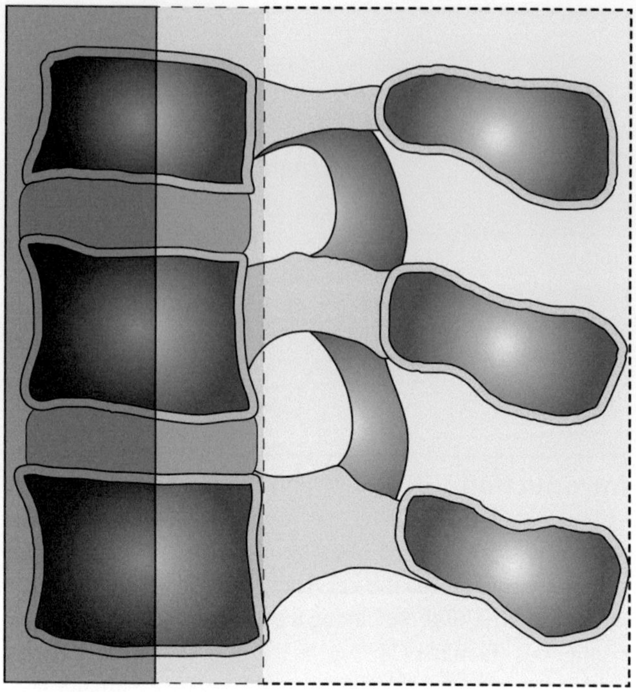

Fig. 1 Diagram according to Denis classification showing anterior, middle and posterior columns

The Thoracolumbar Injury Classification and Severity Score (TLICS) was proposed in 2005 in an attempt to provide a more clear construct that would also better help guide treatment decisions [14]. The three components of the system are: (1) injury morphology; (2) status of the posterior ligamentous complex (PLC- ligamentum flavum, facet joint capsules, interspinous and supraspinous ligaments; and (3) neurologic status of the patient. Injury morphologies include (from least to most severe): compression/burst, rotation/translation and distraction injuries (Fig. 3). The PLC is described as intact, indeterminate or disrupted based primarily on imaging findings. Point values are assigned to each category and the total is then used to direct therapy. A similar system has been developed for the cervical spine: the Subaxial Cervical Spine Injury Classification System (SLIC) [15].

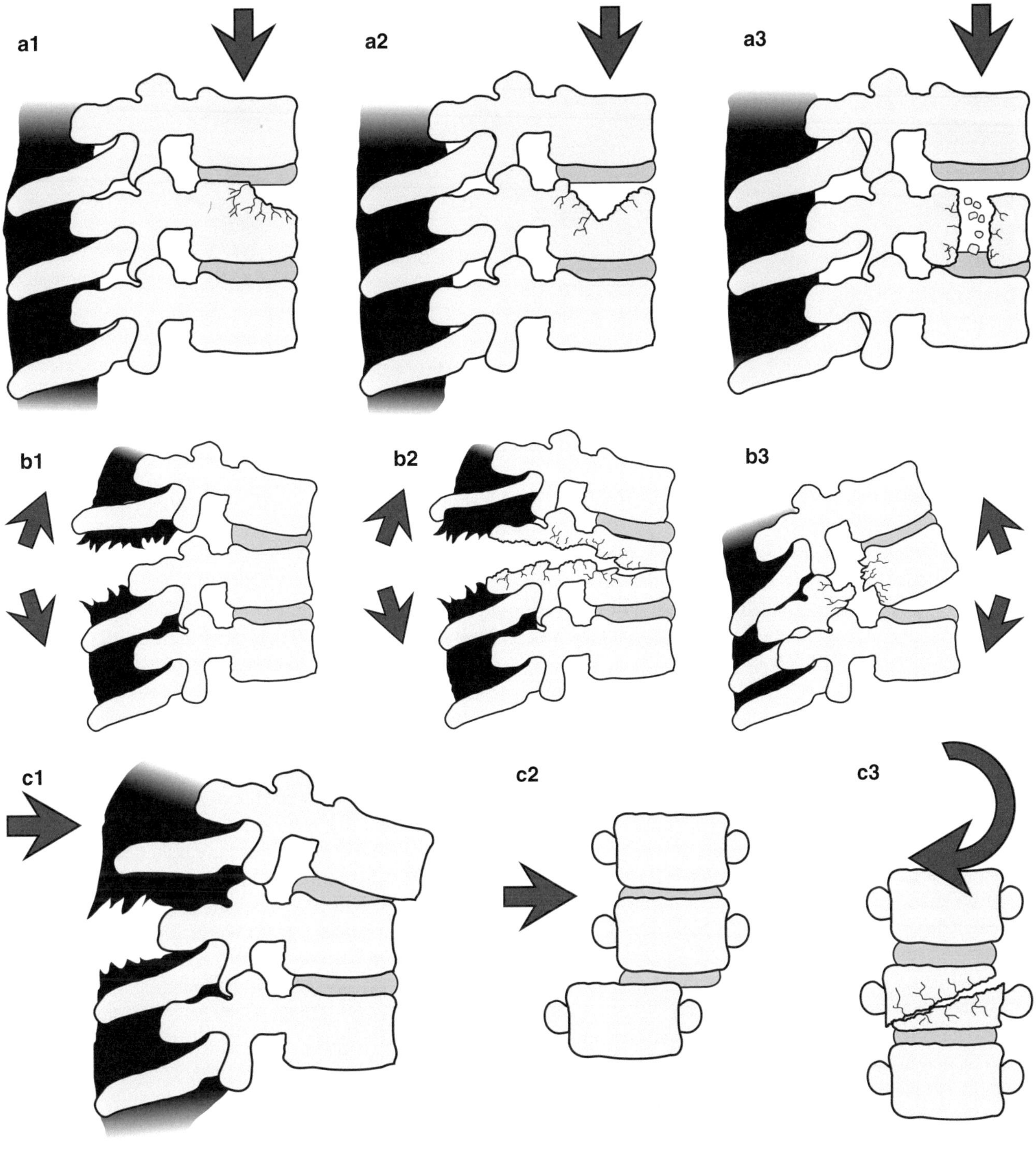

Fig. 2 Basic categories of the AO spine trauma classification system

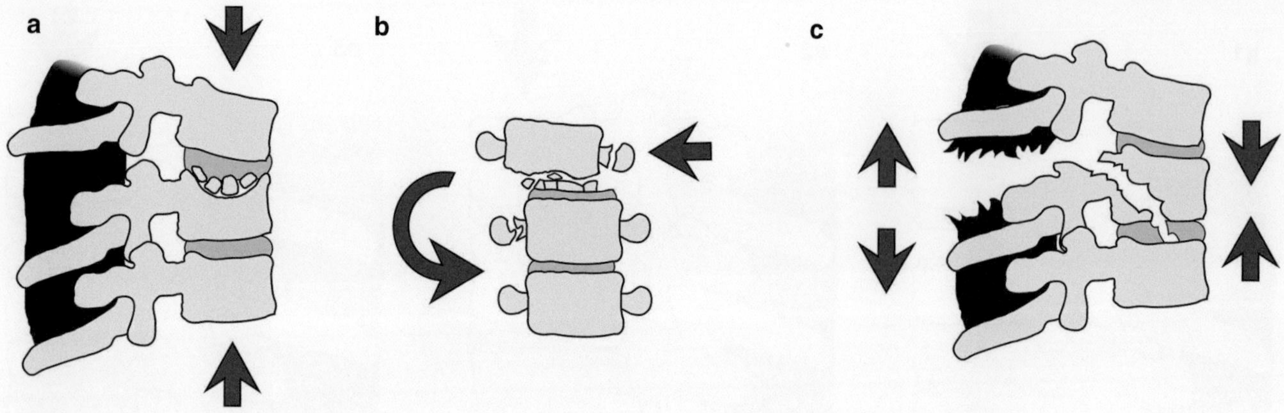

Fig. 3 Basic categories of the TLICS classification system (**a**) compression/burst (**b**) rotation/translation and (**c**) distraction

Cervical Spine

Introduction

Cervical spine injuries are common and fractures of the C1-C2 complex account for about 25% of these injuries with nearly two thirds of these involving odontoid fractures [16, 17].

Cervical spine trauma is often associated with cord and nerve root injury that can be catastrophic if not diagnosed early or if missed. Cervical spine trauma incurs huge health care costs, estimated to be two-fold over an equivalent fracture in the thoracic and lumbar spine [18].

C1-C2 Region

Atlanto-axial dissociations are usually fatal. The diagnosis is made on lateral radiographic findings of displacement and increased distance between the basion and dens.

Occipital condyle fractures are best demonstrated on coronal reformatted CT images. An alar ligament avulsion fracture is the most common type in this region.

At C1, bilateral fractures through the neural arch are most common and result from hyperextension of the head which compresses the neural arch of C1 between the occipital condyles and arch of C2.

A comminuted burst fracture of C1 (Jefferson fracture) is usually due to an axial load to the vertex of the head.

C1-C2 atlantoaxial dissociation may be seen after traumatic rupture of the transverse ligament or in patients with rheumatoid arthritis or Downs syndrome. Imaging reveals an increase in the width of the predental space. Rotary atlanto-axial deformities may result from trauma or torticolis subluxation in children or adolescents. Radiographs show asymmetry of the C1-dens distance, and rotation of the spinous processes may be observed.

The C2 hangman's fracture refers to bilateral fractures of the pars interarticularis, usually due to a hyperextension injury or to hyperflexion and axial compression in some cases. These fractures are not usually associated with cord compression or injury due to the favorable size of the canal at this level and also because the bilateral fractures decompress the cord. Hangman's fracture classification proposed by Effendi consists of three types. Type 1 (commonest form) is a hairline fracture of the C2 ring without displacement. Type 2 is characterized by displacement of the anterior segment with an abnormal C2-3 disc appearance. Type 3 involves anterior displacement of the C2 body in flexion position with disruption of the facet joints.

Fractures of the dens can be difficult to detect, and if missed are associated with high morbidity and mortality. The Anderson and D'Alonzo dens classification describes three types. Type 1 is an oblique fracture through the tip of dens. Type 2 (Figs. 1 and 4) is a transverse fracture through its base that is unstable with the potential for motion and associated complications. Non-union and poorer outcomes have been reported to range as high as 35–40%, especially in the subgroup with atlantoaxial subluxation [19, 20]. Vertebral artery involvement may also occur [17, 21]. A type 3 dens fracture is an oblique fracture extending into the body of the dens and is considered to be a stable lesion with good potential for healing.

Of note, more C1-2 fractures are being documented in the elderly [22]. These are associated with higher morbidity (often associated with non-union) and mortality compared to other fractures. Accurate diagnosis may be compromised by the coexistence of extensive degenerative change and associated deformities. Comorbidities in this frail group also affect survival [17, 19, 20].

Subaxial Cervical Spine

A hyperextension tear drop fracture typically involves C2 resulting in a triangular fragment, though it may involve more than one level and occur in the lower cervical spine. This type of injury often occurs in the elderly with osteoporosis.

A hyperflexion tear drop fracture results from severe flexion and axial loading and produces a characteristic triangular fracture fragment at the anterior inferior margin of the affected vertebral body. It is commonly associated with cord injury producing an anterior cord syndrome or permanent quadriplegia. The anterior and posterior longitudinal ligaments and intervertebral disc are disrupted and there is associated subluxation or dislocation of the facet joints, with a focal kyphosis above the level of injury.

Anterior wedge compression fractures and occasional burst fractures may occur at the C6 or C7 levels. Burst fractures are associated with multiple often displaced fracture fragments that may impinge on the anterior cord. Vertebral widening or a split fracture line may be seen on a frontal radiograph. Vertical split fractures may occasionally occur due to compression in the sagittal plane and may involve more than two contiguous vertebral bodies.

Facet joint injury may result in fracture, subluxation, perching or locking. Bilateral facet dislocation is due to flexion trauma combined with distraction and rotation. Dislocation of the facet joints results in the superior vertebral body being displaced anteriorly by at least 50% over the vertebral body below. Anterior displacement of one vertebral body over another of 25% or 4–5 mm usually reflects a unilateral facet joint dislocation, resulting in the "bow-tie" sign or "messy roof tile" sign (Fig. 5). Dislocation is present when the inferior facet of the vertebra above is located anterior to the superior facet of the subjacent vertebra.

Hyperflexion sprain of the cervical spine is due to disruption of all the posterior ligaments of two adjacent vertebral bodies, with the anterior longitudinal ligament remaining intact. Hyperkyphosis and widening of the posterior elements may be evident although these injuries can quite subtle and initially missed. These are unstable lesions and require surgical fixation.

Hyperextension sprain/dislocation, usually occurs in the elderly though may affect a younger patient as the result of a high speed motor vehicle accident. The anterior longitudinal ligament is disrupted and avulses the disc from the adjacent superior vertebral body at the level of injury. A thin sliver of an avulsed fragment may be seen which differentiates this from an extension tear drop fracture which is more triangular and larger in height. There may also be posterior longitudinal ligament stripping and the cord may be compressed resulting in associated hematomyelia and central cord syndrome. Extensive soft tissue swelling may be evident.

Posterior element fractures are common, occurring in some 20% of all patients with cervical spine fractures any may include fractures of a spinous process, pillar, facet, lamina or transverse process. An avulsion fracture of a spinous process in the lower cervical spine is called a clay shoveler's fracture. Radiculopathy suggests pillar fracture. Laminar fractures usually occur in association with other fractures. Transverse process fractures may extend to the transverse foramen placing the adjacent nerve root and vertebral artery at risk (Fig. 6).

Cervical spine trauma can be associated with whiplash injury. This remains a contentious subject although sub end-plate fractures, ligamentous tears and facet fractures as well as soft tissue muscle injuries have been implicated.

SCIWORA, spinal cord injury without radiographic abnormality, may occur in young children without evidence of fracture or dislocation. Spinal cord injury occurs due to elasticity of the vertebral column in the young, with more spinal cord lesions being evident in children under 8 years. The prognosis is often very guarded.

Spinal cord injury may be evident early after trauma on MRI, with the presence of focal cord hematoma having poorer outcome than diffuse signal change or contusion. Delayed findings include intra or extramedullary cysts, syringomyelia, cord tethering or atrophy.

Common sources of diagnostic error relate to which imaging modality is used, the presence of normal variants such as ossicles and coexisting degenerative disease. The reported incidence of second level spinal fracture is dependent on the imaging modality used. These are reported to be 5–7% for radiographs, (with some reports as high as 20%) [16, 23, 24], 15–17% for CT, and 50% with MR. Normal variants can be a source of error [25]. Being aware of the common C1 and C2 variants (Fig. 7) is useful since these may mimic a fracture.

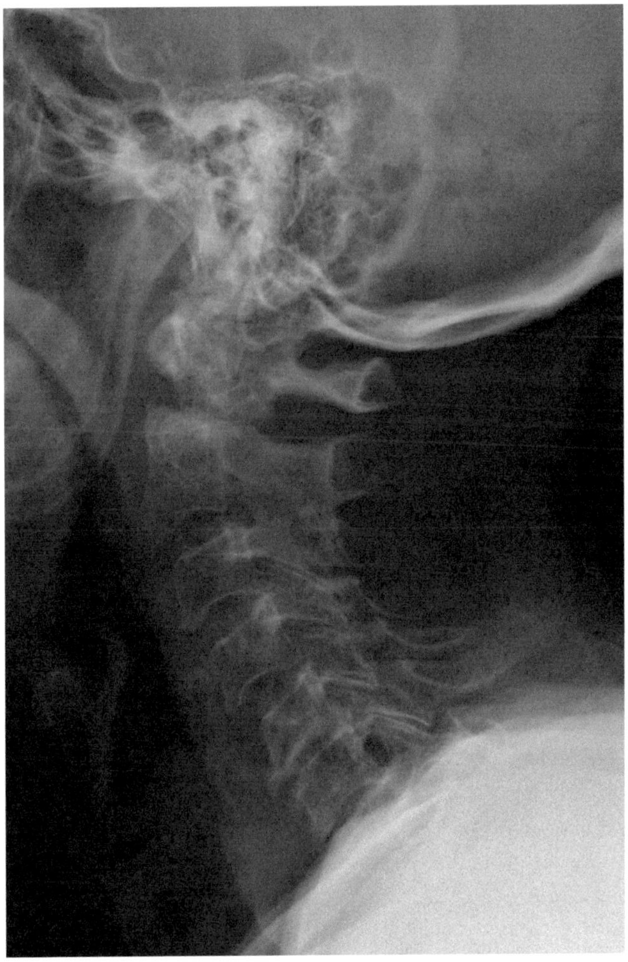

Fig. 4 Lateral radiograph of an 80 year old female patient after a minor fall and feeling "not quite right," shows type 2 dens fracture

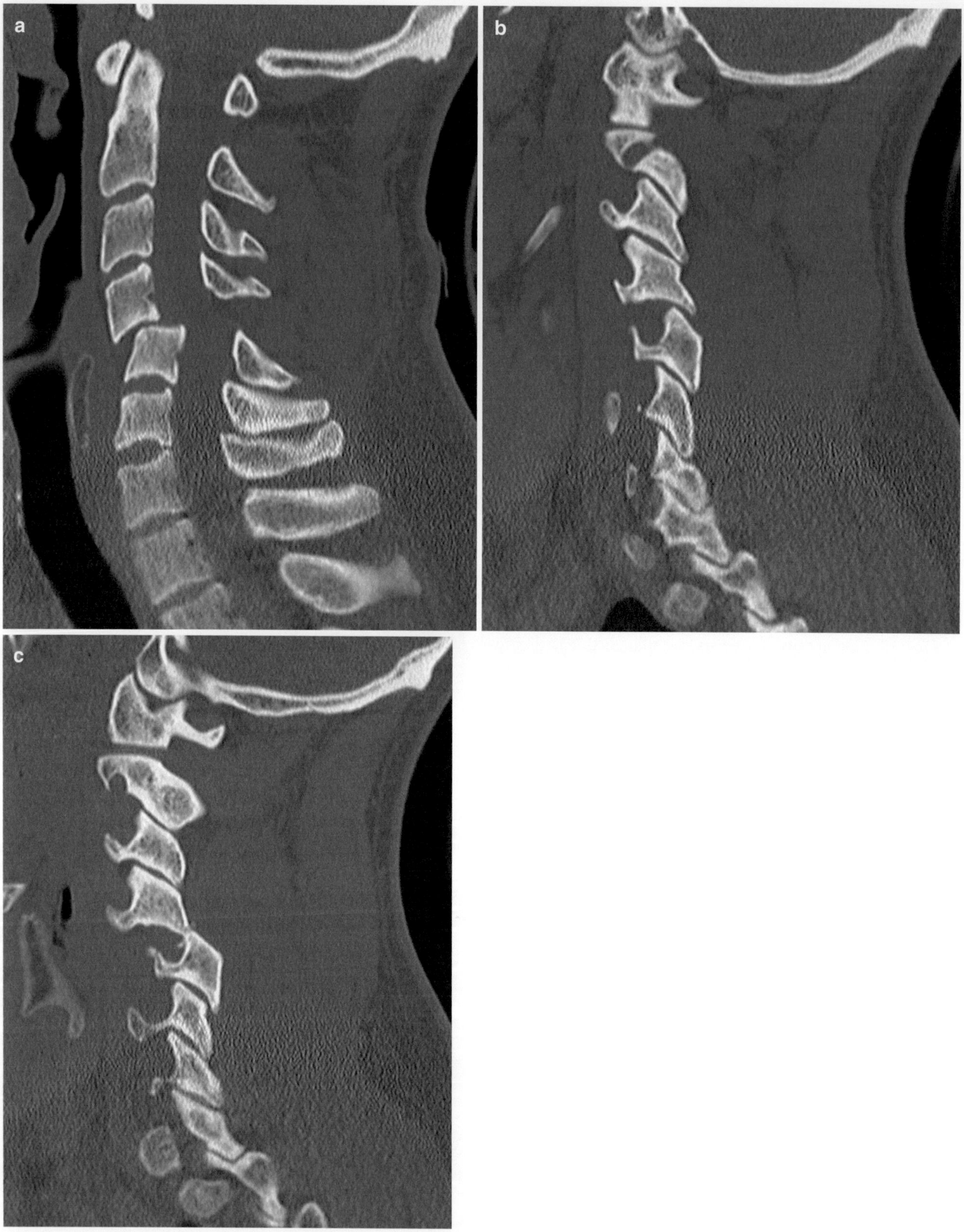

Fig. 5 30 year old male footballer sustained an acute injury during a tackle. CT bone reconstructed sagittal plane images shows (**a**) C4-5 fracture dislocation with (**b**) facet fracture dislocation on one side and (**c**) subluxated facet on the other side

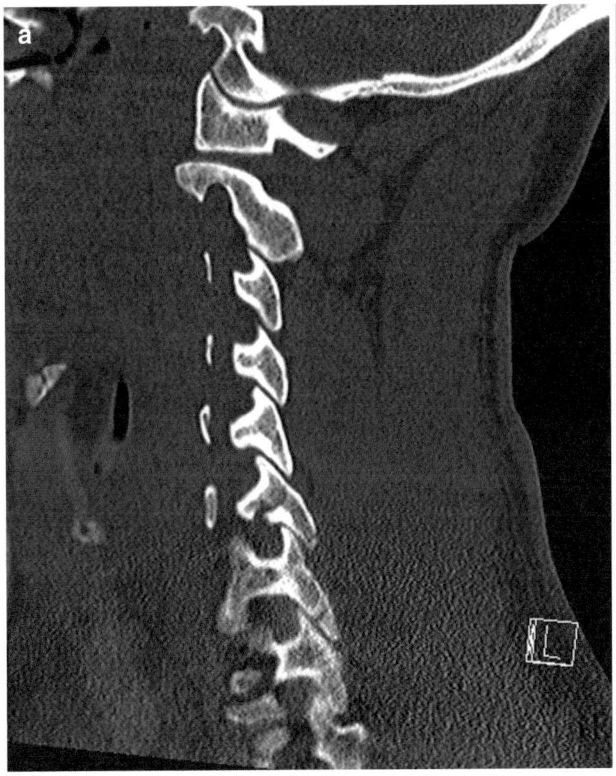

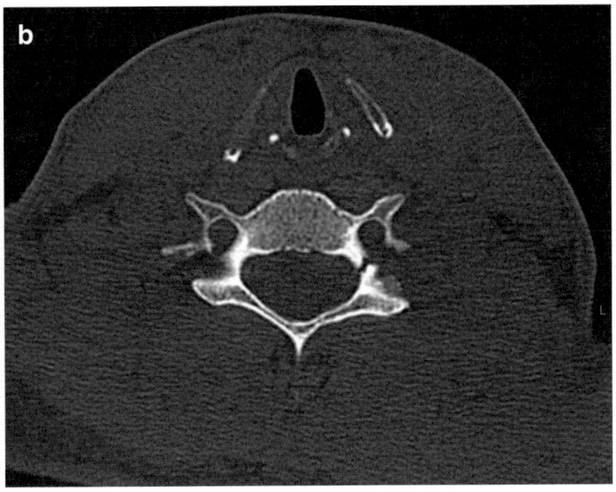

Fig. 6 25 year old male surfer who sustained a neck injury. (**a**) Sagittal CT reconstruction reveals left lateral mass fractures at C6 and C7. (**b**) Axial image demonstrates an additional left pedicle fracture extending into the left foramen transverse foramen raising concern for a vertebral artery injury, however a CT angiogram of the neck showed no arterial injury

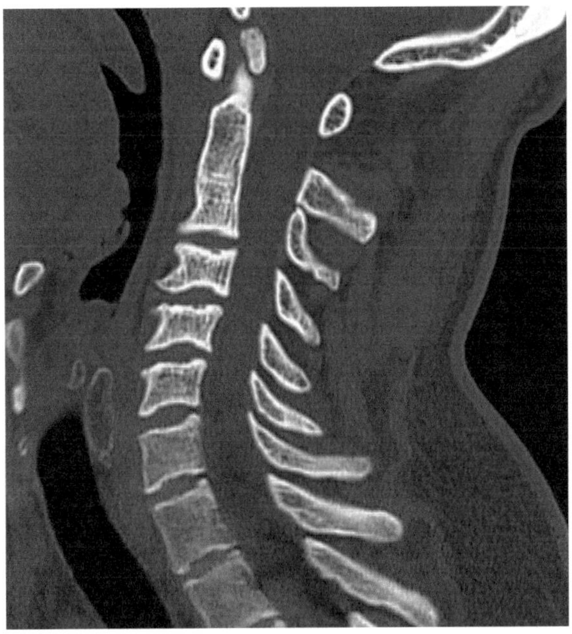

Fig. 7 25 year old patient after minor trauma and concern for fracture. CT sagittal bone window reconstruction shows os odontoideum, a normal C2 ossification variant and no fracture. Note also the congenital fusion of the C2 and C3 vertebral bodies

Thoracolumbar Spine

Most injuries in the thoracic and lumbar spine occur near the thoracolumbar junction. This is likely because it is the area of greatest motion in the thoracolumbar spine and the transition point besteen the first nine vertebrae, which are relatively stable because of the ribcage, and the more mobile lumbar and lower thoracic vertebrae (which have only "floating" ribs). Injuries above the thoracolumbar junction are less common, but are associated with a higher incidence of neurologic injury, probably because of the higher forces required to overcome the inherent stability of the ribcage in this region [26, 27].

Numerous thoracolumbar injury classification systems have been proposed, as discussed above, many of which are so complex as to become mind-numbing! As such, the most important role for the imager is to be aware of what information is most important to the surgeon as well as what basic injury patterns are shared among the systems and how to recognize these on radiographs and cross-sectional imaging studies.

Compression Fracture

A "simple" compression fracture is related to axial and/or flexion forces that affect only the anterior column of the affected vertebra. These most commonly involve anterior wedging of the superior endplate, but more severe injuries may involve both endplates, or even produce a coronal-oriented split in the mid vertebral body. These are considered to be stable lesions and are treated conservatively.

Radiographs demonstrate anterior vertebral wedging without involvement of the posterior wall, but it's important to note that these can be difficult to differentiate from a more severe burst fracture or flexion-distraction injury. In fact, up to 20% of burst fractures may be mis-categorized as simple compression fractures on radiographs, emphasizing the need to consider obtaining a follow-up cross-sectional imaging in many of these patients [28]. On CT, fracture lines will be evident in the anterior 2/3 of the vertebral body with sparing of the middle column (Fig. 8). MR imaging will demonstrate associated edema-like signal intensity within the marrow. Absence of this abnormal signal intensity within a deformed vertebra differentiates an old, healed fracture from an acute injury.

Burst Fracture

A burst fracture is also related to axial and/or flexion forces and involves the middle column, usually along with the anterior column. As such, these involve the posterior vertebral wall and may result in retropulsed bony fragments that may injure adjacent neural structures. Several forms of burst fractures have been described including incomplete burst, pincer type, or complete burst [13].

Radiographic findings include vertebral wedging and disruption of the posterior vertebral cortex with or without retropulsed fragments, although this can be difficult to delineate on radiographs alone. CT will better demonstrate all of these findings and provide an accurate depiction of canal compromise (Fig. 9). MR imaging can better evaluate any cord or nerve root injury as well as any soft tissue causes of canal compromise such as an extruded disc or epidural hematoma.

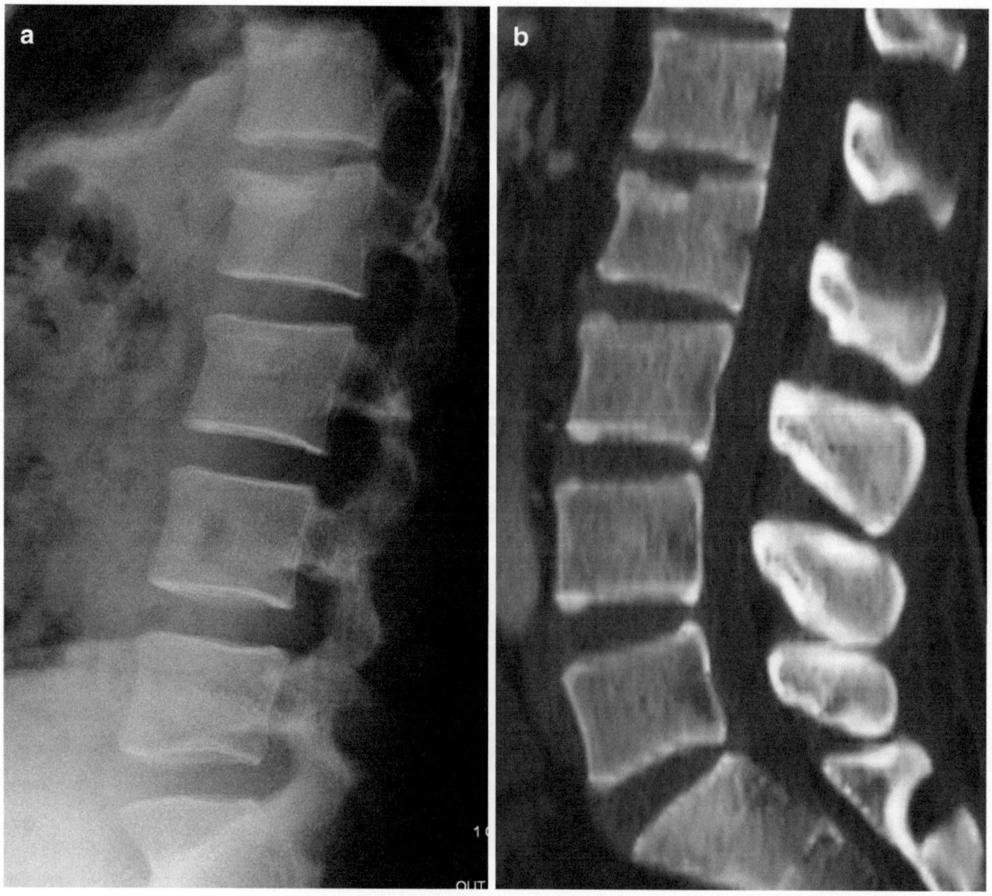

Fig. 8 25 year old male who fell 25 ft while rock climbing. (**a**) Lateral radiograph displays anterior wedging of the L2 vertebral body. (**b**) Sagittal reformatted CT image reveals that the compression fracture involves only the anterior column. The middle column including the posterior vertebral cortex is intact

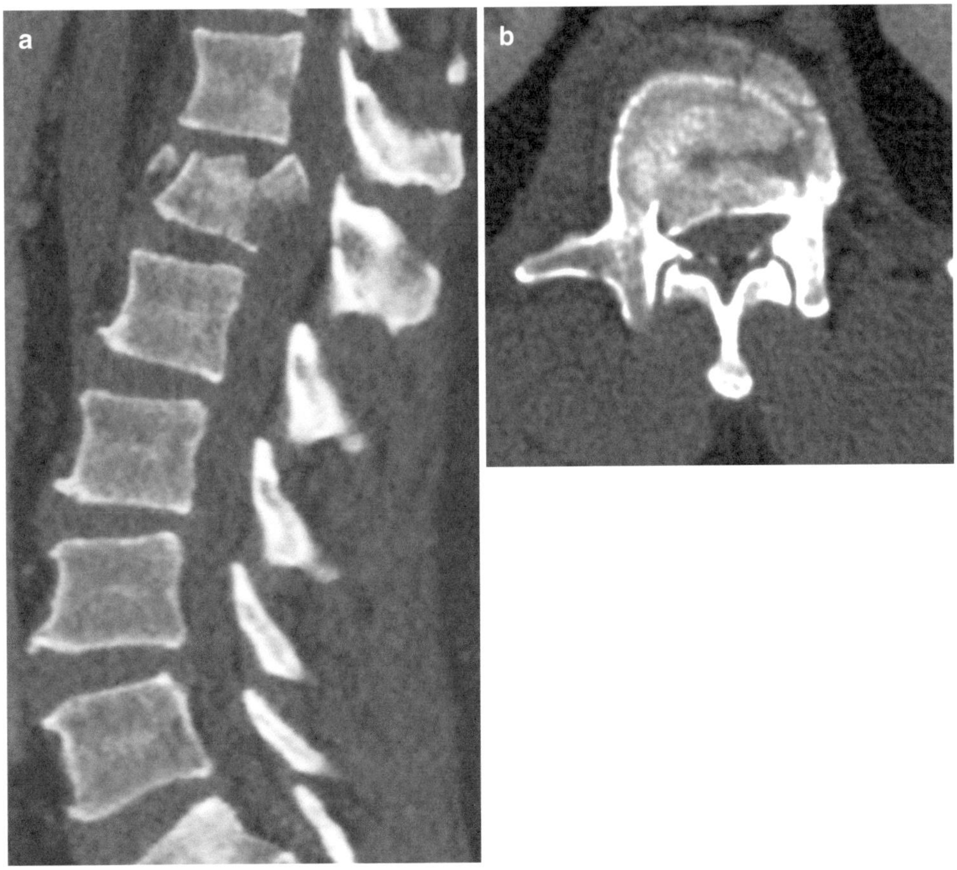

Fig. 9 48 year old male who fell 20 ft and presented with lower extremity weakness. (**a**) Sagittal reformatted CT image shows a comminuted burst fracture of L1 with retropulsion of fragments. (**b**) Axial CT image demonstrates the severe degree of resulting canal stenosis at that level

Distraction Injuries

A distraction injury results in disruption of the spinal column and dissociation of the vertebral elements along its vertical axis. The classic distraction injury is the "Chance" or "seatbelt" fracture which results from hyperflexion of the spine over a lap seatbelt or other object which moves the fulcrum of rotation from its typical location along the vertebral column to a position anterior to the body, which produces markedly increased posterior tensile forces and posterior column fractures or ligament disruption. These injuries typically involve all three columns and are considered unstable.

Similar distraction injuries may occur anteriorly when a hyperextension mechanism disrupts the anterior longitudinal ligament and anterior annulus fibrosus.

On radiographs, findings suggestive of a posterior distraction injury include interspinous widening or fractures through the posterior elements along a predominantly axial plane. Close scrutiny of the pedicles on a frontal radiograph is important since disruption of a pedicle "ring" may be the only clue that he posterior elements are involved. A hyperextension distraction injury is suggested by anterior disc space widening at a level. These are very common in the elderly in which case even a "normal" appearing disc may suggest this type of injury if the other discs in that region are severely narrowed.

There is some evidence that damage from posterior distraction injuries begins in the facet joints and then extends to involve the interspinous and supraspinous ligaments and ultimately the ligamentum flavum [29]. CT is excellent for defining the full extent of these injuries, and is especially useful for demonstrating subluxation/diastasis, dislocation

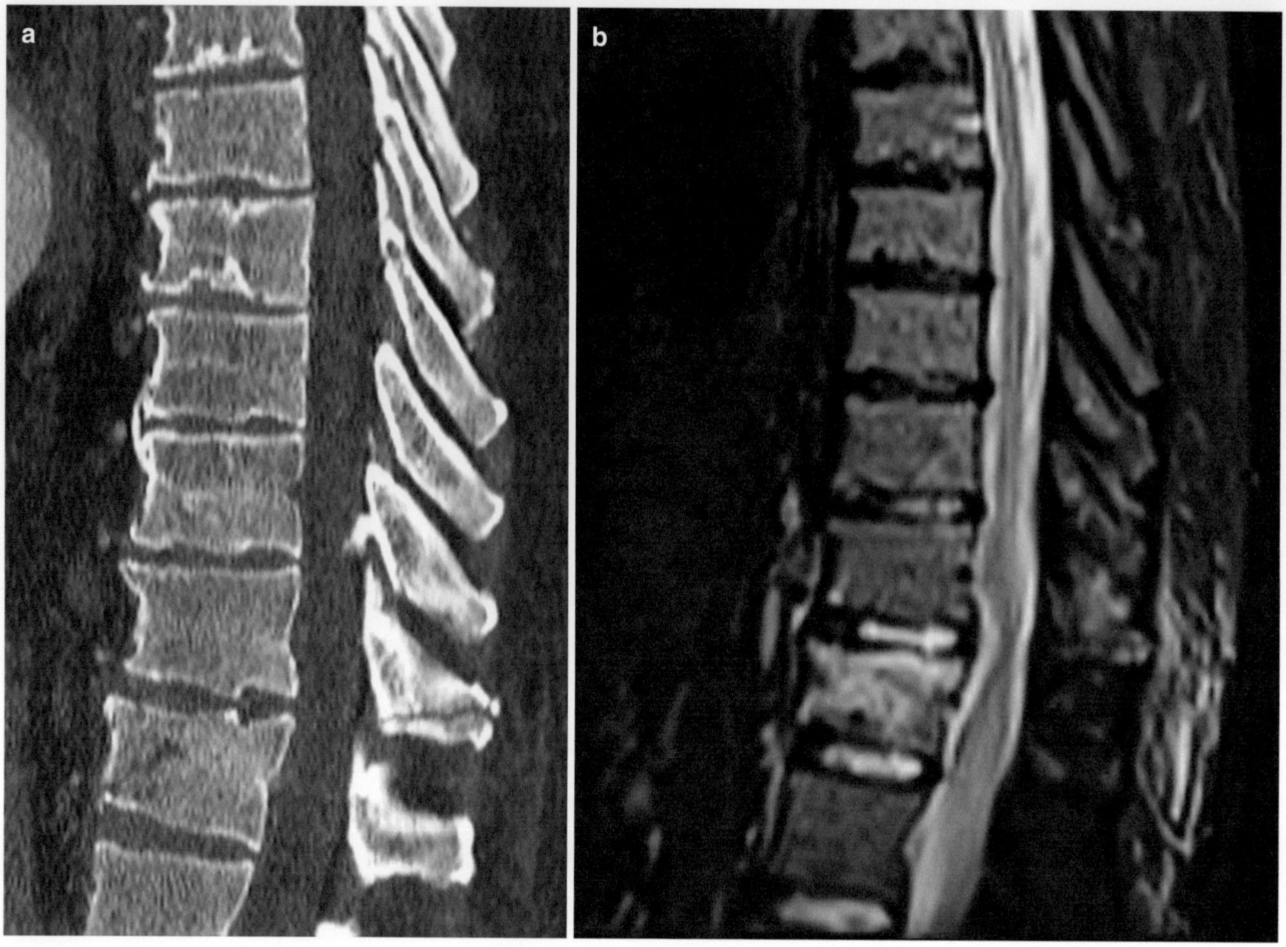

Fig. 10 56 year old male who fell 15 ft from a tree stand while deer hunting. (**a**) Sagittal reformatted CT image reveals compression of a lower thoracic vertebra with fracture lines extending through the anterior and middle columns as well as through the spinous process. (**b**) Sagittal STIR MR image shows edema within the marrow at the fracture sites and additional edema in the posterior soft tissues related to ligament injury

or fractures of the facet joints which are important stabilizing structures [30] (Fig. 10).

The status of the PLC (ligamentum flavum, facet joint capsules, interspinous and supraspinous ligaments), sometimes called the "posterior tension band" is one of the major criteria in the TLICS classification system. Although injuries to these structures can be inferred from radiographic and CT findings, MR imaging is able to directly display these ligaments and has been extensively investigated in this regard. While some authors have touted the accuracy of MR imaging for this purpose [31, 32] others have reported lower than expected specificity and positive predictive values and have suggested MR imaging not be used in isolation for this purpose [33–35].

Rotation/Translation Injuries

These injuries result from rotational and/or shear forces occurring with flexion or extension and typically produce a fracture/dislocation. The result is abnormal displacement or rotation of a portion of the spine at the level of injury. These three column injuries are highly unstable.

Translation injuries are recognized by subluxation of the spine in a medial/lateral or anterior/posterior direction while rotational injuries are suggested by offset of the spinous processes on a frontal view or an abrupt change in the posterior vertebral line at a certain level on a lateral image. These features are more easily detected on CT or MR images (Fig. 11).

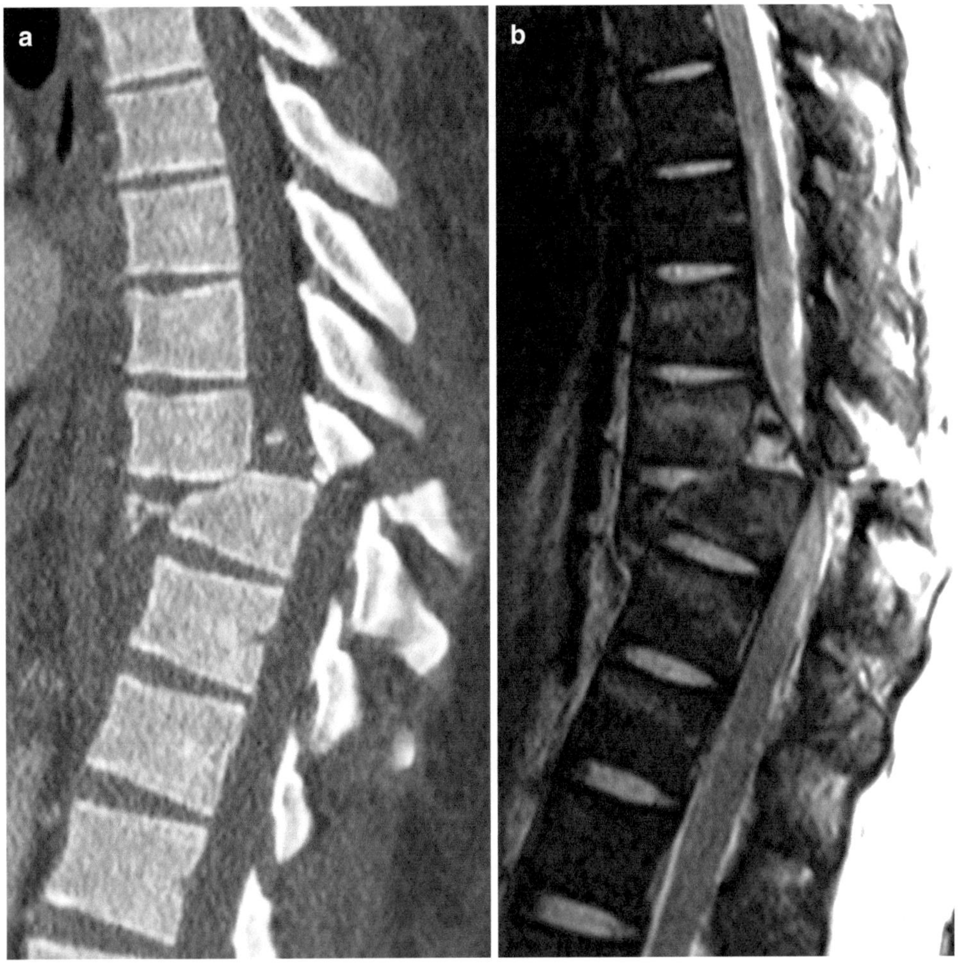

Fig. 11 26 year old male who presented with complete neurologic deficit below the T7 level after a motor vehicle accident. (**a**) Sagittal reformatted CT images displays a comminuted fracture dislocation in the mid thoracic spine with anterior subluxation of the upper thoracic vertebral column. (**b**) Corresponding sagittal STIR MR images demonstrates the fracture dislocation as well as stripping of the posterior longitudinal ligament, essentially transection of the cord and posterior ligament disruption

References

1. Nelson DW, Martin MJ, Martin ND, Beekley A (2013) Evaluation of the risk of noncontiguous fractures of the spine in blunt trauma. J Trauma Acute Care Surg 75:135–139
2. Saltzherr TP, Jin FK, Beenen LFM, Vandertop WP, Goslings JC (2009) Diagnostic imaging of cervical spine injuries following blunt trauma: a review of the literature and practical guideline. Injury 40:795–800
3. Hoffman JR, Mower MR, Wolfson AB, Todd KT, Zucker MI (2000) Validity of a set of clinical criteria to rule out injury to the cervical spine in patients with blunt trauma. N Engl J Med 343:94–99
4. Stiell IG, Wells GA, Vandemheen KL et al (2001) The Canadian c-spine rule for radiography in alert and stable trauma patients. JAMA 286:1841–1848
5. Duane TM, Young A, Mayglothling J et al (2013) CT for all or selective approach? Who really needs a cervical spine CT after blunt trauma. J Trauma Acute Care Surg 74:1098–1101
6. Hanson JA, Blackmore CC, Mann FA, Wilson AJ (2000) Cervical spine injury: a clinical decision rule to identify high-risk patients for helical CT screening. AJR 174:713–717
7. Holmes JF, Akkinepalli R (2005) Computed tomography versus plain radiography to screen for cervical spine injury: a meta-analysis. J Trauma 58:902–905
8. Holmes J, Mirvis SE, Panacek EA, Hoffman JR, Mower WR (2002) Variability in computed tomography and magnetic resonance imaging in patients with cervical spine injuries. J Trauma 53:524–530
9. Plumb JOM, Morris CG (2012) Clinical review: spinal imaging for adult obtunded blunt trauma patient: update from 2004. Intensive Care Med 38:752–771
10. Tomycz ND, Chew BG, Chang YF et al (2008) MRI is unnecessary to clear the cervical spine in obtunded/comatose trauma patients: the four-year experience of a level I trauma center. J Trauma 64:1258–1263
11. Como JJ, Diaz JJ, Dunham M et al (2009) Practice management guidelines for identification of cervical spine injuries following trauma: update from the eastern association for the surgery of trauma practice management guidelines committee. J Trauma 67:651–659

12. Denis F (1983) The three column spine and its significance in the classification of acute thoracolumbar spinal injuries. Spine 8:817–831
13. Magerl F, Aebi M, Gertzbein SD, Harms J, Nazarian S (1994) A comprehensive classification of thoracic and lumbar injuries. Eur Spine J 3:184–201
14. Vaccaro AR, Lehman RA, Hulbert RJ et al (2005) A new classification of thoracolumbar injuries. The importance of injury morphology, the integrity of the posterior ligamentous complex, and neurologic status. Spine 30:2325–2333
15. Vaccaro AR, Hulbert RJ, Patel AA et al (2007) The subaxial cervical spine injury classification system. A novel approach to recognize the importance of morphology, neurology, and integrity of the disco-ligamentous complex. Spine 32:2365–2374
16. Keller S, Bieck K, Karul M et al (2015) Lateralized odontoid in plain film radiography: sign of fractures? A comparison study with MDCT. Rofo 187:801–807
17. Mead LB, Millhouse PW, Krystal J, Vaccaro AR (2016) C1 fractures: a review of diagnoses, management options, and outcomes. Curr Rev Muscoskelet Med 9:255–262
18. Aras EL, Bunger C, Hansen ES, Sogaard R (2016) Health-care costs of conservative management of spine fractures in trauma patients. Eur Spine J [Epub ahead of print]
19. Evaniew N, Yarascavitch B, Madden K et al (2015) Atlantoaxial instability in acute odontoid fractures is associated with nonunion and mortality. Spine 15:910–917
20. Joestl J, Lang NW, Tiefenboeck TM, Hajdu S, Platzer P (2016) Management and outcome of dens fracture nonunions in geriatric patients. J Bone Joint Surg Am 98:193–198
21. Payabvash S, McKinney AM, McKinney ZJ, Palmer CS, Truwit CL (2014) Screening and detection of blunt vertebral artery injury in patients with upper cervical fractures: the role of cervical CT and CT angiography. Eur J Radiol 83:571–577
22. Delcourt T, Begue T, Saintyves G, Mebtouche N, Cottin P (2015) Management of upper cervical spine fractures in elderly patients: current trends and outcomes. Injury 46(Suppl 1):S24–S27
23. Cassar-Pullicino VN, Imhof H (eds) (2006) Spinal trauma—an imaging approach. Thieme, New York
24. Roger LF (ed) (2001) Radiology of skeletal trauma. Churchill Livingstone, Philadelphia
25. Rao RD, Tang S, Lim C, Yoganandan N (2013) Developmental morphology and ossification patterns of the C1 vertebra. J Bone Joint Surg Am 95:e1241–e1247
26. Brandser EA, El-Khoury CY (1997) Thoracic and lumbar spine trauma. Radiol Clin N Am 35:533–537
27. Frontijne WP, de Klerk LW, Braakman R et al (1992) CT scan prediction of neurological deficit in thoracolumbar burst fractures. J Bone Joint Surg Br 74:683–685
28. Ballock RT, Mackersie R, Abitbol JJ, Cervilla V, Resnick D, Garfin SR (1992) Can burst fractures be predicted from plain radiographs? J Bone Joint Surg Br 74:147–150
29. Pizones J, Izquierdo E, Sanchez-Mariscal F, Zuniga L, Alavarez P, Gomez-Rice A (2012) Sequential damage assessment of the different components of the posterior ligamentous complex after magnetic resonance imaging interpretation. Spine 37: E662–E667
30. Pitzen R, Lane C, Goertzen D et al (2003) Anterior cervical plate fixation: biomechanical effectiveness as a function of posterior element injury. J Neurosurg 99:984–990
31. Lee HW, Kim HS, Kim DJ, Suk KS, Park JO, Kim HK (2000) Reliability of magnetic resonance imaging in detecting posterior ligament complex injury in thoracolumbar spinal fractures. Spine 25:2079–2084
32. Haba H, Taneichi H, Kotani Y et al (2003) Diagnostic accuracy of magnetic resonance imaging for detecting posterior ligamentous complex injury associated with thoracic and lumbar fractures. J Neurosurg Spine 99:20–26
33. Dai LY, Ding WG, Wang XY, Jiang LS, Jiang SD, Xu HZ (2009) Assessment of ligamentous injury in patients with thoracolumbar burst fractures using MRI. J Trauma 66:1610–1615
34. Vaccaro AR, Rihn JA, Anderson DG et al (2009) Injury of the posterior ligamentous complex of the thoracolumbar spine. A prospective evaluation of the diagnostic accuracy of magnetic resonance imaging. Spine 34:E841–E847
35. Rihn JA, Yang N, Fisher C et al (2010) Using magnetic resonance imaging to accurately assess injury to the posterior ligamentous complex of the spine: a prospective comparison of the surgeon and radiologist. J Neurosurg Spine 12:391–396

Ultrasonography: Sports Injuries

Jon A. Jacobson and Ian Beggs

Upper Extremity

Introduction

Ultrasound is an effective imaging method for evaluation of upper extremity sports injuries. For evaluation of the shoulder, ultrasound is ideal in evaluation of the rotator cuff, the biceps brachii tendon, and the subacromial-subdeltoid bursa. Evaluation of the cartilaginous structures of the shoulder is significantly limited and therefore MRI and preferably MR arthrography are considered in this scenario. An algorithm based on patient age is often used, where patients over the age of 40 years often are evaluated with ultrasound, and patients under 40 years are evaluated with MRI or MR arthrography. This algorithm is used as patients under the age of 40 years will often have articular-sided partial-thickness rotator cuff tears and concomitant labral pathology, both of which are ideally evaluated with MRI [1]. Beyond the shoulder, ultrasound is most accurate when the indication for imaging is targeted and the structure imaged is superficial. Last, ultrasound complements MRI given its ability to dynamically assess pathology of the upper extremity. Given the superficial location of soft tissue abnormalities, a linear transducer of greater than 12 MHz is preferred, and a small footprint probe is used for the most distal aspects of the upper extremity.

J.A. Jacobson (✉)
Department of Radiology, University of Michigan,
Ann Arbor, MI 48109-0326, USA
e-mail: jjacobsn@umich.edu

I. Beggs
Royal Infirmary of Edinburgh,
Edinburgh, Scotland EH12 4 SU, UK
e-mail: ianbeggs@doctors.org.uk

Shoulder

The rotator cuff is the most commonly imaged tendon using ultrasound, where its accuracy in the diagnosis of cuff pathology is equal to MRI. Unlike the distal aspects of the upper extremity, a protocol-based evaluation with ultrasound is recommended as symptoms do not always directly correlate with pathology, and symptoms may also be multifactorial in etiology [2]. Each individual rotator cuff tendon (supraspinatus, infraspinatus, subscapularis, teres minor) is imaged in short and long axis. Given the curvature of the humeral head and the overlying supraspinatus, care must be taken to not misinterpret artifactual hypoechogenicity from anisotropy as tendon abnormality. Pathology of the rotator cuff, similar to other tendons, include tendinosis and tendon tear. The term tendinosis is used rather than tendinitis as inflammation diminishes after the first week after a tendon injury [3]. Tendinosis refers to mucoid degeneration and chondroid metaplasia of the involved tendon [4, 5]. At ultrasound, tendinosis will appear as abnormal hypoechogenicity with possible increased in tendon thickness [6]. Tendon tear will appear as a well-defined hypoechoic or anechoic defect in the normal hyperechoic fibrillar tendon architecture. Such tendon tears may be partial-thickness and only involve the articular surface (Fig. 1), bursal surface, or may be intrasubstance (or interstitial) not contacting either the articular or bursal surface of the tendon, although isolated greater tuberosity extension is common. A full-thickness tear will extend from the articular to bursal surface of the tendon. Of note, most supraspinatus tendon tears extend to the greater tuberosity footprint, which creates the cortical irregularity as a very important indirect sign in such tears in patients over the age of 40 years [6, 7]. Once a tear is identified, the short and long axis dimensions, as well as percent tear depth (in the case of partial-thickness tears) are measured and included in the imaging report. Chronic and large full-thickness tears, especially those involving the anterior aspect of the supraspinatus, are associated with tendon retraction and subsequent infraspinatus and supraspinatus fatty infiltration and possible

J. Hodler et al. (eds.), *Musculoskeletal Diseases 2017-2020*, DOI 10.1007/978-3-319-54018-4_22

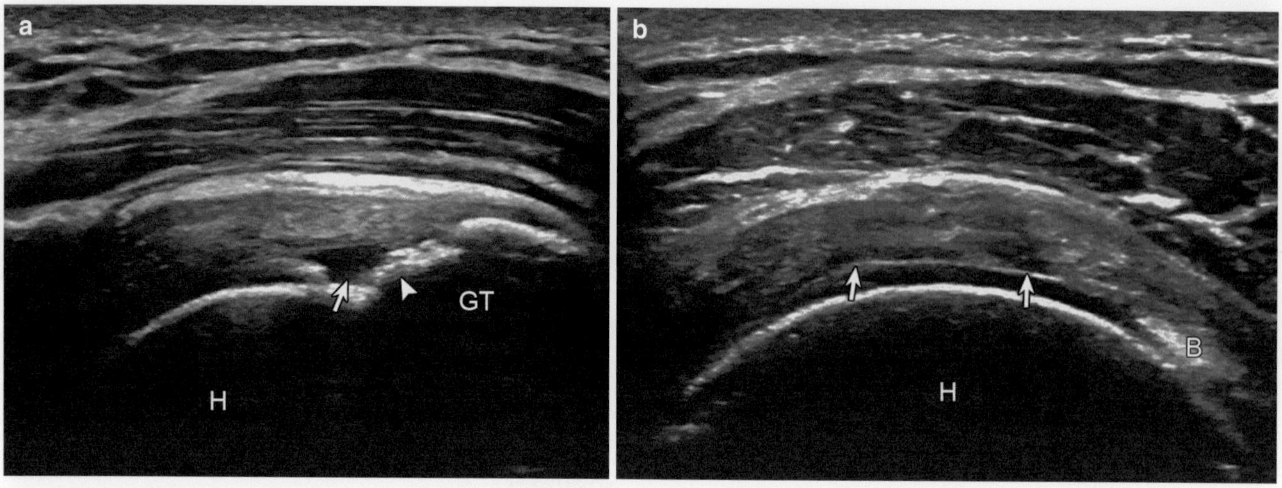

Fig. 1 Supraspinatus tear: articular side partial-thickness. Ultrasound images long axis (**a**) and short axis (**b**) to supraspinatus tendon shows hypoechoic tendon tear (*arrows*) extending to the articular surface of the humeral head (H). Note cortical irregularity (*arrowhead*) of greater tuberosity (GT). B, biceps brachii long head tendon in rotator interval

muscle atrophy [8]. This information should be included in the imaging report as muscle atrophy is associated with poor outcomes after surgical repair of a rotator cuff tear [9].

Another structure commonly imaged with ultrasound is the biceps brachii long head tendon. While the most proximal aspect of the biceps brachii long head tendon at the labrum is not visible with ultrasound, the segment in the bicipital groove and more proximally into the glenohumeral joint are well seen, with the latter best seen with the shoulder in the modified Crass position. Fluid distention of the biceps brachii long head tendon sheath is most commonly from extension of a glenohumeral joint effusion. Heterogeneous or focal distention with hyperemia and focal symptoms would suggest true tenosynovitis. Tendinosis will appear as abnormal hypoechogenicity and possible increased tendon thickness, partial-thickness tears will appear as surface irregularity and hypoechoic or anechoic clefts, and full-thickness tear will show complete tendon discontinuity [10]. The thin hyperechoic aponeurotic expansion of the supraspinatus should not be confused with a longitudinal split of the biceps brachii [11]. Unlike a longitudinal split, the aponeurotic expansion characteristically is located anterior the tendon and blends into the supraspinatus tendon when imaging proximally. Ultrasound may also be used to dynamically assess for biceps brachii tendon subluxation and dislocation, and guide percutaneous tendon sheath injection [12].

Another common structure that is abnormal with overuse injuries is the subacromial-subdeltoid bursa. This composite bursa is quite extensive located deep to the deltoid and covering portions of the supraspinatus, infraspinatus, subscapularis, biceps brachii long head, and proximal humerus. Distention of the bursa may range from anechoic fluid to hypoechoic or hyperechoic synovial hypertrophy [13]. To diagnose subacromial impingement with ultrasound, the arm is abducted and ultrasound will reveal gradual distention of the subacromial-subdeltoid bursa at the edge of the acromion; however, this finding may be found in asymptomatic individuals and clinical correlation is required [14]. Ultrasound may also be used to guide percutaneous bursal injection.

Elbow

The distal biceps brachii tendon may show findings of tendinosis (hypoechoic enlargement), partial-thickness tear (anechoic clefts), and full-thickness tear (complete tendon discontinuity) (Fig. 2) associated with sports injuries [15]. Ultrasound imaging of the distal biceps brachii tendon is often difficult given the oblique course of the distal tendon and resulting anisotropy. Imaging the biceps tendon from a medial or pronator window approach, with possible elbow flexion, is often helpful [16]. Partial-thickness biceps tears may involve one of the two heads, commonly the more superficial short head, which can create refraction shadowing artifact possibly obscuring the deeper long head tendon. In differentiating partial-thickness from full-thickness tendon tear, the use of dynamic evaluation is helpful, either imaging from a medial or lateral approach [17]. With supination and pronation, lack of tendon movement to the same degree as radial tuberosity rotation is indirect evidence of full-thickness tear. Often full-thickness distal biceps brachii tendon tears will be associated with significant tendon retraction.

Distal triceps brachii tendon tear are also effectively evaluated with ultrasound. Partial-thickness tears often involve the superficial combined long and lateral heads, associated with an avulsed enthesophyte bone fragment (Fig. 3) [18]. The deeper medial head is often intact but may be erroneously interpreted as torn given that the medial head tendon is very short. Tendinosis may uncommonly involve the distal

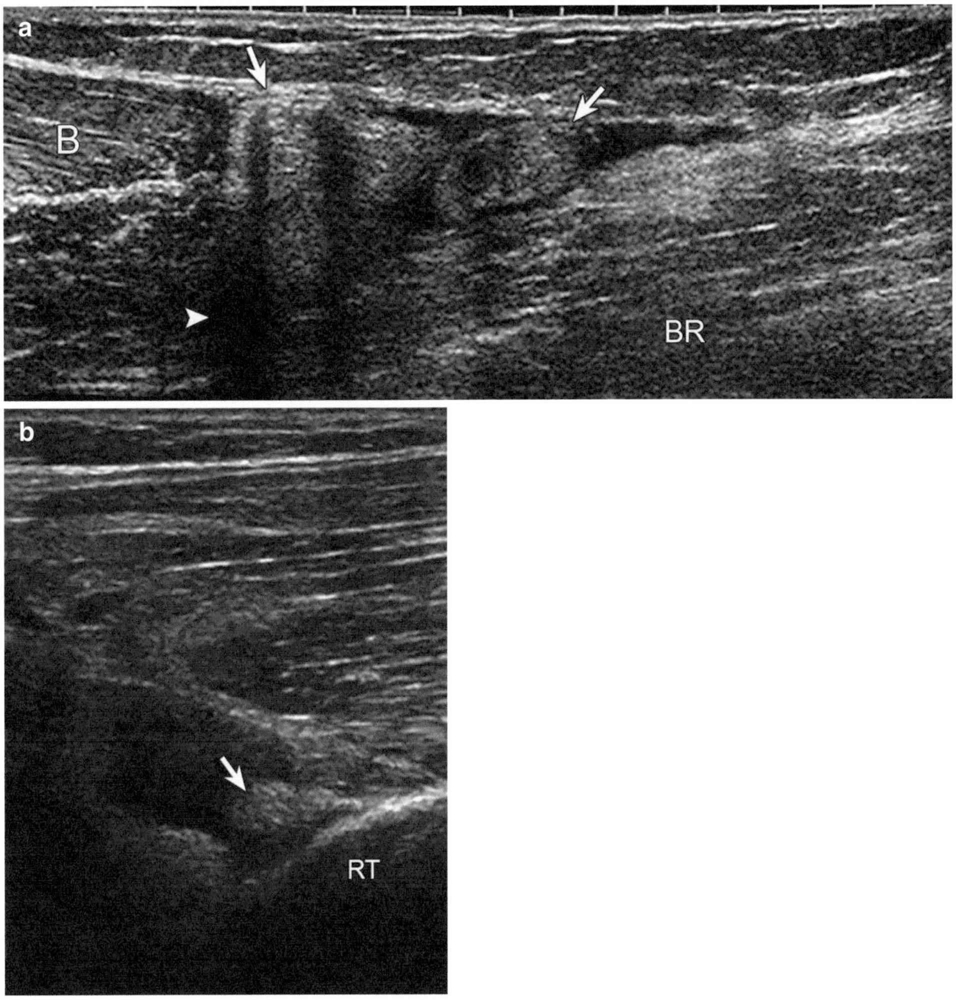

Fig. 2 Biceps Brachii: full-thickness tear. Ultrasound images shows (**a**) proximal and (**b**) distal stumps of the torn and retracted biceps brachii (*arrows*). Note refractions shadowing (*arrowhead*) deep to recoiled proximal stump in (**a**). B, biceps brachii muscle; BR, brachialis muscle; RT, radial tuberosity

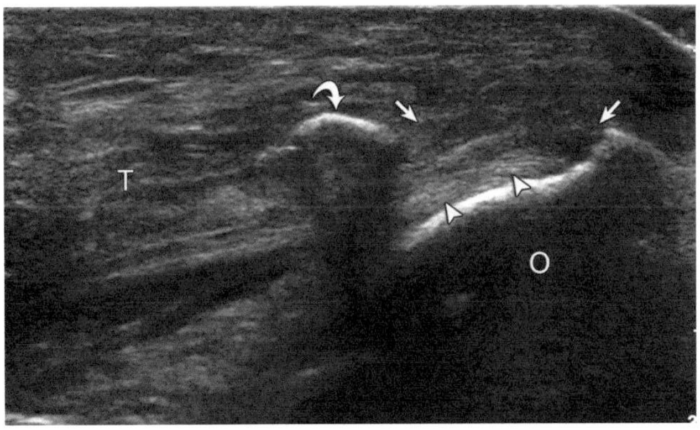

Fig. 3 Triceps Brachii: partial-thickness tear. Ultrasound image long axis to triceps brachii (T) shows retracted tear of superficial combined lateral and long head tendons (between *arrows*) with hyperechoic and shadowing enthesophyte avulsion fragment (*curved arrow*). Note intact deep medial head of triceps brachii (*arrowheads*). O, olecranon process

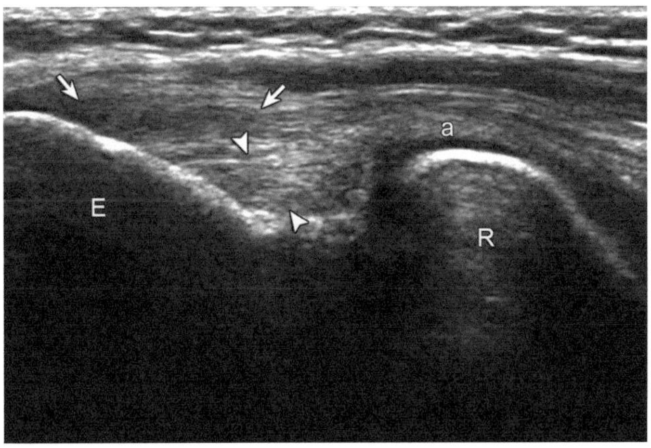

Fig. 4 Common extensor tendon abnormality (lateral epicondylitis). Ultrasound image long axis to common extensor tendon shows hypoechoic tendinosis (*arrows*). Note radial collateral ligament proper (*arrowheads*). E, lateral epicondyle; R, radial head; a, annular ligament

triceps brachii tendon, as well as distention of the overlying olecranon bursa.

Epicondylitis may also be diagnosed with ultrasound. With lateral (tennis elbow) more common than medial (golfer's elbow), the term "epicondylitis" is a misnomer in that it is not a primary epicondyle problem and is not inflamed [19]. The underlying pathology, similar to other tendons, represents tendinosis, interstitial tear, or uncommonly full-thickness tear (Fig. 4). The presence of hyperemia on color Doppler imaging correlates with symptoms and represents neovascularity rather than an indirect sign of inflammation.

The ulnar collateral ligament is evaluated dynamically with ultrasound, and complements MR arthrography where the accuracy in diagnosis of tear is highest when both imaging methods are used [20]. With the elbow flexed at least 30 degrees, valgus stress is placed across the elbow. Asymmetric widening of the medial joint space between the humerus and ulna with valgus stress can indicate ligament tear [20].

Wrist and Hand

Sports injuries of the hand and wrist are often ligamentous or related to the triangular fibrocartilage complex, which are best evaluated with MR or preferably MR arthrography; however, ultrasound can be used to evaluate focal tendon abnormalities. For example, intersection syndrome will appear as asymmetric hypoechoic swelling, edema, and possible hyperemia where the first extensor wrist compartment muscles (extensor pollicis longus and abductor pollicis brevis) cross over the second extensor wrist compartment (extensor carpi radialis longus and brevis) [21]. Full-thickness tendon tears are often associated with tendon retraction. Related to the extensor tendons, sagittal band injury at the level of the metacarpophalangeal joints is diagnosed when abnormal hypoechogenicity is seen with asymmetric location of the extensor tendon, best seen dynamically with flexion at the metacarpophalangeal joints, termed Boxer's knuckle [22]. Related to the flexor tendons of the fingers, ultrasound is effective in evaluation of the pulleys of the digits. Non-visualization of a pulley can indicate injury; however, the finding of tendon bowstringing is an important indirect sign of pulley injury, which appears as an abnormal position of the flexor tendon not approximated to the phalanx (Fig. 5). Bowstringing is evaluated dynamically with active finger flexion against resistance where a distance between the flexor tendon and phalanx greater than 1 mm indicates pulley injury; a distance greater than 3 mm indicates a complete A2 pulley tear and a distance of 5 mm indicates a combined complete tears of A2 and A4 pulleys [23].

One ligament that is ideally evaluated with ultrasound is the ulnar collateral ligament of the thumb [24]. Injury to this ligament, termed skier's or gamekeeper's thumb, can range from sprain (hypoechoic swelling), partial tear (partial anechoic defect), and complete tear (discontinuous ligament), with the latter either being non-displaced or displaced [25]. A displaced ulnar collateral ligament tear with an interposed adductor aponeurosis is termed a Stener lesion. Ultrasound is able to diagnose a Stener lesion with 100% accuracy [24]. Key to evaluation is correct placement of the transducer in the coronal plane relative to the thumb with visualization of the characteristic bone contours at the expected attachments of the ulnar collateral ligament. The adductor aponeurosis is identified as a thin hypoechoic structure that normally overlies the intact ulnar collateral ligament, where flexion and extension at the interphalangeal joint causes isolated movement of the aponeurosis, which aides in its identification. The distal aspect of the displaced ulnar collateral ligament is identified as a hypoechoic round abnormality proximal to the metacarpal joint (Fig. 6), with a possible hyperechoic and shadowing avulsion bone fragment. The end of the torn ligament may be seen superficial to the adductor aponeurosis, or may be seen along the distal metacarpal shaft with the ligament coursing proximal.

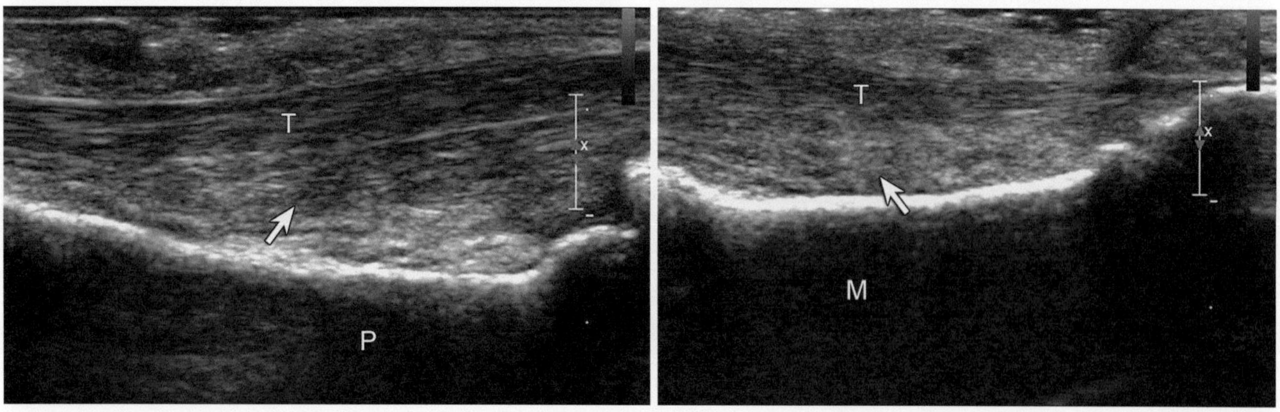

Fig. 5 Pulley injury. Ultrasound image long axis to the flexor tendons (T) of the finger shows abnormal volar displacement or bowstringing of the tendons (*arrows*) opposite the proximal (P) and middle (M) phalanges indicating A2 and A4 pulley tears, respectively

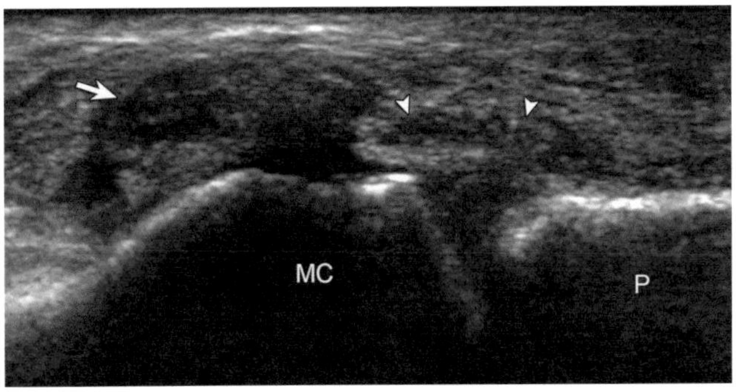

Fig. 6 Ulnar collateral ligament tear of the thumb (Skier's thumb). Ultrasound image long axis to the ulnar collateral ligament of the thumb shows torn and proximally displaced ligament (*arrow*) with interposed, hypoechoic and thickened adductor aponeurosis (*arrowheads*). MC, metacarpal; P, proximal phalanx

Lower Extremity

Introduction

Ultrasound can be an effective imaging tool to evaluate sports injuries of the lower extremity; however, ultrasound is most effective when performed by an experienced sonographer for a focused or precise indication [26]. For example, the scenario of "evaluate for Achilles tendon tear" is preferred over an indication, such as "hip pain." As a general rule, ultrasound performs best when assessing superficial structures, where resolution is optimized with higher frequency transducers (greater than 10 or 12 MHz). Resolution and accuracy decreases with deeper structures, such as about the hip, where MR imaging is often indicated, especially in the face of a negative ultrasound examination. Ultrasound does have the advantages of portability, accessibility, and the ability to correlate directly with patient symptoms and comparison to the contralateral asymptomatic side. The purpose of this syllabus is to briefly review the ultrasound findings of some of the more common lower extremity sports injuries.

Hip

Ultrasound can be effective to evaluate the tendons about the hip, although there is limited evaluation of deeper structures that may require further imaging with MRI. One such indication is evaluation of the adductor tendons at the pubic symphysis for injury. Findings include hypoechoic tendinosis, cortical irregularity and calcification, anechoic interstitial tears, and complete retracted full-thickness tendon tear. Related to the proximal adductor tendons is the subject of groin pain in the athlete. While the exact cause of "sports hernia" is often multifactorial, a proposed theory

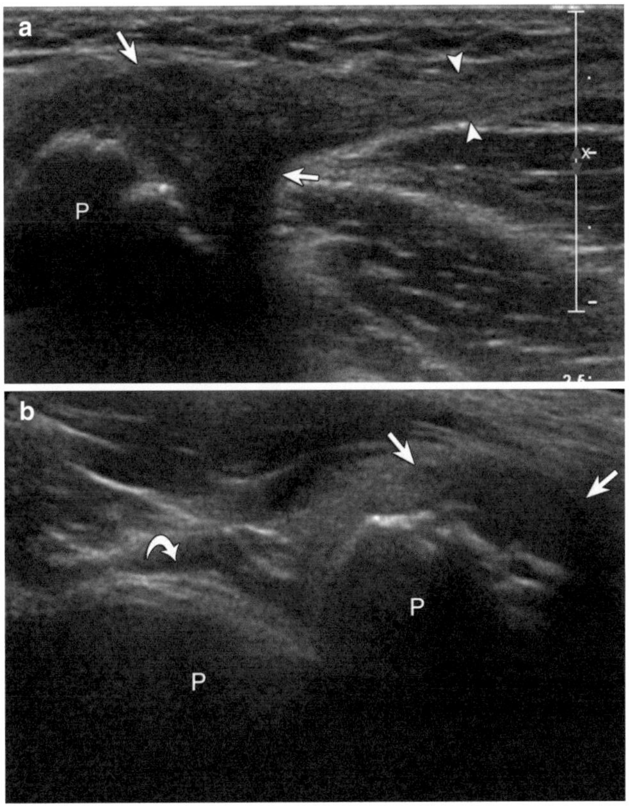

Fig. 7 Common aponeurosis injury at pubis ("sports hernia"). Ultrasound images (**a**) long axis and (**b**) short axis to proximal adductor longus tendon show (*arrows*) abnormal hypoechoic tendinosis and bone irregularity of common aponeurosis between rectus abdominis and adductor longus over pubis (P). Note normal contralateral common aponeurosis (*curved arrow*)

includes hypoechoic injury to the common aponeurosis over the pubis between the rectus abdominis and adductor longus tendon [27] (Fig. 7). Abnormalities of the pubic symphysis, such as joint fluid and cortical irregularity, may also be seen.

Other tendon abnormalities of the hip region with sports injuries include the rectus femoris anteriorly and the hamstring origin posteriorly. An additional tendon effectively evaluated with ultrasound is the iliopsoas, which specifically includes dynamic evaluation for iliopsoas tendon snapping. The cause of iliopsoas snapping is temporary entrapment of the medial aspect of the iliacus between the psoas major tendon and the superior pubic ramus, lateral to the iliopectineal eminence [28]. Moving the patient from a flexed externally rotated, and abducted hip position to full extension is one maneuver that often produces the abnormal finding of abrupt snapping of the iliopsoas complex. In addition, the patient can be simply asked to reproduce the symptoms while imaging under ultrasound. Another form of snapping hip syndrome involves abrupt movement of the iliotibial band (or tract) and/or gluteus maximus over the greater trochanter.

Ultrasound evaluation of this condition involves placing the probe short axis to the femur directly over the greater trochanter with the patient laying on the side while flexing and extending the hip.

Ultrasound can also effectively evaluate the hip joint for effusion and other intra-articular processes. While evaluation of the labrum is limited due to depth of this structure and inability to comprehensively assess, ultrasound can show a labral tear as a well-defined hypoechoic or anechoic cleft within or at the base of the normal hyperechoic fibrocartilage labrum. The finding of an anterior labrum tear and abnormal bone contour at the femoral head-neck can indirectly suggest the diagnosis of femoroacetabular impingement. A paralabral cyst may also be identified with ultrasound, which commonly appears as multilocular and hypoechoic in direct connection to the acetabular labral tear [29].

Knee

Ultrasound evaluation of the knee is primarily limited to the superficial tendons and ligaments, as well as joint effusion and various bursa about the knee [30]. While the peripheral aspects of the menisci can show anechoic or hypoechoic tears similar to the hip labrum, a comprehensive evaluation is not possible. In addition, sports injuries of the knee often involve an array of structures, many of which are not adequately assessed with ultrasound (such as the ACL and PCL) and therefore MR imaging is typically indicated; nonetheless, ultrasound can be effective in evaluation of many structures such as the extensor mechanism of the knee.

One common pathology that involves the extensor mechanism of the knee is termed Jumper's knee, where the proximal patellar tendon can show hypoechoic tendinosis, anechoic interstitial or partial-thickness tears, and potential neovascularity on color and power Doppler imaging (Fig. 8). Various bursa, such as the prepatellar, superficial infrapatellar, deep infrapatellar, and pes anserinus bursa can be evaluated with ultrasound, which may show distention with anechoic fluid and heterogeneous complex fluid or synovial proliferation. In the older athlete, distention of the semimembranosus-medial gastrocnemius bursa, or Baker cyst, may be identified by ultrasound with its characteristic neck extending to the knee joint between the tendons of the semimembranosus and medial head of the gastrocnemius. Ultrasound can also evaluate for Baker cyst rupture and other causes of calf symptoms, such as deep venous thrombosis.

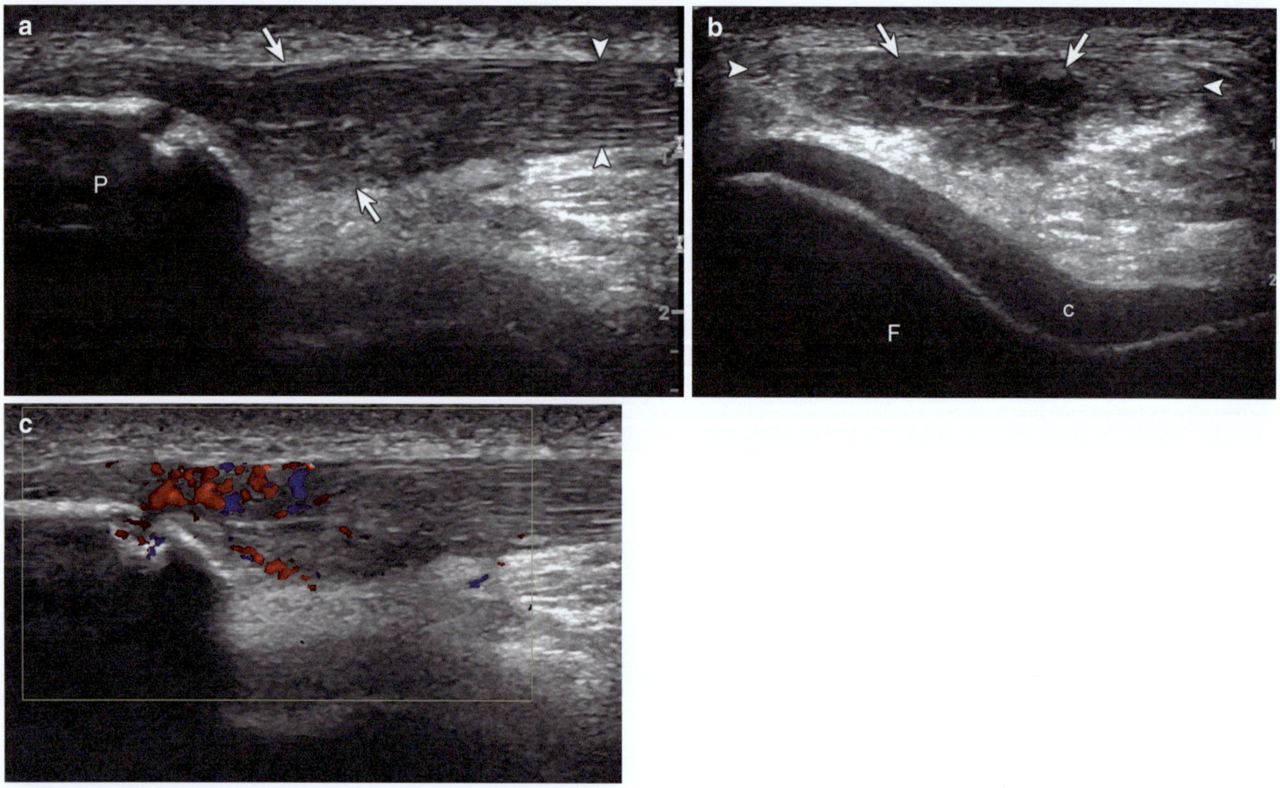

Fig. 8 Patellar tendon tendinosis (Jumper's knee). Ultrasound images (**a**) long axis and (**b**) short axis to the patellar tendon (*arrowheads*) shows hypoechoic tendinosis (*arrows*) and bone irregularity of the patella (P). Note hyperemia from neovascularity on (**c**) color Doppler image (F, femur; c, articular cartilage)

Ankle and Foot

Ultrasound is an ideal imaging method to evaluate various structures about the ankle and foot given the superficial location of many structures [31]. Ultrasound performs well in evaluation of structures such as tendons and ligaments, whereas MR imaging is required to evaluate bone marrow and the articular surfaces of the ankle joint. There are several structures of the calf and posterior ankle that are commonly involved with sports injuries. Injury of the distal medial head of the gastrocnemius, also termed tennis leg, will appear as hypoechoic or anechoic disruption of the distal tendon at its aponeurosis attachment (Fig. 9). Injury to the plantaris tendon will appear as a tubular sagittal-oriented fluid collection in the expected location of the plantaris tendon located between the muscle bellies of the medial head of the gastrocnemius and soleus muscles. Injuries to the plantaris and medial head of the gastrocnemius commonly coexist. While injury and hematoma to the soleus may occur with sports injuries, the finding of an isolated hematoma in the soleus muscle should raise concern for potential underlying malignant tumor in the absence of a bleeding disorder or anti-coagulants.

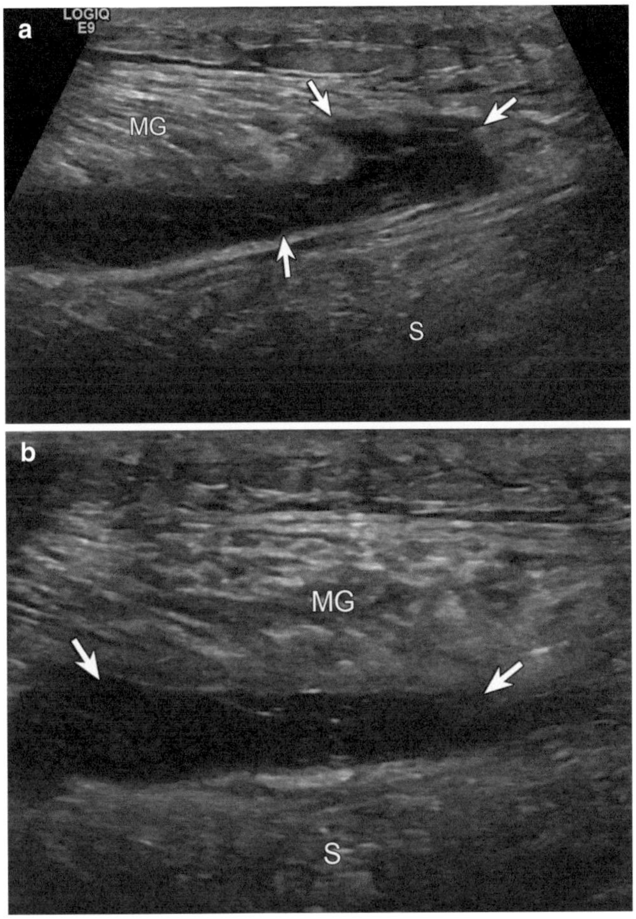

Fig. 9 Medial gastrocnemius tear ("tennis leg"). Ultrasound images (**a**) long axis and (**b**) short axis to the distal medial head of gastrocnemius (MG) show hypoechoic tear at distal aponeurosis (*arrows*) (S, soleus)

Injuries may involve tendons about the foot and ankle, which commonly include the Achilles, tibialis posterior, and peroneal tendons. With respect to the Achilles, abnormalities commonly involve a segment of tendon 2–6 cm proximal to its calcaneal attachment, although distal abnormalities at the calcaneus may also occur [32] (Fig. 10). Potential findings at ultrasound include hypoechoic tendinosis, anechoic interstitial tears, partial-thickness tears, and full-thickness tears. Since there is no surrounding synovial sheath, the term peritendinitis is often used to describe abnormal hypoechoic injury or inflammation surrounding the Achilles tendon. Distention of the retrocalcaneal or retro-Achilles bursa may also be seen. In evaluation for Achilles tendon tear, the use of dynamic imaging with dorsiflexion and plantar flexion of the foot will help differentiate partial-thickness from full-thickness tendon tear. A partial-thickness tear will show tendon fiber continuity with movement of the entire tendon during dynamic imaging, while a full-thickness tear will show lack of tendon translation across the abnormal tendon segment and retracted torn tendon stump. Other tendons about the ankle may also show tenosynovitis, tendinosis, and various types of tendon tears, usually where a tendon changes course near an osseous structure such as the malleoli. With regard to the peroneal tendons, a common tear is the longitudinal split of the peroneus brevis. Dynamic imaging with the foot in dorsiflexion and eversion is helpful to demonstrate possible peroneal tendon subluxation and dislocation in the setting of a peroneal retinaculum tear or fibula avulsion.

The ligaments of the ankle can be visualized with ultrasound [33]. Laterally, the anterior talofibular ligament is

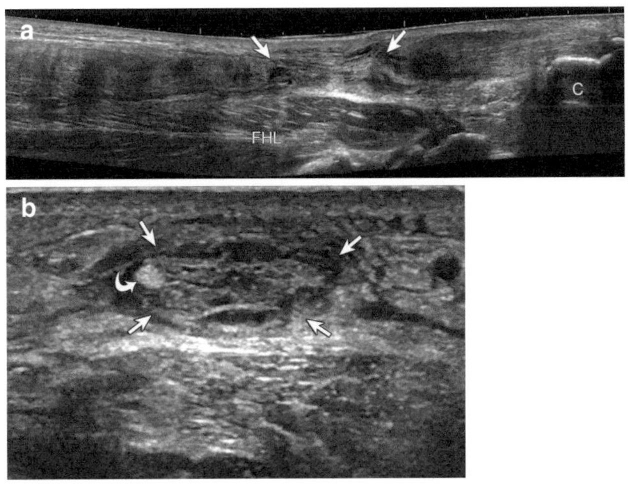

Fig. 10 Achilles tendon: full-thickness tear. Ultrasound images (**a**) long axis and (**b**) short axis to the Achilles tendon show heterogeneous hypoechoic tendon disruption with tendon retraction (between *arrows*). Note intact plantaris tendon (*curved arrow*) at medial aspect (FHL, flexor hallucis longus; C, calcaneus)

most commonly injured, followed by the calcaneofibular ligament. An abnormal ligament can appear as hypoechoic swelling or frank discontinuity with possible hyperechoic avulsion fracture fragment. Evaluation of the anterior inferior tibiofibular ligament is important in the setting of high ankle sprain, where further evaluation of the interosseous membrane and proximal fibula is important to exclude Maisonneuve injury. Medially, the deltoid ligament can also be evaluated for injury. Lastly, a fracture can be identified by ultrasound as a cortical step-off that correlates with point tenderness, with variable echogenic callous depending on the chronicity of the injury.

References

1. Schaeffeler C, Mueller D, Kirchhoff C, Wolf P, Rummeny EJ, Woertler K (2011) Tears at the rotator cuff footprint: prevalence and imaging characteristics in 305 MR arthrograms of the shoulder. Eur Radiol 21(7):1477–1484
2. Jacobson JA (2011) Shoulder US: anatomy, technique, and scanning pitfalls. Radiology 260(1):6–16
3. Galloway MT, Lalley AL, Shearn JT (2013) The role of mechanical loading in tendon development, maintenance, injury, and repair. J Bone Joint Surg Am 95(17):1620–1628
4. Buck FM, Grehn H, Hilbe M, Pfirrmann CW, Manzanell S, Hodler J (2010) Magnetic resonance histologic correlation in rotator cuff tendons. J Magn Reson Imaging 32(1):165–172
5. Kjellin I, Ho CP, Cervilla V, Haghighi P, Kerr R, Vangness CT, Friedman RJ, Trudell D, Resnick D (1991) Alterations in the supraspinatus tendon at MR imaging: correlation with histopathologic findings in cadavers. Radiology 181(3):837–841
6. Jacobson JA, Lancaster S, Prasad A, van Holsbeeck MT, Craig JG, Kolowich P (2004) Full-thickness and partial-thickness supraspinatus tendon tears: value of US signs in diagnosis. Radiology 230(1): 234–242
7. Wohlwend JR, van Holsbeeck M, Craig J, Shirazi K, Habra G, Jacobsen G, Bouffard JA (1998) The association between irregular greater tuberosities and rotator cuff tears: a sonographic study. AJR Am J Roentgenol 171(1):229–233
8. Araki D, Miller RM, Fujimaki Y, Hoshino Y, Musahl V, Debski RE (2015) Effect of tear location on propagation of isolated supraspinatus tendon tears during increasing levels of cyclic loading. J Bone Joint Surg Am 97(4):273–278
9. Park JS, Park HJ, Kim SH, Oh JH (2015) Prognostic factors affecting rotator cuff healing after arthroscopic repair in small to medium-sized tears. Am J Sports Med 43(10):2386–2392
10. Skendzel JG, Jacobson JA, Carpenter JE, Miller BS (2011) Long head of biceps brachii tendon evaluation: accuracy of preoperative ultrasound. AJR Am J Roentgenol 197(4):942–948
11. Moser TP, Cardinal E, Bureau NJ, Guillin R, Lanneville P, Grabs D (2015) The aponeurotic expansion of the supraspinatus tendon: anatomy and prevalence in a series of 150 shoulder MRIs. Skelet Radiol 44(2):223–231
12. Hashiuchi T, Sakurai G, Morimoto M, Komei T, Takakura Y, Tanaka Y (2011) Accuracy of the biceps tendon sheath injection: ultrasound-guided or unguided injection? A randomized controlled trial. J Shoulder Elb Surg 20(7):1069–1073
13. van Holsbeeck M, Strouse PJ (1993) Sonography of the shoulder: evaluation of the subacromial-subdeltoid bursa. AJR Am J Roentgenol 160(3):561–564
14. Daghir AA, Sookur PA, Shah S, Watson M (2012) Dynamic ultrasound of the subacromial-subdeltoid bursa in patients with shoulder impingement: a comparison with normal volunteers. Skelet Radiol 41(9):1047–1053
15. Lobo Lda G, Fessell DP, Miller BS, Kelly A, Lee JY, Brandon C, Jacobson JA (2013) The role of sonography in differentiating full versus partial distal biceps tendon tears: correlation with surgical findings. AJR Am J Roentgenol 200(1):158–162
16. Smith J, Finnoff JT, O'Driscoll SW, Lai JK (2010) Sonographic evaluation of the distal biceps tendon using a medial approach: the pronator window. J Ultrasound Med 29(5):861–865
17. Kalume Brigido M, De Maeseneer M, Jacobson JA, Jamadar DA, Morag Y, Marcelis S (2009) Improved visualization of the radial insertion of the biceps tendon at ultrasound with a lateral approach. Eur Radiol 19(7):1817–1821
18. Downey R, Jacobson JA, Fessell DP, Tran N, Morag Y, Kim SM (2011) Sonography of partial-thickness tears of the distal triceps brachii tendon. J Ultrasound Med 30(10):1351–1356
19. Potter HG, Hannafin JA, Morwessel RM, DiCarlo EF, O'Brien SJ, Altchek DW (1995) Lateral epicondylitis: correlation of MR imaging, surgical, and histopathologic findings. Radiology 196(1):43–46
20. Roedl JB, Gonzalez FM, Zoga AC, Morrison WB, Nevalainen MT, Ciccotti MG, Nazarian LN (2016) Potential utility of a combined approach with US and MR arthrography to image medial elbow pain in baseball players. Radiology 279(3):827–837
21. De Maeseneer M, Marcelis S, Jager T, Girard C, Gest T, Jamadar D (2009) Spectrum of normal and pathologic findings in the region of the first extensor compartment of the wrist: sonographic findings and correlations with dissections. J Ultrasound Med 28(6):779–786
22. Lopez-Ben R, Lee DH, Nicolodi DJ (2003) Boxer knuckle (injury of the extensor hood with extensor tendon subluxation): diagnosis with dynamic US—report of three cases. Radiology 228(3):642–646
23. Klauser A, Frauscher F, Bodner G, Halpern EJ, Schocke MF, Springer P, Gabl M, Judmaier W, Zur Nedden D (2002) Finger pulley injuries in extreme rock climbers: depiction with dynamic US. Radiology 222(3):755–761
24. Melville D, Jacobson JA, Haase S, Brandon C, Brigido MK, Fessell D (2013) Ultrasound of displaced ulnar collateral ligament tears of the thumb: the Stener lesion revisited. Skelet Radiol 42(5): 667–673
25. Ebrahim FS, De Maeseneer M, Jager T, Marcelis S, Jamadar DA, Jacobson JA (2006) US diagnosis of UCL tears of the thumb and Stener lesions: technique, pattern-based approach, and differential diagnosis. Radiographics 26(4):1007–1020
26. Jacobson JA (2002) Ultrasound in sports medicine. Radiol Clin N Am 40(2):363–386
27. Robinson P, Bhat V, English B (2011) Imaging in the assessment and management of athletic pubalgia. Semin Musculoskelet Radiol 15(1):14–26
28. Guillin R, Cardinal E, Bureau NJ (2009) Sonographic anatomy and dynamic study of the normal iliopsoas musculotendinous junction. Eur Radiol 19(4):995–1001
29. Mervak BM, Morag Y, Marcantonio D, Jacobson J, Brandon C, Fessell D (2012) Paralabral cysts of the hip: sonographic evaluation with magnetic resonance arthrographic correlation. J Ultrasound Med 31(3):495–500
30. Lee MJ, Chow K (2007) Ultrasound of the knee. Semin Musculoskelet Radiol 11(2):137–148
31. Khoury V, Guillin R, Dhanju J, Cardinal E (2007) Ultrasound of ankle and foot: overuse and sports injuries. Semin Musculoskelet Radiol 11(2):149–161
32. Calleja M, Connell DA (2010) The Achilles tendon. Semin Musculoskelet Radiol 14(3):307–322
33. Peetrons P, Creteur V, Bacq C (2004) Sonography of ankle ligaments. J Clin Ultrasound 32(9):491–499

Wrist Imaging: The "Top 5" Classic Diagnoses

Robert D. Boutin

Remember, if you ever need a helping hand, you'll find one at the end of your arm. As you grow older, you will discover that you have two hands: one for helping yourself, the other for helping others.

—Sam Levenson

Introduction

The wrist and hand have evolved elegantly over millions of years to become the most important method for interacting with our environment. While our evolution was driven by the need to optimize gripping and throwing [1], our daily digital demands have expanded into multitudinous applications—including manual labor, sport, art, music, "body language", and computer interactions.

Our imaging technologies also have evolved. As radiologists, our professional survival depends on mastery of our imaging tools, including radiography (XR), fluoroscopy, arthrography, computed tomography (CT), magnetic resonance imaging (MRI), and ultrasonography (US) [2]. All of these techniques can add value—narrowing the broad "universal differential diagnosis" of disease categories taught to medical students with the mnemonic "**VINDICATE**" (**V**ascular, **In**flammatory/Infectious, **N**eoplastic, **D**egenerative, **I**diopathic/Iatrogenic, **C**ongenital/Anatomic, **A**utoimmune, **T**raumatic, **E**ndocrine/Metabolic). (Most of these disease categories are covered elsewhere in this book, including arthritis, infection, neuropathies, pediatric conditions, and metabolic conditions. Musculotendinous and neurovascular derangements also are detailed elsewhere.)

In this chapter on the wrist, we review the anatomic structures that are common indications for imaging. Specifically, the focus here is on the "Top 5" classic problems targeting the wrist: (1) fractures (e.g., scaphoid), (2) avascular necrosis (AVN) (e.g., lunate), (3) carpal instability (e.g., scapholunate and lunotriquetral ligament tears), (4) triangular fibrocartilage complex (TFCC) injuries, and (5) common soft-tissue masses.

Osteoarticular Structures

Blunt wrist trauma is commonplace. In the Emergency Department setting, XRs are often positive for fractures (frequency > 30–40%) [3]. *Which patients should receive XRs after trauma to the wrist?* Similar to the "Ottawa Rules" that guide the appropriate ordering of ankle XRs, the "Amsterdam Wrist Rules" [4] are being implemented in some institutions to select appropriate patients for wrist XRs—using a free smart phone application!

To err is human. Although some fractures are radiographically-occult, more than two-thirds are identifiable at a second review. This fact is particularly problematic for patients in Emergency Departments, where the wrist is the anatomic area with the highest percentage of missed extremity fractures (>20%)—most often involving the distal radius, scaphoid, hamate, trapezium, and metacarpal bases [5]. Therefore, even if initial XRs are interpreted as negative, follow-up XRs or cross-sectional imaging may be helpful in the appropriate clinical setting. Unfortunately, advanced imaging often is not performed expeditiously, and delayed diagnosis of wrist fractures is a common medical malpractice claim [6]. Of these, scaphoid fractures are the single most expensive source of claims, and are detailed in the next section.

Fracture—Scaphoid

Scaphoid fractures are notorious because they can be difficult to diagnose and result in adverse outcomes [7, 8]. On clinical examination, "snuff box" tenderness is no better than 85% sensitive and 40% specific [7].

R.D. Boutin
Department of Radiology, University of California, Davis, 4860 Y St., Ste. 3100, Sacramento, CA 95817, USA
e-mail: rdboutin@ucdavis.edu

J. Hodler et al. (eds.), *Musculoskeletal Diseases 2017-2020*, DOI 10.1007/978-3-319-54018-4_23

Imaging Algorithm & Accuracy. With imaging, the sensitivity varies substantially for XR (~70%), CT (~80–95%), and MRI (>95%) [7, 8]. Expert opinions regarding the best diagnostic algorithm vary, too.

- According to the *American College of Radiology* guidelines [8], patients with suspected scaphoid fractures and negative XRs should undergo an early follow-up ***MRI*** examination in order to establish a prompt definitive diagnosis.
- According to the new German interdisciplinary, evidence- and consensus-based *S3 Guidelines* [7], however, ***CT*** is recommended in this setting. These experts argue that CT is superior to MRI because of better spatial resolution for showing fracture patterns and better diagnostic specificity (>95% versus 80–90%, respectively).
- Regardless, in the setting of suspected scaphoid fractures and negative XRs, both CT and MRI are cost-effective for reducing both costs and morbidity [9].

Fracture Patterns & Treatment. Scaphoid fractures are most common at the waist (>60%), but also can occur at the proximal third (15%), distal third (15%), or distal tubercle (<10%) [7] (Fig. 1). Surgery with a headless cannulated compression (e.g., Acutrak®) screw is generally recommended for all proximal fractures and for fractures displaced >1 mm. It is these fracture patterns that place the scaphoid at higher risk of non-union and AVN of the proximal fragment.

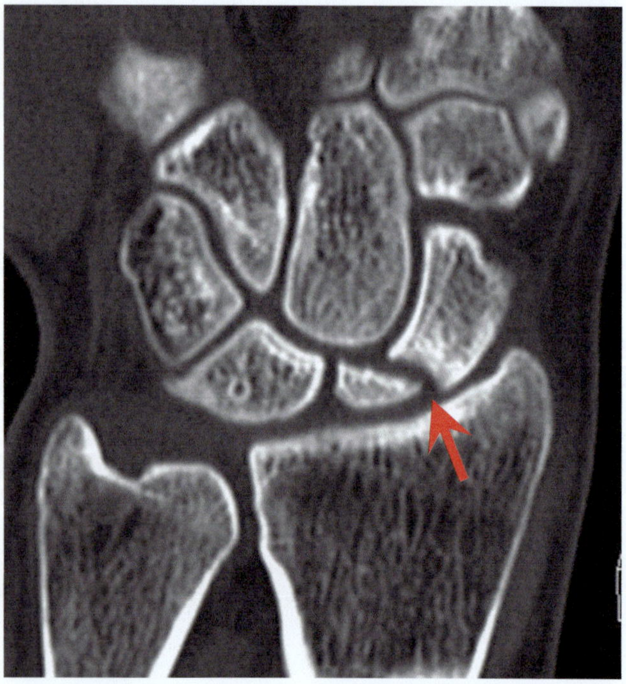

Fig. 1 Scaphoid fracture. 18-year-old soccer player with chronic wrist pain since falling on an outstretched hand 1 year earlier. Wrist radiographs at that time were interpreted as normal (not shown). Coronal CT shows nonunion of a proximal pole scaphoid fracture (*arrow*)

With CT and MRI, the assessment of scaphoid fractures should include evaluation for apex dorsal angulation at the scaphoid waist ("humpback deformity", diagnosed when the intrascaphoid angle is >45°) and *ad latus* (sideways) displacement >1 mm (especially with longitudinally-oriented fractures in the proximal scaphoid).

Follow-up Imaging. With normal healing, the fracture line may widen during the first 4 weeks, and periosteal callus should not be expected. Of note, some proximal pole osteosclerosis is a common finding during the healing process. By week 6–12, cancellous bone bridging usually should be evident (e.g., >8 oblique-sagittal CT slices of 0.5-mm thickness) [7]. Even after fracture healing, a peripheral radiolucent cleft may remain; patients with more than 50% union are generally cleared to resume normal activities.

- *Delayed union* of a scaphoid fracture may be diagnosed on CT scans after 3 months if there is <25% union, cystic change, and resorption along the fracture.
- *Non-union* may be diagnosed after 6 months in the presence of a pseudarthrosis (prevalence, 5–10%), with or without complications of periscaphoid osteoarthritis (e.g., scaphoid nonunion advanced collapse or "SNAC" wrist) and proximal pole AVN.
- *AVN* on MRI is diagnosed in the proximal pole when there is decreased signal on T1-weighted images and contrast enhancement is less than the distal pole [10].

AVN—Lunate

The lunate resembles the shape of a crescent moon, and is the "keystone" intercalated segment withstanding high loads in the central column of the proximal carpal row. AVN of the lunate, commonly known as Kienböck disease, is the topic of abundant recent literature [11] summarized here.

Clinical. Clinically, the stereotypical patient is 20–40 years old. Less commonly, adolescent and elderly patients also can be seen. Patients typically present with non-specific dorsal pain aggravated by wrist use (especially in extension), limited wrist motion, and reduced grip strength.

Pathogenesis. The etiology of Kienböck disease is considered multifactorial. Causative factors may include both vascular factors that compromise bone perfusion (e.g., variations in arterial supply or venous drainage, such as single vessel arterial supply) and biomechanical factors that can concentrate loads at the proximal-radial aspect of the lunate. Specific anatomic features with a possible association with Kienböck disease development or progression include negative ulnar variance, decreased radial inclination, and type I lunate morphology. Knowledge of these anatomic features may improve diagnostic accuracy and affect therapeutic decisions (e.g., negative ulnar variance may be treated with a radial shortening osteotomy).

Imaging. After XR findings are visible, XRs can show progression along a spectrum from osteosclerosis, to bone collapse, malalignment, and premature osteoarthritis. Although the traditional Lichtman staging system was developed based on XR findings, CT can be helpful for early diagnosis and shows a higher stage than XR in two-thirds of cases. MRI also helps with diagnosis of early (XR-occult) Kienböck disease, and can be used to diagnose "nonfunctional articular surfaces" caused by bone collapse or arthritis (e.g., criteria used in the Bain and Begg classification system).

With MRI, T1 images show decreased signal intensity in the bone marrow for all stages of Kienböck disease (Fig. 2). On fat-sat T2 images, the signal intensity can be variable; it is generally *hyper*intense in areas of ischemic (viable) bone marrow containing edema and *hypo*intense in areas that are necrotic. Early stress reaction may be seen at the proximal-radial lunate; later, a coronally-oriented fracture may propagate across the lunate.

After contrast administration, MRI enhancement patterns have been described that may correlate with the potential for lunate revascularization and therefore prognosis (***A***, normal homogeneous bone enhancement, associated with a good prognosis; ***B***, inhomogeneous enhancement, with viable distal lunate and necrotic proximal lunate, associated with an intermediate prognosis; ***C***, no enhancement owing to complete necrosis, with a poor prognosis).

Differential Diagnosis. The MRI differential diagnosis for focal signal alteration in the lunate may include bone edema from other causes, such as cartilage loss (e.g., chondrosis/arthritis) and macrotrauma (e.g., contusion, fracture). Lunate AVN is usually easy to distinguish from *ulnar (ulnocarpal) impaction syndrome*, which is characterized by a triad of findings: positive ulnar variance, TFCC perforation, and chondrosis with subchondral reactive changes at the ulnar head and proximal-ulnar aspect of the lunate (Fig. 3). With end stage (stage IV) Kienböck disease, the pattern of malalignment and OA can resemble scapholunate dissociation with advanced collapse ("SLAC" wrist).

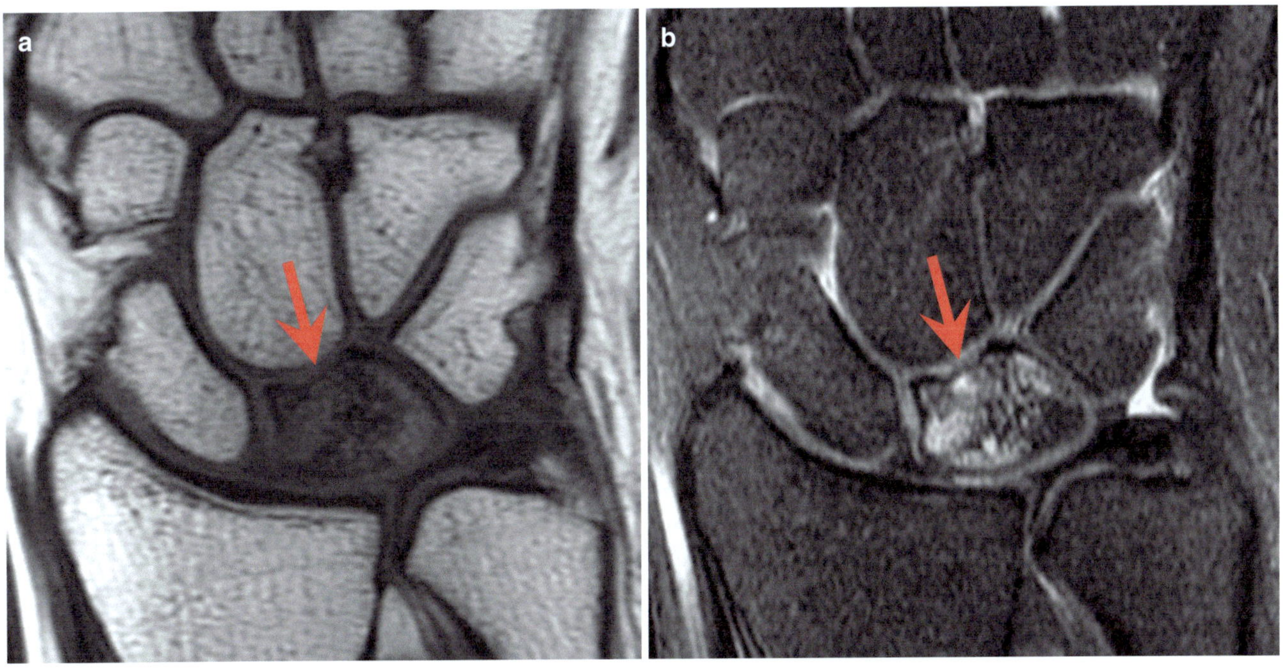

Fig. 2 Kienböck disease. 16-year-old girl with wrist pain for 6 months and history of negative radiographs. Coronal T1-weighted (**a**) and fat-suppressed intermediate-weighted (**b**) MR images show abnormal signal (*arrow*) in the lunate (with relative sparing of the proximal-ulnar corner) characteristic of Kienböck disease

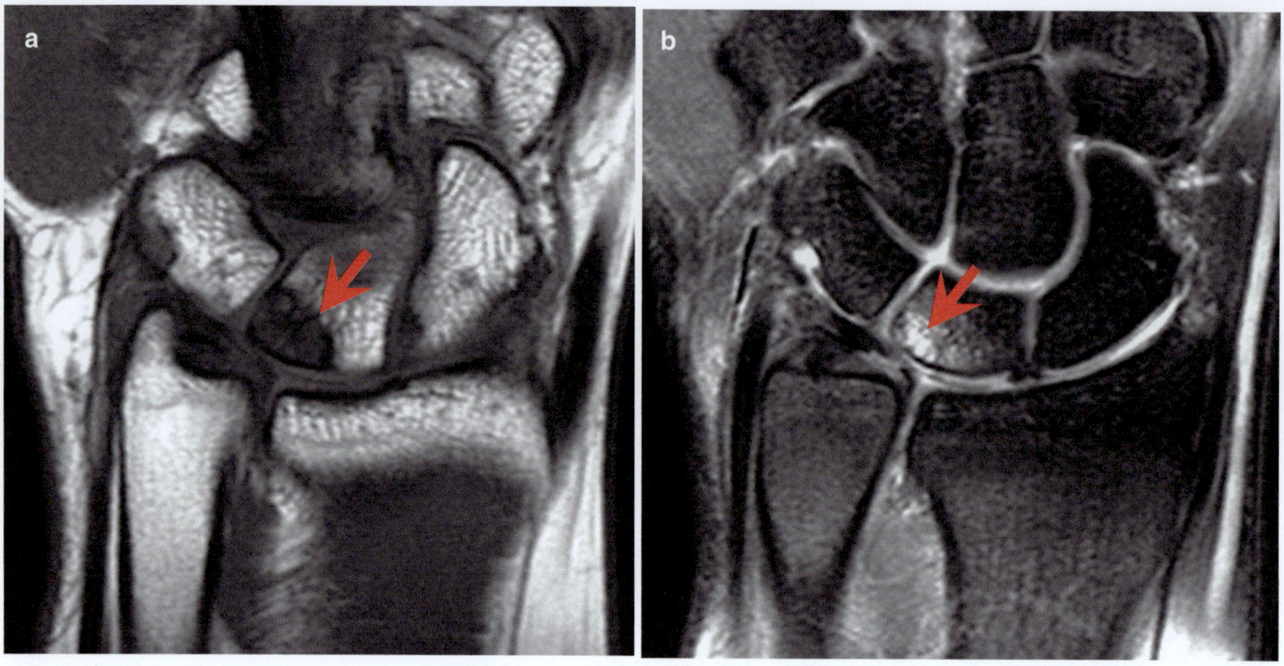

Fig. 3 Ulnar impaction syndrome. 54-year-old woman with ulnar-sided wrist pain and "osteosclerosis" reported on radiographs. Coronal T1-weighted (**a**) and fat-suppressed intermediate-weighted (**b**) MR images demonstrate abnormal signal (*arrow*) centered in the subchondral bone at the proximal-ulnar margin of the lunate. This appearance is accompanied by characteristic findings of overlying lunate chondrosis, mild ulnar positive positioning, and a tiny full-thickness perforation in the triangular fibrocartilage

Ligamentous Structures

A fundamental objective of wrist imaging is the diagnosis of injuries to wrist ligaments. Wrist ligaments are categorized as *extrinsic* (attaching to carpal bones and adjacent structures) or *intrinsic* (attaching only to carpal bones). In patients with acute wrist trauma and bone injury on MRI, there are high rates of injury in both the extrinsic (85%) and intrinsic (67%) ligaments [12]. Highlights from several recent reports [12–17] on this topic are summarized below.

Extrinsic Ligaments

The extrinsic ligaments are considered important "secondary stabilizers". Indeed, if the extrinsic ligaments are intact, even a complete intrinsic ligament tear may not result in carpal instability.

Extrinsic ligaments are named logically according to the bones to which they attach [16]. Although there are numerous extrinsic ligaments, there are arguably four that should be evaluated routinely on MRI or US.

- *Volarly*, the two most important extrinsic ligaments are the *radioscaphocapitate* and *long radiolunate* (also known as the *radiolunotriquetral*) ligaments.
- *Dorsally*, the two most important extrinsic ligaments are the *dorsal radiocarpal ligament* (also known as the *dorsal radiotriquetral ligament*) and the *dorsal intercarpal ligament* (also known as the *dorsal scaphotriquetral ligament*).

Intrinsic Ligaments

Of the intrinsic ligaments, the two most important "primary stabilizers" are the *scapholunate (SL) ligament* and the *lunotriquetral (LT) ligament*. These two ligaments transfer opposing flexion and extension moments to the lunate, which keeps the lunate in neutral alignment.

Carpal instability varies in severity from *static* (severe, non-reducible), to *dynamic* (visible only with clenched fist or ulnar deviation), to *pre-dynamic* (early, normal imaging). SL ligament insufficiency is associated with *dorsal* lunate tilt ("DISI"); this condition is much more common than LT ligament insufficiency, which is associated with *volar* lunate tilt ("VISI").

Anatomy. Both the SL and LT ligaments are "C-shaped" structures with three segments. While the *central* "membranous" segment is composed of fibrocartilage that commonly perforates incidentally with advancing age, the *dorsal* and *volar* segments are composed of biomechanically important collagen. Biomechanically, the dorsal segment is most important for SL stability, while the volar segment is most important for LT stability.

Imaging. The imaging diagnosis of SL instability is characterized by malalignment, generally defined by a wide SL space (>3 mm) or wide scapholunate angle (>60°). LT ligament insufficiency may be associated with abnormal volar flexion of the lunate (scapholunate angle <30° and capitolunate angle >30°). The SL angle measurements are generally similar on XR, CT, and MRI [18].

Normally, with MRI, ligaments appear as linear, hypointense structures. MRI diagnosis of a tear is made by observing hyperintense T2 signal, attenuation, or discontinuity in a ligament (Fig. 4). Injuries are commonly graded according to severity:

1. Mild sprain (periligamentous edema and/or increased intrasubstance signal),
2. Partial-thickness tear (focal fluid-like signal intensity involving a portion of the cross section of the ligament; or abnormal morphologic features such as fraying, irregularity, indistinctness, or abnormal caliber), or
3. Full-thickness tear (focal fluid-like signal or discontinuity extending across the ligament cross section).

With MRI of the intrinsic ligaments, tears in the dorsal and volar segments are best seen on axial images, and usually

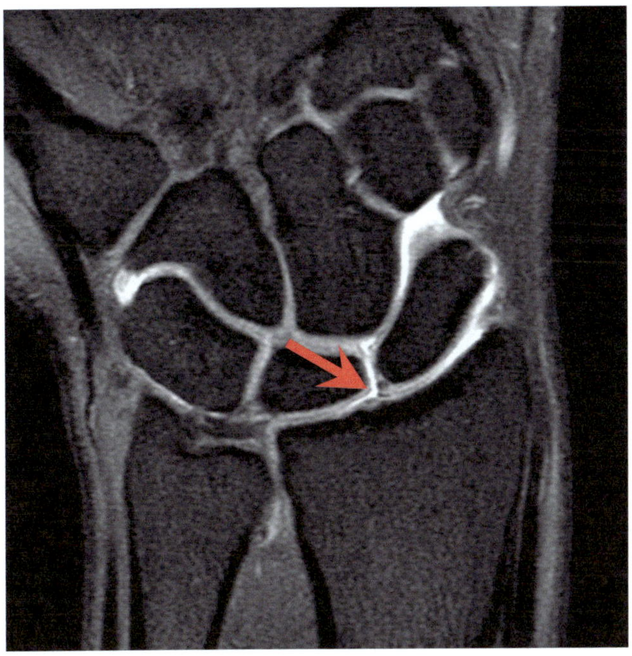

Fig. 4 Scapholunate ligament tear. Coronal fat-suppressed intermediate-weighted image shows hyperintense signal (*arrow*) traversing the membranous portion of the scapholunate ligament indicating a full-thickness tear

are combined with membranous tears [19]. Full-thickness perforation in the dorsal segment of the SL ligament can be associated with a small dorsal ganglion cyst. Such cysts may be "clinically occult" to palpation, but can cause substantial pain by compressing a terminal branch of the posterior interosseous nerve.

Triangular Fibrocartilage Complex (TFCC)

The TFCC helps stabilize the ulnocarpal and distal radioulnar joints and, when injured, may be a source of ulnar-sided wrist pain [20–22]. Given that ulnar-sided wrist pain is so common—and potentially difficult to diagnose and manage—it is sometimes referred to as the "low back pain of the wrist". Although there are numerous etiologies in the clinical differential diagnosis of ulnar-sided pain, the most common pain generators include TFCC injury, osteoarticular damage, and peritendinitis.

Anatomy. The TFCC is the hammock-shaped complex of structures supporting the ulnar-side of the wrist. Although the nomenclature varies, key structures in the TFCC include the:

- Articular disk (triangle-shaped fibrocartilage),
- Distal radioulnar ligaments (both the volar and dorsal ligaments have superficial and deep laminae that bifurcate into styloid and foveal attachments, and are major stabilizers of the DRUJ,
- Tendon sheath of the extensor carpi ulnaris,
- Ulnocarpal (lunotriquetral and ulnolunate) ligaments, and
- Meniscus homologue, blending with the ulnar joint capsule.

Imaging. TFCC derangements are divided into two broad categories: traumatic and degenerative. Additional subclassification is based on the anatomic location (Fig. 5). Similar to the knee meniscus, the TFCC is relatively vascular peripherally (and therefore may be amenable to repair), but is relatively avascular elsewhere (and therefore has less potential for healing).

- A *communicating defect* (full-thickness tear) is diagnosed when a fluid-filled gap extends through the TFCC to both articular surfaces.
- A *non-communicating defect* (partial-thickness tear) is diagnosed when fluid signal contacts only one articular surface of the TFCC.

Clinical correlation is important in assessing the significance of morphologic defects. While TFCC perforations should not be seen before the age of 30, degenerative changes with disk perforation is present half of all individuals after

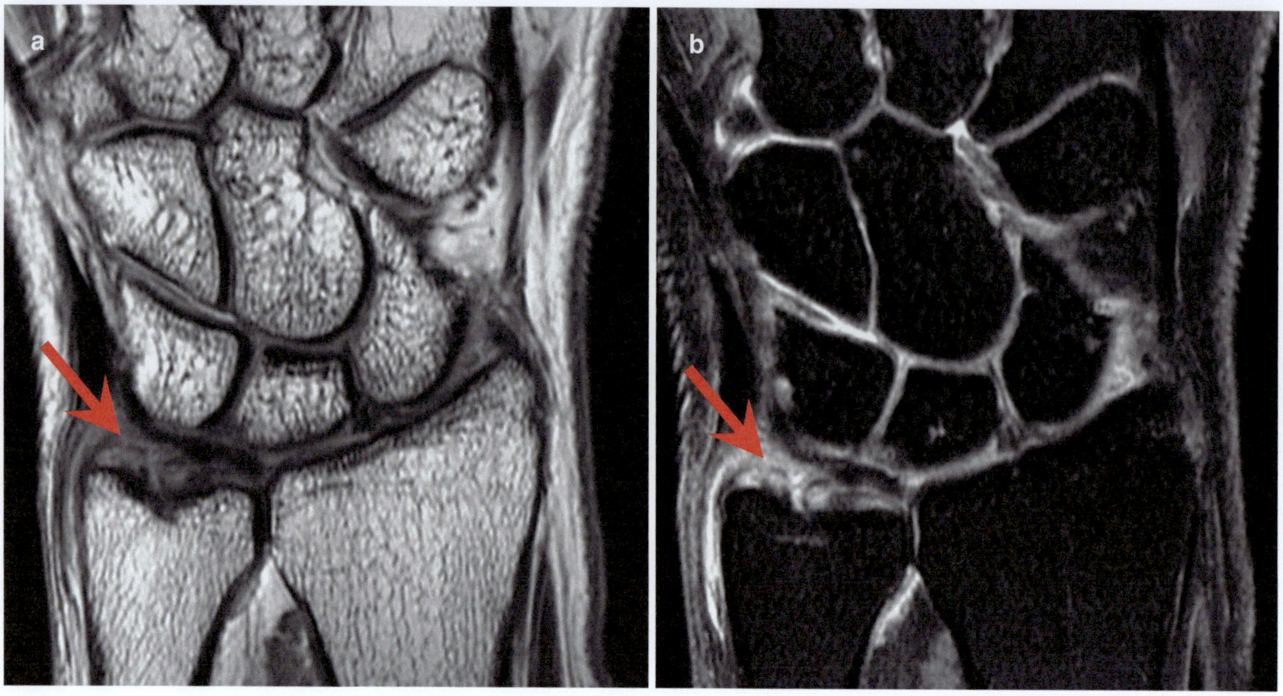

Fig. 5 TFCC tear. Coronal intermediate-weighted (**a**) and fat-suppressed intermediate-weighted (**b**) MR images show increased signal (*arrow*) at the ulnar styloid and foveal attachments. A tear was proven at arthroscopy

age 60–70 years [23, 24]. Interestingly, partial-thickness tears can have a more reliable association with symptoms than full-thickness defects. This phenomenon has been observed particularly with partial-thickness tears in the proximal lamina of the TFCC near the ulnar attachment [25]. There is also increasing interest in longitudinal split tears of the lunotriquetral ligament (usually best seen on axial images) [14].

Potential diagnostic pitfalls are well described, including the false positive diagnosis of TFCC tears owing to fluid in the prestyloid recess (mistaken for an ulnar-sided tear) and intermediate signal articular cartilage at the radial attachment of the TFCC (mistaken for an radial-sided tear).

How Accurate are MRI and CT?

The accuracy of imaging can vary substantially, depending the imaging technique, the location of the disorder, and the severity of the derangement.

- MRI diagnostic accuracy is generally higher with 3 T (vs. <1.5 T), with full-thickness defects (vs. partial-thickness defects), and with TFCC central and radial-sided defects (vs. peripheral and ulnar-sided defects).
- With conventional MRI, the diagnostic accuracy is higher for SL ligament tears (sensitivity >70–80%, specificity >90%) than for LT ligament tears (sensitivity >60–70%, specificity >90%).
- With MR arthrography (compared to conventional MRI), the sensitivity and specificity are generally higher (>90%) for assessment of the intrinsic ligaments and TFCC.
- Wrist MR arthrography with axial traction may further improve the detection of some internal derangements [26].

Regarding the extrinsic ligaments, further work is warranted to optimize reliable correlation between MRI and arthroscopy. One diagnostic challenge relates to the detection of non-acute injuries, because these "capsular" ligaments often heal with hypointense fibrotic tissue that is similar to the signal intensity of native ligaments.

Compared to MRI, CT arthrography allows for higher spatial resolution, less motion artifact, and can have a diagnostic accuracy of >95% for tears of the intrinsic ligaments and TFCC [19]. However, MRI techniques are generally favored as the imaging test of choice after XR, because CT techniques are insensitive to abnormalities in the marrow and periarticular soft tissues. Evolving CT and MRI techniques may change utilization in the future, including the use of spectral CT and kinematic "4D" (3D space +1 D time) imaging [27].

Soft-Tissue Masses

The Good, The Bad, & The Ugly. Soft-tissue masses in the wrist and hand are a frequent indication for advanced imaging. These masses are categorized broadly as "non-neoplastic", "benign neoplastic", and "malignant neoplastic". As in many areas in life, there is a lot of good news and a bit of bad news here.

- *Good news*—Most soft-tissue masses are non-neoplastic. In my practice, approximately 75% of masses fall into this category, and the most common single diagnosis is a cyst (60%). Sonography is sufficient for evaluating typical cysts, while MRI is most helpful for patients with atypical lesions, neurologic symptoms, and for preoperative assessments [28].
- *More good news*—Of all the neoplastic tumors, benign lesions are more than twice as common as malignant lesions.
- *Now for the bad news*—Imaging features may not reliably differentiate benign versus malignant tumors, and therefore histopathologic diagnosis is often appropriate.

Top 3 Considerations. Although patient referral patterns vary geographically and the masses can have a wide differential diagnosis, here are the "top 3" pearls of wisdom that can be helpful in the wrist and hand [29].

- Non-cystic "indeterminate" lesions classified as non-neoplastic include heterotopic ossification, nodular fasciitis, and inflammatory (or reactive) soft-tissue masses.
- Benign neoplastic lesions may include tenosynovial giant cell tumors (commonly referred to as giant cell tumor of the tendon sheath), benign peripheral nerve sheath tumors (i.e., neurofibromas and schwannomas), and lesions containing fibrous tissue (i.e., superficial fibromatosis [Dupuytren contracture], deep fibromatosis, fibroma of the tendon sheath).
- Malignant neoplastic lesions that are considered most commonly in the hand are undifferentiated pleomorphic sarcoma, synovial sarcoma, and epithelioid sarcoma.

In summary, the wrist has intricate anatomy that can be "dissected" non-invasively with imaging. Imaging interpretations can be accomplished comprehensively and efficiently by using a systematic "checklist" approach to these anatomic structures (e.g., osteoarticular, ligamentous, musculotendinous, neurovascular). Most importantly, astute radiologists succeed by mastering the problems certain to appear in their patients. In the wrist, the recurring "classic" disorders worth knowing about include fractures (e.g., scaphoid), AVN (e.g., lunate), carpal instability (e.g., scapholunate and lunotriquetral ligament tears), TFCC injuries, and common soft-tissue masses.

References

1. Young RW (2003) Evolution of the human hand: the role of throwing and clubbing. J Anat 202:165–174
2. American College of Radiology (2014) ACR–SCBT-MR–SPR–SSR practice parameter for the performance of magnetic resonance imaging (MRI) of the wrist [Internet]. https://www.acr.org/~/media/ACR/Documents/PGTS/guidelines/MRI_Wrist.pdf. Accessed 1 Jan 2017
3. van den Brand CL, van Leerdam RH, van Ufford JH et al (2013) Is there a need for a clinical decision rule in blunt wrist trauma? Injury 44:1615–1619
4. Walenkamp MM, Bentohami A, Slaar A et al (2015) The Amsterdam wrist rules: the multicenter prospective derivation and external validation of a clinical decision rule for the use of radiography in acute wrist trauma. BMC Musculoskelet Disord 16:389
5. Wei CJ, Tsai WC, Tiu CM et al (2006) Systematic analysis of missed extremity fractures in emergency radiology. Acta Radiol 47:710–717
6. Ring J, Talbot C, Price J et al (2015) Wrist and scaphoid fractures: a 17-year review of NHSLA litigation data. Injury 46:682–686
7. Schmitt R, Rosenthal H (2016) Imaging of scaphoid fractures according to the new S3 guidelines. Rofo 188:459–469
8. Bruno MA, Weissman BN, Kransdorf MJ et al (2013) Expert panel on musculoskeletal imaging. ACR Appropriateness criteria® acute hand and wrist trauma. American College of Radiology (ACR), Reston, VA. https://acsearch.acr.org/docs/69418/Narrative. Accessed 1 Jan 2017
9. Karl JW, Swart E, Strauch RJ (2015) Diagnosis of occult scaphoid fractures: a cost-effectiveness analysis. J Bone Joint Surg Am 97:1860–1868
10. Fox MG, Wang DT, Chhabra AB (2015) Accuracy of enhanced and unenhanced MRI in diagnosing scaphoid proximal pole avascular necrosis and predicting surgical outcome. Skelet Radiol 44:1671–1678
11. Lichtman DM, Bain GI (eds) (2016) Kienbock's disease. Springer, Switzerland, pp 1–332
12. Taneja AK, Bredella MA, Chang CY et al (2013) Extrinsic wrist ligaments: prevalence of injury by magnetic resonance imaging and association with intrinsic ligament tears. J Comput Assist Tomogr 37:783–789
13. Cockenpot E, Lefebvre G, Demondion X et al (2016) Imaging of sports-related hand and wrist injuries: sports imaging series. Radiology 279:674–692
14. Ringler MD, Murthy NS (2015) MR imaging of wrist ligaments. Magn Reson Imaging Clin N Am 23:367–391
15. Kamal RN, Starr A, Akelman E (2016) Carpal kinematics and kinetics. J Hand Surg Am 41:1011–1018
16. Gitto S, Messina C, Mauri G et al (2017) Dynamic high-resolution ultrasound of intrinsic and extrinsic ligaments of the wrist: how to make it simple. Eur J Radiol 87:20–35
17. Ramamurthy NK, Chojnowski AJ, Toms AP (2016) Imaging in carpal instability. J Hand Surg Eur 41:22–34
18. Tan S, Ghumman SS, Ladouceur M et al (2014) Carpal angles as measured on CT and MRI: can we simply translate radiographic measurements? Skelet Radiol 43:1721–1728
19. Lee RK, Ng AW, Tong CS et al (2013) Intrinsic ligament and triangular fibrocartilage complex tears of the wrist: comparison of MDCT arthrography, conventional 3-T MRI, and MR arthrography. Skelet Radiol 42:1277–1285
20. Kakar S, Garcia-Elias M (2016) The "four-leaf clover" treatment algorithm: a practical approach to manage disorders of the distal radioulnar joint. J Hand Surg Am 41:551–564
21. Tosti R, Shin E (2017) Wrist arthroscopy for athletic injuries. Hand Clin 33:107–117
22. Pidgeon TS, Waryasz G, Carnevale J et al (2015) Triangular fibrocartilage complex: an anatomic review. JBJS Rev 3:e1
23. Mikić ZD (1978) Age changes in the triangular fibrocartilage of the wrist joint. J Anat 126(Pt 2):367–384
24. Chan JJ, Teunis T, Ring D (2014) Prevalence of triangular fibrocartilage complex abnormalities regardless of symptoms rise with

age: systematic review and pooled analysis. Clin Orthop Relat Res 472:3987–3994

25. Zanetti M, Linkous MD, Gilula LA, Hodler J (2000) Characteristics of triangular fibrocartilage defects in symptomatic and contralateral asymptomatic wrists. Radiology 216:840–845
26. Lee RK, Griffith JF, Ng AW et al (2016) Wrist traction during MR arthrography improves detection of triangular fibrocartilage complex and intrinsic ligament tears and visibility of articular cartilage. AJR Am J Roentgenol 206:155–161
27. Boutin RD, Buonocore MH, Immerman I et al (2013) Real-time magnetic resonance imaging (MRI) during active wrist motion—initial observations. PLoS One 8:e84004
28. Freire V, Guérini H, Campagna R et al (2012) Imaging of hand and wrist cysts: a clinical approach. AJR Am J Roentgenol 199:W618–W628
29. Sookur PA, Saifuddin A (2011) Indeterminate soft-tissue tumors of the hand and wrist: a review based on a clinical series of 39 cases. Skelet Radiol 40:977–989

Hand/Finger Assessment

Christine B. Chung

This syllabus contribution is meant to serve as a foundation and reference for organizing processes that affect the hand/fingers. It begins with a brief review of pertinent anatomy.

Anatomy

Ligament/Supporting Structures: At the metacarpophalangeal (MCP) joint, there are two collateral and two accessory collateral ligaments. The former serve as the major stabilizer of the articulation, and are taut in flexion (limiting lateral motion), and lax in extension, permitting a greater arc of lateral motion [1]. The collateral and accessory collateral ligaments originate from the dorsolateral aspect of the metacarpal head and insert on the lateral base of the proximal phalanx and on the volar plate, respectively. This anatomy is approximated at the thumb and lesser MCP's, though the former is more complex due to the presence of the sesamoids and relationships to other soft tissue attachment sites.

Similarly, at the proximal interphalangeal (PIP) joint, the collateral ligament complex (proper collateral and accessory collateral) plays a critical role in joint stabilization. The proper collateral ligaments are fan-shaped and arise from the proximal and dorsal sides of the concave area of the proximal phalanx and insert in the larger lateral roughened areas of the base middle phalanx. The accessory collateral ligaments arise from the volar side of the proper collateral ligament and can be difficult to distinguish from them. They insert into the lateral side of the base middle phalanx, and have a triangular shape [2].

Flexor tendon: The flexor tendons of the hand and fingers pass through the carpal tunnel of the wrist, separating in the palm to their ultimate sites of attachment in the fingers. Each finger has two flexor tendons, the flexor digitorum superficialis (FDS) more palmar in location and the flexor digitorum profundus (FDP), deep to the FDS, at the level of the palm. The FDS splits at the level of the MCP, passes around the FDP forming a ring aperture and passes to a position deep to the FDP, attaching to the palmar aspect of the middle phalanx (Fig. 1). The flexor

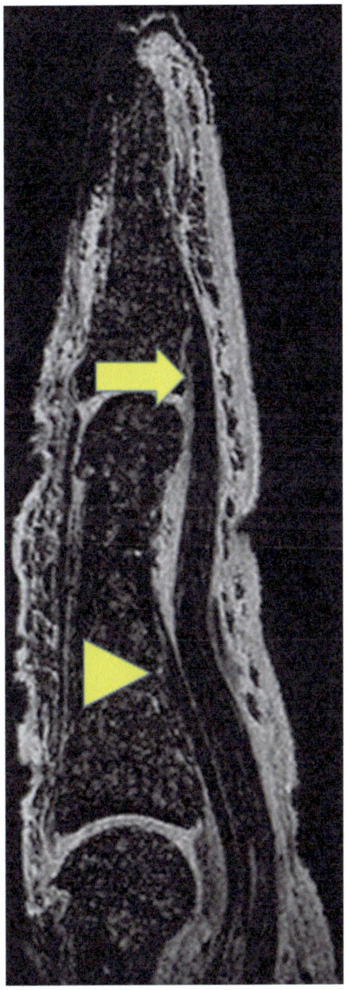

Fig. 1 Sagittal gradient MR image showing the distal attachment sites of flexor digitorum superficialis (*arrowhead*) and flexor digitorum profundus (*arrow*)

C.B. Chung
UCSD Department of Radiology, University of California, San Diego, 9427 Health Sciences Drive, San Diego, CA 92093, USA
e-mail: cbchung@ucsd.edu

J. Hodler et al. (eds.), *Musculoskeletal Diseases 2017-2020*, DOI 10.1007/978-3-319-54018-4_24

tendons are anchored to their osseous counterparts by the pulley system. There are five annular pulleys, fibrous structures that are well-defined thickenings of the tendon sheath located at the MCP (A1), proximal phalanx (A2), PIP joint (A3), middle phalanx (A4), and DIP (A5) (Fig. 2).

Extensor Tendon: At the level of the MCP, the extensor tendon is stabilized by the sagittal bands (SB). The tissue envelopes the extensor tendon with superficial and deep limbs that extend circumferentially around the joint to attach at the palmar volar plate [3]. The extensor tendon divides into three slips distal to the MCP, a central slip (CS) and two lateral slips (Fig. 3). The central slip inserts on the base of the middle phalanx. The lateral slips fuse with the lateral slips of the intrinsic tendons to form conjoined lateral bands. These conjoined lateral bands merge into a single terminal tendon that attaches at the base of the distal phalanx.

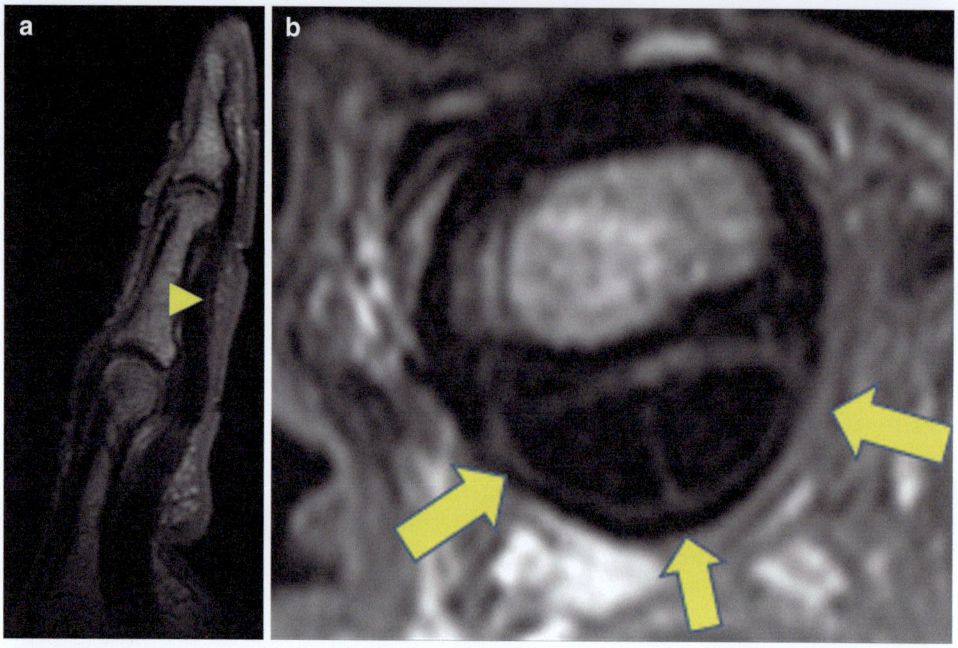

Fig. 2 Sagittal T1-weighted (**a**) and axial PD-weighted (**b**) MR images showing the A4 annular pulley (*arrowheads*) at the level of the middle phalanx

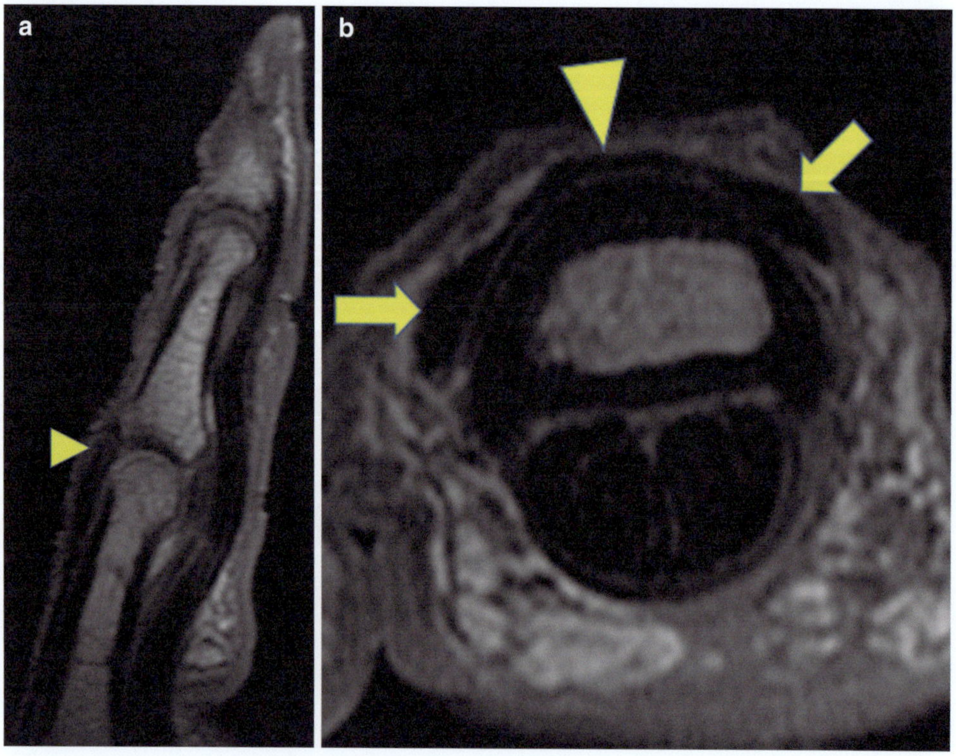

Fig. 3 Sagittal (**a**) and axial (**b**) T1-weighted MR images profile the central slip (*arrowhead*) attachment of the extensor tendon to the base of the middle phalanx, with its two lateral slips (*arrows*)

Pathology

Ligament Pathology

Gamekeeper's thumb: Injuries of the ulnar collateral ligament (UCL) of the thumb are encountered frequently. The most common mechanism is excessive radial deviation of the proximal phalanx, either acutely or through chronic repetitive microtrauma. Rupture of the ligament most often occurs at the ligament's distal insertion on the base of the proximal phalanx. Failure has been reported in the mid-substance, proximal attachment, with an avulsed fragment of bone, and as attritional failure (a thinning of the ligament resulting in laxity) [4].

Stener lesion: Stener described a complication of the UCL injury of the thumb in which the adductor pollicis longus aponeurosis was interpositioned between the distally avulsed ligament and its insertion. Due to the lack of contact between torn ligament and enthesis, he predicted instability would ensue. He further deduced that such lesions represented a surgical repair indication [5].

Collateral ligament injury: While less common that UCL injuries, RCL injuries of the thumb are relatively common. The RCL is important for pinch movements and depression, such as pushing button. The mechanism of injury is forced and sudden adduction of the MCP. Grading systems have incorporated clinical and structural elements: Grade I partial tear with pain but no instability, Grade 2 partial tear with pain and asymmetric laxity, Grade 3 full thickness tear with pain and instability [6].

Injuries to the collateral ligaments of the MCP joints in the fingers are less common than in the thumb. Most reports have described lesions in the RCL of the index finger. The imaging diagnosis can be challenging due to some degree of preexisting "normal" laxity in the joints [7]. The PIP joints are the most common injured articulation in the hand [8]. Grades I and II volar plate and collateral ligament sprains represent the vast majority of PIP joint injuries. The primary indications for surgical treatment include irreducible dislocation or subluxation, or association with a large fracture fragment [9]. Collateral ligament injuries result in instability in the coronal plane, whereas volar plate injuries result in instability in the sagittal plane.

Flexor Tendon Pathology

Injury to the flexor tendon is not as common as injuries to the extensor mechanism. Lesions are broadly categorized as open or closed injuries. In the flexor tendons, pulley lesions are also included.

Flexor tendon lacerations are more common than closed injury. Tendon failure can be partial or complete. Lesions are characterized by zone for identification of point of failure as well as prognostication. The zones are as follows: Zone I from distal FDP to distal FDS insertion, Zone II (no man's land) from distal FDS to distal palmar fold, Zone III from proximal part of A1 pulley (MCP) to distal flexor retinaculum, Zone IV at carpal tunnel, and Zone V forearm proximal to flexor retinaculum. Zone II lesions are the most frequent with the most severe prognosis [10]. Trauma to the four proximal zones implies involvement of both the FDS and FDP and would affect both the PIP and DIP.

In closed injury, avulsion of the FDP is the most common type of failure. It is caused by sudden hyperextension in a flexed finger, and referred to as **'sweater' or 'jersey' finger** [11]. These lesions are characterized by degree of retraction and presence of bone fragment.

Pulley lesion: **Pulley lesions** were recognized with increasing frequency as rock climbing gained popularity as a sport. Flexion of the fingers with MCP joint extension, PIP joint flexion and DIP joint extension results in extensive force at the A2 and A3 pulley, the former being the most common. Injury is reported to begin at eth distal part of the pulley [12]. This injury can be complicated by fibrous scarring and flexion contracture at the PIP.

Extensor Tendon Pathology

Injuries to the extensor tendon apparatus are common. They are superficial and delicate in nature predisposing to both laceration and rupture. As noted above, they are classified as open and closed lesions.

Similar to the flexor tendons, a zonal classification has been proposed for the open extensor tendon injury. Zones 1, 3, 5 and 7 are located at the DIP, PIP, MCP and wrist respectively, with zone 8 at the distal forearm. In total laceration, the tendons do not often show retraction due to the extensive soft tissue network of the extensor hood. Due to the prominent vascularity, complications of lesions can include adhesions [13].

Closed injuries include the mallet finger, central slip avulsion, boutonniere deformity. The **mallet finger** is an avulsion of the terminal tendon from the distal phalanx. If left untreated, this can progress to the swan neck deformity—flexion at the DIP and extension of the PIP due to fibrosis of the extensor hood components. **Central slip** injury is an avulsion of the central slip attachment of the extensor tendon from the base of the middle phalanx. It does not have a functional loss, but if untreated, can progress to the **boutonniere** deformity. Again due to fibrosis and retraction of the extensor hood tissues, this deformity is characterized by flexion at the PIP and hyperextension at the [14].

Miscellaneous Conditions

Soft tissue tumors: There are a host of soft tissue lesions that arise in the hand and can be broadly characterized by tissue of origin with the vast majority benign. These may include cysts, fat, vascular, neurogenic, fibrohistiocytic, pericytic [15].

- Ganglion cyst: thin connective tissue capsule, no true synovial lining
- Lipoma: adipose tumor predilection for thenar or hypothenar eminence
- Giant cell tumor tendon sheath: localized form of pigmented villonodular Synovitis
- Vascular malformation: increased number of vessels characterized by vascular flow
- Peripheral nerve sheath tumor: include schwannoma and neurofibroma
- Glomus tumor: benign hamartomatous lesion (pericytic origin) accounting for 5% of all hand lesions, predilection for the fingertip in the hand

Osseous tumors: Primary bone tumors of the hand are uncommon, and account for 2–5% of all skeletal tumors [16]. The majority of osseous tumors of the phalanges and metacarpal bones are benign, and include:

- Enchondroma: cartilaginous tumor, well marginated arising in medullary cavity with chondroid matrix
- Osteoid osteoma: 12% of all benign bone tumors, infrequent in hand and present with unusual bone marrow edema pattern
- Giant cell tumor: lytic lesion at end of bone, in hand have predilection for Metacarpal

Infectious processes: The hand can be commonly injured, and infected, particularly with penetrating trauma. Host factors can predispose to infection and these can include systemic processes such as diabetes mellitus (higher incidence of mixed and pure gram negatives), immunocompromised state (opportunistic infection such as gonorrhea, candida), IV drug abuse, exposure to sexually transmitted diseases (gonorrhea), and environmental exposures such as tropical fish aquarium (mycobacterium marinum). Common infections include the following [17].

- Paronychia: infection of epidermis bordering nail
- Felon: abscess of distal pulp of fingertip
- Herpetic whitlow: painful infection digit caused by herpes simplex virus
- Pyogenic flexor tenosynovitis: flexor tendon sheath infection
- Fight bite: result of altercation with skin laceration/oral pathogen

References

1. Kataoka T, Moritomo H, Miyake J, Murase T, Yoshikawa H, Sugamoto K (2011) Changes in shape and length of the collateral and accessory collateral ligaments of the metacarpophalangeal joint during flexion. J Bone Joint Surg Am 93(14):1318–1325
2. Chen J, Tan J, Zhang AX (2015) In vivo length changes of the proximal interphalangeal joint proper and accessory collateral ligaments during flexion. J Hand Surg Am 40(6):1130–1137
3. Bellemère P (2015) Treatment of chronix extensor tendons lesions of the fingers. Chir Main 34(4):155–181
4. Baskies MA, Lee SK (2009) Evaluation and treatment of injuries of the ulnar collateral ligament of the thumb metacarpophalangeal joint. Bull NYU Hosp Jt Dis 67(1):68–74
5. Stener B (1962) Displacement of the ruptured ulnar collateral ligament of the metacarpophalangeal joint of the thumb. J Bone Joint Surg Br 44:869–879
6. Edelstein DM, Kardashian G, Lee SK (2008) Radial collateral ligament injuries of the thumb. J Hand Surg Am 33(5):760–770
7. Lutsky K, Levi D, Beredjiklian P (2014) Utility of MRI for diagnosing complete tears of the collateral ligaments of the metacarpophalangeal joints of the lesser digits. Hand N Y 9(1):112–116
8. Clavero JA, Alomar X, Monill JM, Esplugas M, Golanó P, Mendoza M, Salvador A (2002) MR imaging of ligament and tendon injuries of the fingers. Radiographics 22(2):237–256
9. Liss FE, Green SM (1992) Capsular injuries of the proximal interphalangeal joint. Hand Clin 8(4):755–768
10. Ficat C, Hautier S (1975) Wounds of the flexor tendons of the fingers at the level of the hands. Results of primary sutures. J Chir [Paris] 110(6):533–542
11. Leddy JP (1985) Avulsions of the flexor digitorum profundus. Hand Clin 1(1):77–83
12. Marco RA, Sharkey NA, Smith TS, Zissimos AG (1998) Pathomechanics of closed rupture of the flexor tendon pulleys in rock climbers. J Bone Joint Surg Am 80(7):1012–1019
13. Blair WF, Steyers CM (1992) Extensor tendon injuries. Orthop Clin North Am 23(1):141–148
14. Scott SC (2000) Closed injuries to the extension mechanism of the digits. Hand Clin 16(3):367–373
15. Wu JS, Hochman MG (2009) Soft-tissue tumors and tumorlike lesions: a systematic imaging approach. Radiology 253(2): 297–316
16. Melamud K, Drapé JL, Hayashi D, Roemer FW, Zentner J, Guermazi A (2014) Diagnostic imaging of benign and malignant osseous tumors of the fingers. Radiographics 34(7):1954–1967
17. Clarke DC (2003) Common acute hand infections. Am Fam Physician 68(11):2167–2176

Part II

Nuclear Medicine Satellite Course "Diamond"

Imaging of Joints and Joint Prostheses

Anna Hirschmann

Introduction

Various imaging modalities are commonly used in the assessment of painful arthroplasties, including radiographs, ultrasound, computed tomography (CT), magnetic resonance imaging (MRI) and single-photon emission computed tomography/computed tomography (SPECT/CT). Each of these modalities has its own strength and weakness and should be used complementary, if the initially chosen imaging modality is not diagnostic. Periprosthetic complications are commonly encountered in clinical practice with a variety of etiologies including fracture, infection, instability, malposition and malsizing as well as loosening. A profound knowledge of expected normal and pathological appearances of arthroplasties is crucial for every radiologist and nuclear medicine specialist and helps with establishment of the correct diagnosis in those patients.

There are numerous types of arthroplasties available. A basic knowledge about the type of arthroplasty used is essential for the reporting radiologist and nuclear medicine specialist.

This article emphasizes on different imaging modalities of joints and arthroplasties, describes normal postoperative appearances with respect to the modality and highlights the most common pathologies of painful hip and knee replacements.

Imaging Modalities

Radiographs

Radiographs are considered as the first-line imaging modality in the evaluation of painful joints. This is mainly due to the fact, that radiographs are commonly available and less costly than cross-sectional imaging modalities. Generally, radiographs are used as serial follow-up examinations after arthroplasties. In particular, the size and position of a joint prosthesis should be evaluated as well as periprosthetic osteolysis or fractures. Two correctly adjusted orthogonal projections of the joint are mandatory to allow a precise evaluation of the bone-component interface. Comparison with previous radiographs is only feasible in standardized projections. In doubtful cases, comparisons have to be traced back further to the earliest postoperative image or even to preoperative images.

Advanced radiographic investigations of the knee joint include a full-limbs weight-bearing anteroposterior view to assess the mechanical leg alignment. In some cases, stress radiographs are necessary to detect ligament instabilities. These stress radiographs can be performed manually or using a specific stress device such as the TELOS® device. Typically, stress radiographs are performed as anterior and posterior drawer stress radiographs in 90° and 30° flexion to investigate stability of the ligaments and the posterior capsule. Varus and valgus stress radiographs are done in various degrees of knee flexion. In 0° flexion, the posterolateral and posteromedial joint capsule is tested, in 30° flexion, the collateral ligaments are tested and in 90° flexion, flexion instabilities can be detected.

Ultrasound

Ultrasound has the ability to evaluate periarticular soft tissue structures and possible joint effusion. It allows dynamic assessment of the joints. However, in the evaluation of painful arthroplasties, ultrasound plays a minor role. It might be of assistance in imaging-guided biopsies, fluid aspiration or injections.

CT

CT may be beneficial in radiographically suspicious but still unclear cases, especially in the evaluation of periprosthetic osteolysis or fractures. Streaking artifacts may limit the identification of landmark structures. These artifacts are dependent

A. Hirschmann
Department of Radiology and Nuclear Medicine,
University Hospital of Basel, University of Basel, Petersgraben 4,
Basel, BS 4031, Switzerland
e-mail: Anna.hirschmann@usb.ch

J. Hodler et al. (eds.), *Musculoskeletal Diseases 2017-2020*, DOI 10.1007/978-3-319-54018-4_25

on the type and orientation of the prosthesis and not at least on the CT protocol applied. In recent years, technological advances have introduced dual energy CT with the ability of metal artifact reducing algorithms by combining low- and high-energy data and computing monoenergetic images. These monoenergetic images ranging from 40 to 190 kiloelectron volts (kV) and are less susceptible to beam hardening. KV levels between 105 and 133 kV have proven to be beneficial in the evaluation of metal implants [1]. Recently introduced postprocessing artifact correction algorithms such as iterative metal artifact reduction (iMAR) or metal artifact reduction for orthopedic implants (O-MAR) may be advantageous in patients with arthroplasties. An extended Hounsfield unit scale increases the window width and level and aids for further post processing reduction of artifacts. However, most patients have bilateral joint replacements which lead to higher artifacts in the study site. Therefore, appropriate patient positioning is of utmost importance. In CT of the knee joint, we tend to position the opposite knee out of the field of view by flexing the hip and the knee.

SPECT/CT

SPECT/CT as hybrid imaging modality allows a window into the biology of bone remodeling. It combines a 3D bone scan (SPECT) with a conventional CT. Metabolic information is typically obtained in three phases: the perfusion, the bloodpool and the delayed mineral phase. All phases are undertaken with planar scans. A SPECT/CT is performed in the mineral phase at the requested joint region. Ideally, the interpretation of postoperative SPECT/CT images is carried out by a combined radiologist and nuclear medicine expert and the referring orthopedic surgeon.

Metabolic activity may persist several months after the operation and most often depends on the surgical technique and the inserted material. An increased bone tracer uptake is not necessarily associated with pain nor reflects a postoperative complication. Increased bone tracer uptake areas after knee arthroplasty in asymptomatic patients have been described recently [2]. These are located around the tibial stem including the tip, in the medial tibia, the anterolateral tibia, the anteromedial femur and to a lesser extend in the posterior femur [2].

SPECT/CT is an important part of the diagnostic puzzle in painful arthroplasties. However, clearly, it is only one piece of the puzzle.

MRI

MRI has been the gold standard in the evaluation of painful joints and provides an excellent contrast in the assessment of soft tissue structures. MRI of arthroplasties requires special imaging techniques to reduce artifacts. Various parameter modifications can be used with conventional MR sequences such as increasing the receiver bandwidth, decreasing the voxel size, increasing the number of signal averages, using inversion recovery fat saturation and scanning at 1.5 T machines. Advanced metal artifact reduction sequences such as slice encoding for metal artifact correction (SEMAC) or multiacquisition variable resonance image combination (MAVERIC) have proven to be superior to conventional sequences in patients with arthroplasties [3–5]. Particularly focusing on periprosthetic bone and soft tissue structures in close proximity, susceptibility artifacts may obscure these areas and require appropriate advanced imaging techniques. However, every technique has its benefits and drawbacks. Detection of periprosthetic bone marrow edema and osteolysis is improved by using the STIR SEMAC sequence [4, 6]. However, due to a blurring image appearance with this advanced technique, especially in proton density-weighted images, a mixture of advanced and modified techniques to complimentary address bone and soft tissue structures in patients with arthroplasties has been recommended [6]. In painful unicompartimental knee arthroplasties, MRI has the potential benefit in assessing the non-replaced joint compartment.

In hip arthroplasties, MRI allows the assessment of abductor and external rotator tendons at the insertion of the greater trochanter. Evaluation of muscle trophic, which can be divided into grading of fatty muscle infiltration according to Goutallier and muscle atrophy, is best performed on an axial T1-weighted non-fat saturated sequence [7].

Synovitis, extensive bone marrow and soft tissue edema are common findings in the early postoperative period after joint replacements. These findings will reduce as time courses, however, remnants may be apparent in the first postoperative year.

Complications After Arthroplasties

Periprosthetic Fracture

Displaced periprosthetic fractures can confidently be diagnosed on radiographs. In any case of a periprosthetic fracture, subsidence of the component might be an important sign of prosthesis stability. Non-displaced periprosthetic fractures can be difficult to be detected purely on radiographs, in clinically suspected fractures further investigation with CT may be of added value. In patients with severe osteoporosis and extended artifacts, fractures may be missed, even in the use of metal artifact reducing algorithms. In these cases, MRI with non fat-saturated T1-weighted sequences are helpful in the diagnostic workup. The distal and proximal extension of fractures should be included in the scan and provided to the orthopedic surgeon in order to accurately plan the surgical treatment method.

Loosening

Periprosthetic osteolysis, failed osseous integration of a noncemented component, infection, malposition and malsizing are potential causes of hardware loosening. Typically, a thin fibrous membrane surrounds the component. Loosening is seen on radiographs and CT as a linear radiolucency surrounding the component, typically more than 2 mm wide. In MRI, a hyperintense linear signal surrounding the component may reflect a fibrous membrane. Extensive osteolysis tend to be bulky and lobular rather than linear and may be difficult to detect in the intertrochanteric area of hip arthroplasties due to a considerable reduction of trabecula in aged and osteoporotic patients. A well-defined sclerotic rim enhances the less aggressive appearance of this type of osteolysis in comparison to a primary or secondary malignant bone tumor. The osteolysis may have an expansive character with scalloping of the cortices, best alluded in the metadiaphyseal and diaphyseal region, where the cortex is broader. Smooth periosteal reactions may be accompanied. Polyethylene or metal wear may lead to extensive osteolysis. An immune-mediated reaction with histiocytic foreign body response is activated by particulate debris from wear [3]. Accompanying synovitis may break through the joint capsule into the surrounding soft tissue and forming a cystic or solid mass, which is referred to a pseudotumor (Fig. 1) [8]. A pseudotumor may compress

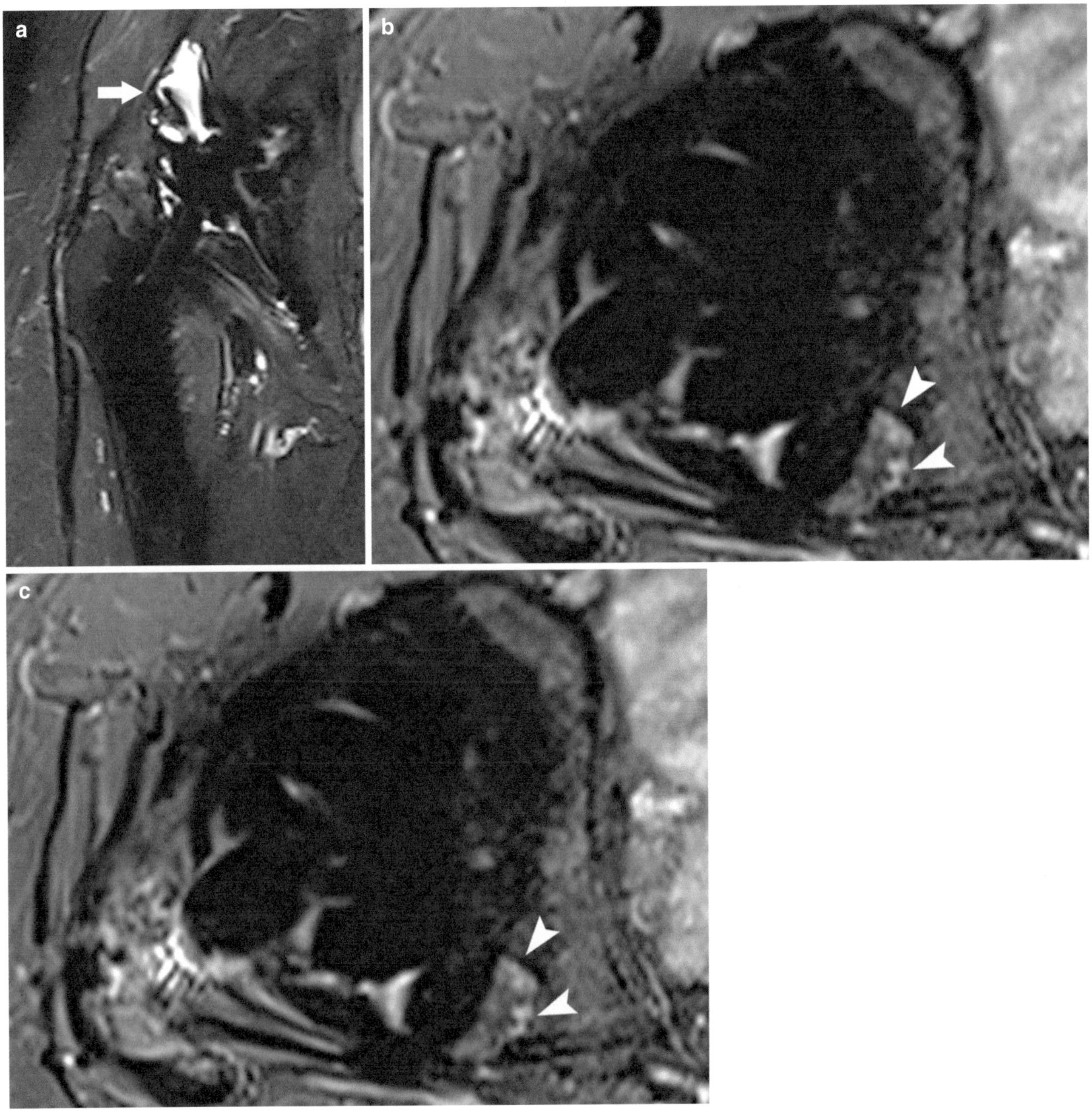

Fig. 1 55-year old female with painful total hip arthroplasty. MRI of the right hip reveals a cyst-like collection in the periarticular soft tissue (*arrow* in **a**), referred to as a pseudotumor. A periprosthetic osteolysis (*arrowheads* in **b** and **c**) with hypointense signal in the axial fluid-sensitive sequence (TIRM WARP; **b**) is evident and consistent with a focal loosening due to wear

neurovascular structures in close proximity to the joint. In patients with severe metal wear, pseudotumors may have focal or diffuse hypointense areas on all sequences due to metal depositions. The presence of a pseudotumor is not necessarily associated with symptoms. Chang et al. [8] reported a high frequency of pseudotumor with 65% in asymptomatic hip arthroplasty patients.

SPECT/CT has the potential benefit of providing structural and metabolic information in periprosthetic loosening. An increased bone tracer uptake surrounding the component reflects loosening. Typical bone tracer uptake patterns are described in patients with total knee arthroplasty (TKA) loosening [9]. Femoral loosening is associated with an increased uptake in the lateral and medial posterior femur, tibial loosening below the tibial TKA and around the stem and tibial pegs [9]. However, often, the increased uptake is only focal and has to be differentiated from other causes, such as malposition, malalignment or even postoperative remodeling of the metal-bone or cement-bone interface. Osteolysis typically show a rim enhancing bone tracer uptake, the central parts are non-enhancing. A small focal osteolysis does not necessarily reflect a loose component, especially if the fixation area of the prosthesis is unremarkable. Care should be taken in the region of the acetabular cup in hip arthroplasties, as large preoperative subchondral cysts may partly remain. In some cases, subsidence of a component may be the only sign for loosening. In any case, comparison with previous examinations are most valuable and will confirm imaging findings.

Malposition and Malsizing

Malposition and malsizing may often be imperceptible, for both, the radiologist and the surgeon and predispose to loosening. As a rule of thumb any arthroplastic component should fit tightly into the osteotomized bone. Familiarity with the type of arthroplasty is crucial for the detection of malsizing and malposition. Malposition of a knee prosthesis can occur in six different degrees of freedom, including flexion, extension, varus, valgus, internal and external rotation. It has been recently shown that flexed and/or internally rotated femoral components of a TKA are seen in symptomatic patients [2]. The various types and usually low degree of malposition require accurate measurement methods, which cannot be precisely addressed on radiographs. However, radiographs provide a first impression and facilitate a comparison with previous images. For knee arthroplasties, the Berger method is a common measurement for rotational alignment [10]. On axial CT images, the femoral component is measured in relation to the epicondylar axis with normal values of 3° (anatomical axis) or 0° (surgical axis) internal rotation. The tibial component is measured in relation to the midpoint of the tibial tuberosity with a normal value of 18° ± 2.6 internal rotation. These measurements on axial images have a wide variability and only address the rotational alignment [11]. Measurements on 3D reconstructed CT images using specialized software yields highly reliable values and is significantly better than axial CT images alone [11]. In particular, all six directions can be addressed with this technique. The full-leg alignment can be measured with additional scans of the hip and ankle joints [12]. SPECT/CT is superior in the assessment of potential malposition of arthroplasties as the degree of malposition can be measured with the CT data and a malposition may demonstrate an increased bone tracer uptake. Flexion of the femoral TKA component typically shows an increased uptake in the region of the posteromedial femur and at the proximal patellar. An internal rotation of the femoral TKA component leads to patellofemoral overloading with an increased bone tracer uptake at the lateral patellar facet and at the posterolateral femur with a lateral lift-off of the femoral condyle from the polyethylene inlay, called mid-flexion instability (Fig. 2) [2, 9]. External rotation of the femoral TKA component shows increased uptake in the posteromedial and posterolateral femur and at the medial patellar facet [9]. An increased posterior tibial slope may show an increased uptake at the posterolateral tibia (Fig. 3). A varus malaligned tibial component typically shows an increased uptake adjacent to the lateral tibial component, a valgus malaligned component on the medial side. Accompanying new bone formation, which is referred to stress-shielding, and in a later stage osteolysis and component subsidence may appear. Values for an optimal TKA position have been reported, however, the range of the position is accepted by each patient individually and does not necessarily account for the patients` symptoms [2].

In hip arthroplasties, radiographic follow ups have the advantage of including the opposite hip on the anteroposterior image for comparison of the leg length and the offset. A small head or an increased ante- or retroversion of the femoral component in hip arthroplasties are prone to dislocation. The anteversion of the femoral stem and the acetabular cup can be measured on axial radiographs or on axial cross sectional images, normal values range for each measurement between 10° and 30° [13, 14]. The tip of the femoral stem is ideally centered in the shaft. Varus or valgus malaligned femoral stems may lead to early loosening (Fig. 4). Retroversion of the acetabular component or an anterior overlap are risk factors for iliopsoas tendinopathy with consistent tendon tearing.

MRI plays a minor role in the assessment of malposition and malsizing in arthroplasties, as the outline of components are not well delineated and the degree of malposition is often very small. Bone marrow edema and cystic changes adjacent to the components may be the only visible sign in a case of malposition.

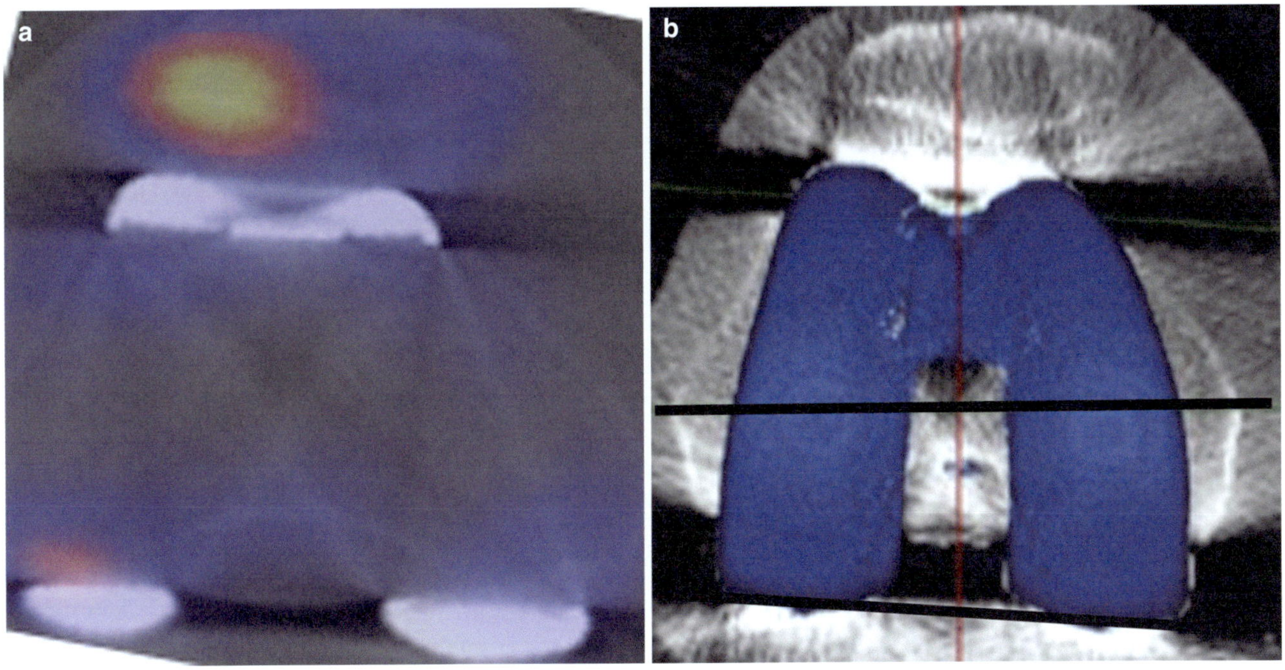

Fig. 2 72-year old female with persistent pain 2 years after total knee arthroplasty. Axial image of the SPECT/CT (**a**) shows increased bone tracer uptake in the lateral patellar facet and posterolateral femur. Measurement of the femoral component alignment (*black* lines in **b**) reveals an internal rotation of 7° accounting the increased bone tracer uptake

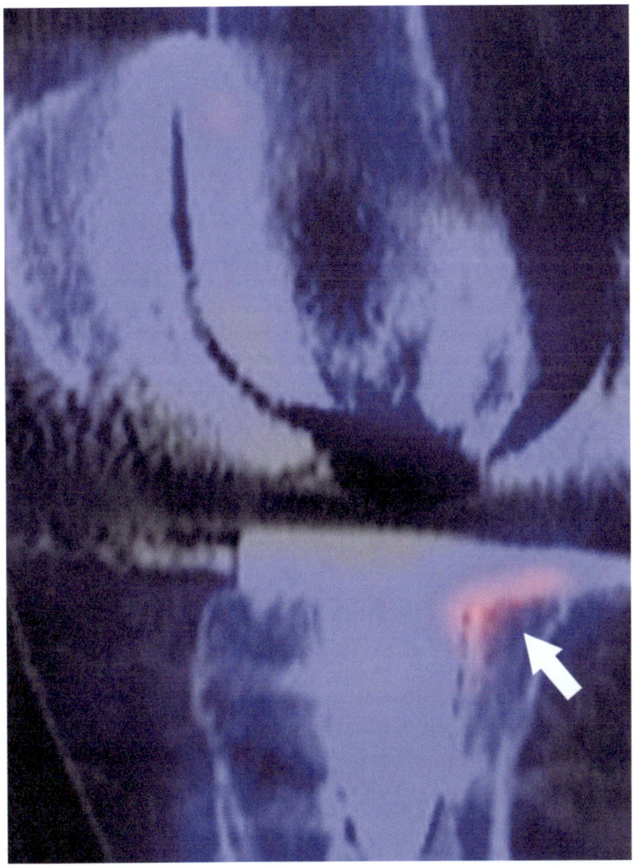

Fig. 3 Sagittal reformatted SPECT/CT image shows an increased bone tracer uptake of the posterior tibia adjacent to the tibial component in a knee arthroplasty due to an increased posterior tibial slope

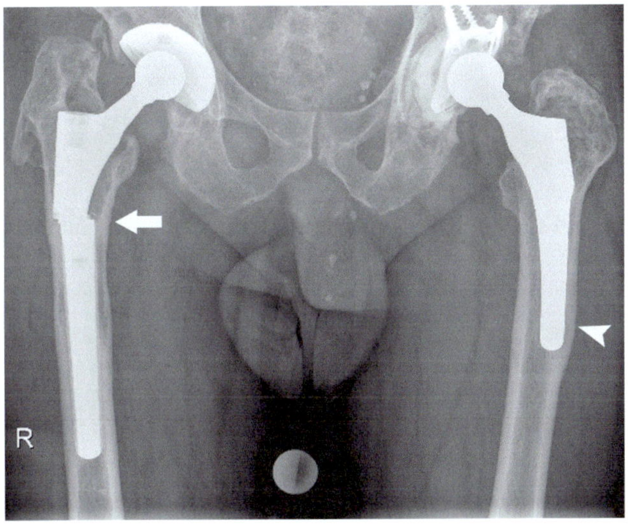

Fig. 4 71-year old male with pain in the right hip. Anteroposterior radiograph reveals a fracture of the femoral component (*arrow*) of the right hip prosthesis and marked periprosthetic osteolysis consistent with component loosening. Varus aligned left femoral component with adjacent stress-shielding of the lateral cortex (*arrowhead*). Note the osteolysis adjacent to the femoral shoulder in the greater trochanter region on the left hip

Instability

Instability after arthroplasty often remains unrecognized. Patients complain of persistent pain, clicking and difficulties while walking. The knee is a complex joint and instability may have various causes. A too thin polyethylene inlay as well as an increased posterior tibial slope in cruciate retaining knee prosthesis may lead to anterior instability. Posterior instability is less common and seen in patients with a torn posterior cruciate ligament in a cruciate retaining prosthesis, in obese patients with hyperlax joints or in patients with a too small femoral component [15]. Varus and valgus instabilities often result in lax or torn collateral ligaments. Clinical and radiological diagnosis of the type and degree of instability remains challenging. Stress radiographs and fluoroscopy are important tools in suspected instabilities, however, up to now, clear threshold values have not been defined. An anteroposterior translation of more than 10 mm is suspicious of a TKA instability [15]. Normal medial and lateral joint space opening during stress examination is below 5° [15]. But again, no diagnostic thresholds have been reported yet, thus, comparison to the contralateral side is mandatory.

Instability after hip arthroplasty is mainly due to insufficiency of the abductor or external rotator tendons or malposition of the components. These tendon insufficiencies may be related to preoperative existing tendon degeneration or the type of surgical access.

MRI may be useful in the evaluation of joint instabilities. The tendons of the hip joint can be well visualized using advanced imaging techniques and may guide therapeutic options. In cruciate retaining TKA, the posterior cruciate ligament should be carefully evaluated in terms of degeneration or tearing. Diagnostics of the medial and lateral collateral ligaments can be challenging, as collateral ligament releases are often performed during surgery, thus, scaring from tearing is often not distinguishable.

SPECT/CT does not play a major role in the evaluation of instabilities, however, certain types of uptake pattern may rise the suspicion for ligament instabilities and have to be further evaluated.

Infection

Infections can be divided into low-grade and high-grade. Early postoperative infections are usually high-grade infections and present in the first weeks after surgery. Radiographs are often unremarkable in this early stage. MRI might be unspecific and findings such as joint effusion, bone marrow and soft tissue edema are difficult to differentiate from reactive changes due to the surgery. Synovitis with a lamellate appearance is a specific finding in these cases [16]. Marked bone tracer uptake in all three phases in SPECT/CT is seen in joint infections, however, a certain differentiation between infection and aseptic loosening is not possible. Antigranulocyte or labelled white blood cell scintigraphies is the current choice for diagnosing periprosthetic infections. However, sensitivity of detecting low-grade infection is low with any imaging modality as well as with laboratory analysis.

Conclusion

Despite imaging modalities have advanced in the past decades, radiographs are still considered the primary imaging modality in the evaluation of painful joints or arthroplasties. Depending on the presumable diagnosis, cross-sectional imaging modalities such as CT and MRI are reasonable. If clinical findings do not correlate with these radiological methods, SPECT/CT may provide additional information. Due to the enhanced understanding of bone tracer uptake pattern in recent years, SPECT/CT has increased in musculoskeletal diagnostics. As a strength, it allows the combination of morphological, structural and functional assessment in patients with painful joints.

References

1. Coupal TM, Mallinson PI, Gershony SL, McLaughlin PD, Munk PL, Nicolaou S et al (2016) Getting the most from your dual-energy scanner: recognizing, reducing, and eliminating artifacts. AJR Am J Roentgenol 206(1):119–128
2. Awengen R, Rasch H, Amsler F, Hirschmann MT (2016) Symptomatic versus asymptomatic knees after bilateral total knee arthroplasty: what is the difference in SPECT/CT? Eur J Nucl Med Mol Imaging 43(4):762–772
3. Burge AJ (2015) Total hip arthroplasty: MR imaging of complications unrelated to metal wear. Semin Musculoskelet Radiol 19(1):31–39
4. Sutter R, Hodek R, Fucentese SF, Nittka M, Pfirrmann CW (2013) Total knee arthroplasty MRI featuring slice-encoding for metal artifact correction: reduction of artifacts for STIR and proton density-weighted sequences. AJR Am J Roentgenol 201(6):1315–1324
5. Fritz J, Lurie B, Potter HG (2015) MR imaging of knee arthroplasty implants. Radiographics 35(5):1483–1501
6. Agten CA, Del Grande F, Fucentese SF, Blatter S, Pfirrmann CW, Sutter R (2015) Unicompartmental knee arthroplasty MRI: impact of slice-encoding for metal artefact correction MRI on image quality, findings and therapy decision. Eur Radiol 25(7):2184–2193
7. Goutallier D, Postel JM, Bernageau J, Lavau L, Voisin MC (1994) Fatty muscle degeneration in cuff ruptures. Pre- and postoperative evaluation by CT scan. Clin Orthop Relat Res 304:78–83
8. Chang EY, McAnally JL, Van Horne JR, Statum S, Wolfson T, Gamst A et al (2012) Metal-on-metal total hip arthroplasty: do symptoms correlate with MR imaging findings? Radiology 265(3):848–857
9. Hirschmann MT, Amsler F, Rasch H (2015) Clinical value of SPECT/CT in the painful total knee arthroplasty (TKA): a prospective study in a consecutive series of 100 TKA. Eur J Nucl Med Mol Imaging 42(12):1869–1882
10. Berger RA, Crossett LS, Jacobs JJ, Rubash HE (1998) Malrotation causing patellofemoral complications after total knee arthroplasty. Clin Orthop Relat Res 356:144–153
11. Hirschmann MT, Konala P, Amsler F, Iranpour F, Friederich NF, Cobb JP (2011) The position and orientation of total knee replacement components: a comparison of conventional radiographs,

transverse 2D-CT slices and 3D-CT reconstruction. J Bone Joint Surg Br 93(5):629–633
12. Hirschmann MT, Konala P, Iranpour F, Kerner A, Rasch H, Friederich NF (2011) Clinical value of SPECT/CT for evaluation of patients with painful knees after total knee arthroplasty—a new dimension of diagnostics? BMC Musculoskelet Disord 12:36
13. Boissonneault AR, Hiranaka T, Roberson JR, Bradbury TL (2017) A validated single-view radiographic alternative to computed tomography for the measurement of femoral anteversion: a method-comparison study. J Arthroplast 32(3):1018–1023
14. Reikeras O, Gunderson RB (2011) Components anteversion in primary cementless THA using straight stem and hemispherical cup: a prospective study in 91 hips using CT-scan measurements. Orthop Traumatol Surg Res 97(6):615–621
15. Hirschmann MT, Becker R, SpringerLink (Online service). The unhappy total knee replacement a comprehensive review and management guide. doi:10.1007/978-3-319-08099-4
16. Li AE, Sneag DB, Greditzer HG, Johnson CC, Miller TT, Potter HG (2016) Total knee arthroplasty: diagnostic accuracy of patterns of Synovitis at MR imaging. Radiology 281(2):499–506

Patterns and Signs in Nuclear Bone and Joint Imaging

Gopinath Gnanasegaran

Introduction

Radionuclide bone scan with 99mTc-MDP is one of the most common nuclear medicine tests used to assess different pathologies relating to bone. Therefore it is important to be aware of various patterns and typical signs while reporting these scans. Increasing knowledge of variants, patterns and signs in nuclear medicine may help in improving the accuracy of clinical reports. Typical patterns and signs will be discussed in the lecture.

Patterns

Pattern recognition is an important aspect in differentiating benign from metastatic disease. On a bone scan, the assessment of tracer uptake within the skull is often challenging. In general, there is low grade tracer uptake in the sutures on a normal bone scan, and it can be more marked in patients with metabolic bone disease [1–3]. Further, increased tracer uptake is often seen at the confluence of sutures, such as at the pterion in the skull, which is a normal variant [1, 2, 4]. Small focal calvarial uptake of tracer is noted in <1% bone scans, which may be due to normal variations such as small cartilaginous rests, sutural foramina, or enlarged pacchionian granulation [5, 6]. Diffuse increased activity in the skull (hot skull), is a normal pattern seen especially in post-menopausal women secondary to post-menopausal hormonal changes in bone metabolism. However, it may also be seen in several other conditions such as hyperparathyroidism, osteomalacia, and post chemotherapy scenarios [7, 8] (Fig. 1). Hyperostosis frontalis interna is seen due to benign irregular thickening of the internal table of the frontal bone in elderly women, which is often seen as diffuse increased uptake in the frontal bone and calvarium on a bone scan [9, 10]. Focal increased uptake in the maxilla or mandible is often seen due to underlying benign dental pathology.

Tracer uptake in the sternum may be variable. A focal area of increased uptake at the angle of Louis is the most common variant on a bone scan. Further, a photon-deficient area above the xiphoid due to sternal foramina and a midline vertical linear area of increased uptake in the sternum are seen in patients who have undergone cardiothoracic surgery with sternotomy (sternal split sign). Occasionally, increased uptake of tracer is seen at the insertion of the iliocostalis thoracis portion of the erector spinae muscles to the ribs (posterior angle of three or more consecutive ribs) known as rib stippling [11] and this should not be confused with sinister malignancy or fractures and caution in interpretation is suggested. In general, multiple foci of tracer uptake throughout the skeleton in a patient with history of cancer are likely to represent widespread skeletal metastases. However, solitary focal uptake is always challenging [12]. The shape of lesions may often help in identifying the etiology, e.g., tracer uptake tracking along the ribs suggests malignant involvement whereas focal increased uptake in multiple ribs in a linear fashion is most likely to be post-traumatic. In general, clinical history of previous trauma or radiotherapy may be useful to may a definitive diagnosis in most cases [1, 2].

Approximately 70% of radiotracer excretion from bone is via the renal system and a focal uptake in a hydrocalyx in the kidney may be confused with uptake in superimposed ribs [1, 2]. Therefore additional oblique image helps in clarifying this potential pitfall. In patients with a renal transplant, ectopic or low lying kidney, one or both kidneys are seen in unusual positions and may be misinterpreted as abnormal uptake in bone [1]. In post-partum females, increased tracer uptake in the pubic symphysis can be seen due to increased stress reaction/pelvic diastases.

The most common site for bone metastases is the spine because of its high vascularisation and presence of red bone marrow [13]. However, this is also a common site for degenerative disease [1]. However, SPECT/CT often provides a unique opportunity combine scintigraphic findings with CT which aids in definitive diagnosis. A common pattern of widespread

G. Gnanasegaran
Department of Nuclear Medicine, Royal Free London NHS Foundation Trust, Pond Street, London NW3 2QG, UK
e-mail: gopinath.gnanasegaran@nhs.net

J. Hodler et al. (eds.), *Musculoskeletal Diseases 2017-2020*, DOI 10.1007/978-3-319-54018-4_26

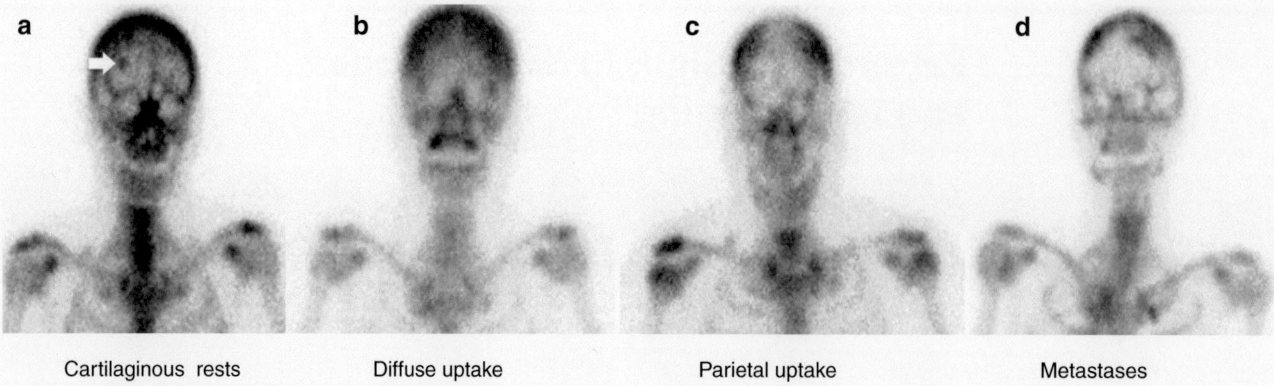

Fig. 1 Different patterns of tracer uptake within the skull on a bone scan: (**a**) Focal tracer uptake may be due to normal variations such as small cartilaginous rests, sutural foramina, or enlarged Pacchionan granulation; (**b**) Diffuse uptake (Hot skull sign) is usually a normal pattern seen usually in post-menopausal women; (**c**) Symmetrical parietal uptake with central photopenia may be seen due to parietal bone thinning; (**d**) Heterogeneous tracer uptake within the skull is usually suggestive of metastases (Image courtesy: Seminars In Nuclear Medicine; Agrawal K, Marafi F, Gnanasegaran G, et al (2015) Pitfalls and limitations of radionuclide planar and hybrid bone imaging. Semin Nucl Med 45(5):347–372)

Table 1 Common reported signs in radionuclide bone imaging [14]

Signs	Diagnosis
Mouse face/Mickey mouse sign	Paget's disease
Pirate sign	Fibrous dysplasia
Abe Lincoln or black beard sign	Paget's disease of mandible
Faint kidney sign	Super scan
Hot patella sign	Non-specific
Tram line/double stripe sign	HPOA
Honda sign	Insufficiency stress fracture involving the pelvis
Yarmulke sign	Paget's disease of skull
Seat belt sign	Rib fractures
Butterfly sign	Thickening of the internal table of the frontal bones
Push up sign	Muscle uptake
Tie sign and striped tie sign	Metabolic bone disease
Saddle sign	Muscle uptake

skeletal metastases in a bone scan is diffuse, generally heterogeneous uptake throughout the skeleton. However, in advanced cases this may present as a "super scan pattern" on a bone scan, which demonstrates markedly increased tracer uptake throughout the whole skeleton with heightened contrast relative to soft tissues and either none or faint tracer activity in the kidneys [1, 2]. A metabolic superscan usually demonstrates more homogeneous distribution of tracer and increased tracer uptake in the skull and long bones unlike a superscan of malignancy.

Signs in Radionuclide Bone Imaging

Nuclear medicine signs have been reported extensively and some specific signs often help in making a definitive diagnosis. Signs is radionuclide bone imaging are briefly described below (Table 1) [14].

References

1. Agrawal K, Marafi F, Gnanasegaran G, Van der Wall H, Fogelman I (2015) Pitfalls and limitations of radionuclide planar and hybrid bone imaging. Semin Nucl Med 45(5):347–372
2. Love C et al (2003) Radionuclide bone imaging: an illustrative review. Radiographics 23:341–358
3. Storey G, Murray IPC (2004) Bone scintigraphy: the procedure and interpretation. In: Ell PJ, Gambhir SS (eds) Nuclear medicine in clinical diagnosis and treatment, vol I, 3rd edn. Churchill Livingstone; Elsevier, New York, NY
4. Gnanasegaran G, Cook G, Adamson K et al (2009) Patterns, variants, artifacts, and pitfalls in conventional radionuclide bone imaging and SPECT/CT. Semin Nucl Med 39:380–395
5. Harbert J, Desai R (1985) Small calvarial bone scan foci—normal variations. J Nucl Med 26:1144–1148
6. Bahk Y-W (ed) (2013) Combined scintigraphic and radiographic diagnosis of bone and joint diseases, 4th edn. Springer, Berlin; New York
7. Ryan PJ, Fogelman I (1997) Bone scintigraphy in metabolic bone disease. Semin Nucl Med 3:291–305
8. Fogelman I, Bessent RG, Cohen HN et al (1980) Skeletal uptake of diphosphonate. Method for prediction of post-menopausal osteoporosis. Lancet 2:667–670
9. She R, Szakacs J (2004) Hyperostosis frontalis interna: case report and review of literature. Ann Clin Lab Sci 34:206–208
10. Senda K, Itoh S (1987) Evaluation of diffusely high uptake by the calvaria in bone scintigraphy. Ann Nucl Med 1:23–26
11. Fink-Bennett D, Johnson J (1986) Stippled ribs: a potential pitfall in bone scan interpretation. J Nucl Med 27:216–218
12. Tumeh SS, Beadle G, Kaplan WD (1985) Clinical significance of solitary rib lesions in patients with extraskeletal malignancy. J Nucl Med 26:1140–1143
13. Even-Sapir E (2005) Imaging of malignant bone involvement by morphologic, scintigraphic, and hybrid modalities. J Nucl Med 47:1356–1367
14. Gnanasegaran G, Sit C, Chen R, Agrawal K, Fogelman I (2015) Interesting signs in nuclear medicine. Semin Nucl Med 45(6):560–590

Pet Imaging of Bone Metastases Using Different Tracers

Einat Even-Sapir

Scintigraphy plays a major role in assessment of malignant bone involvement in cancer patients. Imaging is aimed to identify skeletal involvement as early as possible, to determine the extent of skeletal disease and to monitor response to therapy. Modern scintigraphic systems are integrated with CT. The combined functional-morphological fused data obtained is of clinical relevance for risk stratification detecting complications of bone metastases. Fused data may identify specific disease sites that require attention such as eminent fractures or tumor invasion to the spinal canal with risk for permanent neurologic deficits [1–4].

The concept of personalized medicine in treatment of cancer gave rise to the theranostics paradigm with the assumption that diagnostic test findings can accurately determine whether an individual is likely to benefit from a specific treatment. Nuclear medicine plays an essential role in theranostics by allowing SPECT or PET imaging of labeled molecular targets to assist in selecting patients with scintigraphy-positive disease sites for treatment with the same molecule labeled with high doses of β-emitting tracers [5].

The following chapter describes the role of PET/CT in assessment of malignant skeletal spread using four different PET tracers: ^{18}F-Fluordeoxyglucose (^{18}F-FDG), ^{68}Ga-Somatostatin and ^{68}Ga-Prostate Specific Membrane Antigen (PSMA). The forth tracer ^{18}F-Fluoride is a bone seeking agent high sensitive for detection of bone pathology either benign or malignant. The chapter also discusses the collaboration of PET imaging and treatment of bone metastases based on the teranostics paradigm.

^{18}F-FDG is the most commonly used PET tracer for imaging of various oncologic diseases. ^{68}Ga-Somatostatin is used in patients with neuroendocrine tumors and ^{68}Ga-PSMA PET has been recently introduced for imaging of patients with prostate cancer. All three PET tracers are characterized by direct accumulation by viable tumor cells. With this regard, the most prominent advantage of PET imaging with these tracers is that they accumulate in early marrow-based deposits (Figs. 1, 2 and 3). The vast majority of bone metastases initiate as bone marrow deposit of malignant cells. As the lesion enlarges, the surrounding bone undergoes osteoclastic (resorptive) and osteoblastic (depositional) activity and based on the balance between these two processes, lesions may appear radiographicaly as lytic, sclerotic (blastic) or mixed cortical lesions [1, 2, 6]. ^{99m}Tc-MDP bone scintigraphy (BS) and CT identify cortical metastases thus are insensitive for identification of early metastatic skeletal involvement when the tumor is confined to the marrow. The latter can be identified on PET using the tracers that accumulate in the tumor tissue regardless of the cortical accompanying changes [7].

Numerous publications have addressed the role of ^{18}F-FDG PET-CT in staging and follow up of cancer patients. ^{18}F-FDG PET imaging was shown to be superior to BS omitting the need to perform a separate BS for assessment of skeletal disease. In addition to its ability to detect metastasis confined to the marrow component, ^{18}F-FDG-PET is highly sensitive for detection of lytic type cortical metastases characterized by their high rate of glycolysis and hypoxia while BS is relatively insensitive for detection of this type of cortical lesions (Fig. 1a). Although ^{18}F-FDG-PET has been reported appropriate for detecting all types of bone metastases, it is considered to be somewhat less sensitive for detection of blastic type metastases that are considered generally less aggressive. Detection of the latter can be achieved, however, by reviewing the CT data of PET-CT [1–3, 6–8].

In spite of its proven relevance in various oncologic diseases, ^{18}F-FDG-PET/CT has no place in imaging patients with non-FDG avid tumors. Neuroendocrine tumors (NET) and prostate cancer are examples of basically non-FDG avid tumors for which we now have alternative suitable PET tracers. ^{68}Ga-Somatostatin PET-CT is of value for staging and follow-up of patients with the NET showing high-expression

E. Even-Sapir
Department of Nuclear Medicine, Tel Aviv Sourasky Medical Center, Sackler School of Medicine Tel Aviv University, 6 Weizman St, Tel Aviv, Israel
e-mail: evensap@tlvmc.gov.il

J. Hodler et al. (eds.), *Musculoskeletal Diseases 2017-2020*, DOI 10.1007/978-3-319-54018-4_27

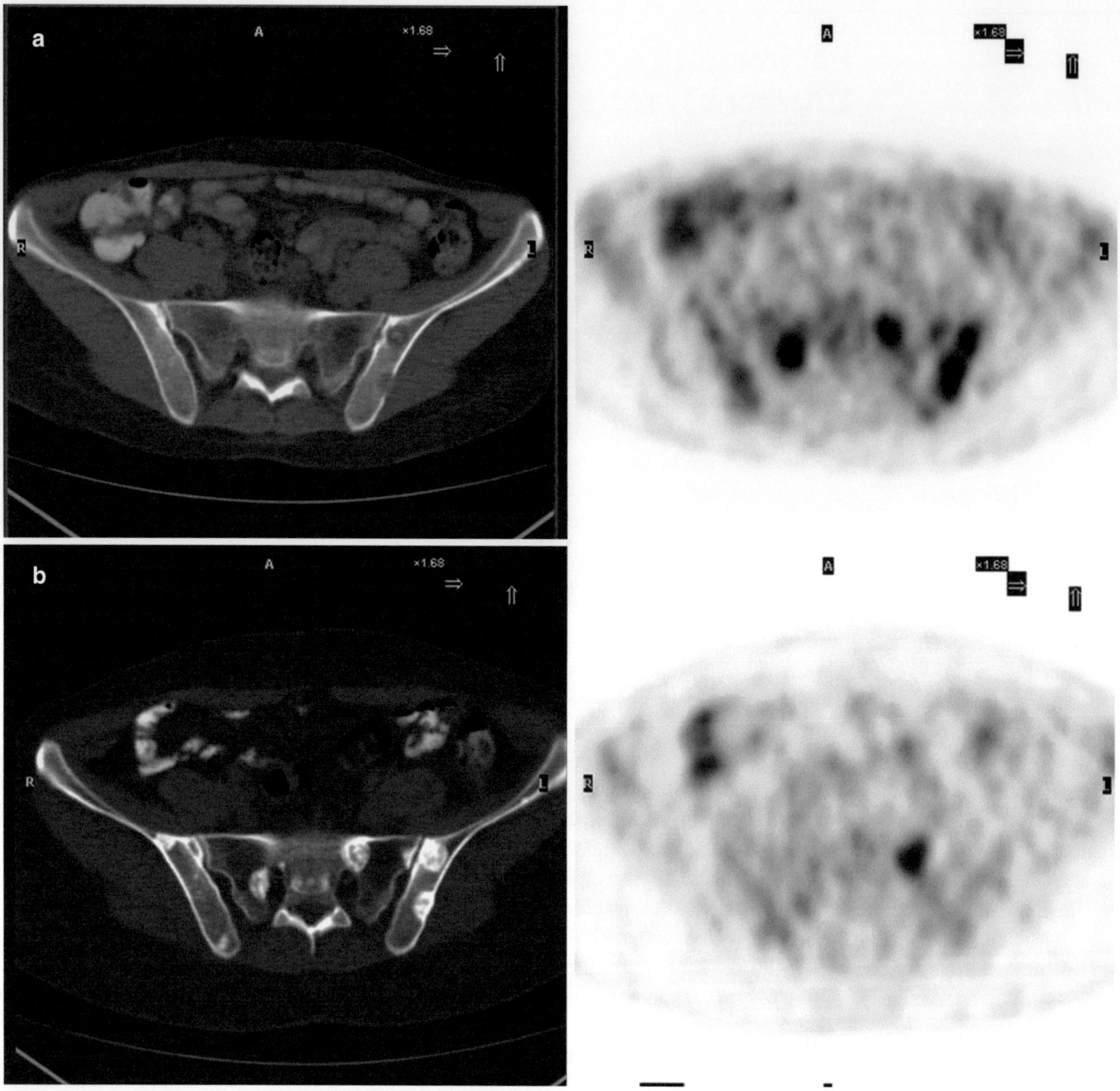

Fig. 1 ^{18}F-FDP identifying lytic and bone-marrow metastases at staging (**a**). After successful therapy the lesions appear sclerotic on CT with no increased uptake except for the lesion in the left sacrum which appears to be active with increased ^{18}F-FDG uptake in spite of the sclerotic changes that indicate repair (**b**)

of Somatostatin receptors. ^{68}Ga is a short lived PET tracer with a half-life of 68 min available from an in house generator of ^{68}Ge with a half-life of 270.8d independent of an onsite cyclotron. Analogues, mostly DOTA-derivatized peptides such as DOTA-Tyr3-octreotide (DOTATOC), show high affinity to Somatostatin receptors with beneficial pharmacokinetic properties. Combined with the better resolution of PET technology, ^{68}Ga-Somatostatin PET was reported to show high performance in assessment of bone involvement (Fig. 2a). It was found to be superior to BS, to CT and to gamma camera imaging with ^{111}In-Somatostatin (SRS). In a study on 89 patients with NET, SPECT STS identified only 72.5% and CT identified only 50% of the skeletal lesions identified by ^{68}Ga-Somatostatin PET [9–11].

PET with PSMA-ligands has gained attention as a promising imaging method in patients with prostate cancer. PSMA is a transmembrane protein with significantly elevated expression in most prostate cancer cells compared to benign prostatic tissue [12]. Comparison of ^{68}Ga-PSMA PET and planar BS for detection of skeletal involvement was the scope of a recently published manuscript. In a cohort of 126 patients with prostate cancer, sensitivity and specificity of PET were 98.7–100% and 88.2–100%, compared to 86.7–89.3% and 60.8–96.1% ($p < 0.001$) for BS, with ranges representing results for 'optimistic' or 'pessimistic' classification of equivocal lesions [13]. It should be noted, however that approximately 8% of prostate cancers do not show PSMA overexpression [14].

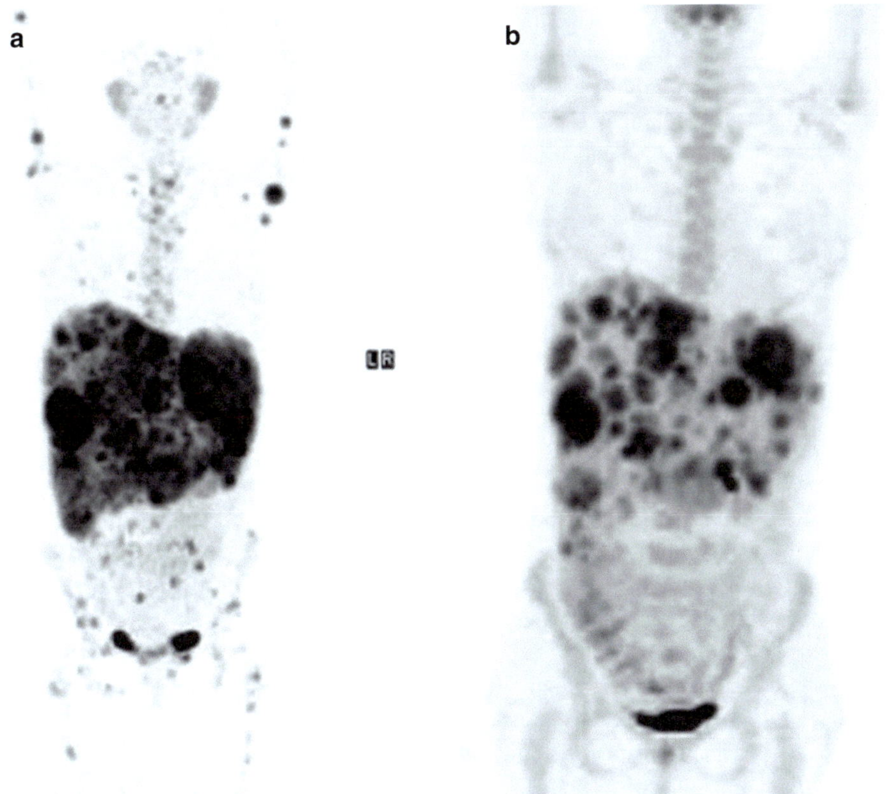

Fig. 2 Metastatic Carcinoid with extensive involvement of liver and bone marrow. ^{68}Ga-Somatostatin before (**a**) and after (**b**) PRRT therapy

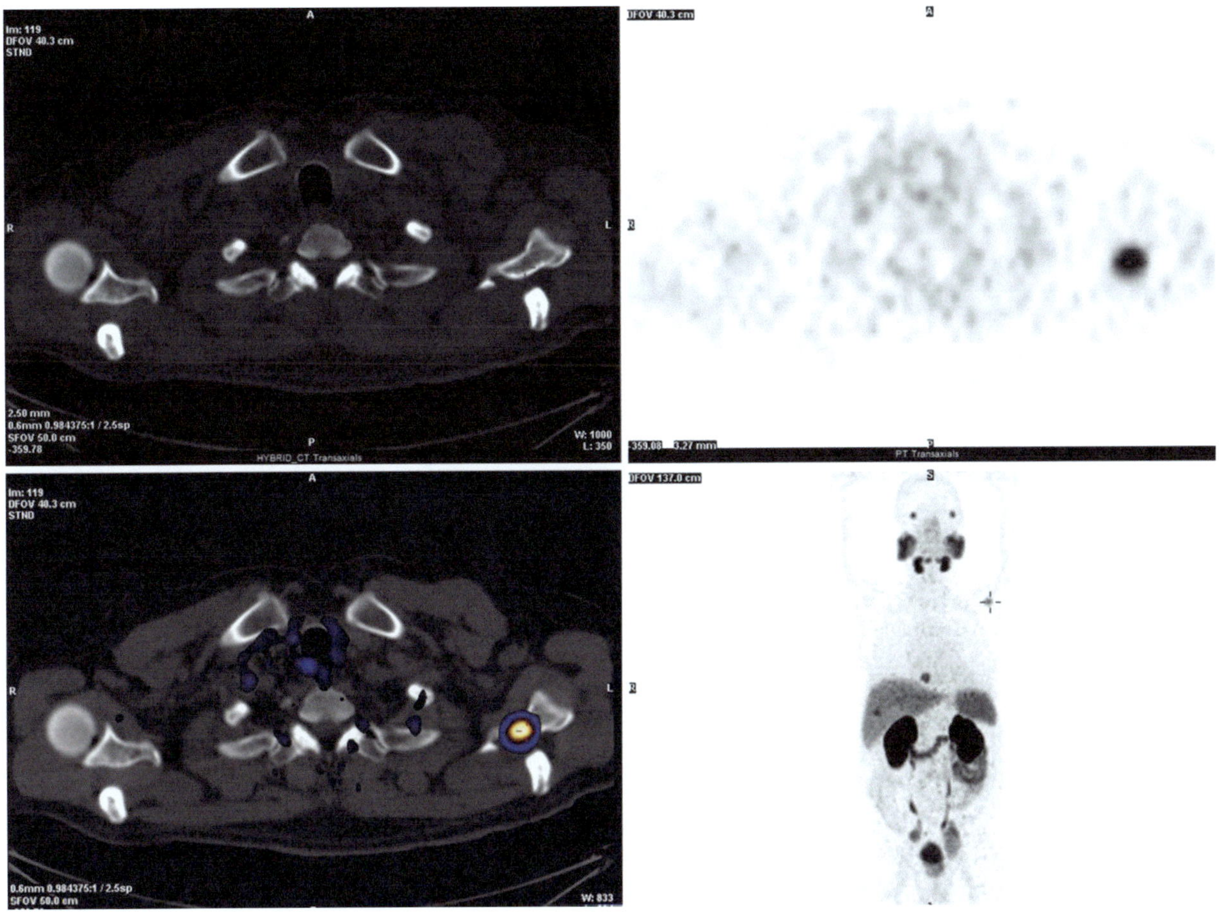

Fig. 3 ^{68}Ga-PSMA PET-CT in a patient with newly diagnosed high-risk prostate cancer identifying early marrow-based bone metastasis in the left scapula with morphological normal bone on CT

Monitoring response of bone metastases to therapy is an on going challenge on follow up imaging. Repair and active tumor may appear similar on BS and on CT, particularly when therapy protocol includes anti-osteoclastic agents such as bisphosphonates which encourage the appearance of sclerotic changes in the healing bone. The latter may remain permanent even when the metastasis is no longer active. ^{18}F-FDG, ^{68}Ga-Somatostatin and ^{68}Ga-PSMA accumulate only in active tumor tissue regardless of its morphologic appearance thus PET using these tracers can assist in separating repair of bone and active bone metastasis (Fig. 1b). Sequential ^{18}F-FDG PET-CT studies performed in patients with breast cancer have shown that ^{18}F-FDG uptake reflects the immediate tumor activity of bone metastases. Response is associated with decrease in intensity of uptake [15, 16]. Similarly, in NET, response of bone metastases after treatment can be evaluated efficiently by SRS or ^{68}Ga-Somatostatin PET (Fig. 2) [13, 14].

Same ligands of Somatostatin and of PSMA can be labeled with either ^{68}Ga for imaging purposes or with ^{177}Lu for therapy following the theranostics paradigm [17]. ^{177}Lu-Somatostatin has been the first of the two to be used starting in the early 1990s. Lessons learned from the studies on treatment of metastatic NETs were that bone marrow suppression, and even myelodysplastic syndrome may be a side effect in patients treated with high dosages of >100 GBq (>3 Gy bone marrow radiation dose), therefore radiation dosimetry after each therapy is essential for individual optimization of future doses [18, 19]. However it should be noted that bone marrow involvement by itself is effectively controlled by PRRT, with long progression-free survival and overall survival [20].

Clinical data on the role of ^{177}Lu-PSMA for treatment of patients with metastatic prostate cancer is being accumulated. It appears that this mode of therapy is effective and safe in patients that are appropriately selected [21]. Diffuse bone marrow involvement is a risk factor for significant myelosuppression but could be identified by ^{68}GA PSMA imaging in advance [22]. It has been shown that as high as 58% with bone metastases treated with ^{177}Lu-PSMA report reduction in bone pain [23].

The forth PET tracer that can be used for assessment of skeletal bone involvement is ^{18}F-Fluoride. In contrast with the three earlier discussed tracers that accumulate directly in the tumor tissue, ^{18}F-Fluoride is a PET bone-seeking agent with uptake mechanism similar to that of ^{99m}Tc-MDP. Fluoride ions exchange with hydroxyl groups in hydroxyapetite crystal bone to form fluoroapatite, and are deposited at the bone surface where bone turnover is greatest. Similarly to ^{99m}Tc-MDP, accumulation of ^{18}F-Fluoride uptake in bone metastases reflects increased regional blood flow and high bone turnover, secondary changes occurring in bone as reaction to the presence of tumor cells. ^{18}F-Fluoride has better pharmacokinetic characteristics compared to those of ^{99m}Tc-MDP. The bone uptake of the former is two-fold higher, in contrast with ^{99m}Tc-MDP it does not bind to protein. The capillary permeability of ^{18}F-Fluoride is higher and its blood clearance is faster resulting in a better target- to-background ratio. Regional plasma clearance of ^{18}F-Fluoride was reported to be 3–10 times higher in bone metastases compared with that in normal bone [7, 24].

^{18}F-Fluoride-PET is very sensitive for detection of not only osteoblastic metastases but also of lytic ones, as the latter even when considered "pure lytic", do have minimal osteoblastic activity which is enough for detection by ^{18}F-Fluoride-PET. It should be borne in mind that ^{18}F-Fluoride is not tumor specific and therefore is a sensitive modality for detection of any bone abnormalities, not only malignant.

When interpreting ^{18}F-Fluoride-PET-CT for assessment of metastatic skeletal spread, the morphologic appearance of the bone should be carefully considered on the CT data for accurate separation of benign and malignant sites of ^{18}F-Fluoride uptake [25–28].

References

1. Cook GJ, Fogelman I (2001) The role of positron emission tomography in skeletal disease. Semin Nucl Med 31:50–61
2. Even-Sapir E (2005) Imaging of malignant bone involvement by morphologic, scintigraphic, and hybrid modalities. J Nucl Med 46:1356–1367
3. Taira AV, Herfkens RJ, Gambhir SS et al (2007) Detection of bone metastases: assessment of integrated FDG PET/CT imaging. Radiology 243:204–211
4. Metser U, Lerman H, Blank A et al (2004) Malignant involvement of the spine: assessment by ^{18}FFDG PET/CT. J Nucl Med 45:279–284
5. Taïeb D, Hicks RJ, Pacak K (2016) Nuclear medicine in cancer theranostics: beyond the target. J Nucl Med 57(11):1659–1660
6. Hamaoka T, Madewell JE, Podoloff DA et al (2004) Bone imaging in metastatic breast cancer. J Clin Oncol 22:2942–2953
7. Grant FD, Fahey FH, Packard AB et al (2008) Skeletal PET with ^{18}F-fluoride: applying new technology to an old tracer. J Nucl Med 49:68–78
8. Cook GJR, Houston S, Rubens R et al (1998) Detection of bone metastases in breast cancer by ^{18}FDG PET: differing metabolic activity in osteoblastic and osteolytic lesions. J Clin Oncol 16(10):3375–3379
9. Maecke HR, Hofmann M, Haberkorn U (2005) 68 Ga-labeled peptides in tumor imaging. J Nucl Med 46(1):172S–175S
10. Putzer D, Gabriel M, Henninger B et al (2009) Bone metastases in patients with neuroendocrine tumor: ^{68}Ga-DOTA-Tyr3-octreotide PET in comparison to CT and bone scintigraphy. J Nucl Med 50(8):1214–1221
11. Gabriel M, Decristoforo C, Kendler D et al (2007) ^{68}Ga-DOTA-Tyr3-octreotide PET in neuroendocrine tumors: comparison with somatostatin receptor scintigraphy and CT. J Nucl Med 48: 508–518
12. Rauscher I, Maurer T, Fendler WP et al (2016) ^{68}Ga-PSMA ligand PET/CT in patients with prostate cancer: how we review and report. Cancer Imaging 16(1):14
13. Pyka T, Okamoto S, Dahlbender M et al (2016) Comparison of bone scintigraphy and ^{68}Ga-PSMA PET for skeletal staging in prostate cancer. Eur J Nucl Med Mol Imaging 43(12):2114–2121
14. Maurer T, Gschwend JE, Rauscher I et al (2016) Diagnostic efficacy of gallium-PSMA positron emission tomography compared to

conventional imaging in lymph node staging of 130 consecutive patients with intermediate to high risk prostate cancer. J Urol 195(5):1436–1443

15. Du Y, Cullum I, Illidge TM et al (2007) Fusion of metabolic function and morphology: sequential [18F]fluorodeoxyglucose positron-emission tomography/computed tomography studies yield new insights into the natural history of bone metastases in breast cancer. J Clin Oncol 25(23):3440–3447
16. Katayama T, Kubota K, Machida Y et al (2012) Evaluation of sequential FDG-PET/CT for monitoring bone metastasis of breast cancer during therapy: correlation between morphological and metabolic changes with tumor markers. Ann Nucl Med 26:426–435
17. Weineisen M, Schottelius M, Simecek J et al (2015) ^{68}Ga- and 177Lu-labeled PSMA I&T: optimization of a PSMA-targeted theranostic concept and first proof-of-concept human studies. J Nucl Med 56(8):1169–1176
18. Forrer F, Krenning EP, Kooij PP et al (2009) Bone marrow dosimetry in peptide receptor radionuclide therapy with [177Lu-DOTA(0),Tyr(3)] octreotate. Eur J Nucl Med Mol Imaging 36(7):1138–1146
19. Kam BL, Teunissen JJ, Krenning EP et al (2012) Lutetium-labelled peptides for therapy of neuroendocrine tumours. Eur J Nucl Med Mol Imaging 39(Suppl 1):S103–S112
20. Ezziddin S, Sabet A, Heinemann F et al (2011) Response and long-term control of bone metastases after peptide receptor radionuclide therapy with 177Lu-octreotate. J Nucl Med 52:1197–1203
21. Baum RP, Kulkarni HR, Schuchardt C et al (2016) 177Lu-labeled prostate-specific membrane antigen Radioligand therapy of metastatic castration-resistant prostate cancer: safety and efficacy. J Nucl Med 57(7):1006–1013
22. Heck MM, Retz M, D'Alessandria C et al (2016) Systemic Radioligand therapy with (177)Lu labeled prostate specific membrane antigen ligand for imaging and therapy in patients with metastatic castration resistant prostate cancer. J Urol 196(2):382–391
23. Kratochwil C, Giesel FL, Stefanova M et al (2016) PSMA-targeted radionuclide therapy of metastatic castration-resistant prostate cancer with 177Lu-labeled PSMA-617. J Nucl Med 57(8):1170–1176
24. Blake GM, Park-Holohan SJ, Cook GJR et al (2001) Quantitative studies of bone with the use of ^{18}F-fluoride and 99mTc-methylene diphosphonate. Semin Nucl Med 31:28–49
25. Even-Sapir E, Metser U, Flusser G et al (2004) Assessment of malignant skeletal disease: initial experience with ^{18}F-fluoride PET/CT and comparison between ^{18}F-fluoride PET and ^{18}F-fluoride PET/CT. J Nucl Med 45:272–278
26. Even-Sapir E, Metser U, Mishani E et al (2006) The detection of bone metastases in patients with high risk prostate cancer: 99mTc MDP planar bone scintigraphy, single and multi field of view SPECT, ^{18}F-fluoride PET and ^{18}F-fluoride PET/CT. J Nucl Med 47:287–297
27. Bortot DC, Amorim BJ, Oki GC, Gapski SB et al (2012) ^{18}F-fluoride PET/CT is highly effective for excluding bone metastases even in patients with equivocal bone scintigraphy. Eur J Nucl Med Mol Imaging 39:1730–1736
28. Even-Sapir E (2014) ^{18}F-fluoride PET/computed tomography imaging. PET Clin 9(3):277–285
29. Cook GJR (2010) PET and PET/CT imaging of skeletal metastases. Cancer Imaging 10:153–160

Pitfalls in Planar and Hybrid Bone and Joint Imaging

Klaus Strobel

Introduction

A big variety of different nuclear medicine imaging modalities are increasingly used to diagnose bone and joint disorders: planar bone scan, leucocyte and antigranulocyte scintigraphy, SPECT and SPECT/CT, FDG-, Fluoride-, Choline-, PSMA-PET/CT and others. Tumors, infection/inflammation, trauma and degenerative diseases are the main reasons to perform nuclear medicine bone and joint imaging. It is crucial to be aware of the various technical, radiopharmaceutical and patient related artifacts that can occur and might lead to misinterpretation. Additionally, uptake in benign tumors, osteoarthritis, inflammation and infection can lead to false positive findings. The following article summarizes potential pitfalls in nuclear medicine bone and joint imaging.

Artifacts

Instrument related artefacts can be false positive photopenic areas due to photomultiplier tube defects or noisy images due to inproper photopeak window settings. Arterial injection (Fig. 1) leads to increased uptake in the upper distal extremity and might imitate inflammatory disease.

Paravasation of radiotracer at the injection site may lead to hot spots that may mask pathologic uptake and might lead to "sentinel nodes" in the axilla (Fig. 2).

Injection through central venous catheter might lead to retention of activity in the plastic tube. Patient movement can lead to false positive and false negative findings by summation or masking of tracer uptake (Fig. 3).

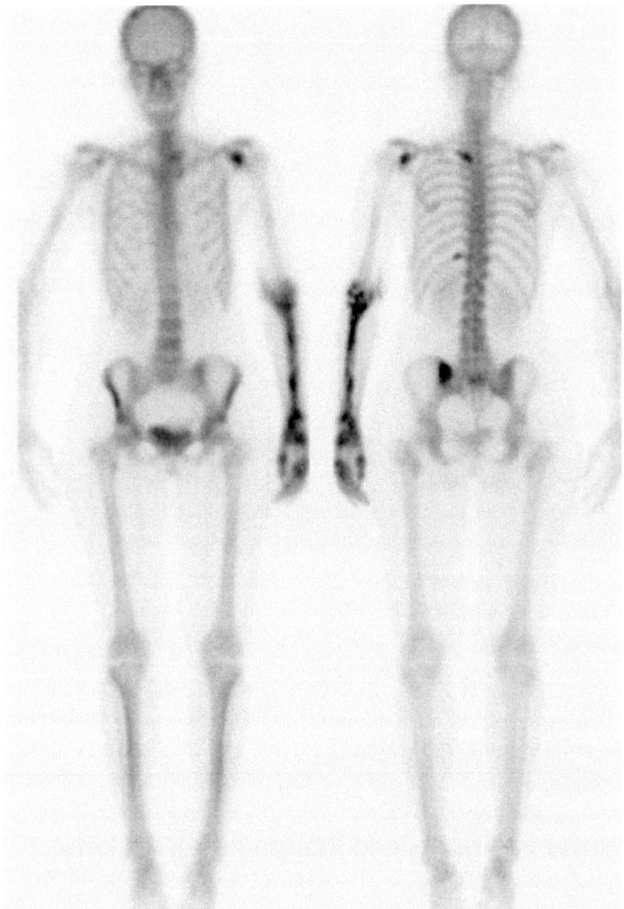

Fig. 1 Patient for breast cancer staging. Besides multiple metastases (scapula, pelvis, spine) the increased uptake in the distal upper extremity is caused by intraarterial radiotracer injection

K. Strobel
Radiologie und Nuklearmedizin, Luzerner Kantonsspital, Spitalstrasse, Luzern, Switzerland
e-mail: klaus.strobel@luks.ch

J. Hodler et al. (eds.), *Musculoskeletal Diseases 2017-2020*, DOI 10.1007/978-3-319-54018-4_28

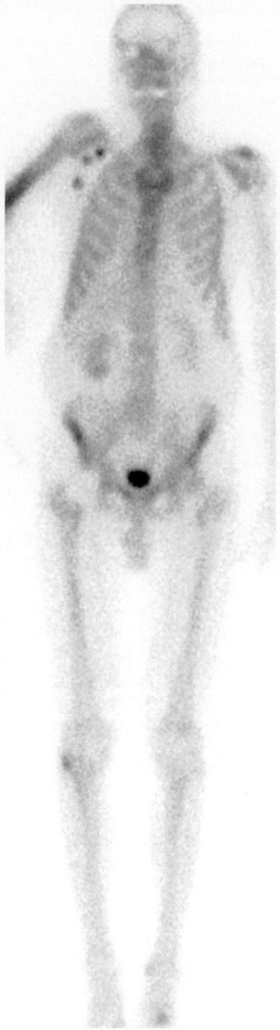

Fig. 2 Patient for prostate cancer staging. No metastases visible. Three focal uptakes in the right axilla representing "sentinel nodes" due to paravasation of radiotracer at the right elbow injection site

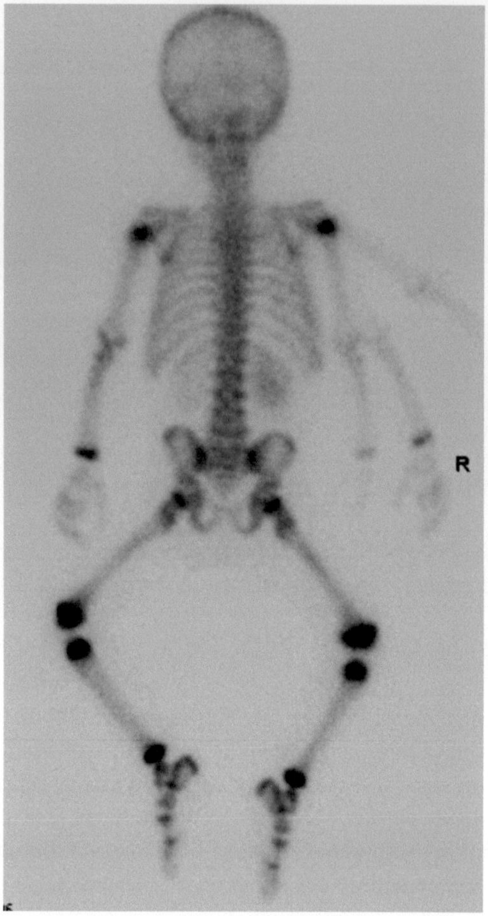

Fig. 3 Posterior planar bone scan in a child for sarcoma staging. Threefold visibility of the right arm due to patient movement

Contamination with urine is a relative common cause of uptake in the pelvis and can be avoided by removal of underwear (Fig. 4). If contamination is suspected cleaning and repetition of spot images or SPECT/CT can be obtained to avoid misinterpretation.

Normal Variants and Benign Pitfall Lesions

Focal uptake in the skull in tumor staging bone scans is often visible and might represent benign incidentally detected lesions like meningioma, osteoma or fibrous dysplasia [1] (Fig. 5).

Increased uptake in the frontal skull is often related to hyperostosis frontalis interna [2]. The typical appearance of these skull lesions in diagnostic CT enables to rule out metastasis in most cases by performing a dedicated SPECT/CT. Increased focal uptake in the jaw is regularly seen on bone scans and FDG PET/CT and most likely represents inflammatory lesions with dental origin or healing processes after dental interventions. Typical sternal midline longitudinal uptake in bone scan and FDG PET/CT is related to

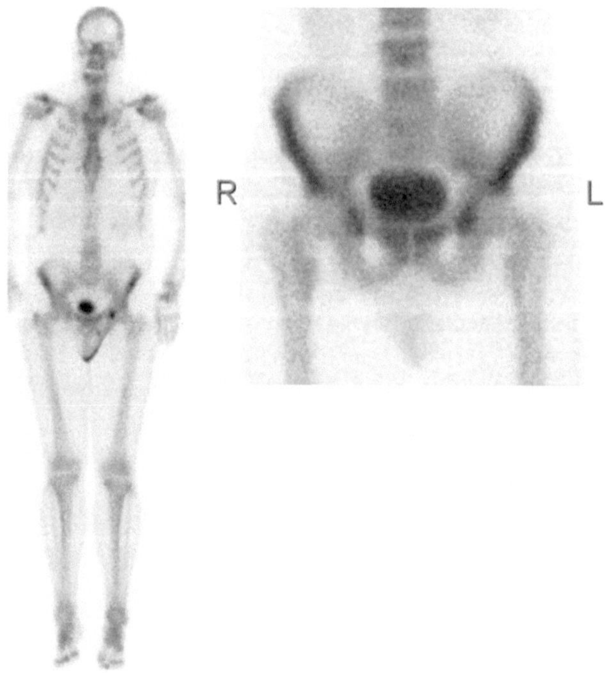

Fig. 4 Patient for prostate cancer staging with focal uptake in the left pelvis. Spot image after removal of underwear confirms urine contamination and excludes metastasis

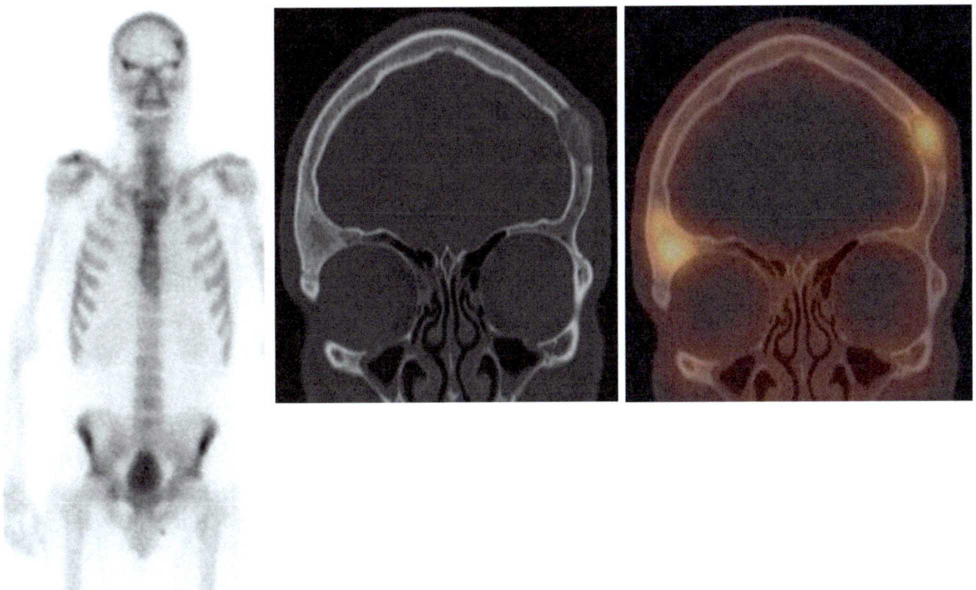

Fig. 5 Patient for prostate cancer staging with incidental uptake in two skull lesions on planar images. SPECT/CT shows typical appearance of fibrous dysplasia (*right side*) and hemangioma (*left side*)

patients after sternotomy due to cardiothoracic surgery. Some uptake in the manubriosternal synchondrosis ist regularly seen in asymptomatic patients and should not be misinterpreted for inflammation or metastasis [3]. The majority of rib lesions on bone scans and to a lesser extent in FDG PET/CT is not caused by metastases but by trauma or benign lesions like enchondroma or fibrous dysplasia. If the clinical history and pattern of uptake is unspecific SPECT/CT can add important information by showing fractures, osteolysis or osteoblastic rib lesions.

While most tracers are excreted through the renal system, pathologies in the urinary tract and urine contamination can lead to various pitfalls like bladder diverticulum, urinoma and renal concrements [4] (Fig. 6).

In children uptake in the physeal and apophyseal growth centers of the long bones is a normal finding in bone scans. Physiologic uptake in the ischiopubic synchondrosis in children should not be mistaken for osteomyelitis, tumor or trauma. Additional x-rays or MR—in doubtful cases—can help to provide the correct diagnosis. Increased uptake at the insertion or origin side of tendons like at ischiac bone (ischiocrural muscle), pubic bone and femur (adductor muscles), ribs (pectoralis muscle), humeral head (deltoid muscle), greater trochanter (abductor muscles), greater tuberculum (supraspinatus muscle) might represent physiologic uptake or enthesopathy and should not be mistaken for metastases [5]. Incidental uptake in the spine in tumor patients is regularly seen and often related to degenerative lesions, especially in the cervical and lumbar spine. If the scintigraphic pattern is unspecific additional imaging with conventional x-rays or SPECT/CT are able to clarify the lesions in the majority of cases [6, 7].

Regarding staging of tumor patients with bone scintigraphy one should be aware of the pitfall, that aggressive osteolytic bone metastases—like in breast cancer—might be invisible due to the absence of osteoblastic tumor components (Fig. 7).

In these cases FDG PET/CT will show intensive uptake. On the other hand FDG PET/CT might show no uptake at all in osteoblastic metastases [8, 9].

Increasing or even new active lesions in the skeleton in tumor patients under systemic therapy, especially some months after initiation of hormonal treatment of prostate cancer metastases should not be interpreted as progression until confirmed by 3 month follow up imaging. This well known "flare phenomenon", which represents healing processes and occurs typically 3–6 months after starting a systemic therapy, might be a sign of good therapy response [10]. In fluoride PET/CT even small degenerative lesions lead to a high lesions to background ratio, so interpretation of active lesions in fluoride PET/CT should always be matched with the underlying morphology in CT to avoid overdiagnosis of bone metastases [11].

FDG uptake in PET/CT studies is not tumor specific. There are various benign tumors which can cause increased FDG uptake in the bone like giant cell tumor, osteoblastoma or fibrous dysplasia [12–14]. On the other hand low grade malignant tumors like chondrosarcoma can have low or no FDG uptake. Incidentally detected focal FDG uptake around the knee with relationship to the synovia might represent giant cell tumor of the tendon sheath or pigmented villonodular synovitis, which can be confirmed with MR or biopsy (Fig. 8) [15].

Uptake in bone scintigraphy or FDG PET/CT around joint arthroplasty in tumour patients is regularly visible and

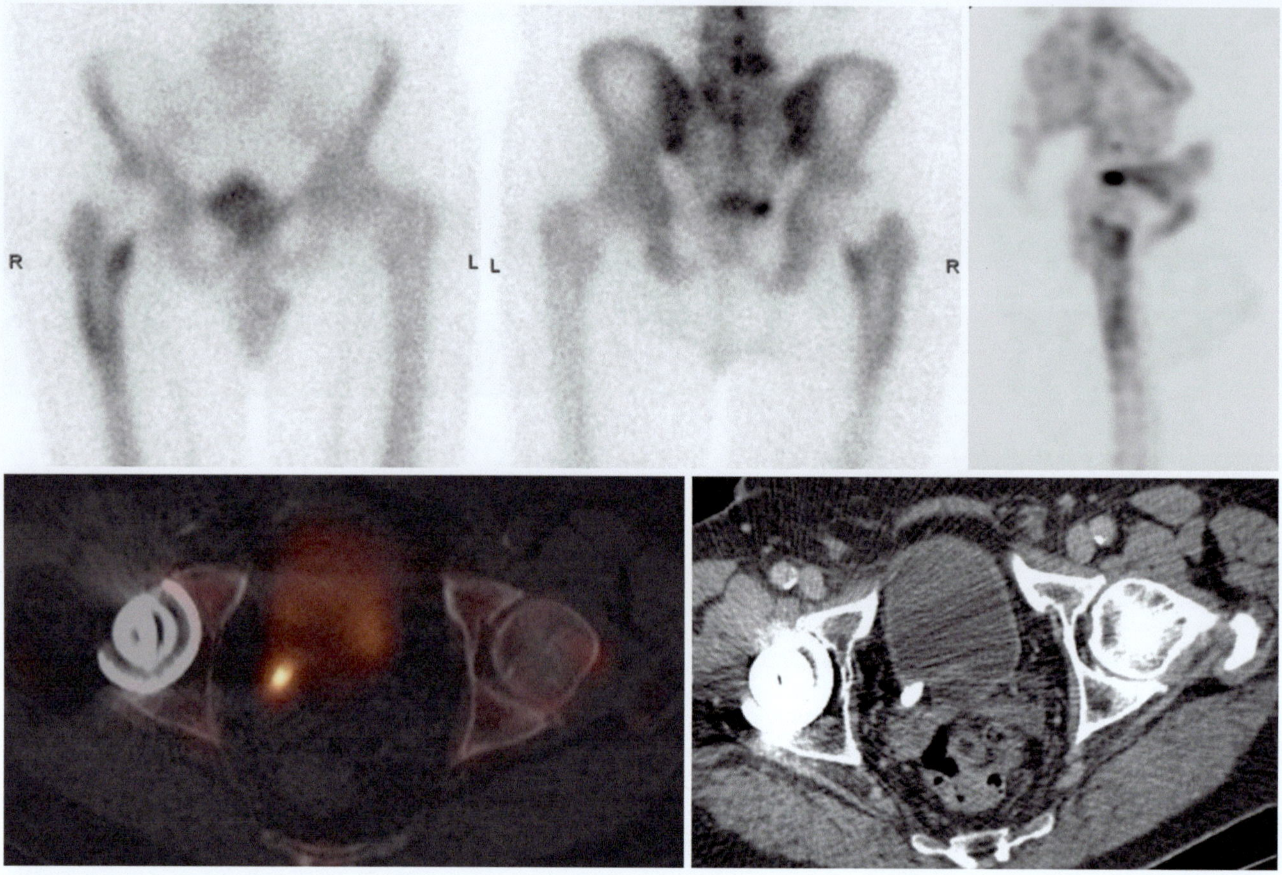

Fig. 6 Patient for prostate cancer staging with focal increased uptake in the right pelvis. Lateral spot image shows that the uptake is probably not in the bone. SPECT/CT comfirms uptake in a distal ureter concrement

often represents physiological inflammation without any clinical importance.

Postoperative Intervention Related Pitfalls

Bone and joint interventions can lead to increased bone seeking tracer or FDG uptake. For the interpretation of hip and knee joint arthroplasty timepoint of joint replacement should be considered for interpretation because physiological uptake due to integration of the foreign body material, especially in uncemented arthroplasties, might take up to 2 years time in the hip and three in the knee [16]. Implantation of bone substitute material like blocks of ceramic made of hydroxyapatite and tricalcium phosphate can cause significant physiologic uptake in bone scans [17]. Even bone marrow biopsies, sometimes performed before FDG PET/CT lymphoma staging might be responsible for some faint uptake in the iliac crest.

Conclusion

There is a wide range of pitfalls in nuclear medicine planar and hybrid bone and joint imaging. Knowledge of patients history, previous treatment and interventions, uptake patterns and CT morphology is crucial for adequate interpretation and prevention of misdiagnosis. For further reading I recommend the article of Agrawal et al. where all pitfalls are systematically summarized and explained [18].

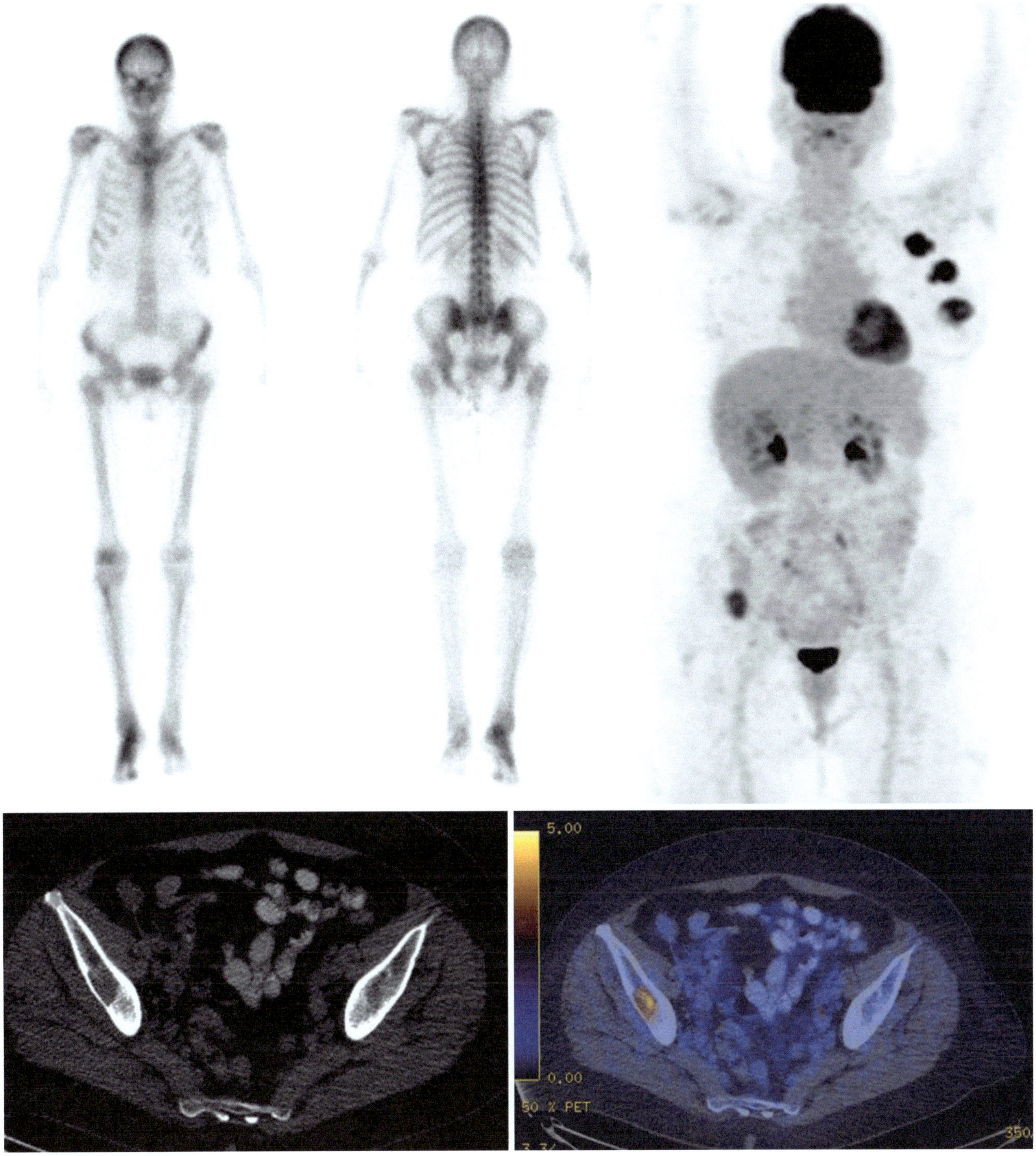

Fig. 7 Patient with breast cancer and normal bone scan. FDG PET/CT shows pathologic FDG uptake in an osteolytic bone metastasis in the right iliac bone and multiple active lymph node metastases in the left axilla

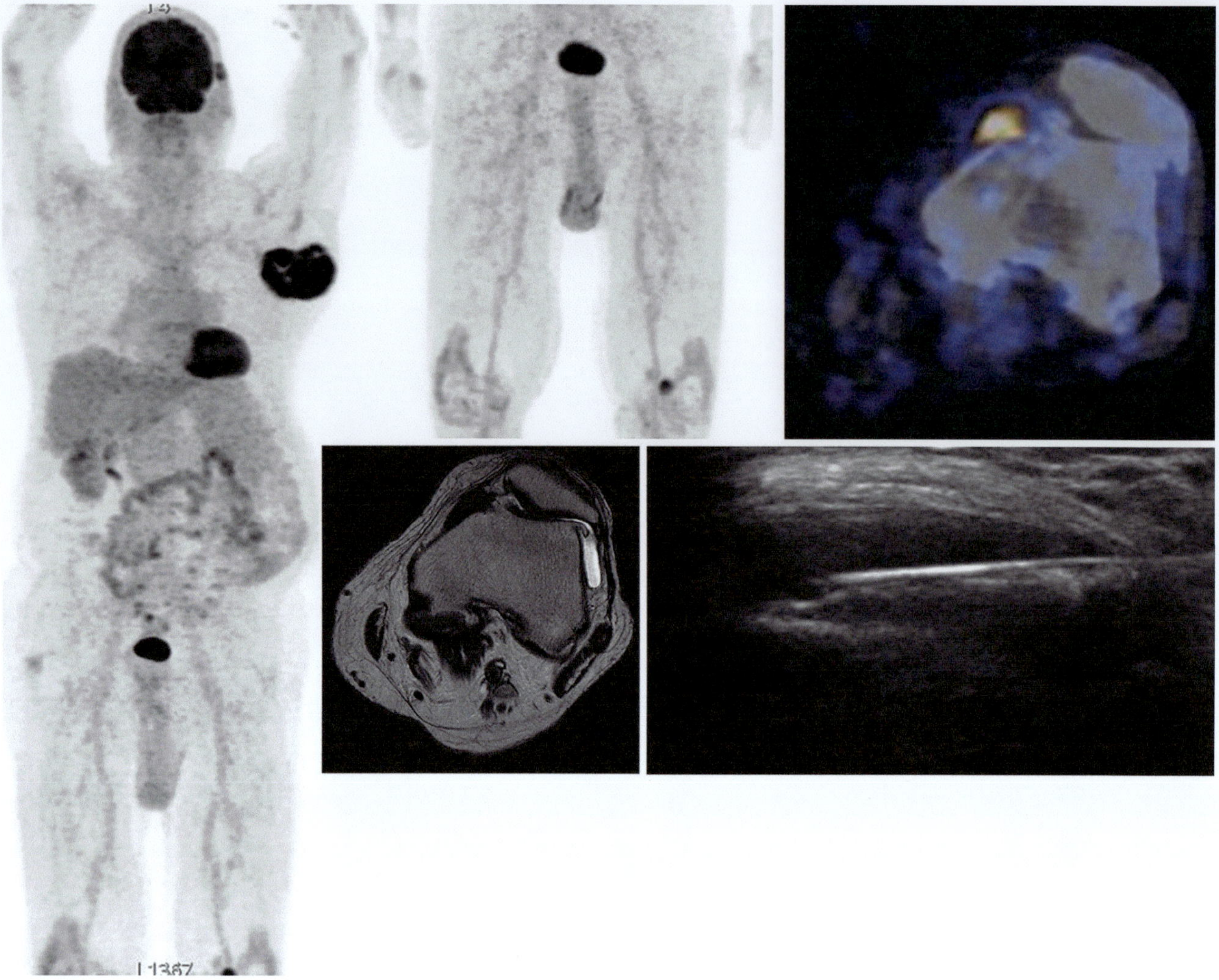

Fig. 8 Patient for melanoma staging. Besides a large axillary lymph node metastasis FDG PET/CT shows focal uptake in the left knee. MR and US guided biopsy confirm a benign giant cell tumor of the tendon sheath

References

1. Harbert J, Desai R (1985) Small calvarial bone scan foci—normal variations. J Nucl Med 26(10):1144–1148
2. Senda K, Itoh S (1987) Evaluation of diffusely high uptake by the calvaria in bone scintigraphy. Ann Nucl Med 1(1):23–26
3. Syed GM, Fielding HW, Collier BD (2005) Sternal uptake on bone scintigraphy: age-related variants. Nucl Med Commun 26(3):253–257
4. Cohenpour M, Simon YC, Zenaty I, Horne T (2002) Unusual urinary bladder accumulation in bone scan. Semin Nucl Med 32(3):231–232
5. Hassan FU, Mohan HK, Gnanasegaran G, Vijayanathan S, Fogelman I (2011) Beware of the focal uptake at the ischium on the bone scan in prostate cancer. Nucl Med Commun 32(4):320–323
6. Romer W, Nomayr A, Uder M, Bautz W, Kuwert T (2006) SPECT-guided CT for evaluating foci of increased bone metabolism classified as indeterminate on SPECT in cancer patients. J Nucl Med 47(7):1102–1106
7. Strobel K, Burger C, Seifert B, Husarik DB, Soyka JD, Hany TF (2007) Characterization of focal bone lesions in the axial skeleton: performance of planar bone scintigraphy compared with SPECT and SPECT fused with CT. AJR Am J Roentgenol 188(5):W467–W474
8. Nakai T, Okuyama C, Kubota T, Yamada K, Ushijima Y, Taniike K et al (2005) Pitfalls of FDG-PET for the diagnosis of osteoblastic bone metastases in patients with breast cancer. Eur J Nucl Med Mol Imaging 32(11):1253–1258
9. Abe K, Sasaki M, Kuwabara Y, Koga H, Baba S, Hayashi K et al (2005) Comparison of 18FDG-PET with 99mTc-HMDP scintigraphy for the detection of bone metastases in patients with breast cancer. Ann Nucl Med 19(7):573–579
10. Cook GJ, Venkitaraman R, Sohaib AS, Lewington VJ, Chua SC, Huddart RA et al (2011) The diagnostic utility of the flare phenomenon on bone scintigraphy in staging prostate cancer. Eur J Nucl Med Mol Imaging 38(1):7–13
11. Even-Sapir E, Metser U, Mishani E, Lievshitz G, Lerman H, Leibovitch I (2006) The detection of bone metastases in patients

with high-risk prostate cancer: 99mTc-MDP planar bone scintigraphy, single- and multi-field-of-view SPECT, 18F-fluoride PET, and 18F-fluoride PET/CT. J Nucl Med 47(2):287–297
12. Aoki J, Watanabe H, Shinozaki T, Takagishi K, Ishijima H, Oya N et al (2001) FDG PET of primary benign and malignant bone tumors: standardized uptake value in 52 lesions. Radiology 219(3): 774–777
13. Strobel K, Bode B, Lardinois D, Exner U (2007) PET-positive fibrous dysplasia—a potentially misleading incidental finding in a patient with intimal sarcoma of the pulmonary artery. Skelet Radiol 36(Suppl 1):S24–S28
14. Strobel K, Merwald M, Huellner M, Zenklusen HR, Kuttenberger J (2013) Osteoblastoma of the mandible mimicking osteosarcoma in FDG PET/CT imaging. Clin Nucl Med 38(2): 143–144
15. Broski SM, Murdoch NM, Skinner JA, Wenger DE (2016) Pigmented villonodular synovitis: potential pitfall on oncologic 18F-FDG PET/CT. Clin Nucl Med 41(1):e24–e31
16. Gemmel F, Van den Wyngaert H, Love C, Welling MM, Gemmel P, Palestro CJ (2012) Prosthetic joint infections: radionuclide state-of-the-art imaging. Eur J Nucl Med Mol Imaging 39(5):892–909
17. Tabouret-Viaud C, Mainta I, Boudabbous S, Amzalag G, Ratib O, Rager O et al (2014) High protracted (99m)Tc-HDP uptake in synthetic bone implants—a potentially misleading incidental finding on bone scintigraphy. Knee 21(6):1284–1287
18. Agrawal K, Marafi F, Gnanasegaran G, Van der Wall H, Fogelman I (2015) Pitfalls and limitations of radionuclide planar and hybrid bone imaging. Semin Nucl Med 45(5):347–372

Scintigraphic Planar and Hybrid Imaging of Primary Bone Tumors

Frédéric Paycha

There is a large variety of tumors and tumorlike lesions that can involve the skeleton. These tumors and tumorlike lesions present a bewildering spectrum of radiologic appearances that all too often can lead to misinterpretations resulting in suboptimal management of patients. Although primary malignancies are relatively rare, they often pose an intriguing diagnostic problem for radiologists, particularly as the pathology is frequently equally challenging.

Skeletal Bisphosphonates-(99mTc) SPECT/multislice CT is a useful problem solving tool that can be utilised selectively to assess the anatomical significance of equivocal areas of tracer uptake on planar whole-body scintigraphy or define the functional significance of indeterminate abnormalities detected on cross-sectional morphological imaging [1]. SPECT/CT is particularly useful for problem solving of indeterminate bone lesions (as opposed to joint lesions).

Likely, but still controversial, mechanisms of uptake of bisphosphonates-(99mTc) are multiple: uptake on organic phase, uptake on mineral phase and/or cellular internalization (osteoclasts and osteoblasts). These tissular- and cellular-levels mechanisms have been lumped together and oversimplified by increased bone vascularization and increased bone turnover.

Bisphosphonates-(99mTc) SPECT/CT and Fluoride-(18F) PET/CT are analysed according a common pathway, because of the similarities of normal and abnormal distribution of these two bone-seekers radiopharmaceuticals of these two cross-sectional hybrid imaging modalities.

Bone tumors and pseudotumors complete phenotyping must incorporate radiological and scintigraphic features.

Uptake of Sclerotic Lesions on Bone Scintigraphy

The case of the solitary sclerotic lesion

- **Metastasis**–rarely solitary: **Increased uptake**
- **Lymphoma (Hodgkin lymphoma++)**: **Increased uptake**
- **Osteoid Osteoma**–cortical location with lucent nidus: **Increased uptake**
- **Osteoblastoma**–similar to OO, but larger: **Increased uptake**
- **Osteosarcoma**–aggressive periosteal reaction and new bone formation: **Increased uptake**
- **Osteoma–Increased uptake**
- **Enchondroma, low grade chondrosarcoma**: **Increased uptake alike**
- **Bone island**–Normal uptake (75% of cases)
- **FD**–ground glass opacity: **Increased uptake (80% of cases)**
- **Bone infarct**–serpiginous: **Increased uptake**
- **Callus, healing fracture**–compare with old films: **Increased uptake** (up to 2 years)
- **Sclerosing OM of Garré: Increased uptake**
- **Paget's**–bone expansion, thick coarse trabeculae: Phases I, II: **Increased uptake**, phase III: normal uptake
- **Bone graft**–well defined dense bone: **Increased uptake**
- **Melorheostosis**–molten wax flowing down the burning candle, sclerotome, may have periosteal new bone formation: **Increased uptake**

F. Paycha
Service de Médecine Nucléaire, Hôpital Lariboisière, Assistance Publique—Hôpitaux de Paris, 2 rue Ambroise Paré, 75010 Paris, France
e-mail: frederic.paycha@wanadoo.fr

J. Hodler et al. (eds.), *Musculoskeletal Diseases 2017-2020*, DOI 10.1007/978-3-319-54018-4_29

Uptake of Lytic Lesions on Bone Scintigraphy

The case of the solitary lytic lesion

- Fibrous dysplasia: **Increased uptake (80% of cases)**
- Osteoblastoma: **Increased uptake**
- Giant cell tumor: **Increased uptake**
- Metastasis/Myeloma: **Increased/heterogeneous uptake** (50% of cases only!)
- Aneurysmal Bone Cyst: No uptake
- Chondroblastoma: **Increased uptake**
- Hyperparathyroidism (brown tumors): **Increased uptake/** Hemangioma: No uptake/Hydatid cyst: No uptake
- Infection: **Increased uptake**
- Non-ossifying Fibroma: No uptake (rarely faint uptake)
- Langerhans cell histiocytosis: **Increased uptake**
- Solitary Bone Cyst: No uptake

Clinical indications of bone hybrid imaging in the setting of a bone tumor or tumorlike lesions are the following ones:

1. Scintigraphic featuring of a bone lesion of undetermined significance on radiological imaging, an increased uptake meaning a growing/aggressive process, a contrario, a normal uptake meaning a slow-growing, a quiescent or burn-out process
2. Enduring bone pain left unexplained (no history of trauma, pain of inflammatory rhythm, at distance of joints)
3. Local, locoregional (skip metastases, neighbouring soft tissues) extension, and systemic (whole skeleton, lungs) extension initial work-up of a biopsy-proved or radiologically highly suspected malignant primitive bone tumor
4. New or follow-up imaging of an untreated long-standing primitive bone tumor purportedly classified as benign because of a suspected complication (malignant transformation, fracture, necrosis…)
5. Follow-up of a treated bone tumor with a high propensity either to local recurrence or to systemic recurrence

Skeletal SPECT/multislice CT gains wider clinical acceptance and can improve lesion localization and characterization, as well as boost diagnostic confidence.

Skeletal Fluoride-(18F) PET/CT has great potential, being more sensitive than planar bone scintigraphy and when PET/CT is performed it is highly accurate for detection of both lytic and sclerotic lesions and to distinguish benign from malignant skeletal findings [2].

To date, no study has compared sensitivity and specificity between bone PET/CT and SPECT/CT.

Imaging pitfalls relate either to a benign appearance abnormality which reflects indeed a malignant condition or to a worrisome appearance abnormality which relates to a benign condition.

Because of exquisite spatial resolution and 3-D imaging of whole spine (SPECT/CT) or whole skeleton (PET/CT), both hybrid imaging modalities have been mainly fraught with overdiagnosis of bone metastases because of inadequate image analysis of artifacts, bone and joint normal variants, incidentalomas ("don't touch lesions") or non-malignant conditions. Rarely, a second pitfall is the overlooking of actual metastases or primitive malignant bone tumours masquerading as a benign lesion appearance or even invisible on SPECT or PET images but identifiable on CT images.

Bisphosphonates-(99mTc) SPECT/CT and Fluoride-(18F) PET/CT are analysed according a common pathway, because of the similarities of normal and abnormal distribution of these two bone-seekers radiopharmaceuticals of two cross-sectional hybrid imaging modalities.

The connecting thread in ascertaining the main diagnostic patterns of a tumor or a tumorlike is the dominant phenotype of the abnormality encountered in bone SPECT/CT or PET/CT imaging: lytic/osteoclastic, sclerotic/osteoblastic, and mixed.

Imaging abnormalities will be then classified according to their anatomical location: axial or peripheral bones.

A carefully entertained scenario is the case of the solitary lesion located in spine because a majority (90%) of metastases occur in this structure [3].

Tactics of interpretation of bone SPECT/CT may be itemized in seven steps:

(a) Epidemiological (incidence and prevalence of main conditions involved in the imaging gamut) and clinical (is the patient painful or not?, is there a medical history of malignancy?) data.
(b) Pathophysiological reminders centered on most frequent bone and joint disorders (e.g., bone metastases, degenerative joint diseases).
(c) Display lay out, mode of exploration of images, 3-D display adjuncts.
(d) Selection of four key features of the lesion, first on metabolic portion then on morphological portion of hybrid imaging (topographic features, type of matrix, margins and limits, periosteal reaction, locoregional extension).
(e) Quantitative measures (SUV, uptake, density) of lesion of concern.
(f) Derivation of the differentials (gamut sketched out according to similar features and epidemiology).
(g) Searching for obvious extra-osseous manifestations (e.g., SKIBO [association of SKIn and BOne lesions] diseases) [4, 5].

Bone SPECT/CT and PET/CT integrative reading is eventually fostered in order to maximize the chances to correctly classify benign and malignant bone tumoral lesions, especially when intermodality discrepancies occur (SPECT+/CT- [or PET+/CT-], SPECT-/CT+ [or PET-/CT+)].

Such discrepant combinations, far from delaying diagnosis, should convey clues to attain the correct diagnosis [5].

Bone SPECT/CT and PET/CT images should be interpreted with the aid of a diagnostic Radiologist or Nuclear Medicine physicians should acquire sufficient experience in CT image interpretation in order to optimise diagnostic benefit from SPECT/CT.

That academic and practical training should not waive the reader to indulge specific drill in fused imaging in order to interpret intermodality mismatching (SPECT (PET) +/CT- or SPECT(PET)-/CT+).

References

1. Gnanasegaran G, Cook G, Adamson K, Fogelman I (2009) Patterns, variants, artifacts, and pitfalls in conventional radionuclide bone imaging and SPECT/CT. Semin Nucl Med 39:380–395
2. Grant FD, Fahey FH, Packard AB, Davis RT, Alavi A, Treves ST (2008) Skeletal PET with 18F-fluoride: applying new technology to an old tracer. J Nucl Med 49:68–78
3. Rodallec MH, Feydy A, Larousserie F, Anract P, Campagna R, Babinet A, Zins M, Drapé JL (2008) Diagnostic imaging of solitary tumors of the spine: what to do and say. Radiographics 28:1019–1041
4. Paycha F, Maia S, Ayachi N, Grossin M, de Vernejoul MC (2007) Quelle Est la signification des anomalies observées en scintigraphie osseuse? Retour Sur les mécanismes de fixation des bisphosphonates-(99mTc) [what is the meaning of abnormalities observed on bone scintigraphy? Bisphosphonates-(99mTc) mechanisms of uptake revisited]. Méd Nucl 31:356–365
5. Paycha F, Girma A, Granier P (2010) Démarche sémiologique en scintigraphie osseuse. Une approche intégrée de l'imagerie hybride [patterns in bone SPECT/CT. An integrative diagnostic pathway in hybrid imaging]. Méd Nucl 34:490–511

Scintigraphy and SPECT/CT in Disease of the Spine

Torsten Kuwert

Introduction

Scintigraphic images acquired early after intravenous injection of the ^{99m}Tc-labeled polyphosphonates provide information on perfusion and floridity of skeletal lesions (for a general review, see [1]). Scintigraphy performed several hours after tracer injection allows insight into bone metabolism or, more specifically, osteoblastic activity, since the polyphosphonates are adsorbed on freshly built bone tissue. Due to the sensitivity of this examination to detect osseous lesions, skeletal scintigraphy has been widely used as screening tool, e.g., for staging malignant disease. In the late 1980s, single-photon emission computed tomography (SPECT) became widely available, allowing three-dimensional visualization of the distribution of radioactivity within the human body. This technology considerably improved the diagnostic accuracy of bone scintigraphy by allowing a better localization of areas exhibiting pathological tracer uptake (for a review, see [2]). Nevertheless, due to limitations in spatial resolution of skeletal SPECT, which ranges from ca. 8–10 mm in the reconstructed images, the specificity of skeletal scintigraphy is still limited. This is, in particular, true when compared to radiological techniques such as X-ray computerized tomography (CT) or magnetic resonance imaging (MRI), the latter technique also allowing visualization of soft-tissue structures associated with bone such as of the tendons, ligaments and cartilage that elude bone scintigraphy for obvious methodological reasons.

For approximately 12 years, hybrid systems integrating a SPECT camera with a CT scanner into one gantry have now been commercially available (for a review, see [3]). These systems allow the acquisition of a CT scan of X-ray density together with a SPECT image of bone metabolism within one patient examination. Since then, numerous studies have demonstrated the diagnostic superiority of SPECT/CT over stand-alone nuclear medical imaging (for a review, see [4]).

T. Kuwert
Clinic of Nuclear Medicine, University of Erlangen-Nürnberg, Ulmenweg 18, 91054 Erlangen, Germany
e-mail: torsten.kuwert@uk-erlangen.de

The present introductory text to the seminar discusses the use of skeletal scintigraphy including SPECT/CT in staging malignant disease with a particular focus on the spine as well as in lower back pain.

SPECT/ CT for Staging Malignant Bone Disease

Skeletal lesions most frequently arise as a result of metastatic disease from primary tumors in other organs. Metastatic disease to the skeleton occurs in about 30% of the oncologic patients, and identification of bone involvement is mandatory for correct staging and subsequent therapy. Bone scintigraphy with the ^{99m}Tc-labeled polyphosphonates, e.g., ^{99m}Tc-methylene diphosphonate (^{99m}Tc-MDP) affords visualization of the entire skeleton with an extremely high sensitivity approaching 100% for breast and prostate cancer (for reviews, see [2, 5]). Purely lytic metastases such as those due to renal carcinoma or plasmocytoma may not increase bone metabolism and thus escape diagnosis by bone scintigraphy. This is also the case of sclerotic neoplastic osseous foci after treatment, e.g., by bisphosphonates, which occasionally are difficult to differentiate from bone islands.

The specificity of bone scintigraphy is rather low, as also benign conditions may be accompanied by an increase in bone metabolism. Pertinent examples are spinal degenerative conditions such as osteochondrosis and spondylarthropathy, as well as osteoporotic fractures of the vertebral bodies. They pose a particular problem as they have a very high incidence in elderly subjects—an age group where malignant disease typically occurs. Additionally, benign primary bone tumors such as enchondromas or fibrous dysplasia, as well as inflammatory diseases such as osteomyelitis may be difficult to differentiate from metastases on the basis of radionuclide bone imaging alone. Its rather low specificity, therefore, often requires further investigation with, e.g., planar X-ray radiography, CT or magnetic resonance imaging (MRI).

J. Hodler et al. (eds.), *Musculoskeletal Diseases 2017-2020*, DOI 10.1007/978-3-319-54018-4_30

In the case of indeterminate bone lesions detected by bone scintigraphy for which a definite diagnosis cannot be reached, SPECT/CT offers the unique opportunity to directly correlate the scintigraphic findings with CT images to improve lesion classification (Fig. 1). Since 2006, the diagnostic value of SPECT/CT for osseous staging of malignant disease has been investigated in several clinical studies: Table 1 gives a rough overview of the characteristics of each

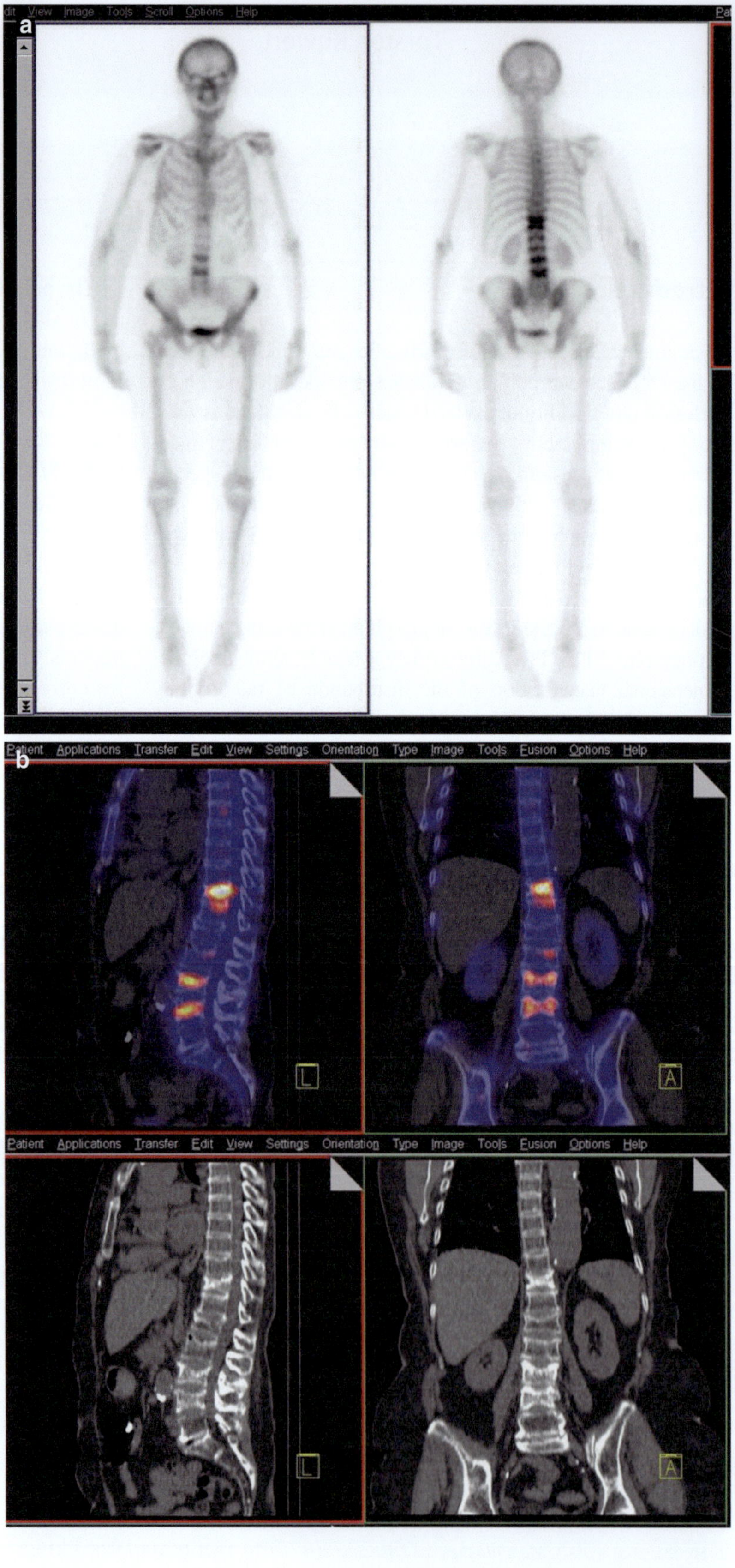

Fig. 1 (**a**) Planar whole-body scintigrams in a patient with lumbar pain 3 years after diagnosis and treatment of breast cancer. (**b**) SPECT/CT fusion images (*upper row*) and matching CT images (*lower row*) of that patient. All foci of increased tracer accumulation correspond to compression fractures of the vertebrae, malignancy can be reliably ruled out in one hybrid imaging session

Table 1 Overview of studies reporting rates of SPECT/CT elucidation of hypermetabolic foci found on skeletal planar/SPECT images in cancer patients

First author	Study design	Independent gold standard?[a]	CT[b]	Number of lesions	% Elucidated by SPECT/CT
Horger [6]	Prospective	Yes	Low-power X-ray tube	104	85
Römer [7]	Retrospective	No	Low-dose spiral-CT (40 mAs)	52[c]	92
Helyar [8]	Retrospective	No	Diagnostic spiral-CT (100 mAs)	50[c]	92
Zhao [9]	Prospective	Yes	Diagnostic spiral CT (140 mA)	37[c]	86.5
Ndlovu [10]	Prospective	Yes	Low-power X-ray tube (2.5 mA)	58[c]	71.1
Sharma [11]	Retrospective	Yes	Diagnostic spiral-CT (100 mAs)	65[c]	95.3
Zhang [12]	Retrospective	Yes	Diagnostic spiral-CT (160 mA)	90[c]	94.4
Sharma [13]	Retrospective	No	Diagnostic spiral-CT (100 mAs)	36 (skull only)	100

[a]Gold standard was in most studies clinical and radiological follow-up, pathological diagnosis was only in erare instances available
[b]All studies use dual-headed SPECT cameras in conjunction with the CT scanners given in this column
[c]Number of lesions reported as equivocal on planar/SPECT imaging

of these different studies and the results obtained. Despite various apparent weaknesses and heterogeneities in study design of the available evidence, the results obtained are remarkably consistent: SPECT/CT enables a definitive diagnosis in between 71.0 and 95.3% of lesions deemed equivocal on planar/ SPECT imaging [7–11]. SPECT/CT with bone-seeking radiopharmaceuticals is becoming a cost-effective standard-of-reference imaging technique in the evaluation of patients with various types of cancer.

Merits of Bone Scintigraphy in Lower Back Pain

Although MRI currently represents the standard of reference for benign orthopedic disease, bone scintigraphy is still frequently used for these indications due to its cost-effectiveness and the high sensitivity to osseous lesions and complete view of the skeleton it provides. However, aside from its inability to visualize the soft-tissue structures of the joints, its major drawback is its low specificity.

SPECT/CT appears to overcome most of the diagnostic limitations of purely nuclear bone scintigraphy, by enabling precise anatomic localization of bone turnover abnormalities.

Lower back pain has a very high incidence in western populations and a vast gamut of differential diagnoses (for a review, see [14]). Disk herniation is not accessible to bone scintigraphy and can only be diagnosed by MRI. Active degenerative disease of the axial skeleton is, however, accompanied by an increase in polyphosphonate uptake and, therefore, amenable to bone scintigraphy (Fig. 2). This applies to osteochondrosis radiologically characterized by disk space narrowing, subchondral sclerosis of the vertebral bodies, osteophytes, and radiological signs of disk degeneration such as the occurrence of gas in the disk—the so-called vacuum phenomenon. More relevant to clinical management is the determination of an active facet's level of osteoarthritis, as this diagnosis and localization helps in directing topical therapies such as a medical branch block or intraarticular instillation of corticosteroids.

Active facet joint disease can be diagnosed by SPECT/CT: Matar and coworkers reported a frequency of 65% for metabolically active facet joint disease in 72 patients referred for SPECT/CT for workup of chronic neck or back pain [15]. In their retrospective study, SPECT/CT identified potential pain generators in 92% of the study population. Makki et al. reported that 91.1% of 486 patients consecutively studied by SPECT/CT for spinal pain over 7.5 years had at least one abnormality visible using SPECT/CT potentially causing the symptoms [16]. They found a prevalence of 42.8% of subjects with increased uptake in at least one zygoapophyseal joint in their cohort. In a further large retrospective study, Lehmann and coworkers analyzed data from 212 patients referred for spinal SPECT/CT to their department over a period of roughly 4 years [17]. 191 of these subjects had been examined for workup of back pain, with suspicion of abnormal facet joint activity being the most frequent indication at 37% of the total. In 50% of the whole group, pathological uptake was described in at least one facet joint. Most noteworthy, 40% of the whole group had undergone SPECT/CT after prior MRI examinations, and 35% of the subjects referred for differential diagnosis of pain had had prior percutaneous interventions with incomplete response. As recorded on the clinical notes of the treating physician, SPECT/CT findings led to a change in clinical management in 79% of patients, impressively documenting the acceptance and utility of hybrid SPECT/CT imaging.

Fig. 2 CT (*left*) and SPECT/CT fusion (*right*) images of ^{99m}Tc-polyphosphonate uptake in the lumbar spine showing increased tracer uptake in active osteochondrosis

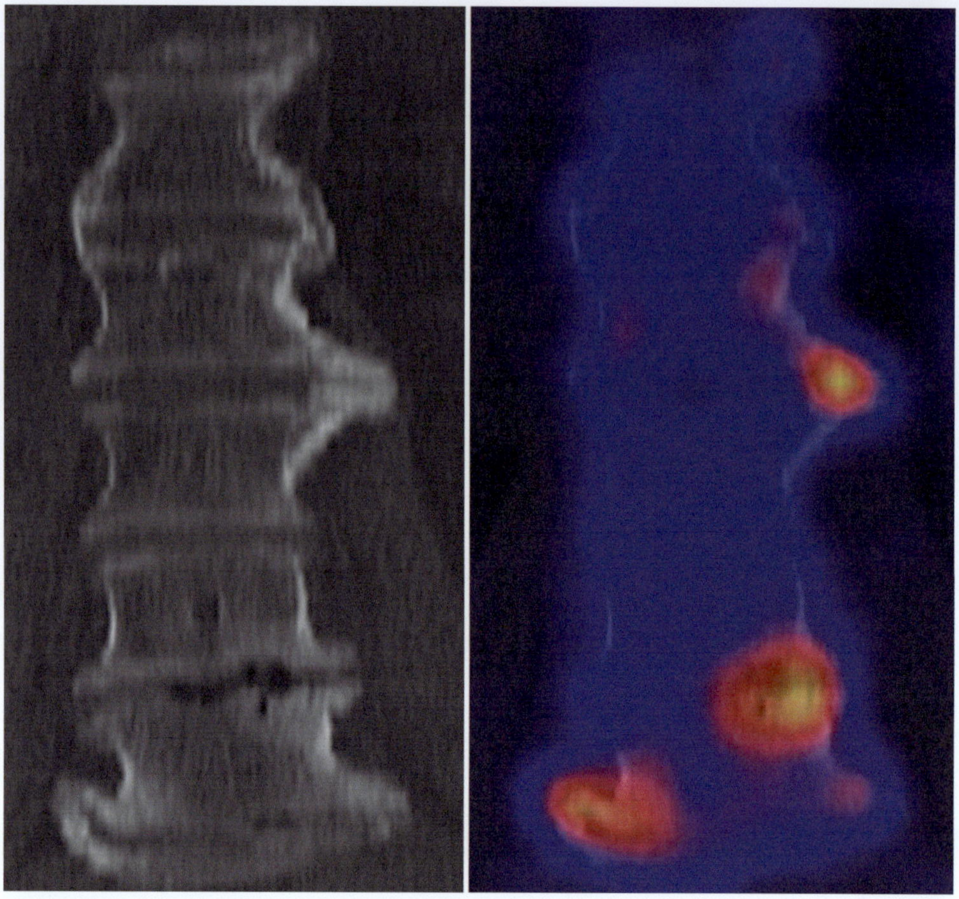

The evidence presented above suggests that skeletal SPECT/CT might have the potential to guide percutaneous therapy of facet joint arthritis. Additional data on the use of stand-alone SPECT point into this direction as well [18–20]. In a further publication, however, Lehmann et al. analyzed the relationship between the localization of abnormal tracer uptake in the facet joint and the joint percutaneously treated in a group of 74 patients [21]. In 70% of these subjects, site of treatment and SPECT/CT abnormality did not coincide. Furthermore, 46% of subjects had a right versus left discrepancy. This shows that the relationship between the scintigraphic abnormality and the occurrence of back pain is not as straightforward as initially expected. Type of treatment also is a variable that should receive consideration in this context: in a prospective double-blinded outcome study, Ackerman and Ahmad showed that SPECT/CT fared better in predicting pain relief after intraarticular injections of cortisone than after medial branch blocks [22]. Clearly, more evidence from further prospective—ideally, double-blinded—investigations with pain relief as outcome variable would be necessary to establish the value of SPECT/CT for planning local therapies of painful facet arthritis.

Another frequent cause of back pain, in particular in the elderly, is osteoporotic compression fracture of vertebral bodies. Within the first year of occurrence, this condition is metabolically active and can thus be visualized by bone scintigraphy. SPECT/CT may help in localization and also in differentiating them from metabolically active osteochondrosis. Vertebral osteoporotic fractures may be treated by percutaneous vertebroplasty. In a recently published prospective study of 33 consecutive patients with this condition, positive SPECT/CT images predicted clinical improvement in 91% of these subjects as induced by this minimally invasive measure [23]. Furthermore, it identified alternative causes of pain in the subgroup of nine patients for whom the therapy in question had then not been performed. Anecdotal evidence lets one surmise that SPECT/CT might also be helpful in acute spinal traumas and, in particular, in diagnosing stress fractures in bilateral pedicles of the spine, as they can occur in athletes [24].

Spinal fusion surgery is performed in patients with severe chronic back pain when segmental instability is believed to cause the symptoms. The rationale for this is that pain relief will be achieved once the fusion restricts motion in the painful segments. An estimated 10–20% of patients develop lumbar pain after lumbar fusion surgery. This may be related to loosening of the metallic implants or failure of a stably implanted graft to immobilize the fused segments. A further differential diagnosis is degenerative disease involving the spinal segments above or below the instrumented region. Differentiation between these conditions has therapeutic consequences: in the first case, a complementary ventral spondylodesis must be considered, in the second an amplification of the instrumentation in cranial or caudal direction. Near metallic implants, CT quality is considerably degraded by streak artefacts and that of MRI by susceptibility phenomena so that the accuracy of these two modalities to differentiate between the above-described causes of pain after spondylodesis is reduced. Bone scintigraphy, which is either not affected by these artefacts or only indirectly via attenuation correction, might thus be of particular value for this purpose [25]. Emerging evidence from SPECT/CT studies indicates that this technology holds much promise in the differential diagnosis of pain recurring or prevailing after lumbar instrumentation [26–29].

Conclusion

Skeletal scintigraphy is one of the most frequent in-vivo procedures in the field of nuclear medicine. By visualizing bone metabolism, it exhibits a fairly high sensitivity for detecting skeletal lesions, but has limitations with regard to specificity and spatial resolution, even when single-photon emission computed tomography (SPECT) is used. Combining SPECT with X-ray computed tomography (CT) helps overcome these limitations. This has, in particular, been shown when diagnosing bone involvement in malignant tumors. Emerging evidence indicates some benefit of hybrid imaging for bone scintigraphy also for workup of lower back pain.

Conflicts of Interest Torsten Kuwert has an ongoing research collaboration with Siemens Molecular Imaging in the field of SPECT/CT. He gives occasional lectures on behalf of Siemens Molecular Imaging pertaining to SPECT/CT research.

References

1. Brenner AI, Koshy J, Morey J, Lin C, DiPoce J (2012) The bone scan. Semin Nucl Med 42(1):11–26
2. Even-Sapir E (2005) Imaging of malignant bone involvement by morphologic, scintigraphic, and hybrid modalities. J Nucl Med 46(8):1356–1367
3. Beyer T, Veit-Haibach P (2014) State-of-the-art SPECT/CT: technology, methodology and applications-defining a new role for an undervalued multimodality imaging technique. Eur J Nucl Med Mol Imaging 41(Suppl 1):S1–S2
4. Mariani G et al (2010) A review on the clinical uses of SPECT/CT. Eur J Nucl Med Mol Imaging 37(10):1959–1985
5. Talbot JN, Paycha F, Balogova S (2011) Diagnosis of bone metastasis: recent comparative studies of imaging modalities. Q J Nucl Med Mol Imaging 55(4):374–410
6. Horger M et al (2004) Evaluation of combined transmission and emission tomography for classification of skeletal lesions. AJR Am J Roentgenol 183(3):655–661
7. Romer W, Nomayr A, Uder M, Bautz W, Kuwert T (2006) SPECT-guided CT for evaluating foci of increased bone metabolism classified as indeterminate on SPECT in cancer patients. J Nucl Med 47(7):1102–1106
8. Helyar V et al (2010) The added value of multislice SPECT/CT in patients with equivocal bony metastasis from carcinoma of the prostate. Eur J Nucl Med Mol Imaging 37(4):706–713
9. Zhao Z, Li L, Li F, Zhao L (2010) Single photon emission computed tomography/spiral computed tomography fusion imaging for the diagnosis of bone metastasis in patients with known cancer. Skelet Radiol 39(2):147–153
10. Ndlovu X, George R, Ellmann A, Warwick J (2010) Should SPECT-CT replace SPECT for the evaluation of equivocal bone scan lesions in patients with underlying malignancies? Nucl Med Commun 31(7):659–665
11. Sharma P et al (2012) Indeterminate lesions on planar bone scintigraphy in lung cancer patients: SPECT, CT or SPECT-CT? Skelet Radiol 41(7):843–850
12. Zhang Y et al (2013) Added value of SPECT/spiral CT versus SPECT in diagnosing solitary spinal lesions in patients with extraskeletal malignancies. Nucl Med Commun 34(5):451–458
13. Sharma P et al (2014) Comparison of single photon emission computed tomography-computed tomography, computed tomography, single photon emission computed tomography and planar scintigraphy for characterization of isolated skull lesions seen on bone scintigraphy in cancer patients. Indian J Nucl Med 29(1): 22–29
14. Balague F, Mannion AF, Pellise F, Cedraschi C (2007) Clinical update: low back pain. Lancet 369(9563):726–728
15. Matar HE et al (2013) Is hybrid imaging (SPECT/CT) a useful adjunct in the management of suspected facet joints arthropathy? Int Orthop 37(5):865–870
16. Makki D, Khazim R, Zaidan AA, Ravi K, Toma T (2010) Single photon emission computerized tomography (SPECT) scan-positive facet joints and other spinal structures in a hospital-wide population with spinal pain. Spine J 10(1):58–62
17. Lehman VT, Murphy RC, Maus TP (2013) 99mTc-MDP SPECT/CT of the spine and sacrum at a multispecialty institution: clinical use, findings, and impact on patient management. Nucl Med Commun 34(11):1097–1106
18. Pneumaticos SG, Chatziioannou SN, Hipp JA, Moore WH, Esses SI (2006) Low back pain: prediction of short-term outcome of facet joint injection with bone scintigraphy. Radiology 238(2): 693–698
19. Dolan AL et al (1996) The value of SPECT scans in identifying back pain likely to benefit from facet joint injection. Br J Rheumatol 35(12):1269–1273
20. Koh WU et al (2011) Value of bone scintigraphy and single photon emission computed tomography (SPECT) in lumbar facet disease and prediction of short-term outcome of ultrasound guided medial branch block with bone SPECT. Korean J Pain 24(2):81–86
21. Lehman VT et al (2014) Frequency of discordance between facet joint activity on technetium Tc99m methylene diphosphonate SPECT/CT and selection for percutaneous treatment at a large multispecialty institution. AJNR Am J Neuroradiol 35(3):609–614
22. Ackerman WE III, Ahmad M (2008) Pain relief with intraarticular or medial branch nerve blocks in patients with positive lumbar facet joint SPECT imaging: a 12-week outcome study. South Med J 101(9):931–934
23. Sola M et al (2011) Value of bone SPECT-CT to predict chronic pain relief after percutaneous vertebroplasty in vertebral fractures. Spine J 11(12):1102–1107
24. Van der Wall H et al (2010) Radionuclide bone scintigraphy in sports injuries. Semin Nucl Med 40(1):16–30
25. Even-Sapir E et al (1994) Assessment of painful late effects of lumbar spinal fusion with SPECT. J Nucl Med 35(3):416–422

26. Damgaard M, Nimb L, Madsen JL (2010) The role of bone SPECT/CT in the evaluation of lumbar spinal fusion with metallic fixation devices. Clin Nucl Med 35(4):234–236
27. Hudyana H et al (2016) Accuracy of bone SPECT/CT for identifying hardware loosening in patients who underwent lumbar fusion with pedicle screws. Eur J Nucl Med Mol Imaging 43(2):349–354
28. Rager O et al (2012) SPECT/CT in differentiation of pseudarthrosis from other causes of back pain in lumbar spinal fusion: report on 10 consecutive cases. Clin Nucl Med 37(4):339–343
29. Sumer J et al (2013) SPECT/CT in patients with lower back pain after lumbar fusion surgery. Nucl Med Commun 34(10):964–970

Part III

Pediatric Radiology Satellite Course "Kangaroo"

Congenital Disorders of the Pediatric Extremities

Rutger A.J. Nievelstein

Introduction

The congenital disorders of the pediatric extremities consist of a broad spectrum of congenital anomalies that present with failure of formation, failure of differentiation, or duplication of one or more bones of the limbs (Table 1) [1, 2]. They are relatively rare with an incidence of approximately 1 in 1300–2000 births, and do occur in isolation or in association with other anomalies. Several classification systems with often confusing and imprecise (historical) terms circulate in the literature. Recently, Gold et al. introduced a new anatomic classification system that includes all possible phenotypes of congenital limb deficiencies (Table 2) [3]. This classification system starts with two main groups, i.e., complete and partial absence of one or more limbs. In case of partial absence the limb disorders are subdivided into three basic types; intercalary, longitudinal, and (terminal) transverse. The intercalary deficiency is characterized by hypo- or aplasia of the middle part of the limb (also known as phocomelia), whereas transverse deficiencies correspond to a partial or complete absence distal to a specified level across the

Table 1 Congenital disorders of the pediatric extremities

Failure of formation
Transverse deficiencies
Intercalary deficiencies
Longitudinal deficiencies
Failure of differentiation
Humeroradial and radioulnar synostosis
Carpal and tarsal coalition
Syndactyly
Symphalangism
Duplication
Dimelia of the long bones
Polydactyly
Brachydactyly

Table 2 Anatomic classification of limb deficiencies (based on Gold NB et al. [3])

Complete absence			
Partial absence	Intercalary deficiencies		
	Transverse deficiencies	Upper arm	With or without nubbins
		Forearm	
		Wrist	
		Mid-hand	
		MCP joints	Digits 2–5, 1–4 or 1–5
	Longitudinal deficiencies	Preaxial	Radius and digit 1
			Radius and digits 1–2
			Digit 1
			Digits 1–2, or 1–3
		Mesoaxial	Digit 2, or 3, or 4
			Digits 2–3, or 3–4, or 2–4
		Postaxial	Ulna and digit 5
			Digit 5
			Digits 4–5, or 3–5
		Complex	Ulna, radius and digit 1
			Digits 1 and 5
			Digits 2 and 5
			Digit 1 and digits 3–5
			Digits 1–2 and 4–5
			Digits 2–5
			Radius and digit 5
			Radius and digits 1 and 5
			Radius and digits 1–4

R.A.J. Nievelstein
Department of Radiology and Nuclear Medicine, University Medical Center Utrecht, Heidelberglaan 100, Utrecht 3584 CX, The Netherlands
e-mail: r.a.j.nievelstein@umcutrecht.nl

J. Hodler et al. (eds.), *Musculoskeletal Diseases 2017-2020*, DOI 10.1007/978-3-319-54018-4_31

long axis of the limb (also known as congenital amputation). Longitudinal deficiencies are characterized by hypo- or aplasia of one or several bones along the long axis of the limb. They are usually subdivided into preaxial (radial or tibial side), mesoaxial or central, and postaxial (ulnar or fibular side) defects.

Congenital disorders of the extremities usually develop between the third and 8th week of embryogenesis, when outgrowth and spatial patterning of the limbs occur. Many different causes have been identified, including genetic defects (e.g., Fanconi anemia), chromosomal abnormalities (e.g., Trisomy 18), environmental exposures (e.g., Thalidomide), placental pathology (amniotic bands) and prenatal diagnostic procedures. There are more than 120 clinical congenital limb disorders listed in OMIM (Online Mendelian Inheritance in Man; www.ncbi.nlm.nih.gov/omim), but in only 40% of them the molecular basis is known. Moreover, for many of the disorders for which a genetic defect is known, there is evidence for genetic locus heterogeneity, with genes remaining to be discovered.

The diagnostic evaluation of a child with a congenital disorder of the extremities starts with a complete physical examination looking for other congenital malformations [2]. Furthermore, a 3-generation pedigree should be taken and a detailed pregnancy history should be reconstructed including drug use, medications, chorionic villus sampling, diabetes, and illness during the first trimester. In case of a transverse defect radiography of the affected limb is indicated and will help to define the extent of bony deficiency. Placental pathology is helpful to identify the presence of amniotic bands. The longitudinal defects are often part of a syndrome or chromosome abnormality. That is why in these cases usually a skeletal survey is required to detect abnormalities of other parts of the skeleton (pointing to a skeletal dysplasia) instead of imaging restricted to the affected and contralateral limb. Ultrasound (US) and Magnetic Resonance Imaging (MRI) can play a role in selective cases, to detect additional non-ossified (cartilaginous) or ligamentous congenital defects [1, 2, 4, 5]. If the child with a longitudinal limb disorder also presents with neurologic abnormalities, a brain MRI is indicated. Furthermore, the parents should be examined for limb anomalies, as these can be very subtle (e.g., mild thumb hypoplasia). Further chromosome and/or molecular investigations depend on the type of congenital disorder. Table 3 gives an overview of the diagnostic strategy of congenital disorders of the extremities.

In this chapter the most important congenital disorders of the pediatric extremities will be discussed in more detail with a focus on their principal imaging features and correct terminology.

Table 3 Diagnostic strategy for congenital disorders of the extremities (based on Wilcox WR et al. [2])

Physical examination for other anomalies, 3-generation pedigree, pregnancy history	
Transverse deficiencies	Longitudinal deficiencies
Radiography of affected limb Placental pathology US and/or MRI of affected limbs in selected cases	Radiography of affected and contralateral limb, or Skeletal survey US and/or MRI of affected limbs in selected cases Brain MRI in case of neurological signs Physical examination of parents for limb anomalies Chromosomal testing Blood testing, echocardiography (radial deficiency)
	Molecular testing if indicated
Final diagnosis and genetic counseling	

Failure of Formation (Limb Deficiencies)

Transverse Deficiencies ("Congenital Amputations") [1, 2]

Transverse deficiency of the limb is usually a sporadic event that is thought to be the result of a vascular disruption during embryogenesis. The whole limb (amelia) or different segments (e.g., forearm, hand, digits) may be absent, depending on the level of ischemia and stage of limb development at time of disruption (Fig. 1). Most transverse deficiencies are unilateral but they can present bilaterally in rare syndromes, and in association with other skeletal abnormalities or non-skeletal abnormalities (e.g., tetra-amelia (absence of all four limbs), Roberts' syndrome(severe and symmetrical reduction of all four limbs with facial abnormalities) , and toxic embryo fetopathies (thalidomide, valproic acid, hydantoins)). Transverse deficiencies can also be caused by amniotic bands, which are thought to be the consequence of intrauterine rupture of the amnion (amniotic band syndrome). The limbs, digits, or other parts of the fetus become entangled in these fibrous constriction bands resulting in limb or digital amputations, or limb deformities. The risk for amniotic band syndrome is increased after chorionic villus sampling, particularly when performed before 10 weeks of gestation. There is an increased prevalence of club feet, which has been reported as high as 31%. On radiographs, a wide spectrum of asymmetrical abnormalities distal to the level of constriction is seen, including amputation or hypoplasia of the whole or part of the limb or digits, as well as soft tissue thickening (owing to lymphoedema) or thinning. Furthermore, one or several encircling fibrous bands may sometimes be visible on radiographs. Sometimes, MRI might be helpful in identifying

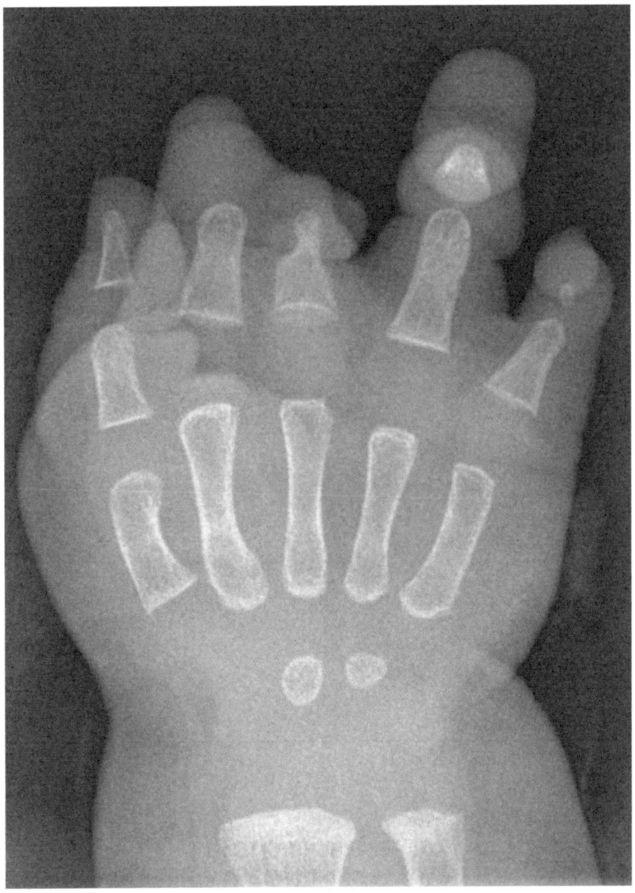

Fig. 1 Amniotic band syndrome of the hand. The digits 2–5 show different levels of amputation, aplasia and deformation of bony structures, as well as constrictions of the skin and soft tissue syndactyly

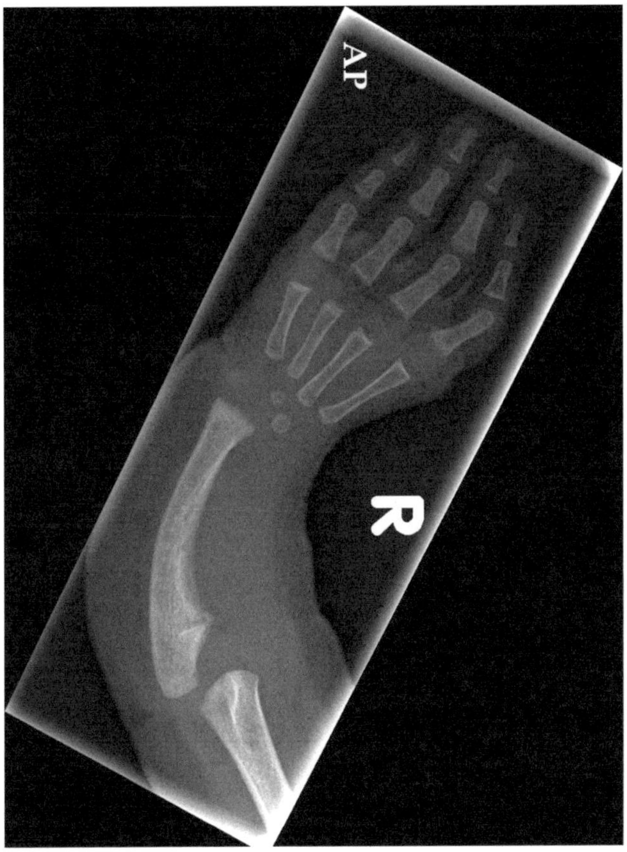

Fig. 2 Radial club hand. There is an aplasia of the radius and thumb as well as a bowing and hypoplasia of the ulna

non-ossified (cartilaginous) structures and soft tissue anomalies, and to detect the course of relevant neurovascular bundles pre-operatively.

Longitudinal Deficiencies

Radial Deficiency [1, 2, 6, 7]

This is the most common (preaxial) longitudinal upper limb deficiency and includes all degrees of hypoplasia or aplasia of the radius (Fig. 2). Radial deficiency occurs bilaterally as frequently as unilaterally and is often associated with hypoplasia or aplasia of the thumb, absent scaphoid and trapezium, and bowing of the ulna (also known as radial club hand). Other upper limb anomalies that might be seen in association with radial deficiency include humeral hypoplasia, proximal radioulnar synostosis, congenital radial head dislocation, as well as coalition of the radial carpal bones. It is commonly associated with other anomalies or syndromes and frequently has a known genetic cause. Children with radial deficiencies often present with or develop hematologic abnormalities (e.g., Fanconi anemia, and thrombocytopenia absent radius (TAR)). Other well-known disorders or syndromes with radial deficiencies include trisomy 18, Brachmann-de Lange syndrome, Holt-Oram syndrome, and the VACTERL association. The acronym VACTERL stands for a non-random association of **V**ertebral anomalies, **A**nal atresia, **C**ardiovascular anomalies, **T**racheoesophageal fistula, **E**sophageal atresia, **R**enal anomalies, and preaxial **L**imb anomalies.

Ulnar Deficiency [1, 2, 6, 7]

This longitudinal upper limb deficiency is 3–10 times rarer than the preaxial upper limb deficiencies. Ulnar deficiency is usual unilateral and nonsyndromic. It can be associated with hypoplasia or aplasia of the ulnar carpal bones (triquetrum, pisiform, and hamatum), and/or the fourth and fifth digits. Humeroradial synostosis, congenital radial head dislocation, radial bowing, and coalition of the ulnar carpal or metacarpal bones may also be seen. Ulnar deficiencies have been described in combination with femoral and fibular deficiencies, and craniofacial malformations.

Cleft Hand [1, 2, 6, 7]

This mesoaxial deficiency presents with the absence of metacarpal bones and/or digits within the central portion of the hand, whereas the radius and ulna are normal (Fig. 3). Due to the lack of second and/or third digits a deep V- or U-shaped central defect (cleft) of the hand occurs, also known as "split hand," "lobster-claw hand," or "extrodactyly". Carpal coalition, pre- or postaxial syndactyly, macrodactyly, pseudo-polydactyly, and supernumerary metacarpal bones can be seen in association. Mesoaxial deficiencies can also occur in the foot, with or without deficiencies of the hand. The typical "cleft hand" is usually bilateral and found in families affected by syndromes such as split hand/split foot syndrome or ectrodactyly-ectodermal dysplasia-cleft lip or palate syndrome.

Proximal Femoral Focal Deficiency (PFFD) [2, 5, 8]

This type of lower limb deficiency is characterized by a simple shortening or minor to total absence of major components of the proximal femur (Fig. 4). PFFD is rare with an incidence of approximately 1 in 50,000 births. It is predominantly unilateral (90% of cases), and up to two thirds of patients have ipsilateral fibular deficiency and a deformity of the foot. PFFD is usually classified according to Aitken, based on the degree of deformity:

- Aitken type A (less severe): a small portion of the proximal femur is absent, but the femoral head and neck are present, there is a normal acetabulum, and there is usually a mild varus alignment;
- Aitken type B: a larger portion of the proximal femur is absent, but the femoral head and neck are still present, the

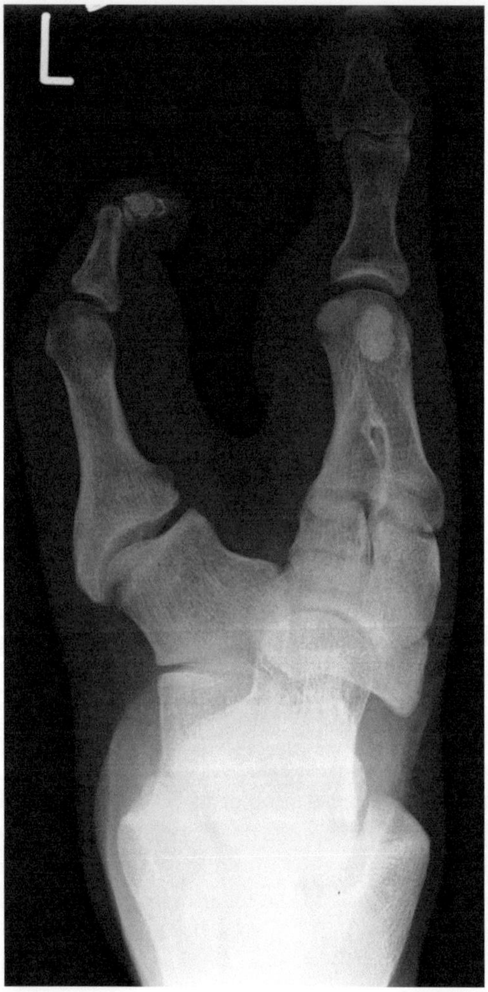

Fig. 3 Cleft foot. There is an absence of the third and fourth metatarsal bones and digits. The second metatarsal bone is fused with the first metatarsal bone and the digits of the second ray are absent. The lateral cuneiform bone is aplastic or hypoplastic and fused with the cuboid bone

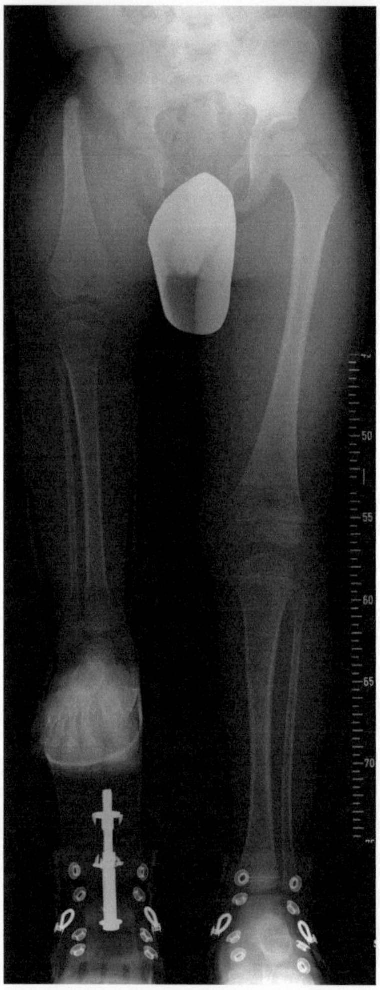

Fig. 4 Proximal femoral focal deficiency (PFFD). A large portion of the proximal femur is absent. The femoral head is present but hypoplastic and the neck shows delayed and fragmented ossification. There is a dysplastic acetabulum. The distal femoral remnant is tapered at its proximal end and migrated upward (PFFD type C)

acetabulum is normal or mildly dysplastic, and there is usually a severe varus alignment or upward migration of the distal femoral remnant;
- Aitken type C: a large portion of the femur is absent, the proximal end of the distal femur is tapered and migrated upwards, the femoral head and neck are missing or severely hypoplastic, and the acetabulum shows severe dysplasia;
- Aitken type D (most severe): the residual femur is very short, deformed and can be fused with the tibia below, whereas the femoral head and neck and the acetabulum are missing.

US and particularly MRI are useful to assess the exact nature of the (fibro-cartilaginous) tissues at the side of loss of continuity. Furthermore, MRI is used to evaluate the hip joint, and the knee joint as aplasia or hypoplasia of the cruciate ligaments can occur in association. PFFD should be distinguished from congenital short femur (CSF) which is characterized by a general hypoplasia of a otherwise anatomically normal femur. In CSF some degree of lateral bowing of the diaphysis and coxa vara may be seen, as well as delayed ossification of the femoral head and neck and flattening or hypoplasia of the condylar complex.

Tibial Deficiency [2, 5, 8]

This lower limb deficiency (also known as tibial hemimelia) is very rare with a reported incidence of approximately 1 in 1,000,000 births. The majority of cases are sporadic and unilateral but it can be bilateral in up to one third of the patients. If bilaterally, it is usually part of complex malformations syndromes (e.g., Split hand/Split foot syndrome, and Short rib polydactyly syndrome type 2 (Majewski type)). Tibial deficiencies are usually classified according to Clément:

- Clément type I (59%): total absence of the tibia;
- Clément type IIa (10%): the (cartilaginous) epiphysis of proximal tibia is present, which may be undetectable on radiographs in young infants because of non-ossification, and additional hypoplasia of the adjacent distal femoral epiphysis is often observed;
- Clément type IIb (24%): the proximal tibia is present including a portion of metaphysis and/or diaphysis, and there is a normal proximal epiphysis and normal growth plate;
- Clément type III (1.5%): only the distal tibia is present;
- Clément type IV (5%): the entire tibia is present but generally hypoplastic or only hypoplastic at its distal end, in the latter the distal end is tapered and sometimes deviates from the distal end of the fibula to articulate with the medial side of the ankle.

The fibula is usually normal in size and appearance, but can be hypoplastic or deformed. The foot may be normal but in varus equinus position. It can also be hypoplastic and deformed, especially on the medial (preaxial) side. In contrast to fibular hemimelia, the femur is often normal. US and in particular MRI can play a role in identifying non-ossified (cartilaginous) remnants of the tibia, tarsal bone abnormalities (such as coalition), ligamentous and muscular abnormalities, and neurovascular anatomy.

Congenital Bowing of the Tibia [2, 5, 8]

As the exact cause of unilateral tibial bowing is not known, it is unclear whether this disorder should be classified as a failure of formation or failure of differentiation. Several reasons have been described such as poor intra-uterine positioning, focal osseous dysplasia, and impaired prenatal vascular development. Congenital posteromedial bowing of the tibia (CPMBT) generally has a good prognosis, usually disappearing in early childhood. It is sometimes associated with club foot. Congenital anterolateral bowing of the tibia has a much poorer clinical prognosis because it is often associated with neurofibromatosis type 1 with the risk of pathological fracture and congenital pseudarthrosis. Prognosis is better for patients who do not have concurrent neurofibromatosis type 1. In general, tibial bowing can be associated with polydactyly, preliminary midtibial duplication, bifid homolateral great toe and hand malformations in the context of a minor tibial duplication. Finally, congenital anteromedial bowing of the tibia usually occurs in combination with fibular hemimelia. Because of this combination, anteromedial bowing of the tibia has a poorer prognosis than CPMBT.

Fibular Deficiency [2, 5, 8–10]

Fibular deficiency or hemimelia is the most common (postaxial) longitudinal deficiency of the long bones with an incidence of 7.4–20 per 1,000,000 births. As in tibial hemimelia, the majority of cases are unilateral and sporadic but it can be bilateral. In the latter, fibula deficiency is often part of complex malformations syndromes (e.g., FFU (Femur-Fibula-Ulna) syndrome, TAR (Thrombocytopenia-Absent Radius) syndrome, and Furhmann syndrome). Fibular deficiencies are usually classified according to Achterman and Kalamchi's:

- Achterman and Kalamchi's type IA: there is a complete but hypoplastic fibula with its proximal end distal to its normal position;
- Achterman and Kalamchi's type IB: the proximal fibula is absent;
- Achterman and Kalamchi's type II: complete aplasia of the fibula with anteromedial bowing of the tibia.

Fibular deficiencies occur often in combination with absence of one or more lateral foot rays, hypoplasia of the lateral aspect of the knee (resulting in genu valgum), and femoral defects (PFFD, CSF). Again, US and in particular MRI can play a role in identifying non-ossified (cartilaginous) remnants of the fibula, tarsal bone abnormalities (such as coalition), ligamentous and muscular abnormalities, and neurovascular anatomy.

Failure of Differentiation

Humeroradial and Radioulnar Synostoses [1, 6, 7]

Congenital synostoses of the arm involve the distal humerus and radius, and less frequently the proximal radius and ulna. The synostosis can be bony (synostosis), fibrous (syndesmosis), or cartilaginous (synchondrosis). Proximal radioulnar synostosis is almost always combined with radial head abnormalities such as hypoplasia, subluxation, or posterior dislocation. It is most often found sporadically and bilaterally, as an isolated finding, but can be seen as part of longitudinal preaxial deficiencies, in association with X chromosome anomalies, or in several syndromes (e.g., Poland's or Cornelia de Lange's syndrome).

Carpal/Tarsal Coalition [1, 11–13]

Carpal coalitions are often asymptomatic and an incidental finding on radiographs (Fig. 5). The terminology is actually a misnomer because it represents failure of normal segmentation of the primitive carpal mesenchyme. Carpal coalition may be isolated or multiple. It can be bony (synostosis), fibrous (syndesmosis), or cartilaginous (synchondrosis). Isolated coalitions usually involve two carpal bones in the same row, with lunotriquetral coalition being by far the most common. In contrast, multiple coalitions usually extend across carpal rows, and are often part of congenital syndromes (e.g., arthrogryposis, Turner's syndrome, Ellis-van Creveld syndrome, multiple synostosis syndrome). Tarsal coalitions, on the other hand, usually present with restricted motion and pain in active adolescents. Again, the coalition can be bony (synostosis), fibrous (syndesmosis), or cartilaginous (synchondrosis). Up to 90% are calcaneonavicular or talocalcaneal, whereas other types are rare. 50–60% of tarsal coalitions are bilateral. They are usually isolated but can be associated with other congenital anomalies (e.g., tibial and fibular hemimelia, PFFD) or syndromes (e.g., Apert syndrome). As the coalitions can be fibrous or cartilaginous, US

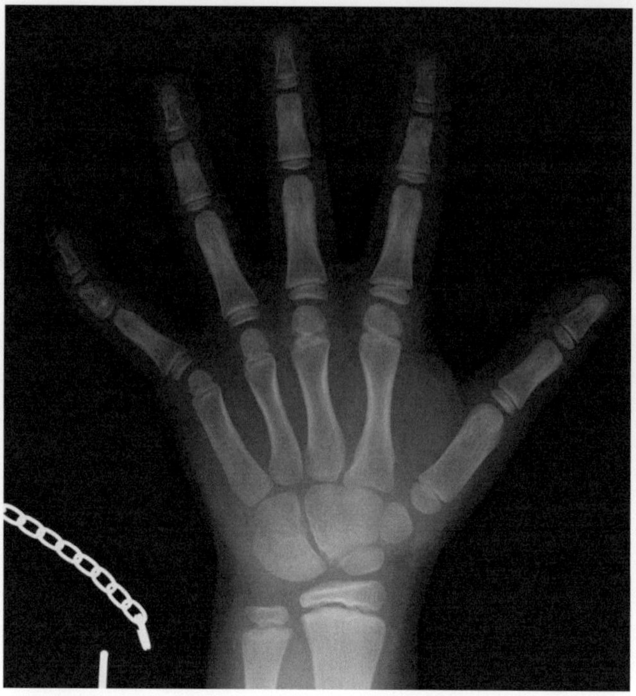

Fig. 5 Carpal coalition. There is a congenital fusion of the trapezoid and capitate bone, and of the hamate, triquetrum and lunate bone

and MRI can play a role in the diagnosis especially if operative resection is considered (as in symptomatic tarsal coalition), whereas CT might be indicated in the preoperative planning of bony (tarsal) coalitions.

Syndactyly [1, 14]

This is one of the commonest congenital disorders of the hand or foot caused by a failure in the process of digital separation and web space formation that normally occurs by apoptosis at the end of embryonic life. The resulting fusion of digits can involve only the soft tissues (membranous or simple syndactyly) (Fig. 6), or both the soft tissues and bony structures (osseous syndactyly or complex syndactyly). The syndactyly may be complete or incomplete and may affect two digits only (most commonly the ring and middle fingers) or several digits. They are classified as preaxial, postaxial, or mesoaxial syndactyly, and do occur in combination with polydactyly (synpolydactyly). Most syndactylies are isolated and bilateral. They do occur sporadically, usually with an autosomal dominant inheritance pattern, and can involve both hands and feet. Syndactylies can also be secondary to an amniotic band syndrome (Fig. 1), or occur as part of certain syndromes like Poland's syndrome or acrocephalosyndactylies (Apert syndrome).

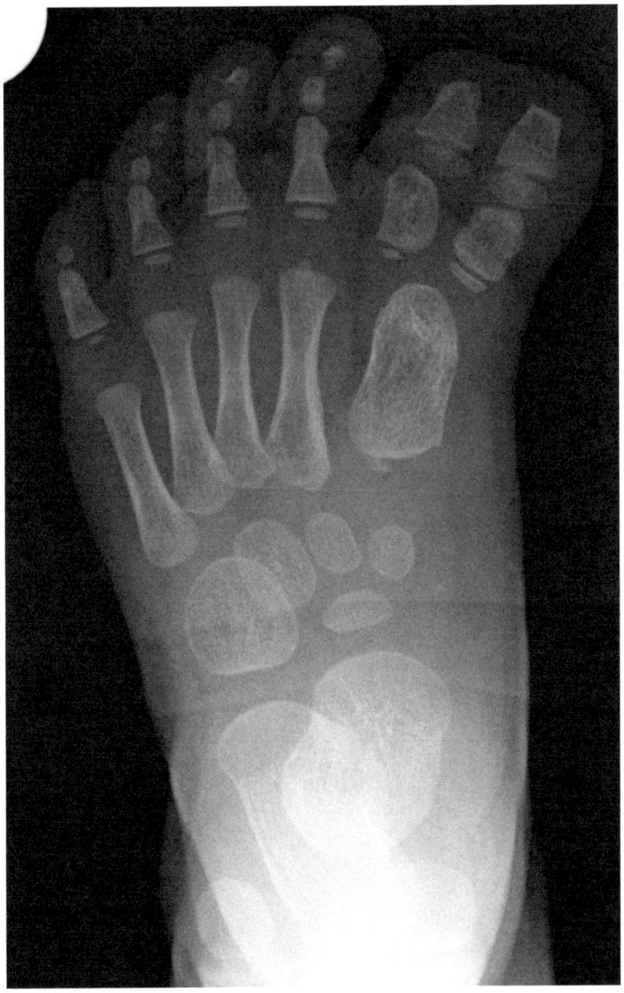

Fig. 6 Preaxial polydactyly and syndactyly of the foot. There is a duplication of the phalanges of the first digit in combination with a syndactyly of the soft tissues. The first metatarsal bone is enlarged, most likely due to congenital osseous fusion of a duplicated first metatarsal bone

Symphalangism [1]

This is a peculiar condition in which an interphalangeal joint (usually the proximal interphalangeal joint of the fifth finger or toe) fails to differentiate. The fusion can be bony or fibrous resulting in finger stiffness. Symphalangism is usually familial, inherited in an autosomal dominant pattern, but can be associated with other anomalies.

Duplication

Duplication of the Long Bones [1, 8]

Duplication (or dimelia) of the long bones is extremely rare. Ulnar dimelia (also known as "mirror hand") is characterized by duplication of the ulna, absence of preaxial structures (radius, radial carpal bones, and preaxial fingers), and postaxial polydactyly with a variable degree of symmetry across the midline. It is usually unilateral and isolated, but in bilateral cases Laurin-Sandrow syndrome (mirror hands and feet with nose anomalies) must be suspected. Radiographs of the whole upper limb are required as duplication of the proximal humerus, hypoplasia of the scapula, and congenital dislocation of the shoulder are associated with ulnar dimelia. In femoral dimelia the femur almost always bifurcates at its distal end. It results in a more or less pronounced shortening of the thigh with an unusually wide and sometimes triangular shaped distal part. On radiographs a partial to complete duplication of the distal end of the femur can be seen, dividing into two separate distal ends, the most lateral articulating with the fibula. Femoral dimelia is often associated with other bone malformations of the homolateral limb, such as tibial hemimelia and/or ectrodactyly (Gollop-Wolfgang complex). Isolated cases of femoral dimelia are rare.

Polydactyly [1, 14–16]

This common congenital disorder of hands and feet refers to the presence of supernumerary digits (Fig. 6). Polydactyly is classified as preaxial, postaxial, mesoaxial, or complex. The duplication can occur at any level of the finger and usually involves bony duplication but a rudimentary pedunculated nubbin is also possible. It can be combined with syndactyly in complex cases. Polydactyly is usually isolated, transmitted with an autosomal dominant pattern, but may be part of numerous syndromes (e.g., short rib-polydactyly syndromes, Ellis Van Creveld syndrome, oculodentodigital syndrome, Pallister-Hall syndrome, Greig's cephalopolysyndactyly syndrome).

Brachydactyly [1, 17]

Children with brachydactyly present with shortening of one or several fingers or toes. Brachydactyly can occur either as an isolated malformation or as part of a complex malformation syndromes. Furthermore, it may be accompanied by other malformations of hands and/or feet such as syndactyly, polydactyly, or symphalangism. Brachydactylies are classified according to Bell's classification into five types (from A to E) and different subtypes, depending on the involved skeletal segment or the affected finger/toe. A very common type of brachydactyly is the shortening of the middle phalanx of the little finger, often considered an normal variant (Brachydactyly type A3). It can be responsible for additional clinodactyly (finger deviation in the coronal plane). Brachydactyly type E (i.e., shortening of the metacarpals) is seen in conditions such as pseudohypoparathyroidism (Albright's hereditary osteodystrophy) and Turner's syndrome.

References

1. Aucourt J, Budzik JF, Manouvrier-Hanu S, Mézel A, Cotton A, Boutry N (2012) Congenital malformations of the hand and forearm in children: what radiologists should know. Semin Musculoskelet Radiol 16:146–158
2. Wilcox WR, Coulter CP, Schmitz ML (2015) Congenital limb deficiency disorders. Clin Perinatol 42:281–300
3. Gold NB, Westgate M-N, Holmes LB (2011) Anatomic and etiological classification of congenital limb deficiencies. Am J Med Genet A 155:1225–1235
4. Laor T, Jaramillo D, Hoffer EA, Kasser JR (1996) MR imaging in congenital lower limb deformities. Pediatr Radiol 26:381–387
5. Bedoya MA, Chauvin NA, Jaramillo D, Davidson R, Horn BD, Ho-Fung V (2015) Common patterns of congenital lower extremity shortening: diagnosis, classification, and follow-up. Radiographics 35:1191–1207
6. Bednar MS, James MA, Light TR (2009) Congenital longitudinal deficiency. J Hand Surg Am 34:1739–1747
7. Bauer AS, Bednar MS, James MA (2013) Disruption of the radial/ulnar axis: congenital longitudinal deficiencies. J Hand Surg Am 38:2293–2302
8. Bergèrea A, Amzallag-Bellengera E, Lefebvreb G et al (2015) Imaging features of lower limb malformations above the foot. Diagn Interv Imaging 96:901–914
9. Yoong P, Mansour R (2014) Internal derangement of the knee in fibular hemimelia: radiographic and MRI findings. Knee 21:749–756
10. Hamdy RC, Makhdom AM, Saran N, Birch J (2014) Congenital fibular deficiency. J Am Acad Orthop Surg 22:246–255
11. Pruszczynski B, Saller J, Rogers KJ, Holmes LJ, Ty JM (2016) Incidence of carpal coalition in the pediatric population. J Pediatr Orthop 36(8):e106–e110
12. Newman JS, Newberg AH (2000) Congenital tarsal coalition: multimodality evaluation with emphasis on CT and MR imaging. Radiographics 20(2):321–332
13. Lawrence DA, Rolen MF, Haims AH, Zayour Z, Moukaddam HA (2014) Tarsal coalitions: radiographic, CT, and MR imaging findings. HSS J 10(2):153–166
14. Kozin SH, Zlotolow DA (2015) Common pediatric congenital conditions of the hand. Plast Reconstr Surg 136(2):241e–257e
15. Faust KC, Kimbrough T, Oakes JE, Edmunds JO, Faust DC (2015) Polydactyly of the hand. Am J Orthop 44(5):E127–E134
16. Malik S (2014) Polydactyly: phenotypes, genetics and classification. Clin Genet 85(3):203–212
17. Temtamy SA, Aglan MS (2008) Brachydactyly. Orphanet J Rare Dis 3:15

Infections and Inflammatory Musculoskeletal Disorders in Children

Peter J. Strouse

Infection and inflammatory disease in children varies from that seen in adults. The disease processes are different and manifest differently due to the growing skeleton and immature tissues. The sequelae of infection and inflammation in children may affect growth and development of structures. As such, proper diagnosis is imperative for prompt and appropriate treatment. In this essay, the commoner infectious and inflammatory processes in the pediatric musculoskeletal system are emphasized.

Infection

Infection can occur in bone (osteomyelitis), joints (septic arthritis), muscle (pyomyositis) or soft tissues (cellulitis, necrotizing fasciitis). Morbidity varies with site, organism, age and the adequacy of host response. Distinction of the type of infection by imaging guides work-up and treatment.

Osteomyelitis

Sources of osteomyelitis in children include hematogenous seeding, adjacent joint or soft tissue infection or direct implantation via surgery, trauma or a foreign body. Risk factures include a history of trauma (in one third), prematurity, umbilical catheterization, urinary tract infection, immunodeficiency, and pre-existing disease [1].

Acute osteomyelitis occurs due to bacterial seeding of a metaphysis or metaphyseal equivalent. Slow flow in sinusoidal end vessels and the local environment promote seeding and bacterial growth in the metaphysis [1–4]. In infants less than 18-months old, transphyseal vessels also promote spread of infection from metaphysis to epiphysis. Epiphyseal and secondary joint infections are therefore more common in infants.

The diagnosis of osteomyelitis is made by positive blood cultures or, if blood cultures are negative, imaging findings consistent with infection with abnormal white blood cell count (WBC), elevated erythrocyte sedimentation rate (ESR) and C-reactive protein (CRP). Blood cultures are positive in 30–75% of cases [3]. *Staphylococcus aureus* is the most common organism. Methicillin-resistant *Staphylococcus aureus* (MRSA) is now seen in 3–40% of cases and is increasing in incidence [5, 6]. *Kingella kingae* is seen in young children [1].

The earliest finding of osteomyelitis on radiography is soft tissue swelling. Bone changes are not seen until the second week, at the earliest (Fig. 1). Ultrasound may show soft tissue swelling, periosteal thickening and subperiosteal abscess [7]. MRI is the preferred modality for detection and characterization including demonstration of abscess (Figs. 1 and 2) [1, 3, 4]. Gadolinium aids in identifying intraosseous abscess, identifying necrotic bone and delineating soft tissue extension. Nuclear medicine bone scans become positive by showing increased activity 24–48 h after symptom onset. Bone scans have a sensitivity of 90–95% and specificity of 60–70% of bone scans for osteomyelitis [1, 4]. Differential diagnosis on bone scans includes trauma, tumors and bone infarcts (sickle cell disease). Occasionally, "cold defects" may be seen. Nuclear medicine is now less commonly used with advances in MRI. PET is not widely used for pediatric osteomyelitis but may show increased metabolic activity with an infection [1]. Whole body MRI is increasingly being used in lieu of bone scan to find infection when symptoms do not localize [4].

Seventy percent of patients with *Staphylococcus aureus* osteomyelitis have a complication, which include subperiosteal abscess, pyomyositis, deep venous thrombosis/septic thrombophlebitis and septic arthritis [1, 3]. MRSA often manifests as aggressive disease with complications (Fig. 1) [5, 6]. Other long term complications may include chronic osteomyelitis, bone infarction, pathologic fracture, joint destruction, growth plate fusion, deformity and leg length difference.

P.J. Strouse
Section of Pediatric Radiology, C. S. Mott Children's Hospital, Department of Radiology, University of Michigan Health System, 1540 E. Hospital Drive, Ann Arbor, MI 48109-4252, USA
e-mail: pstrouse@umich.edu

J. Hodler et al. (eds.), *Musculoskeletal Diseases 2017-2020*, DOI 10.1007/978-3-319-54018-4_32

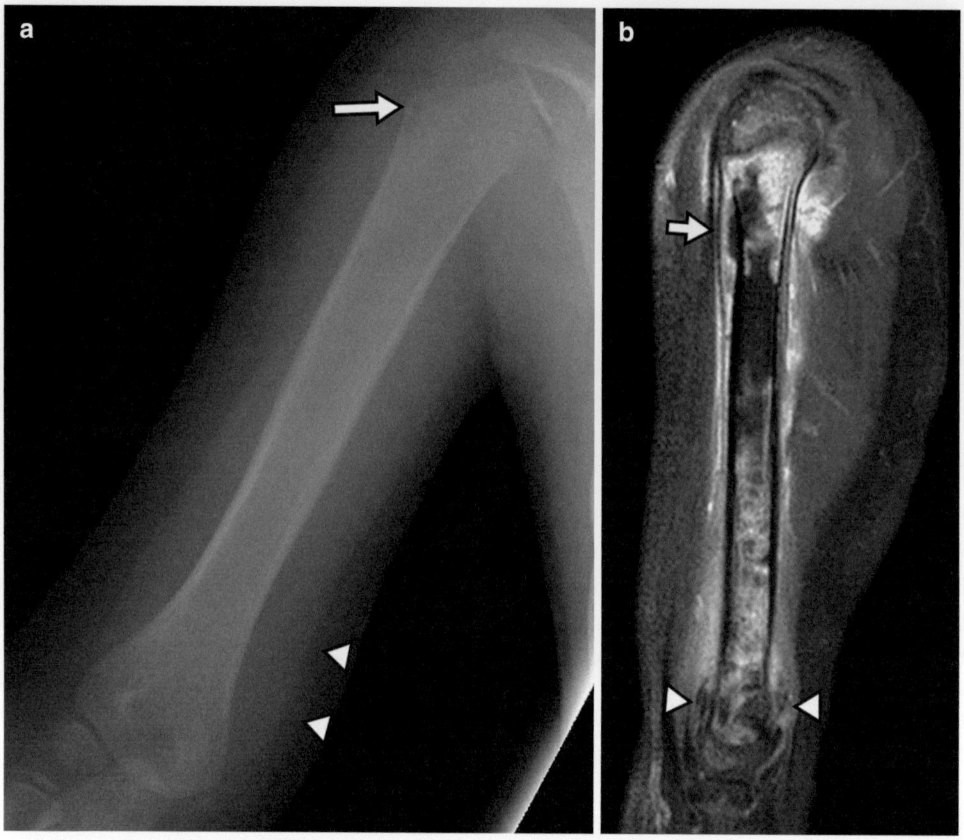

Fig. 1 Three year-old boy with methicillin resistant staph aureus (MRSA) osteomyelitis. The patient presented with arm swelling, pain and fever. MRSA was found on blood culture prior to imaging. (**a**) Anteroposterior radiograph shows a subtle lucency within the proximal humeral metaphysis (*arrow*). At most, there is subtle abrnomality of diaphyseal bone. Soft tissue swelling is most prominent medially, near the elbow (*arrowheads*). (**b**) Fat-saturated sagittal T1-weighted MR image after gadolinium-based contrast (TR 628 ms, TE 15 ms) shows diffuse abnormality of the marrow space extending from proximal metaphysis to distal metaphysis. Areas of increased enhancement and areas of absent enhancement (abscess, necrosis) are seen throughout. A small superiosteal abscess is seen at the anterior aspect of the proximal humeral metaphysis (*arrow*). Synovial enhancement is partially seen at the elbow (*arrowheads*). Enhancement is seen within adjacent soft tissues

Spinal osteomyelitis occurs due to seeding of the metaphyseal equivalent of vertebral body endplates. In distinction, disciitis is infection of the disc space and vertebral body endplate. Imaging findings overlap. MRI is performed with spinal osteomyelistis to define the extent of disease and to exclude epidural abscess.

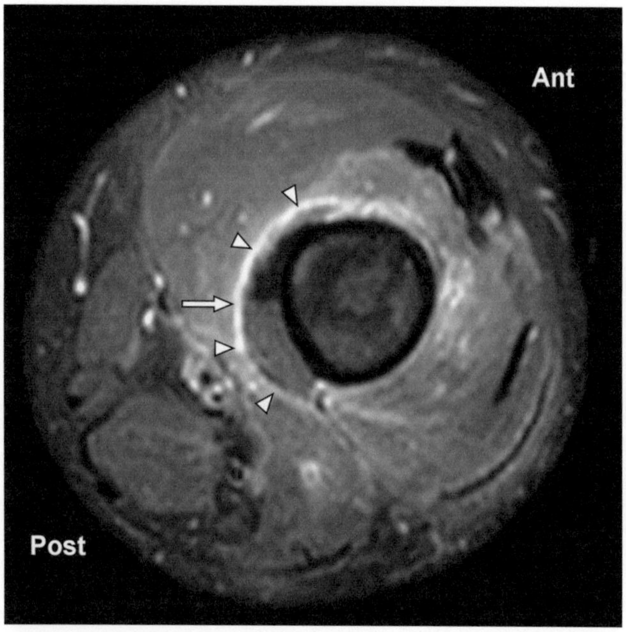

Fig. 2 Thirteen year-old girl with acute osteomyelitis of the distal femur. The girl had a preceding viral illness two weeks prior and questionable trauma to the knee area one week prior. She presented with pain worse with movement, swelling and fever. White blood count, erythrocyte sedimentation rate and C-reactive protein were all markedly elevated. Axial fat-saturated T1-weighted MR image after gadolinium-based contrast (TR 600 ms, TE 18 ms) shows a subperiosteal abscess at the posterior aspect of the distal femoral metaphysis (*arrowheads*). Low signal extruded fat is seen anteriorly within the subperiosteal abscess delineated by a fluid/fluid level (*arrow*). Periosteal and adjacent soft tissue enhancement is noted. *Ant* anterior, *Post* posterior

Pelvic osteomyelitis occurs as metaphyseal equivalents—adjacent to the sacroiliac joints, triradiate cartilage, pubic symphysis, ischiopubic synchondrosis and iliac apophyses [2, 8]. MRI is used to assess the site and extent of infection—osteomyelitis verses septic arthritis verses pyomyositis. With osteomyelitis, MRI is necessary to assess for intrapelvic extension [8].

Neonatal osteomyelitis is often indolent or masked by other medical issues. Delayed diagnosis is common. In neonates, group B streptococcus, *Escherichia coli* and Enterobacter are more frequent with a lesser incidence of *Staphylococcus aureus* than in older children [4]. More epiphyseal and joint disease also portends a worse prognosis.

Patients with **sickle cell disease** have a higher incidence of infection with encapsulated organisms including Salmonella due to decreased splenic function with relative immunosuppression [9]. Infection with *Staphylococcus aureus* is also common. Differentiation of infection from bone marrow infarction is challenging but may be suggested by high signal on fat-saturated unenhanced T1-weighted MR images [9]. There is a higher incidence of diaphyseal disease with sickle cell disease, likely related to seeding of bone marrow infarcts.

Subacute osteomylelitis is due to a less virulent organism and a partial host response which walls off the infection. On imaging, a well-defined lucent lesion (Brodie abscess) is seen in a metaphysis or metaphyseal equivalent (Fig. 3) [1, 3].

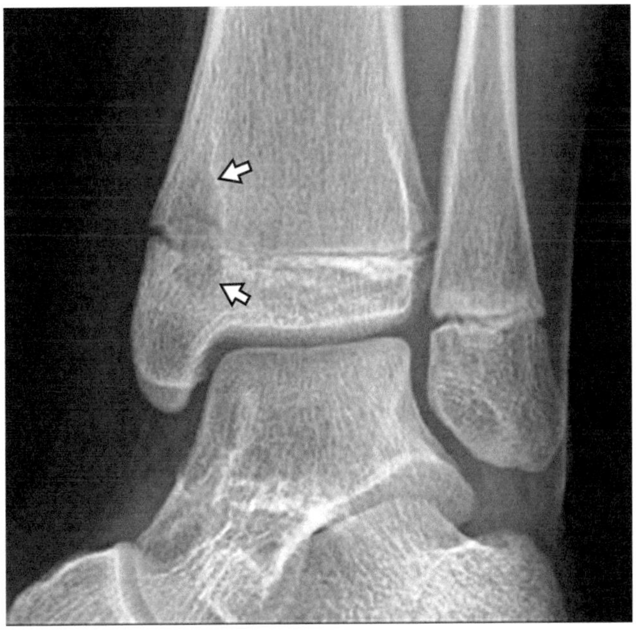

Fig. 3 Twelve year-old girl with subacute osteomyelitis (Brodie abscess). The patient presented with ankle pain and swelling for one month, but no fever. Mortise view of the left ankle shows a well-defined ovoid lucency with faintly sclerotic margins bridging the medial distal tibial growth plate (*arrows*)

A tract may be seen to the adjacent physis and, occasionally into epiphysis. Adjacent sclerosis and non-aggressive periosteal new bone may be seen. Rarely, a similar lesion occurs within an epiphysis. Children with subacute osteomyelitis present with less severe and insidious symptoms, less fever and marginally abnormal laboratory tests.

Chronic osteomyelitis is variably defined as osteomyelitis persisting for longer than 4–6 weeks [1, 4]. It is due to inadequately treated acute or subacute osteomyelitis. Chronic osteomyelitis is characterized by sequestra (fragments of necrotic bone within the infection), involucrum (cloaking periosteal new bone) and cloaca (draining sinus) [1]. Chronic osteomyelitis may complicate open fractures.

Septic Arthritis

Septic arthritis may occur due to hematogenous seeding of the synovium, extension of adjacent osteomyelitis or soft tissue infection, or by direct inoculation (trauma, surgery, iatrogenic) [10]. As previously noted, in infants less than 18-months old there is an increased association between osteomyelitis and septic arthritis due to transphyseal extension of infection.

Septic arthritis is most commonly due to *Staphylococcus aureus* [11]. Other organisms include group B streptococcus *and Escherichia coli* (particularly in neonates), *Pseudomonas aeruginosa*, *Streptococcus pneumoniae*, *Kingella kingae* (3-months to 3-years old), and *Neisseria gonorrhoeae* (neonates, sexually active teen). Peak presentation is 2–3 years of age. Lower extremity joints are more frequently involved than upper extremity joints. The hip and knee are most common with ankle and elbow less frequent. Symptoms are fever, localized joint pain and overlying warmth, erythema, soft tissue swelling, limp and refusal to bear weight.

ESR and WBC are increased. Blood cultures may be positive. Criteria for diagnosis on arthrocentesis are positive culture, positive gram stain or joint fluid WBC > 50,000/μL [10]. In approximately 30% of cases, an organism is not identified.

Depending on the joint involved, radiographs may show evidence of a joint effusion or adjacent soft tissue swelling, but are often normal. At the elbow, radiographs suffice to evaluate for effusion. Ultrasound is used at the hips to assess for effusion [7]. Ultrasound cannot distinguish infected for uninfected effusion from; however, abundant debris, synovial thickening or hyperemia on Doppler evaluation raises concern for infection (Fig. 4) [7]. On MR, increased signal (edema) and enhancement is seen in adjacent soft tissues and mildly increased adjacent bone marrow increase signal and enhancement may be seen. Distinction of reactive edema/enhancement from osteomyelitis may be difficult.

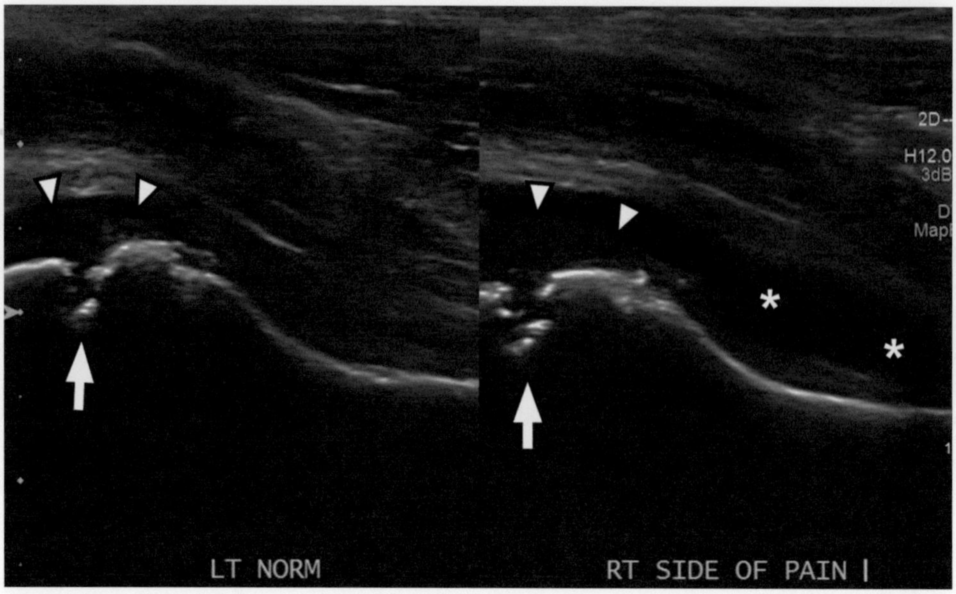

Fig. 4 Four year-old boy with transient synovitis of the right hip. The patient presented with a complaint of intermittent hip pain for 1 month, worsening in the last 24 h. He had some difficulty bearing weight, but full range of motion on exam. He was afebrile, with normal white blood count and C-reactive protein. Erythrocyte sedimentation rate was minimally elevated. Sagittal ultrasound images show a normal left (*LT NORM*) hip without effusion and a moderate him effusion on the right (*RT*, *asterisks*). Note that the effusion is most prominent anterior to the femoral neck and tapers over the femoral head. Femoral head cartilage is marked by *arrowheads* on each side. *Arrows* indicate the proximal femoral growth plates. The patient was treated conservatively without joint aspiration

The differential diagnosis for septic arthritis includes Lyme disease, viral infection, tuberculosis, Legg-Perthes disease, juvenile idiopathic arthritis (JIA), rheumatic fever and transient synovitis [10]. JIA is discussed later in this article. Rheumatic fever occurs post group A streptococcal infection with polyarthritis, carditis, erythema and subcutaneous nodules [11]. It is diagnoses with a strept test. Lyme disease is due to *Borrelia burgorferi* via tick bite [11]. Lyme disease simulates oligoarthritic JIA or septic arthritis. Lyme disease usually affects the knee or less commonly the hip, ankle and elbows. Patients with Lyme disease may also have myositis and lymph node enlargement.

Transient synovitis is the chief differential diagnosis for septic arthritis of the hip in young children. Transient synovitis often occurs after an upper respiratory tract infection. Patients have joint pain, mild fever and mildly increased ESR. Transient synovitis may be unilateral or bilateral. Treatment is conservative. Symptoms may recur.

Clinical factors may be used to distinguish septic arthritis from transient synovitis and guide management [12, 13]. Criteria include temperature (>38.5°C), WBC (>12 × 10^9/L), ESR (≥40 mm/h), CRP (≥20 mg/L) and weight bearing status. If all are abnormal, septic arthritis is certain—operative incision and drainage is indicated. If all are normal, septic arthritis is very unlikely—management may be conservative without joint aspiration (Fig. 4). It is patients in whom some criteria are positive and others not or with marginal abnormality who benefit most from joint aspiration to evaluate for infection [12, 13]. Depending on the joint, aspiration can be performed without or with imaging guidance (ultrasound or fluoroscopy).

Soft Tissue Infections

Pyomyositis is defined as a bacterial infection within muscle [7, 14]. Frank abscesses may form. Pyomyositis is most commonly seen in the pelvis. Care must be taken to exclude underlying osteomyelitis with extension into muscle and soft tissues. Prominent soft tissue findings may draw attention away from subtler bone findings.

Cellulitis is defined as a non-necrotizing infection limited to subcutaneous tissues, hypodermis and superficial fascia without muscle or deep fascial involvement [7, 14]. Imaging, principally ultrasound, is used to assess for fluid collection (abscess) or deeper extension. **Necrotizing fasciitis** is a rapidly progressive infection of deep fascia and adjacent soft tissues with areas of necrosis (which lack enhancement) [7, 14]. Fortunately, necrotizing fasciitis is uncommon in children. Differentiation of necrotizing fasciitis from pyomyositis and cellulitis may be challenging. Expedient surgical debridement is indicated for necrotizing fasciitis [14].

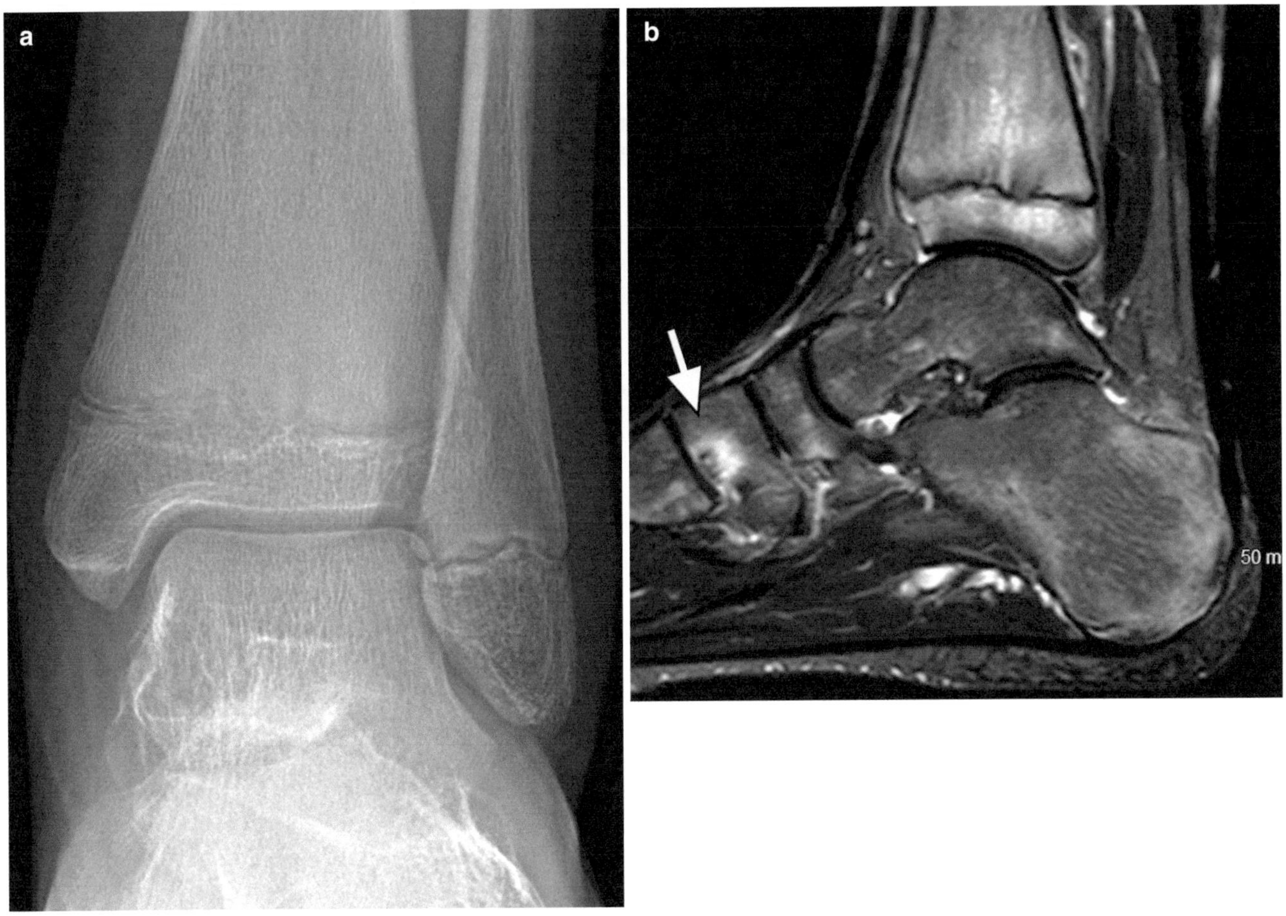

Fig. 5 Fifteen year-old boy with chronic recurrent multifocal osteomyelitis. The boy complained of chronic intermittent bone pain in his lower extremities. Erythrocyte sedimentation rate and C-reactive protein were mildly elevated. Multiple sites of disease were found on imaging. (**a**) Anteroposterior view of the right ankle shows ill-defined sclerosis in the distal tibial metaphysis with ill-defined lucencies near the growth plate. Mild soft tissue swelling is noted. (**b**) Sagittal inversion recovery MR image (TR 418 ms, TE 60 ms, TI 140 ms) shows increased signal within the distal tibial metaphysis and epiphysis, increased signal within the posterior calcaneus and a focal lesion with the medial cuneiform (*arrow*)

Chronic Recurrent Multifocal Osteomyelitis (CRMO)

CRMO is a disorder uncertain cause that has features of infections and inflammatory process and not infrequently mimics an osseous neoplastic process in presentation [15, 16]. The disease is related to sternoclavicular hyperostosis/SAPHO (synovitis, acne, pustulosis, hyperostosis and osteitis) syndrome and HLA-B27 related diseases. CRMO is characterized by recurrent episodes of swelling and pain, low grade fever, leukocytosis and elevated ESR. On biopsy, no infectious agent is found and no neoplastic cells are found; rather, there are non-specific, chronic appearing inflammatory changes highlighted by the presence of plasma cells. The disease is characterized by exacerbations and recurrences.

On imaging, the appearance of CMRO is protean [15, 16]. Disease is most common in metaphyses and metaphyseal equivalents with mixed, ill-defined lucent and sclerotic lesions abutting the physis (Fig. 5). Periosteal reaction, if present, is non-aggressive in appearance. Characteristic locations include lower extremity metaphyses, the clavicles and pelvic metaphyseal equivalents. Multifocality is characteristic. On MRI, lesions have ill-defined increased signal and enhancement (Fig. 5). Whole body MRI is useful for delineation of sites of disease [17].

Inflammatory Disease

Juvenile idiopathic arthritis (JIA) is not a single disease, but rather a heterogeneous spectrum of diseases characterized by inflammation of the synovium [11, 18–21]. On histology, JIA affected joints show inflammatory cells, fibrin, collagen. Similar pathology findings can be seen with other

Table 1 Juvenile idiopathic arthritis (JIA)—International League of Associations for Rheumatology (ILAR) classification [18–20]

Disorder	Percentage of JIA patients (%)	Criteria
Systemic-onset JIA	4–17	≥1 joint; with or preceded by fever; with one or more of: rash, lymph node enlargement, hepatosplenomegaly, serositis
Oligoarticular JIA	27–56	1–4 joints during first 6 months Persistent: not >4 joints affected throughout course of disease Extended: >4 joints affected after first 6 months
Polyarticular JIA—RF-positive	2–7	≥5 joints during first 6 months RF-positive
Polyarticular JIA—RF-negative	11–28	≥5 joints during first 6 months RF-negative
Enthesis related arthritis (ERA)	3–11	Arthritis + enthesitis or arthritis or enthesitis with at least two of: sacroiliac tenderness or lumbosacral pain, HLA-B27 antigen positive, new arthritis in male > 6-years-old, acute anterior uveitis, history of ankylosing spondylitis, ERA, IBD with sacroiliitis, Reiter syndrome or acute anterior uveitis in a first-degree relative
Juvenile psoriatic arthritis	2–11	Arthritis + psoriasis; or arthritis with at least two of: dactylitis, nail pitting or onycholysis, psoriasis in first-degree relative
Undifferentiated arthritis	11–21	Fulfills criteria for none of the above OR fulfills criteria in ≥2 of the above

IBD inflammatory bowel disease, *RF* rheumatoid factor

arthopathies including some infections (i.e. *Mycobacterium tuberculosis*, Coccidiomycosis). JIA is a diagnosis of exclusion. It is of unknown cause. JIA is defined as having onset before 16-years of age and symptoms greater than 6 months in duration [18]. JIA is classified by the International League of Associations for Rheumatology (ILAR) classification (Table 1) [18].

Systemic-onset JIA (Still disease) accounts for 5–10% of JIA [19] Incidence is near equal in boys and girls. Extra-articular manifestations may precede joint disease. The diagnosis is defined by having fever for greater than two weeks with one or more of: rash, hepatosplenomegaly, lymph node enlargement or serositis [18, 19, 21, 22]. Systemic symptoms may mask and/or precede joint symptoms. Early, there a little or no radiographic changes [11]. Joint disease tends to be late-onset, symmetric and polyarticular. One third to one half of patients proceed to a chronic destructive arthritis. Greater overall morbidity is seen with systemic disease. Macrophage activation syndrome (MAS) is a potentially fatal complication characterized by pancytopenia, disseminated intravascular coagulation (DIC), liver dysfunction, sustained fever, and, eventually, multi-organ failure [21].

Oligoarticular JIA is the most common form of JIA [19, 21]. Oligoarticular JIA (formerly "pauciarcitular") is defined as less than five joints involved within the first six months of disease. Oligoarticular JIA is divided into persistent oligoarticular disease (≤four joints; 75% remission [= good prognosis]) and extended oligoarticular disease (more joints involved after 6 months, 12% remission [= worse prognosis]). Peak incidence oligoarticular JIA is in young childhood (2–4-years-old) with girls more often affected than boys. The classic presentation of oligoarticular JIA is in the knee or ankle of a preschool girl [21].

Polyarticular JIA is less severe than systemic JIA and is defined by five or greater joints involved in the first six months of disease [18, 19, 21]. It is more common in girls. Polyarticular JIA is subclassified into rheumatoid factor (RF)-positive and RF-negative. RF-positive polyarticular JIA tends to occur in later childhood or adulthood; often the small joints of the hand and feet are symmetrically affected in adolescent girls; disease is adult rheumatoid arthritis-like with erosive joint destruction; outcomes are generally worse [21]. Patients with RF-negative polyarticular JIA may any age but tend to be younger; presentation and prognosis are more heterogeneous [21].

Radiographs in JIA are non-specific early [20, 21]. Juxta-articular soft tissue swelling, joint effusion and osteopenia may be seen (Figs. 6 and 7). Osteopenia is periarticular early and diffuse later (in part due to steroid treatment). Periosteal reaction may be seen on phalanges, metacarpals and metatarsals. Periarticular calcifications may occur with unclear pathophysiology. Cartilage in growing joints limits radiographic evaluation. Joint space narrowing takes time to be seen (usually > 2 years). Joint space narrowing may be seen early with polyarticular RF-positive or systemic-onset JIA. Bone erosions are not seen in young children due to the cartilaginous model. Erosions can occur anywhere within a joint, but are more common at synovial reflections and ligamentous insertions where there is less overlying protective cartilage [21].

Later, radiographs may show osteopenia, deformed epiphyses (overgrowth), larger erosions (cyst-like), abnormal angular carpal bones, carpal ankylosis, wrist subluxation, premature fusion (brachydactyly, shortening), contractures, squaring of the knee and patella, coxa magna/coxa valga, protrusio acetabulae, early degenerative joint disease, cervical ankylosis, cervical spine subluxation, and temporomandibular joint (TMJ) deformity with micrognathia [20, 21]. Avascular necrosis of the hip may occur due to steroid therapy.

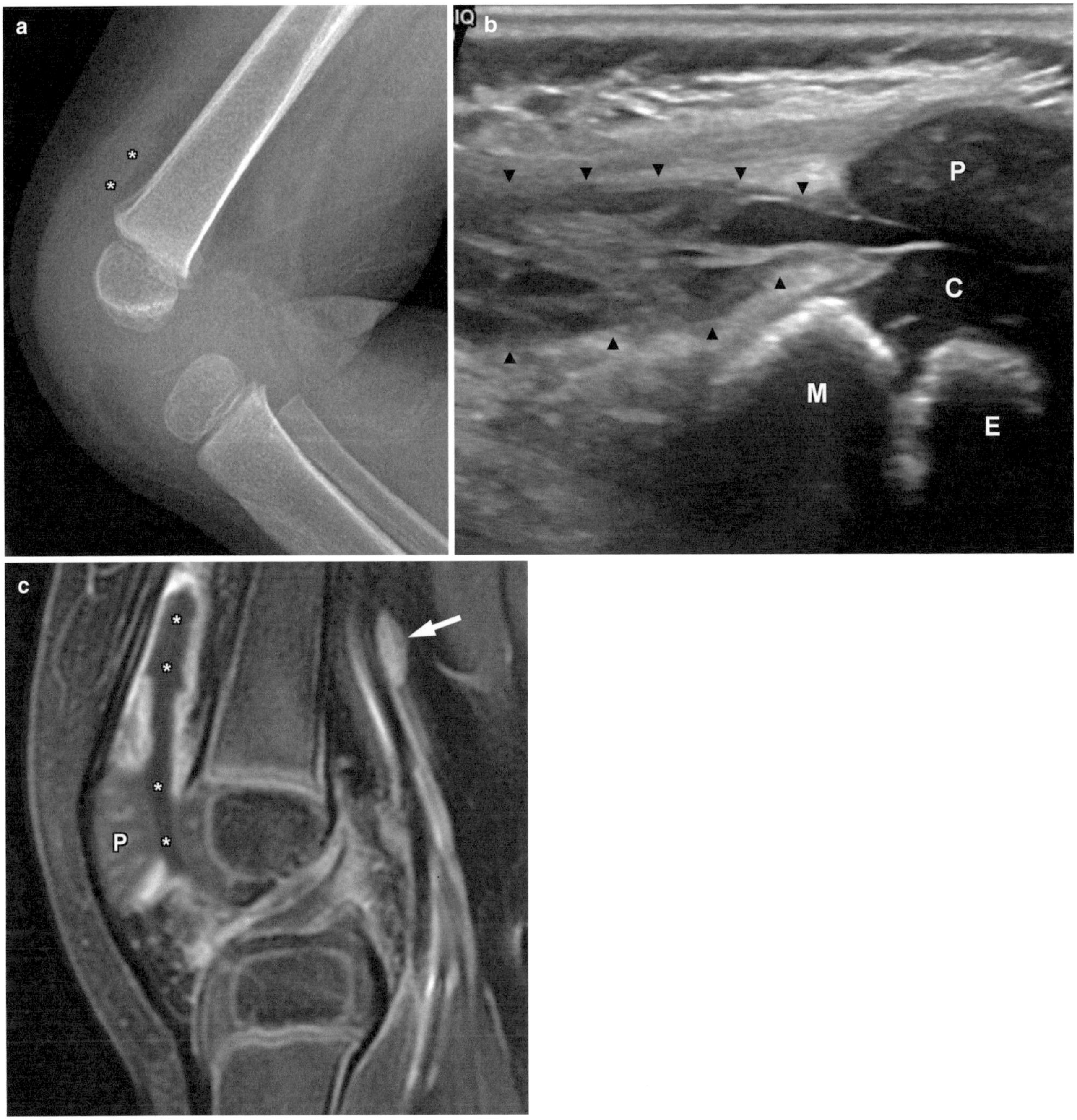

Fig. 6 Nineteen month-old girl with oligoarticular juvenile idiopathic arthritis. The girl presented with knee swelling and refusal to bear weight. (**a**) Lateral radiograph shows a knee joint effusion (*asterisks*). Diffuse periarticular soft tissue swelling is seen, most notable in the infrapatellar region. (**b**) Sagittal ultrasound shows a complex effusion within the suprapatellar pouch (*arrowheads*) with debris, septations and synovial thickening. *P* patella, *M* distal femoral metaphysis, *E* distal femoral epiphysis, *C* distal femoral epiphyseal cartilage. (**c**) Sagittal fat-saturated T1-weighted MR image after gadolinium-based contrast (TR 617 ms, TE 17 ms) shows the effusion (*asterisks*) and marked enhancement of thickened synovium throughout the joint. Striated enhancement is seen within the patellar cartilage (*P*). Similar "spokewheel" enhancement was seen within the distal femoral and proximal tibial epiphyses (not shown). A reactive lymph node is seen posteriorly (*arrow*)

Ultrasound may show synovial thickening/hypertrophy, joint effusion, synovial cysts, pannus, rice bodies (small fragments of free floating synovial proliferation indicative of chronic inflammation) involving the joints, tendon sheathes and bursa (Figs. 6 and 7) [19–21]. Hyperemia on color/power Doppler indicates inflammation. Ultrasound is particularly helpful for evaluation of small joints of the hands and feet and of tendon sheaths.

Roles of MRI for imaging of JIA are to diagnose and differentiate from other disorders, to assess severity of disease, to guide treatment, to monitor disease activity and assess the efficacy of treatment and to detect complications [11, 19, 21,

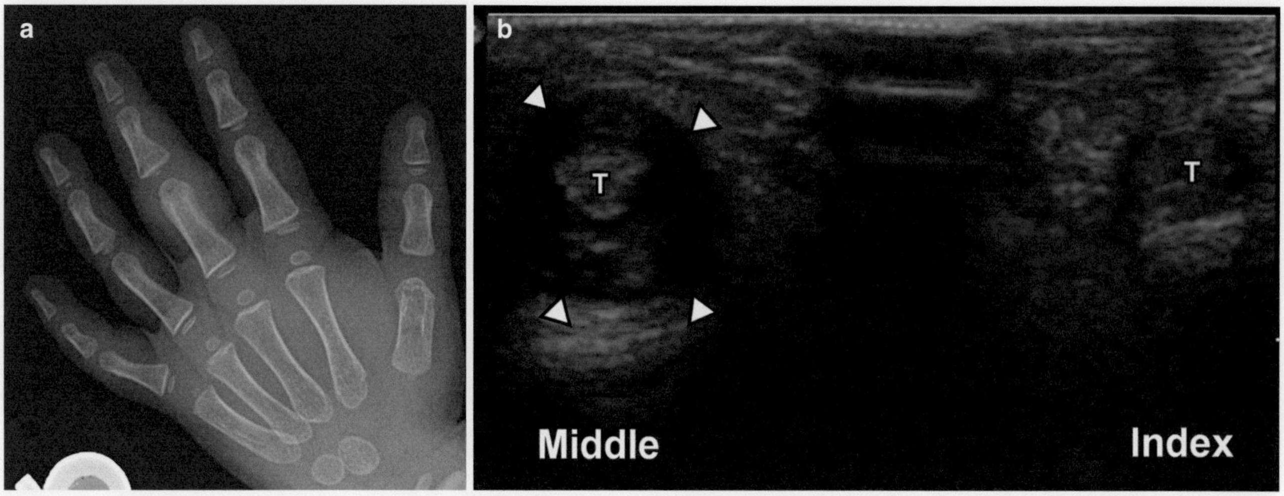

Fig. 7 Seventeen month-old girl with polyarticular rheumatoid factor-negative juvenile idiopathic arthritis. (**a**) Posteroanterior radiograph of the left hand shows soft tissue swelling of the middle finger. Mild swelling of other fingers is not well appreciated. Paradoxically, the epiphysis of the middle phalanx of the index finger appears small. (**b**) Palmar transverse ultrasound image shows synovial hypertrophy of the middle finger flexor tendon sheath (*arrowheads*). The flexor tendon sheath of the index finger is normal. *T* flexor tendons

22]. Cartilage sensitive sequences are performed to assess the integrity of articular cartilage. T2-weighted, inversion recovery and gadolinium-enhanced images will show the degree of inflammation. Early post-gadolinium images are used to differentiate synovitis verses effusion. Imaging should be performed within 10 min of contrast injection otherwise contrast will diffuse into joint fluid and epiphyseal cartilage. Advanced MRI techniques include subjective, semi-quantitative grading of joint inflammation, dynamic enhancement curves, synovial volume quantification, cartilage mapping, and diffusion weighted imaging (DWI) [11, 19, 22].

MRI shows effusion, synovial proliferation, pannus, cartilage destruction and erosion, bone erosion (Fig. 6) [11]. Bone marrow edema is a pre-erosive sign, and indication for initiation of treatment [21]. Bone marrow edema is a misnomer—histologically, it is a true osteitis with an inflammatory infiltrate [22].

At the knee, MRI findings of JIA also include joint effusion, synovial proliferation and enhancement, rice bodies, popliteal cysts, meniscal hypoplasia/atrophy, hemosiderin (differential diagnosis: pigmented villonodular synovitis, hemophilia, post-traumatic, venous malformation), widened femoral notch and reactive popliteal lymph nodes (Fig. 6). Characteristic sites for pannus are infrapatellar and adjacent to the cruciate ligaments. In young children, spoke-wheel enhancement may be seen within the cartilaginous epiphyses and patella due to hyperemia [21]. Bone erosions are rare in young and increase in incidence with age. Reactive changes may be seen in adjacent bone marrow (edema vs. osteitis). Adjacent soft tissue changes may include tenosynovitis, myositis, fasciitis, edema, bursa and ganglia.

The hands and wrists are frequently involved in JIA [20, 21]. Early changes include soft tissue swelling and periarticular osteopenia (Fig. 7). With more advanced disease, findings include joint space loss, erosions, periosteal new bone, soft tissue calcification, advanced maturation, shortening of the carpus and carpal fusion (Fig. 8). Erosions preferentially occur at non-articular regions of the metacarpal and metatarsal heads and bases which are devoid of cartilage.

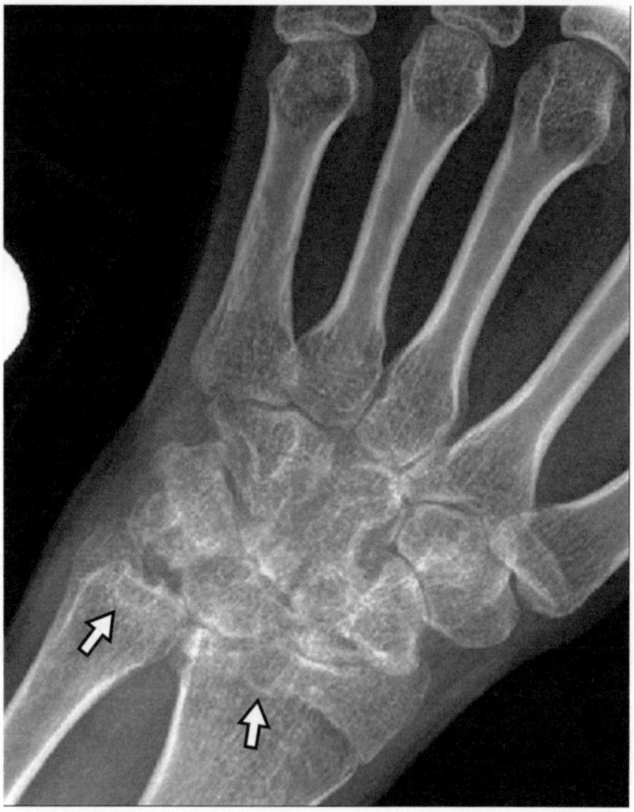

Fig. 8 Fifteen year-old girl with longstanding polyarticular rheumatoid factor-positive juvenile idiopathic arthritis. Posteroanterior view of the left wrist shows diffuse osteopenia and diffuse narrowing of all joint spaces within the wrist. The carpal bones are irregular and perhaps partially fused. Large erosions are seen within the distal radius and ulna (*arrows*)

Ultrasound can be used to look at small joints and tendon sheaths in the hands and wrists. On MRI, care must be taken not to mistake normal carpal undulations for erosions [23]. Bone marrow edema, cartilage destruction and synovial enhancement suggest erosions.

Patients with JIA involvement of the cervical spine present with neck stiffness and decreased range of motion. Disease may progress to ankyloses [20, 21]. C2/C3 is most affected but disease is often multilevel. With fusion before skeletal maturation, the vertebra bodies appear hypoplastic with decreased disc spaces. Odontoid erosions may be associated with C1/C2 ligamentous instability.

The temporomandibular joints (TMJs) are involved in a substantial portion of JIA patients, probably over 50% of patients [21]. Outcomes may be aesthetic and functional. Symptoms often underestimate the severity involvement and may even be absent. Radiographs show chronic deformity and erosions. US is not helpful, especially early, and is challenging. Contrast-enhanced MRI shows joint effusion, synovial enhancement, bone marrow edema and indicative of the need for treatment (steroid injection) [21]. MRI also shows the TMJ disc, internal derangement and condylar deformities. CT is limited to showing osseous deformity.

Enthesis Related Arthritis (ERA)

ERA disorders are characterized by a positive family history, enthesitis, sacroileiits (usually later in children) and normal RF [11, 18, 24]. Diagnosis of ERA is by arthritis and/or enthesitis with any two of five criteria: sacroiliac or spinal pain, HLA-B27 positivity, acute anterior uvietitis; arthritis onset in boy > 6-years-old or positive family history [18, 19]]. ERA includes juvenile ankylosing spondylitis and reactive arthritis and occurs in boys more frequently than girls, usually in later childhood or adolescence [11]. Enthesitis characteristically occurs at the Achilles insertion, plantar tendons/fascia, the knee (quadriceps and patellar tendons) and within the pelvis. Other manifestations include peripheral arthritis (usually asymmetric), tendonitis, dactylitis, uveitis and sacroileitis (in approximately 30%) [11, 21], spondylitis, and extra-articular manifestations (psoriasis, inflammatory bowel disease [IBD]). Asymmetric involvement of the hip is common at presentation [21]. Spinal involvement is late (very uncommon in children). On MRI, sacroiliitis is characterized high signal on T2-weighted images with adjacent bone marrow edema or osteitits, erosions and synovial enhancement [21, 25]

Juvenile ankylosing spondylitis is characterized by sacroiliitis and spondylitis [11, 20, 21, 24]. Extra-axial involvement is most common at the hip, knee and ankle. Significant spinal disease is uncommon in children. Dactylitis can affect the fingers and toes. Characteristic presentation is an adolescent male with acute anterior uveitis and hip arthritis [21].

Reactive arthritis (Reiter syndrome) may be provoked by infection, most often in the genitourinary or gastrointestinal tract [11, 20]. Patients are HLA-B27 positive. It is defined as reactive arthritis with conjunctivitis and urethritis. Enthesitis and whiskered periosteal new bone in the foot are characteristic [20].

Juvenile psoriatic arthritis is more common in females than males [26]. Presentation peaks in early adolescence [26]. It is defined as psoriasis with arthritis or arthritis with two of dactyliits, nail pitting/oncholysis, or psoriasis in a first degree relative [18, 26]. It is more common for arthritis to precede skin disease in children than adults. Associated joint disease is bilateral and tends to be asymmetric and pauciarticular early. However, any number of joints may be involved. Large or small joints may be affected with most frequent involvement of small joints of hands and feet, the knee or the sacroiliac joints [11]. Tendon sheaths may be affected. Changes in fingers are characteristic with tenosynovitis causing "sausage digits" [11]. In a study by Lee et al. [26], MR findings in descending order of frequency were synovial enhancement, joint effusions, bone marrow edema/osteitis, soft tissue edema/enhancement, tendon abnormality (including "sausage digit") and bone erosions. Bone marrow abnormality in juvenile psoriatic arthritis may appear similar to CRMO [26].

Arthritis associated with inflammatory bowel disease may accompany ulcerative colitis or, less prevalently, Crohn disease. Joint involvement is pauciarticular, involves peripheral larger joints, most commonly affecting the sacroiliac joints or the lower extremities. Arthritis is similar to other types of ERA.

Radiographs in ERA are normal early. Soft tissue swelling, joint effusion, osteopenia, decreased joint space, erosions, late fusion (rare), whiskered periosteal new bone may be seen [11, 20, 21]. Rarely, there is rapid destruction of a joint. Dactylitis may be seen. With enthesitis, there is local osteopenia, erosions and later osteophytes at characteristic locations (Achilles, plantar, patella). Sacroiliitis is seen as joint indistinctness, psuedowidening and reactive sclerosis (iliac > sacral). CT and MR are good for evaluating the sacroiliac joints. Radiography of the SI joints is challenging with significant variability (Fig. 9) [25]. Anteroposterior and bilateral Ferguson oblique views are obtained (tube angled 30° cephalad). Sacroiliac joint MRI may be positive before symptoms. Vertebral changes on radiography are uncommon in pediatric patients.

MRI in patients with ERA may also show bone marrow edema/osteitis, erosions and syndovial enhancement. Contrast is useful to look for synovitis, capsulitis and enthesitis. Whole body MRI has been used to identify and follow sites of disease [27].

Undifferentiated arthritis is an arthritis that does not fulfil criteria of a specific arthritis or fulfils criteria of two or more types of arthritis.

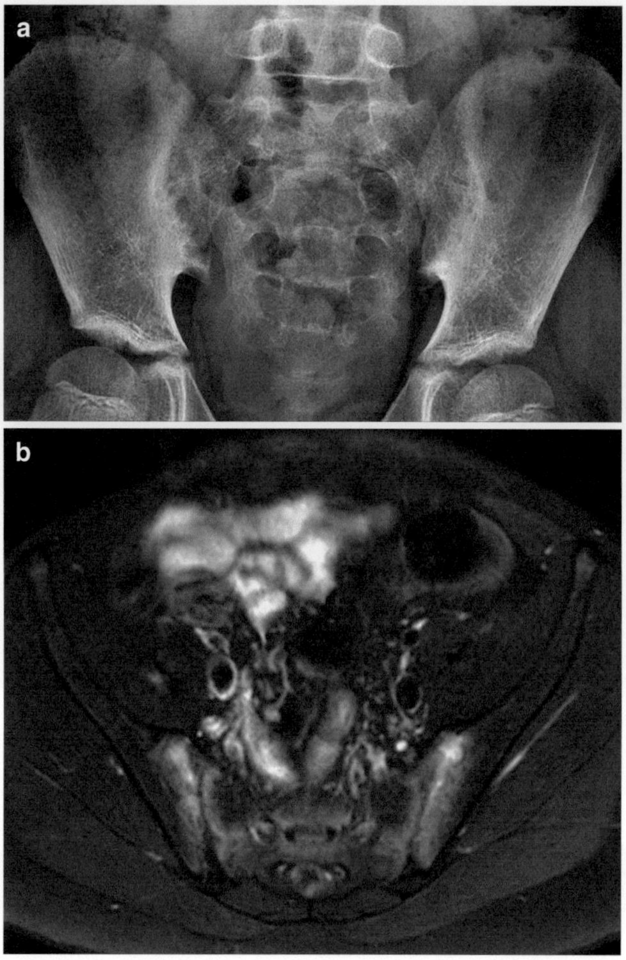

Fig. 9 Twelve year-old boy with juvenile spondyloarthritis. (**a**) Anteroposterior radiograph shows symmetric widening and ill definition of the sacroiliac joints. Mild sclerosis is seen on the iliac side of each joint. (**b**) Axial T2-weighted MR image (TR 3,403 ms, TE 65 ms) shows synovial hypertrophy in both sacroiliac joints with irregularity and adjacent bone marrow edema

Other Autoimmune Conditions

Dermatomyositis is an autoimmune disease of muscle and skin. Charactaristically, the gluteal muscles and adductors are most affected with relative sparing of the hamstring muscles [28]. Active disease will show signal on T2-weighing and STIR. Contrast is not necessary. MRI is helpful for confirming disease, delineating extent, guiding biopsy and for assessment of treatment reponse [28]. Dermal, subcutaneous and muscle calcifications are seen late and evident on radiography.

Musculoskeletal findings in systemic lupus erythematosus (SLE) are uncommon in children. Most patients have articular symptoms. Findings include soft tissue swelling, tenosynovitis, joint subluxation/dislocation without erosions or joint space loss and hip avascular necrosis [11]. Scleroderma and mixed connective tissue disorder rarely manifest in children.

Hemophilic Arthropathy

Hemophilia is an X-linked hereditary condition with deficient clotting factors (A–factor VIII; B–factor IX). It occurs in approximately 1 of 10,000 boys [19]. With modern treatment (clotting factor replacement regimens), hemophilic arthropathy is much less common than in the past. The knee, elbow and ankle are most frequently affected with the hip and shoulder less common [22, 29]. Arthropathy may be post-traumatic or spontaneous. Recurrent hemarthrosis leads to joint inflammation and synovial hypertrophy (inflammation/proliferation), in turn leading to cartilage and bone erosions (cartilage destruction, joint space loss), in turn leading to degenerative changes [29]. Hyperemia leads to epiphyseal overgrowth and premature physeal fusion.

Radiographic findings can be staged by the Arnold-Hilgartner system (stages 0–5) [22, 29]. Radiographic findings include osteopenia, increased density effusion, enlarged epiphyses, subchondral cysts, late joint space loss and late osteoarthritis [11, 20]. MRI shows blood, hemosiderin, synovial thickening, enhancement, cartilage loss (focal early and diffuse late with decreased joint space), bone erosions and subchondral cysts [11, 20, 22]. At the knee, the femoral notch is wide and the femoral condyles and patella are squared. At the elbow, the radial head is enlarged, the distal humerus is broad and the olecranon fossa is enlarged.

Other manifestations of hemophilia include intraosseous bleeds leading to pseudotumor and intramuscular bleeds.

Intra-Articular Venous Malformation

Intra-articular vascular malformations are associated with soft tissue and cutaneous vascular malformations, recurrent hemarthrosis and arthropathy [20]. Diagnosis is often delayed. Synovial lesions may be venous, venolymphatic or arteriovenous malformation. On MRI, venous lesions enhance inhomogeneously and lymphatic lesions are microcystic with peripheral enhancement. Hemorrhage and thrombosis leads to heterogeneity and hemosiderin deposition [20].

Pigmented Villonodular Synovitis (PVNS)

The extra-articular, localized, nodular form of PVNS is called giant cell tumor of the tendon sheath or bursa. The diffuse form of PVNS, involving all of the synovium of the involved joint, is most commonly seen at the knee (80%), and less commonly at the hip, shoulder, ankle or elbow [22]. There is an association with Noonan syndrome.

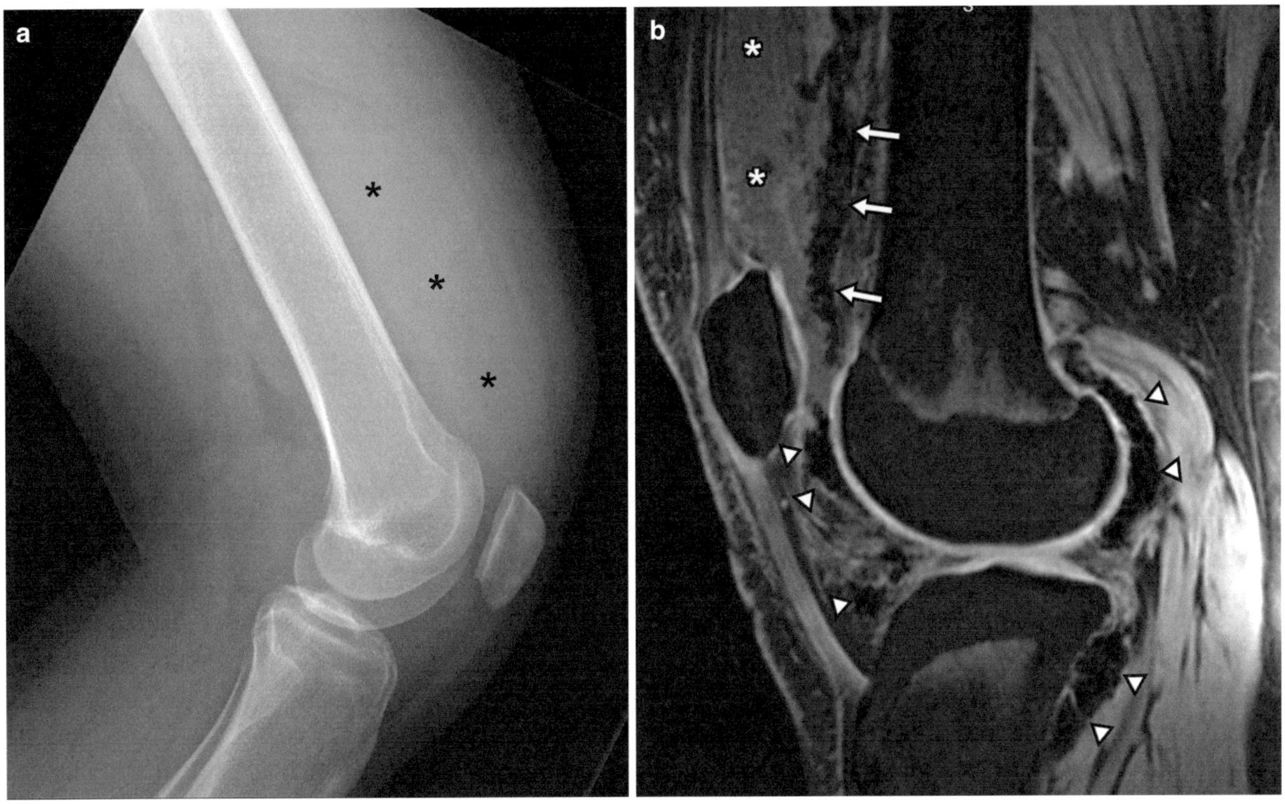

Fig. 10 Sixteen year-old girl with pigmented villonodular synovitis of the knee. The patient had a 1–2 year history of increasing knee swelling and pain. (**a**) Lateral radiograph shows a very large effusion within the suprapatellar pouch (*asterisks*). (**b**) Sagittal water selective (WATS) gradient echo MR image (TR 22 ms, TE 11 ms) shows a complex knee effusion (*asterisks*) with synovial proliferation (*arrows*). Low signal is seen with the synovium throughout the joint consistent with hemosiderin deposition (*arrowheads*)

Synovial proliferative change is seen with ultrasound or MRI. Hemosiderin deposition is characteristic and best seen on gradient echo MRI sequences (Fig. 10) [30]. Radiographs show soft tissue swelling, erosions, subchondral cysts and effusion.

Synovial Osteochondromatosis

Synovial osteochondromatosis is due to a metaplastic transformation of synovium with formation of osteocartilaginous foci [20, 22]. The knee is most commonly affected, and less commonly the elbow, hip, shoulder or small joints (interphalangeal, TMJ, acromioclavicular). Secondary degenerative changes occur. Synvial osteochondromatosis may be primary or secondary to osteochonditis dissecans, avascular necrosis, trauma, neuropathic joint, osteoarthritis or other joint disease. One third of patients have no calcification (synovial chondromatosis).

Synovial osteochondromatosis is a disorder of unknown etiology. There are three phases: (1) active intrasynovial chondral proliferation without loose bodies; (2) transitional intrasynovial osteochondral proliferation with intra-articular loose bodies; (3) quiescent multiple intra-articular loose bodies without intrasynovial proliferation [22].

Neruopathic Joint

Neuropathic arthropathy occurs due to myelomeningocele, synrinx, familial dysautonomia/congenital insensitivity to pain or diabetes (a rare cause in child). Neuropathic arthopathy is characterized by the 4 D's—distension (effusion), degeneration (articular surfaces/fragmentation), debris, dislocation/fracture [11]. Meniscal and ligament disruption occurs. Widening of adjacent growth plates may represent associated neuropathic fractures.

Conclusion

Musculoskeletal infection and inflammatory disease in children are myriad and overlapping in clinical presentation. Imaging plays an important role in diagnosis, delineation of extent, identification of complications, guidance of treatment and monitoring of disease and response to treatment.

References

1. Ranson M (2009) Imaging of pediatric musculoskeletal infections. Semin Musculoskelet Radiol 13:277–300
2. Nixon GW (1978) Hematogenous osteomyelitis of metaphysel-equivalent locations. AJR Am J Roentgenol 130:123–129
3. Guillerman RP (2013) Osteomyelitis and beyond. Pediatr Radiol 43:S193–S203
4. Jaramillo D (2011) Infection: musculoskeletal. Pediatr Radiol 41:S127–S134
5. Browne LP, Mason EO, Kaplan SL et al (2008) Optimal strategy for community-acquired *Staphylococcus aureus* musculodeletal infections in children. Pediatr Radiol 38:841–847
6. Pendleton A, Kocher MS (2015) Methicillin-resistant *Staphylococcus aureus* bone and joint infections in children. J Am Acad Orthop Surg 23:29–37
7. Robben SGF (2004) Ultrasonography of musculoskeletal infections in children. Eur Radiol 14:L65–L77
8. Connolly SA, Connolly LP, Drubach LA et al (2007) MRI for detection of abscess in acute osteomyelitis of the pelvis in children. AJR Am J Roentgenol 189:867–872
9. Delgado J, Bedoya MA, Green AM et al (2015) Utility of unenhanced fat-suppressed T1-weighted MRI in children with sickle cell disease–can it differentiate bone infarcts from acute osteomyelitis? Pediatr Radiol 45:1981–1987
10. Horowitz DL, Katzap E, Horowitz S, Barilla-LaBarca M-L (2011) Approach to septic arthritis. Am Fam Physician 84:653–660
11. Dalrup-Link HE, Steinbach L (2009) MR imaging of pediatric arthritis. Magn Reson Clin N Am 17:451–467
12. Sultan J, Hughes PJ (2010) Septic arthritis or transient synovitis of the hip in children: the value of clinical prediction algorithms. J Bone Joint Surg Br 92:1289–1293
13. Kocher MS, Zurakowski D, Kasser JR (1999) Differentiating between septic arthritis and transient synovitis of the hip in children: an evidence-based clinical prediction algorithm. J Bone Joint Surg Am 81:1662–1670
14. Hayeri MR, Ziai P, Shehata ML et al (2016) Soft-tissue infections and their imaging mimics: from cellulitis to necrotizing fasciitis. Radiographics 36:1888–1910
15. Khanna G, Sato TSP, Ferguson P (2009) Imaging of chronic recurrent multifocal osteomyelitis. Radiographics 29:1159–1177
16. Falip C, Alison M, Boutry N (2013) Chronic recurrent multifocal osteomyelitis (CRMO): a longitudinal case series review. Pediatr Radiol 43:355–375
17. Fritz J, Tzaribatchev N, Claussen CD et al (2009) Chronic recurrent multifocal osteomyelitis: comparison of whole-body MR imaging with radiography and correlation with clinical and laboratory data. Radiology 352:842–851
18. Petty RE, Southwood TR, Manners P (2001) International League of Associations for Rheumatology classification of juvenile idiopathic arthritis: second revision, Edmonton, 2001. J Rheumatol 31:390–392
19. Damasio MB, Malattia C, Martini A, Tomà P (2010) Synovial and inflammatory diseases of childhood: role of new imaging modalities in the assessment of patients with juvenile idiopathic arthritis. Pediatr Radiol 40:985–998
20. Ranson MDE, Babyn PS (2008) The joints. In: Slovis TL (ed) Caffey's pediatric diagnostic imaging. Mosby, Philadelphia, PA, pp 3037–3072
21. Sheybani EF, Khanna G, White AJ, Dmertzis JL (2013) Imaging of juvenile idiopathic arthritis: a multimodality approach. Radiographics 33:1253–1273
22. Kim HK, Zbojniewicz AM, Merros AC et al (2011) MR findings of synovial disease in children and young adults: part 1. Pediatr Radiol 41:495–511
23. DFM A, Müller L-SO, Rosendahl K (2016) Erosion of normal variant? 4-year MRI follow-up of the wrists in healthy children. Pediatr Radiol 46:322–330
24. Burgos-Vargas R (2002) The juvenile-onset spondyloarthritides. Rheum Clin NA 28:531–560
25. Bollow M, Braum J, Biedermann T et al (1998) Use of contrast-enhanced MR imaging to detect sacroiliitis in children. Skelet Radiol 27:606–616
26. Lee EY, Sundel RP, Kim S et al (2008) MRI findings of juvenile psoriatic arthritis. Skelet Radiol 37:987–996
27. Aquino MR, Rse SM, Gupta S et al (2015) Whole-body MRI of juvenile spondyloarthritis: protocols and pictorial review of characteristic patterns. Pediatr Radiol 45:754–762
28. Hernandez RJ, Sullivan DB, Chenevert TL, Kiem DR (1993) MR imaging in children with dermatomyositis: musculoskeletal findings and correlation with clinical and laboratory findings. AJR Am J Roentgenol 161:359–366
29. Arnold WD, Hilgarner MW (1977) Hemophilic arthropathy. J Bone Joint Surg Am 59:287–305
30. Eckhardt BP, Hernandez RJ (2004) Pigmented villonodular synovitis: MR imaging in pediatric patients. Pediatr Radiol 34:943–947

Pediatric Bone Marrow Imaging

Diego Jaramillo

Introduction

The evaluation marrow disorders in children relies primarily on MR imaging and to a lesser extent PET imaging and scintigraphy. On T1-weighted MR images, fatty marrow, which has a fatty component of 80% or more, is of high signal intensity (SI), similar to subcutaneous fat. Hematopoietic marrow, which contains 40% fat, has a signal intensity that is higher than adjacent muscle on T1-weighted images. Hematopoietic marrow has a higher water content in infants and tends to be of low SI on T1-weighted images and high SI on water sensitive images [1]. The composition of the marrow changes significantly in the first two decades of life. For this reason, it is important to become intimately familiar with the sequence of normal marrow transformation to be able to diagnose marrow abnormalities.

Normal Marrow Transformation

At birth, the entire skeleton is hematopoietic. The transformation to fatty marrow begins in the epiphyses (Fig. 1). The epiphyseal ossification centers become fatty on MR imaging approximately 6 months after the radiographic appearance of these centers. For example, the proximal femoral epiphysis becomes ossified around 5–6 months of age, and therefore the marrow should have a fatty appearance by 1 year of age. The second segment of the bones to transform is the diaphysis, followed by the metaphyses. In each extremity, marrow transformation also occurs from the periphery to the center, that is, beginning at the fingers and toes and ending in the shoulders and hips [2, 3].

In the axial skeleton, the marrow remains hematopoietic throughout life, but the fat component increases with age. In infants younger than 1 year of age, the SI of the marrow is lower than the adjacent disc on T1-weighted images. Between 1 and 5 years of age, the SI is isointense or hyperintense relative to the disc, and over 5 years of age the vertebral body is hyperintense relative to the disc [4].

Hematopoietic marrow is highly cellular and well perfused whereas fatty marrow is poorly perfused [5, 6]. Hence, blood-borne diseases such as infection or metastatic disease tend to affect hematopoietic marrow, whereas fatty marrow is more often affected by ischemia. After gadolinium administration, hematopoietic marrow shows marked enhancement, whereas fatty marrow enhances poorly. On diffusion weighted imaging, the high cellularity of hematopoietic marrow results in restricted diffusion [7]. On FDG PET/CT or PET/MRI, hematopoietic marrow has an uptake that is less than that of the liver [8].

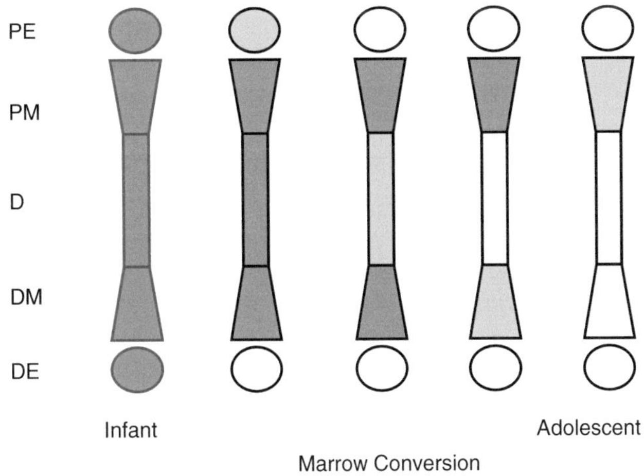

Fig. 1 Sequence of marrow transformation as seen on T1-weighted images, where hematopoietic marrow is depicted as *dark gray*, marrow undergoing transformation as *light gray*, and fatty marrow as *white*. PE: proximal epiphysis; PM: proximal metaphysis; D: diaphysis; DM: distal metaphysis; and DE: distal epiphysis. Marrow conversion begins in the epiphyses followed by diaphysis and metaphyses. Conversion also follow a distal to proximal sequence

D. Jaramillo
Department of Radiology, Miami Children's Hospital, 3100 S.W. 62nd Ave, Miami, FL 33155, USA
e-mail: Diegjar1@gmail.com

J. Hodler et al. (eds.), *Musculoskeletal Diseases 2017-2020*, DOI 10.1007/978-3-319-54018-4_33

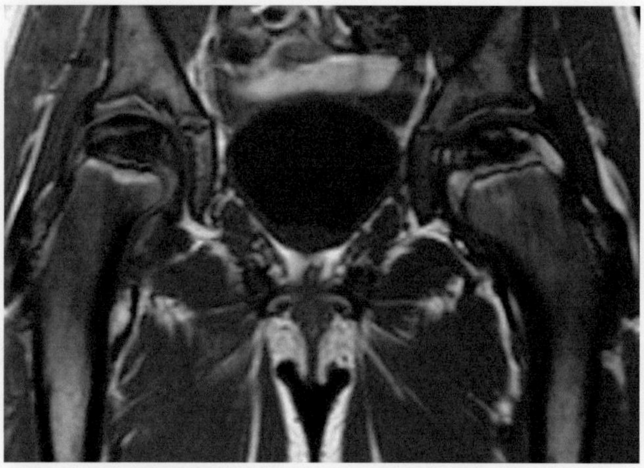

Fig. 2 12-year-old with sickle cell disease. There is increased hematopoietic marrow in the proximal femurs because of the anemia. The SI in the epiphyses, which should be high because of fat, is very low because of bilateral avascular necrosis

Hyperactive Marrow

Hyperplasia of the hematopoietic marrow occurs in diseases that produce anemia such as Thalassemia or sickle cell disease (Fig. 2). Granulocytic-colony stimulating factor also results in very active marrow, as does hypoxia, polycythemia vera and smoking. Hyperactive marrow can simulate metastatic disease, particularly in patients with a malignancy who are receiving granulocytic colony stimulating factor. Out-of-phase MR imaging helps differentiate between the two, as the signal intensity drops considerably with hematopoietic marrow (due to its fatty component) whereas it does not with metastatic disease.

Ischemia

Avascular necrosis is most often seen in the epiphysis of the proximal femur. Legg-Calvé-Perthes disease is an idiopathic condition affecting mostly boys 4–8 years of age. Radiographically the head undergoes sclerosis, collapse, fragmentation and ultimately healing. In order to heal appropriately, the femoral epiphysis must be well contained by the acetabulum. Radiographically, the degree of collapse of the lateral pillar of the femoral head is an important prognostic sign. Reperfusion occurs around the physis (periphyseal), which is important so that the physis does not close prematurely. Lucencies developing in the juxtaphyseal metaphysis are of bad prognosis, and they are associated with transphyseal reperfusion (instead of periphyseal reperfusion) and premature closure of the physis. MR imaging shows decreased SI on the femoral epiphysis on T1-weighted images, increased SI on T2-weighted images, absent enhancement after gadolinium administration, and increased ADC on diffusion-weighted images.

There are other causes of epiphyseal ischemia in children including steroids, sickle cell disease (Fig. 2), and Gaucher disease. An important subpopulation is the group of patients who are treated for leukemia. These patients have multiple infarcts throughout the bones, but the degree of subchondral involvement in the epiphysis determines the degree of pain. Early marrow inhomogeneity with a linear pattern in these high-risk patients is associated with subsequent development of infarcts.

Infarcts can occur in the metaphysis and diaphysis. Stagnant blood can result in high signal intensity on fat-suppressed T1-weighted images. Acute infarcts are also associated with increased marrow signal on T2-weighted images, and with subperiosteal fluid and surrounding soft tissue edema. Thus, it is difficult to differentiate between infection and infarction in conditions such as sickle cell disease. The difficulty in differentiating between these two conditions is aggravated by the fact that infection can develop in areas of pre-existing infarction.

Marrow Infiltration and Deposition

Extensive infiltration of marrow by malignant cells is seen in leukemic children or in children with diffuse metastatic disease such as neuroblastoma or neuroblastoma (Fig. 3). On

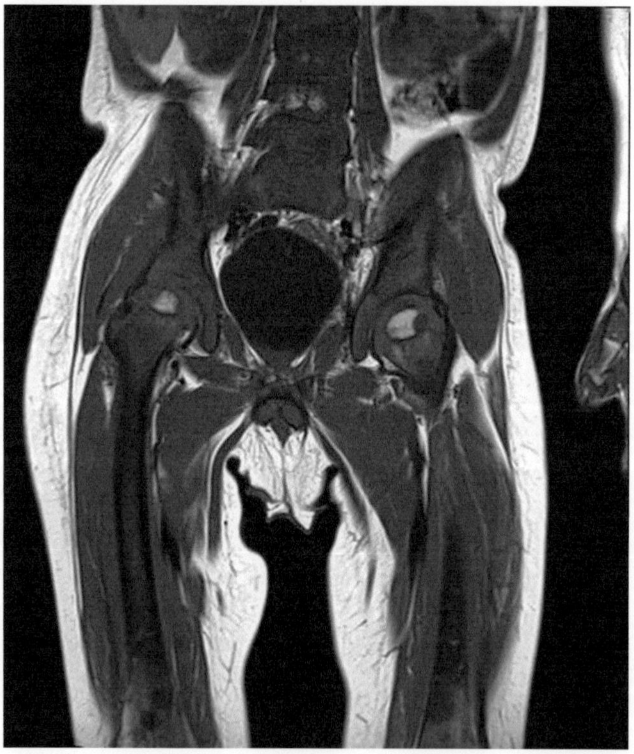

Fig. 3 2-year-old boy with metastatic neuroblastoma. Coronal T1-weighted image shows uniformly decreased marrow in the pelvis and femurs. The femoral epiphysis on the left is partially involved

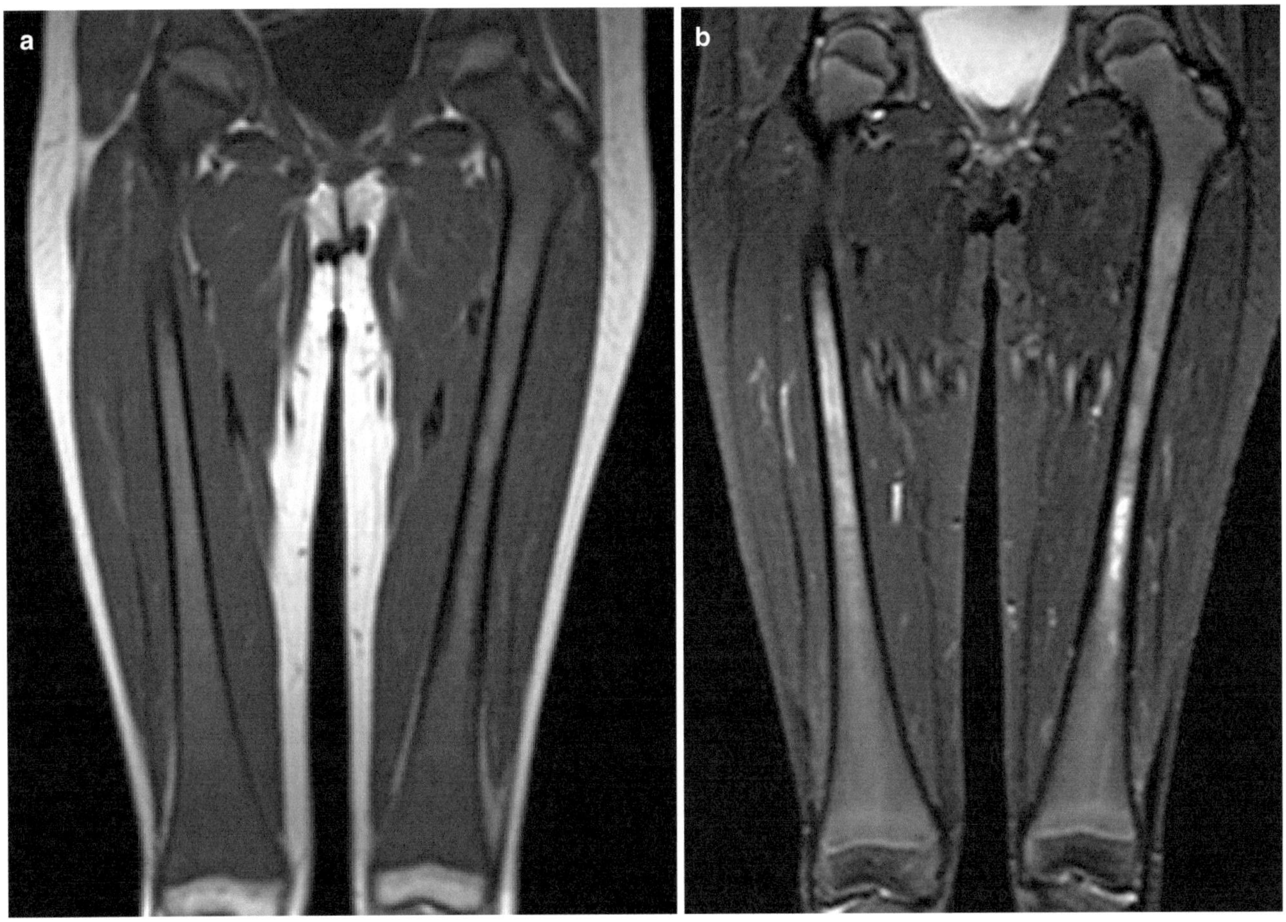

Fig. 4 7-year-old boy with Gaucher disease. (**a**) Coronal T1-weighted image shows diffuse decrease in the SI of the marrow of the metaphyses and diaphysis. (**b**) Coronal STIR image shows that the SI remains relatively low in the metaphyses. This helps differentiate the disease from leukemia or metastatic disease, in which the SI from the marrow would be much higher

MR images, infiltrated marrow is of very low SI on T1-weighted images on high SI on STIR or T2-weighted images, the so-called "flip-flop phenomenon". Children with acute lymphoblastic leukemia show a very homogenous pattern of infiltration whereas other leukemias and metastatic processes tend to be more patchy.

In Gaucher disease the marrow is infiltrated by macrophages laden with glucocerebrosides. The marrow is of diffuse low SI on T1-weighted images, but is of relatively low SI on T2-weighted images, which helps differentiate this disease from cellular infiltration (Fig. 4). When the involvement is less severe, the abnormality of Gaucher disease follows the same distribution of hematopoietic marrow and it can be difficult to differentiate hyperactive marrow from Gaucher's disease. Patients are treated with enzyme replacement therapy. This results in an increase in the fat fraction of the marrow. Response to therapy can be assessed by quantifying this fat fraction by either Dixon methods or spectroscopy [9].

Deposition of iron in the reticulo-endothelial system results in low SI on both T1- and T2-weighted images. Patients with excessive iron in the marrow will also have increased iron in other cells of the reticulo-endothelial system such as the spleen and liver.

Marrow Depletion

Aplastic anemia can result in decreased cellularity of the marrow and thus increased SI on T1-weighted images due to increased marrow fat. Radiation therapy also results in fatty marrow which follows the configuration of the radiation portal (Fig. 5).

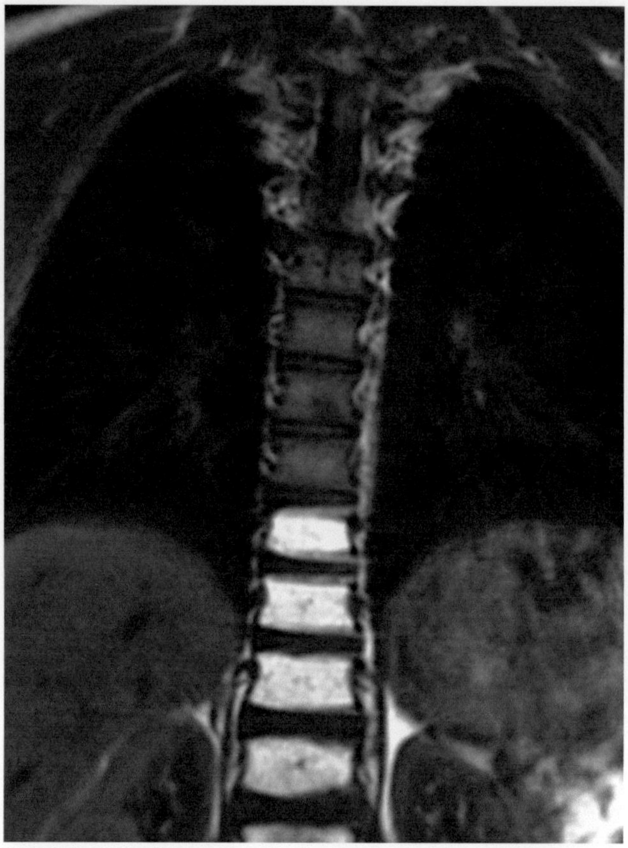

Fig. 5 12-year-old with post-radiation therapy change. Coronal T1-weighted image shows that the SI of the marrow is very high on the vertebral bodies of the lower thoracic spine and lumbar spine consistent with fatty replacement. The absence of hematopoietic marrow with a geometric border is typical of the effect of radiation therapy

Other Marrow Abnormalities

Scurvy and anorexia can result in gelatinous transformation of the marrow, which is seen as areas of low SI on T1-weighted images and high T2 SI in the metaphysis. In scurvy all the metaphyses are involved and there can be subperiosteal hemorrhages.

Marrow Edema

Marrow edema, resulting in increased water, is seen with trauma, infection or infarction. It is also seen in association with certain benign tumors such as osteoid osteoma, chondroblastoma and osteoblastoma.

Conclusion

In order to diagnose and characterize marrow disorders in children, it is fundamental to know the pattern of normal marrow transformation. It is also important to know the patterns of diffuse and focal bone marrow abnormalities.

References

1. Bracken J, Nandurkar D, Radhakrishnan K et al (2013) Normal paediatric bone marrow: magnetic resonance imaging appearances from birth to 5 years. J Med Imaging Radiat Oncol 57: 283–291
2. Burdiles A, Babyn PS (2009) Pediatric bone marrow MR imaging. Magn Reson Imaging Clin N Am 17:391–409, v
3. Laor T, Jaramillo D (2009) MR imaging insights into skeletal maturation: what is normal? Radiology 250:28–38
4. Sebag GH, Dubois J, Tabet M et al (1993) Pediatric spinal bone marrow: assessment of normal age-related changes in the MRI appearance. Pediatr Radiol 23:515–518
5. Bedoya MA, Jaimes C, Khrichenko D et al (2014) Dynamic gadolinium-enhanced MRI of the proximal femur: preliminary experience in healthy children. AJR Am J Roentgenol 203: W440–W446
6. Dwek JR, Shapiro F, Laor T et al (1997) Normal gadolinium-enhanced MR images of the developing appendicular skeleton: Part 2. Epiphyseal and metaphyseal marrow. AJR Am J Roentgenol 169:191–196
7. Ording Muller LS, Avenarius D, Olsen OE (2011) High signal in bone marrow at diffusion-weighted imaging with body background suppression (DWIBS) in healthy children. Pediatr Radiol 41: 221–226
8. Shammas A, Lim R, Charron M (2009) Pediatric FDG PET/CT: physiologic uptake, normal variants, and benign conditions. Radiographics 29:1467–1486
9. Jaramillo D, Bedoya MA, Wang DJ et al (2015) Quantification of bone marrow involvement in treated gaucher disease with proton MR spectroscopy: correlation with bone marrow MRI scores and clinical status. AJR Am J Roentgenol 204:1296–1302

Scoliosis or Back Pain in Children: What to Consider

Sonia F. Calloni, Thierry A.G.M. Huisman, and Bruno P. Soares

Introduction and Clinical Approach

The complaint of back pain in children should always be taken seriously, particularly when the pain is persistent. Back pain is often but not always the manifestation of a benign self-limited process. Pain that occurs at night and awakens the child may be associated with tumors or infection [1]. Clinicians must be aware of alerting symptoms that include pain in prepubertal children, acute trauma, progression of symptoms over time, functional/neurological disability, pain lasting more than 4 weeks, history of malignancy or tuberculosis exposure, recurrent or worsening pain, radicular pain, night pain that disrupts sleep, limp or altered gait [2].

Childhood scoliosis is a common clinical entity with numerous causes. Scoliosis is usually defined as a lateral curvature of the spine of >10°, and it is estimated that 2% of children are affected at some stage of their life [3].

The etiology of the spinal deformity may be idiopathic (80% of cases), particularly in adolescents. It may however also be associated with underlying systemic syndromes, secondary to a neuromuscular condition (10% of cases), skeletal dysplasia, or secondary to congenital spinal deformity in 10% of cases [4]. Bone tumors and intraspinal neoplasms may also present with back pain and associated scoliosis [5].

There is significant etiological and clinical overlap between scoliosis and back pain. Spinal asymmetry or scoliosis is a major risk factor for back pain.

Imaging Indications and Protocols for Back Pain and Scoliosis

Children with back pain of short duration, normal physical examination, and no history of trauma do not require further laboratory or imaging evaluation [6]. Imaging should be reserved for children with persistent back pain and concerning clinical/neurological and laboratory findings.

Clinicians must be mindful of the amount of radiation exposure associated with conventional radiography and CT. Alternative imaging tests like MRI and in select cases ultrasonography (US) should be considered.

CT is widely accepted as the gold standard for the evaluation of osseous structures, acute trauma, and to monitor fracture healing, but may fail in detecting early or subtle stress injuries. CT may also be non-diagnostic in children with Spinal Cord Injury Without Radiographic Abnormalities (SCIWORA) where injury is confined to non-osseous structures. To limit dose exposure, CT imaging should be restricted to the region of interest and use modern dose reduction techniques [7]. MRI directly visualizes the spinal cord, ligaments and intervertebral discs. It is optimal in the evaluation of paraspinal or intraspinal disorders. T2-weighted imaging with fat suppression techniques are optimal to assess bone marrow edema and paraspinal pathology. Fat suppressed T2 and contrast-enhanced T1-weighted MR imaging sequences are ideal for evaluation of infectious and neoplastic disease involving the vertebrae, discs, paraspinous soft tissues and spinal cord. The decision to perform an MRI examination should consider cost and the possible need to sedate young children [8]. Tc-99 m whole body bone scan has high sensitivity of to detect stress fractures and most lytic bone lesions [9].

S.F. Calloni
Università degli Studi di Milano,
Postgraduation School in Radiodiagnostics,
Milan 20122, Italy

Division of Pediatric Radiology, Russell H. Morgan Department of Radiology and Radiological Science, Section of Pediatric Neuroradiology, The Johns Hopkins University School of Medicine, 1800 Orleans St, Baltimore, MD 21287, USA
e-mail: sonia.calloni@unimi.it

T.A.G.M. Huisman • B.P. Soares (✉)
Division of Pediatric Radiology, Russell H. Morgan Department of Radiology and Radiological Science, Section of Pediatric Neuroradiology, The Johns Hopkins University School of Medicine, 1800 Orleans St, Baltimore, MD 21287, USA
e-mail: thuisma1@jhmi.edu; bruno.soares@jhmi.edu

J. Hodler et al. (eds.), *Musculoskeletal Diseases 2017-2020*, DOI 10.1007/978-3-319-54018-4_34

Common Causes of Back Pain in Children

Spondylolysis and Spondylolisthesis

Lumbar spondylolysis and spondylolisthesis are common causes of low back pain in children older than 10 years [10]. Spondylolysis is a stress injury/fracture of the pars interarticularis. It is more frequent in young males and athletes, and the vast majority of osseous defects occur at the L5 level (85–95%). With continued biomechanical stress, spondylolysis can progress to spondylolisthesis characterized by anterior displacement of the affected vertebral body, possibly complicated by stenosis of the spinal canal and/or neuroforamen.

Plain radiographs acquired in oblique projection show a focal band-like lucency with adjacent sclerosis or elongation of the pars interarticularis. MRI shows the bone defect as linear hypointensity on T1-weighted images. Marrow edema in the adjacent pars or pedicles is seen in the acute phase as hyperintense signal on T2-weighted images. CT is the most reliable modality to depict the pars interarticularis fracture, and when performed should be focused to the region of interest (Fig. 1).

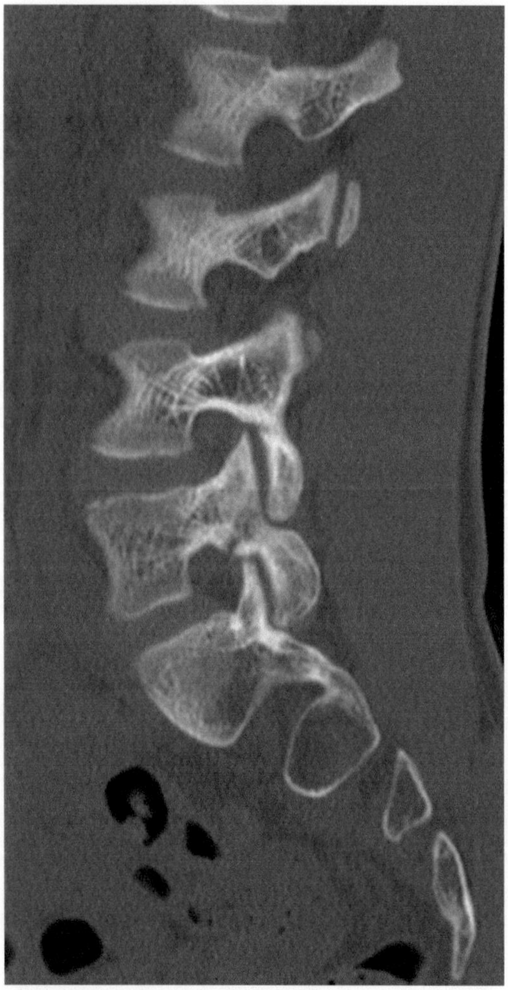

Fig. 1 Spondylolysis. Sagittal CT image shows a fracture of the right L5 pars interarticularis

Trauma and Degenerative Conditions

Dislocations, ligamentous injuries, epiphyseal detachments, and lesions of the ossification centers are more frequent than fractures in young children [11]. Cervical fractures and craniocervical ligamentous injuries occur more frequently in younger children, while thoracolumbar fractures are more common in older children and adolescents [6].

Intervertebral disc herniation in children is often accompanied by a fracture of the adjacent vertebral end plate. MRI is the imaging of choice to assess intervertebral disc disease [6].

Scheuermann's disease is an osteochondrosis presenting in late childhood and early adolescence and is characterized by a slowly progressive, fixed or stiff kyphotic deformity of the thoracic or thoracolumbar spine. Radiographic criterion for diagnosis is more than five of anterior wedging of at least three adjacent vertebral bodies [6].

Infectious and Inflammatory Diseases

Back pain in children can be caused by various inflammatory and infectious disorders of the spine, spinal cord, nerve roots, meninges, vertebrae, discs, and epidural space [12].

Disorders primarily involving the spinal cord include inflammatory/auto-immune disorders and infectious disorders of bacterial, viral, fungal, or parasitic etiology.

Acute Transverse Myelitis (ATM) is an inflammatory condition associated with rapidly progressive motor, sensory and autonomic dysfunction, most commonly seen between ages 10–19 years [13]. Etiology includes idiopathic forms and entities such as acute disseminated encephalomyelitis (ADEM), neuromyelitis optica (NMO), multiple sclerosis, and ischemic, paraneoplastic, and post-radiation myelitis. MR imaging criteria for myelitis include normal or slightly expanded spinal cord showing diffuse or patchy hyperintensity on T2-weighted images, which may be associated with contrast enhancement. The conus medullaris is frequently involved [14] (Fig. 2a, b). Diffusion weighted imaging typically reveals vasogenic edema.

Infectious discitis and vertebral osteomyelitis are particularly common in children between the ages of 2–12 years and mostly affect males (M:F of 3:1) [15]. It most often results from hematogenous spread. Staphylococcus aureus is by far the most common agent. Spinal tuberculosis is another important cause of back pain and subsequent scoliosis or kyphotic deformity.

CT findings depend on the phase of infection and include cortical erosion, sclerosis, disc hypodensity, reduced disc height and gas within the disc. MR imaging is the gold standard due to its high sensitivity in detecting early abnormal signal within the disc or bone marrow. In

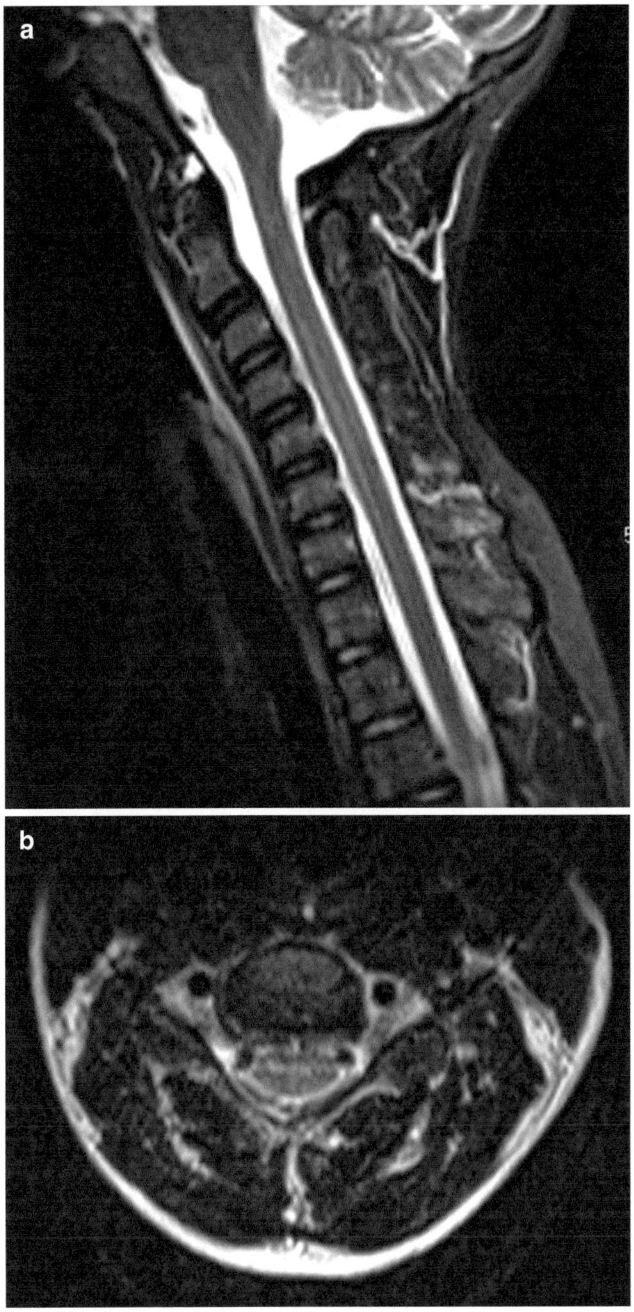

Fig. 2 Myelitis secondary to Enterovirus D68 infection. (**a**) Sagittal STIR MR image shows mild hyperintense signal and minimal swelling of the cervical spinal cord. (**b**) Axial T2-weighted MR image confirms the presence of abnomal hyperintense signal involving the anterior spinal cord

the early stages of infection, imaging studies show decreased disc height and abnormal T2 hyperintense signal, with enhancement after contrast administration. With advancing disease, the endplates and vertebrae become T2 hyperintense. Later, infection may spread into the epidural space forming a phlegmon or abscess with thecal sac compression.

In children with symptoms suggestive of infection but negative biopsy and/or cultures, one differential diagnosis to consider in children is Chronic Recurrent Multifocal Osteomyelitis (CRMO), a sterile skeletal inflammation that in the spine typically shows thoracic vertebral involvement with sparing of the intervertebral discs [16].

Neoplasms

Vertebral and spinal cord neoplasms are overall rare in children. Suggestive clinical features include persistent and localized back pain, progressive scoliosis, motor weakness, gait disturbance, and paraspinal muscle spasm.

Benign neoplasms of the vertebrae include osteoid osteoma, osteoblastoma, and aneurysmal bone cyst. Malignant neoplasms include Ewing sarcoma, lymphoma, neuroblastoma, Langerhans cell histiocytosis, and metastatic disease. Over 40% of all malignancies affecting the pediatric population arise in the lymphoreticular system [17].

Intrinsic spinal cord tumors include astrocytomas and ependymomas and are most commonly located in the cervical spinal cord [18]. Intradural extramedullary tumors include meningioma, nerve sheath tumors and drop metastasis from CSF spread of malignancy (Fig. 3).

Osteoid osteoma and osteoblastoma are usually located within the lumbar spine involving the lamina or pedicle. Patients typically report back pain at night, relieved by NSAIDs and aspirin. Plain radiographs and CT imaging typically show a radiolucent nidus surrounded by sclerosis, while MR better depicts the surrounding bone marrow edema.

The most frequent tumors of the spinal cord are the pilocytic and anaplastic astrocytomas (60%) and ependymomas (30%). Ependymomas are rare before the first

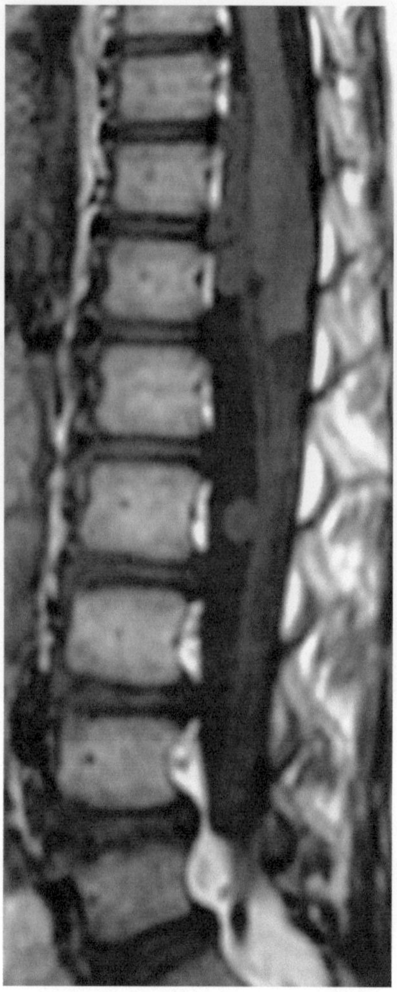

Fig. 3 Drop metastases. Sagittal T1-weighted MR image shows several nodular lesions anterior to the conus medullaris and adherent to the cauda equina

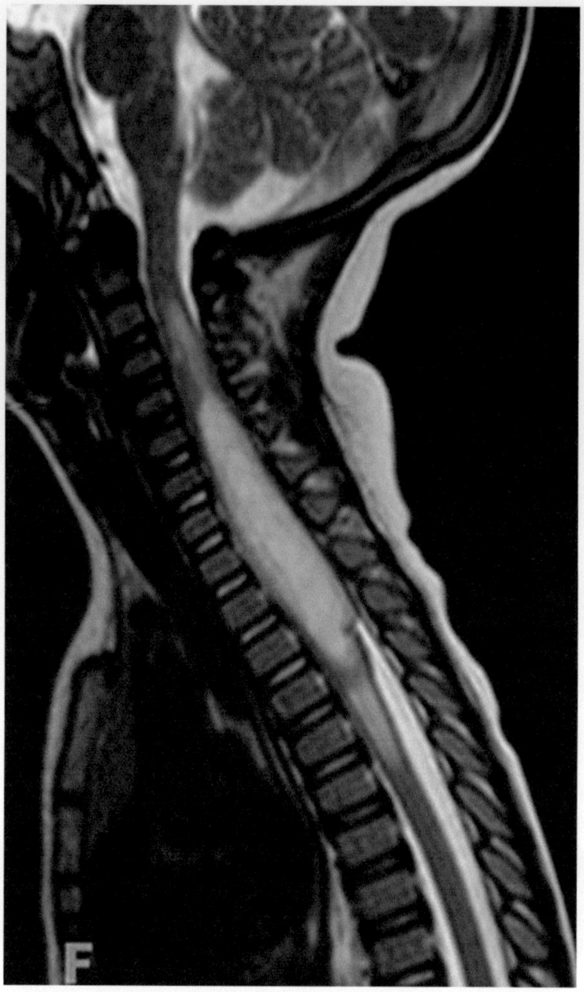

Fig. 4 Astrocytoma. Sagittal T2-weighted MR image shows a homogeneously hyperintense intramedullary mass expanding the lower cervical and upper thoracic spinal cord. Note the mild expansion of the spinal canal. Caudal and cranial segments of hyperintense signal may represent vasogenic edema or infiltrative tumor

decade, whereas astrocytomas are most common in early childhood. Astrocytomas are most common at the cervicothoracic junction [19]. Neoplastic tissue usually extends beyond the solid enhancing component (Fig. 4). On MRI, astrocytomas are seen as T2 hyperintense lesions with poorly defined margins due to their infiltrative morphology. Ependymomas are slow growing and less infiltrative than astrocytomas, are typically located around the central canal at the cervical spinal cord and tend to compress and displace the adjacent spinal cord tissue. Peritumoral cysts are seen in up to 80% of ependymomas. Ependymomas may be highly vascular with multiple small feedings vessels and intense contrast enhancement. A rim of T2 hypointense signal around the mass, reflecting chronic hemorrhage, is more suggestive of an ependymoma (Fig. 5).

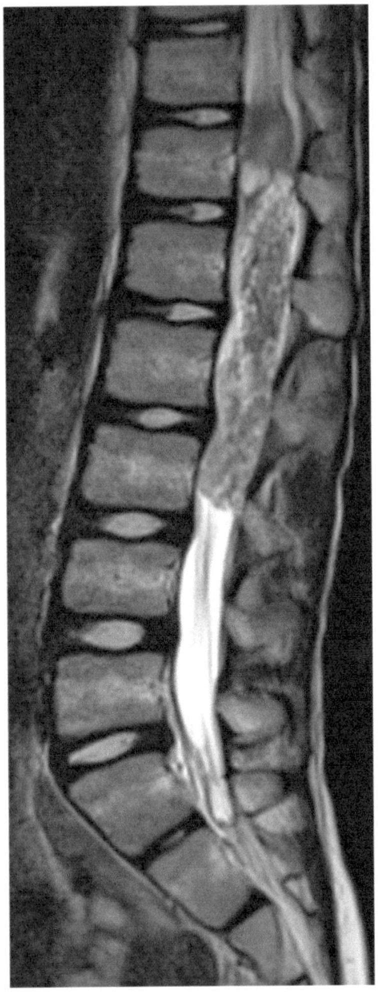

Fig. 5 Mixopapillary ependymoma. Sagittal T2-weighted MR image shows a heterogenous intraspinal mass involving the conus medullaris and proximal cauda equina

Other Conditions

Langerhans cell histiocytosis (LCH) is a disorder secondary to overproduction and accumulation of histiocytes. In the spine, it most commonly involves the thoracic vertebrae and spares the posterior elements. LCH is the most frequent cause of solitary vertebra plana in young people, particularly boys [20]. MRI shows vertebral disc preservation and epidural soft-tissue extension (Fig. 6).

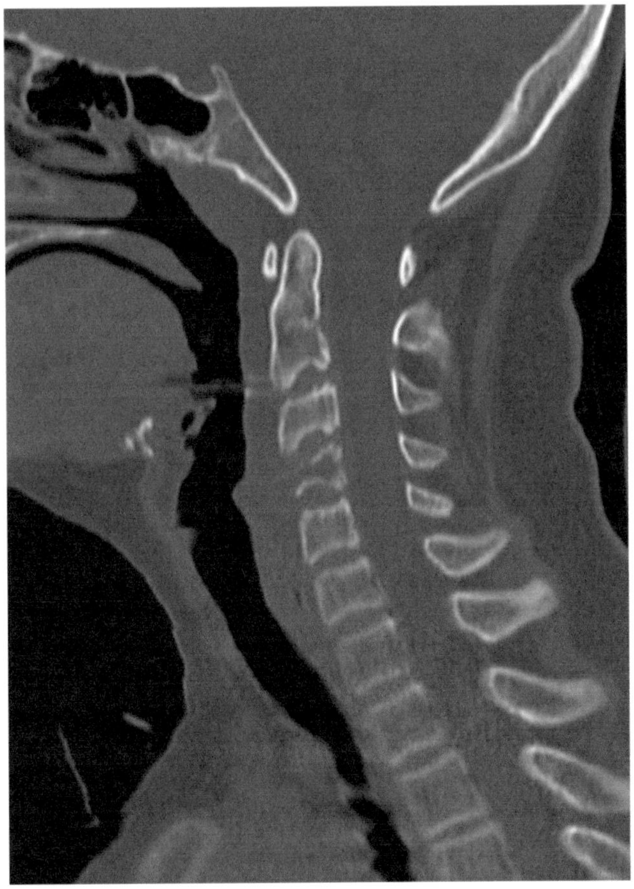

Fig. 6 Langerhans cell hystiocytosis. Sagittal CT image shows a C4 lytic lesion with areas of cortical disruption and loss of vertebral body height. The posterior elements are spared

Neurofibromatosis type 1 commonly presents with scoliosis and back pain. Neurofibromas may occur in the intraspinal or paraspinal compartments (Fig. 7). The classic curve pattern is short-segment, sharp angular kyphoscoliosis of the upper thoracic spine [21].

Bone marrow infarctions may cause acute back pain in children with sickle cell disease.

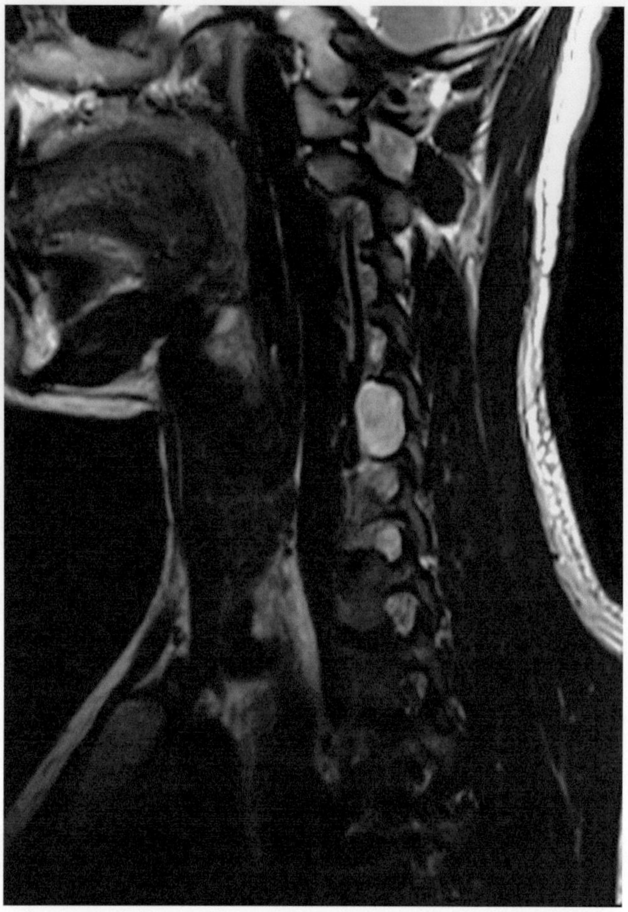

Fig. 7 Neurofibroma. Sagittal T2-weighted MR image shows a rounded hyperintense lesion expanding the C6–C7 neural foramen

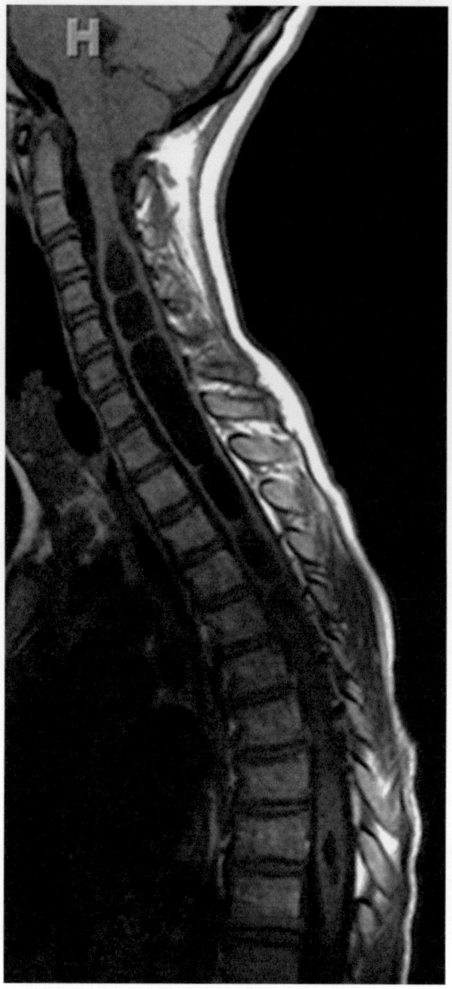

Fig. 8 Syringohydromyelia. Sagittal T1-weighted MR image shows marked cystic dilatation of the spinal cord in this child with Chiari I deformity

Types of Scoliosis in Children

Adolescent Idiopathic Scoliosis

Adolescent idiopathic scoliosis (AIS) is classified by age of onset as infantile before 3 years of age, juvenile between three and 10 years of age or puberty, and adolescent when detected after the age of ten or post puberty. Back pain can be present, and lung function may be affected with more severe curves. The most common type of curve in AIS is a right thoracic, left lumbar sigmoid curve.

Congenital Scoliosis

Congenital scoliosis may be the result of developmental abnormalities of the spine that are present at birth [22]. Chiari 1 malformation is the most common incidental finding when children with AIS are imaged. MRI is the gold standard imaging to detect both tonsillar descent and the presence of a hydromyelia and/or syringomyelia (Fig. 8).

Spinal segmentation anomalies can present as scoliosis or kyphosis or both. Vertebral anomalies can range from hemivertebrae, block vertebrae, wedge shaped or butterfly vertebrae. Patients with vertebral segmentation anomalies are at higher risk of having neural axis abnormalities.

Open spinal dysraphism is characterized by a neural placode exposed through a midline skin defect on the back, in level with the cutaneous surface (myelocele) or with a sac containing cerebrospinal fluid and neural elements protruding above the adjacent (myelomeningocele). Myelomeningocele is by far the most common spinal

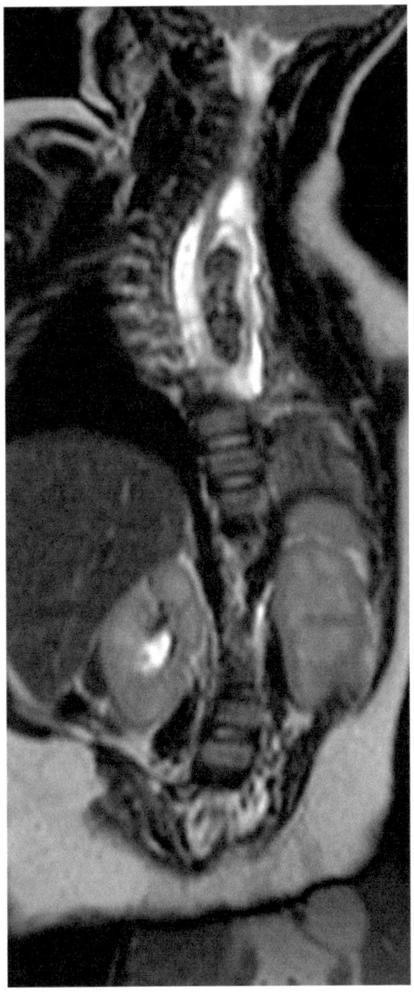

Fig. 9 Diastematomyelia. Coronal T2-weighted MR image shows a large cervicothoracic osseous spur splitting the spinal canal in this child with scoliosis

dysraphism. Scoliosis often develops in children with myelomeningocele, particularly if the dysraphism is extensive. MR is the imaging of the choice in assessing the degree of associated hindbrain herniation and in evaluating the spinal cord anatomy. Skin covered or closed spinal dysraphisms have better prognosis because the neural tissue is covered by skin and subcutaneous tissue.

Another condition associated with congenital scoliosis is diastematomyelia, present in up to 20% patients with congenital scoliosis. In over 80% of the cases the osseous or fibrous septum is located in the lumbar region. MRI depicts the septum and details the anatomy of the spinal cord and canal (Fig. 9).

Congenital scoliosis is frequently associated with abnormalities involving other organ systems such as VACTERL association or horizontal gaze palsy with progressive scoliosis [23].

Other Conditions

Neuromuscular scoliosis (NMS) can result from a variety of neuropathic or muscular disorders (e.g., cerebral palsy, myelodysplasia, muscular dystrophy). Skeletal dysplasias may result in scoliosis as a result of abnormal bone formation. These include achondroplasia, osteogenesis imperfecta and osteopetrosis. Connective tissue disorders, such as Marfan and Ehlers-Danlos syndrome, also commonly present with associated scoliosis.

References

1. Slipman CW, Patel RK, Botwin K, Huston C, Zhang L, Lenrow D et al (2003) Epidemiology of spine tumors presenting to musculoskeletal physiatrists. Arch Phys Med Rehabil 84:492–495
2. Jackson C, McLaughlin K, Teti B (2011) Back pain in children: a holistic approach to diagnosis and management. J Pediatr Health Care 25(5):284–293
3. Cheng JC, Castelein RM, Chu WC, Danielsson AJ, Dobbs MB (2015) Adolescent idiopathic scoliosis. Nat Rev Dis Primers 1:15030
4. Van Goethem J, Van Campenhout A, van den Hauwe L, Parizel PM (2007) Scoliosis. Neuroimaging Clin N Am 17(1):105–115
5. Janicki JA, Alman B (2007) Scoliosis: review of diagnosis and treatment. Paediatr Child Health 12(9):771–776
6. Rodriguez DP, Poussaint TY (2010) Imaging of back pain in children. AJNR Am J Neuroradiol 31(5):787–802
7. Nahle IS, Hamam MS, Masrouha KZ, Afeiche NE, Abdelnoor J (2016) Back pain: a puzzle in children. J Paediatr Child Health 52(8):802–808
8. Rodriguez DP, Poussaint TY (2010) Imaging of back pain in children. AJNR Am J Neuroradiol 31(5):787–802
9. Hospach T, Langendoerfer M, von Kalle T, Maier J, Dannecker GE (2010) Spinal involvement in chronic recurrent multifocal osteomyelitis (CRMO) in childhood and effect of pamidronate. Eur J Pediatr 169(9):1105–1111
10. King HA (1999) Back pain in children. Orthop Clin North Am 30(3):467–474, ix
11. Huisman TA, Wagner MW, Bosemani T, Tekes A, Poretti A (2015) Pediatric spinal trauma. J Neuroimaging 25(3):337–353
12. Rossi A (2015) Pediatric spinal infection and inflammation. Neuroimaging Clin N Am 25(2):173–191
13. Transverse Myelitis Consortium Working Group (2002) Proposed diagnostic criteria and nosology of acute transverse myelitis. Neurology 59(4):499–505
14. Tartaglino LM, Croul SE, Flanders AE, Sweeney JD, Schwartzman RJ (1996) Idiopathic acute transverse myelitis: MR imaging findings. Radiology 201(3):661–669
15. Karabouta Z, Bisbinas I, Davidson A, Goldsworthy LL (2005) Discitis in toddlers: a case series and review. Acta Paediatr 94:1516–1518
16. Khanna G, Sato TS, Ferguson P (2009) Imaging of chronic recurrent multifocal osteomyelitis. Radiographics 29(4):1159–1177

17. Vázquez E, Lucaya J, Castellote A, Piqueras J, Sainz P (2002) Neuroimaging in pediatric leukemia and lymphoma: differential diagnosis. Radiographics 22(6):1411–1428
18. Davis PJ, Williams HJ (2008) The investigation and management of back pain in children. Arch Dis Child Educ Pract Ed 93:73–83
19. Merhemic Z, Stosic-Opincal T, Thurnher MM (2016) Neuroimaging of spinal tumors. Magn Reson Imaging Clin N Am 24(3):563–579
20. Huang WD, Yang XH, Wu ZP, Huang Q, Xiao JR (2013) Langerhans cell histiocytosis of spine: comparative study of clinical, imaging features, and diagnosis inchildren, adolescents, and adults. Spine J 13(9):1108–1117
21. Holt RT, Johnson JR (1989) Cotrel-Dubousset instrumentation in neurofibromatosis spine curves. Clin Orthop 245:19–23
22. Janicki JA, Alman B (2007) Scoliosis: review of diagnosis and treatment. Paediatr Child Health 12(9):771–776
23. Basu PS, Elsebaie H, Noordeen MH (2002) Congenital-spinaldeformity: a comprehensive assessment at presentation. Spine 27:2255–2259

Part IV

Breast Imaging Satellite Course "Pearl"

High-Risk Multimodality Screening

Ulrich Bick

Population-based mammography screening programs primarily aim at postmenopausal women, where the incidence of breast cancer in normal-risk women is highest. These programs are not adequate for high-risk women such as BRCA1 or BRCA2 mutation carriers, in whom breast cancer not only occurs much more frequently, but also much earlier, sometimes even before the age of 30 [1]. It is well known that sensitivity of mammography is substantially lower in premenopausal women with dense breasts [2] and therefore additional imaging modalities such as breast ultrasound and contrast-enhanced MRI breast cancer are of increasing importance in these women. Several countries have now introduced structured high-risk screening programs, usually starting at an age of 25–30 [3–6]. The cornerstone of these programs is an annual contrast-enhanced MRI of the breast, which by far has the highest sensitivity for breast cancer [3, 4], especially in young premenopausal women. Due to the higher radiation risk in younger women [7], mammography is usually not added before the age of 40 and may find some additional cancers occult on MRI, predominantly in-situ cancers associated with microcalcifications. Clinical breast exam and breast ultrasound usually do not contribute to the detection of additional cancers if a high-quality MRI is available, but may—if performed after and in full knowledge of the MRI—improve patient satisfaction and compliance by offering the possibility to discuss the MRI results directly with the patient. In addition, they can be helpful to correlate non-specific findings on the MRI and reduce false-positives e.g. due to common benign findings such as lymph nodes and fibroadenomas. Even though high-risk MRI-based screening programs may find breast cancer at a very early stage in a large proportion of patients, it is important to realize and discuss with the patients, that screening can never prevent breast cancer for occurring. Some cancers, especially triple negative cancers, will be dangerous even if found early and may require aggressive chemotherapy with all its side effect. Therefore especially in BRCA1 mutation carriers, in whom triple-negative breast cancers are very common, primary surgical prevention through bilateral prophylactic mastectomy should be offered as a viable alternative to screening.

U. Bick
Department of Radiology, CCM, Charité—Universitätsmedizin, Berlin 10117, Germany
e-mail: Ulrich.Bick@charite.de

Selecting Women for High-Risk Screening

Almost all current guidelines now agree that women with a known pathologic mutation in the BRCA1 or BRCA2 gene should be offered MRI-based high-risk screening. Cumulative lifetime risk for breast cancer in these women will be as high as 60% for BRCA1 and 55% for BRCA2 mutation carriers [1]. More than half of these women will develop breast cancer before the age of 50 [1]. However, even among BRCA1/2 carriers, individual breast cancer risk will vary substantially based on existence of genetic modifiers in the family [1] as well as lifestyle factors [8]. The group of women without a known mutation in one of the high penetrance genes, who will benefit from high-risk screening, is much more difficult to define. Usually a lifetime risk for breast cancer above a threshold of between 20 and 30% is used to select women for high-risk screening. However, it is well known, that the estimated lifetime risk may vary substantially depending on the algorithm used for the risk calculation [9].

How Long and How Often to Screen

Based on the age-specific incidence of breast cancer in BRCA1/2 carriers [1, 10], high-risk MRI-based screening should be offered to these women at least from age 30 [11]. It is much more difficult to decide for how long to continue the MRI-based screening. Most will agree, that the MRI-based screening should be continued at least until the age of 50 [12]. However, breast cancer incidence remains high in postmenopausal BRCA1/2 carriers and there is increasing evidence, that the benefit of MRI over mammography and ultrasound is rela-

J. Hodler et al. (eds.), *Musculoskeletal Diseases 2017-2020*, DOI 10.1007/978-3-319-54018-4_35

tively independent of age [13]. Therefore it appears feasible to continue MRI-based screening beyond the age of 50, at least in women, who continue to have a higher breast density on mammography. Especially for BRCA1 mutation carriers with a high incidence of aggressive, fast-growing triple-negative breast cancers, the usual annual screening frequency may not be sufficient to prevent advanced-stage interval cancers. In these women, additional breast ultrasound in the 6-month interval should be considered. Another option for patients over the age of 40 is to alternate MRI and mammography every 6 months.

Magnetic Resonance Imaging

Breast MRI is by far the most sensitive screening modality in high-risk women. More than 30% of breast cancers detected at high-risk screening will be primarily found by MRI [3, 4]. These cancers will either be completely occult on mammography and ultrasound or visible only on tailored imaging in knowledge of the MRI findings. Since breast cancer detection on MRI is based on the increased contrast uptake in the area of the cancer compared to the normal surrounding breast parenchyma, sensitivity and specificity of MRI will be influenced by the background activity of the breast parenchyma. In premenopausal women, MRI should therefore preferably be scheduled in the second week of the menstrual cycle [14], when parenchymal background activity is lower. Use of oral contraceptives (especially if taken continuously) as well hormone replacement therapy may negatively impact diagnostic accuracy of MRI and lead to false-positive findings (Fig. 1). If this is the case, a short-term follow-up exam after discontinuation of the hormone medication may be necessary.

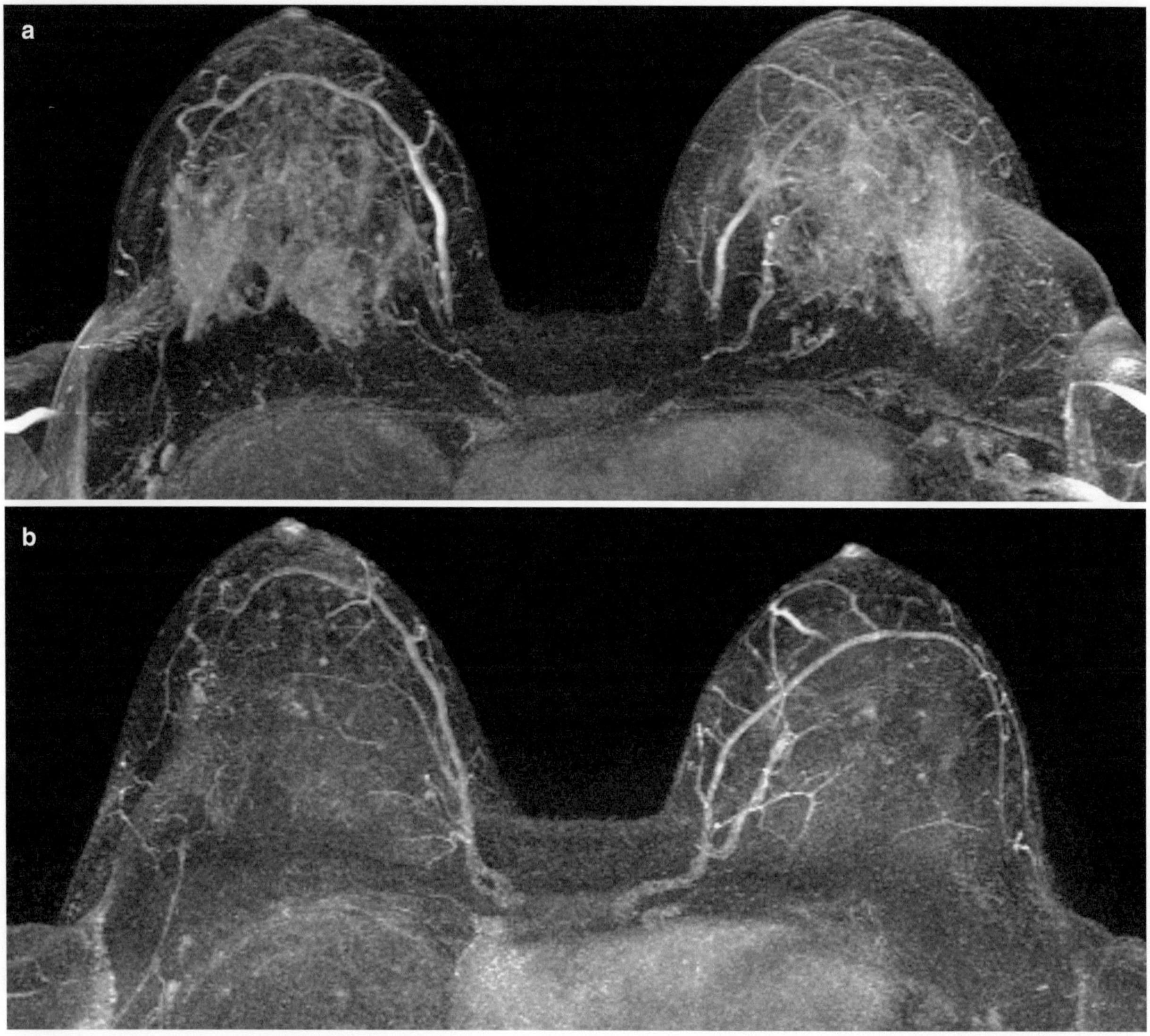

Fig. 1 32-year-old asymptomatic female with a known pathologic BRCA1 mutation attending high-risk multimodal screening. MRI performed during oral contraceptive use (**a**) shows very strong bilateral background parenchymal enhancement, limiting the diagnostic capabilities of MRI. On a short-term follow-up exam 6 months later after discontinuation of oral contraceptive use (**b**), the background parenchymal enhancement has almost completely subsided

For screening high-risk women, a standard contrast-enhanced dynamic imaging protocol at 1.5 or 3 T with a scan duration of at least 5 min post contrast and a good compromise between spatial resolution (<1 × 1 mm in-plane) and speed (e.g. around 1 min or less per series) should be used. Typically a T1-weighted, in-phase, 3D gradient echo sequence with or without fat saturation is used for the dynamic scanning. The addition of a high-resolution, preferably not fat-saturated, T2-weighted sequence may improve specificity and facilitate correlation with the other imaging modalities, especially ultrasound. To maximize sensitivity and specificity in high-risk patients, abbreviated protocols should be avoided in this situation.

Sufficient time resolution not only improves specificity but is also important to increase sensitivity by providing a better separation between the usually more rapid enhancement of malignant lesions and the slower parenchymal background enhancement.

The most important predictors of malignancy in enhancing mass lesions on MRI are irregular or spiculated margins (regardless of type of enhancement curve) as well as strong and fast enhancement in the inital phase (even in lesions with a relatively circumscribed margin), especially when combined with later washout or rim enhancement. Further clues regarding the type of lesion may be obtained from the T2-weighted images (e.g. fatty hilum in intramammary lymph nodes and lobular composition with predominantly high signal intensity on T2-weigthed images in fibroadenomas). With a combination of these morphological and contrast-enhancement criteria most enhancing mass lesions with a size of more than 5 mm can usually be characterized reliably on MRI. It is important to realize however, that morphological criteria are less reliable in smaller lesions due to the limited spatial resolution of MRI. This is especially true for lesions 5 mm or less in size. Obviously this cutoff will vary somewhat with the spatial resolution of the employed imaging sequence. In order to avoid a delay in diagnosis, small enhancing masses on MRI which are clearly new or increased in size compared to the prior exam usually will require histological confirmation through biopsy, even if no corresponding correlate is found on mammography or second-look ultrasound. This is especially true for BRCA1 mutation carriers, in whom an otherwise non-descript small enhancing mass lesion may represent an aggressive triple-negative breast cancer.

Characterization of non-mass enhancement on MRI is much more difficult, since the overlap of malignant lesions with physiological and benign changes in the breast is much bigger. In this situation careful second-look correlation with clinical exam, ultrasound and mammography (presence of microcalcifications?) is important to improve the specificity of MRI, since a non-mass enhancement on MRI with a correlating finding on another modality, even if the correlating finding by itself is considered non-specific, will have a higher probability of malignancy [15] (Fig. 2). If no correlating finding is found for a non-mass enhancement on MRI, short-term follow-up may be considered instead of immediate MRI-guided biopsy. If the non-mass enhancement persists (or even increases in size) on short-term follow-up, MRI-guided biopsy is usually indicated.

Despite the fact, that contrast-enhanced MRI is usually considered a very safe procedure [16], appropriate safeguards (e.g. single-dose protocols, use of low NSF-risk contrast media and screening for renal function impairment) should be put in place considering the repeated nature of the exam in screening. This has become even more important after the recent reports of Gadolinium depositions in the brain after repeated contrast-enhanced MRI's.

In some patients, MRI cannot be performed e.g. due to prior adverse reactions to contrast media, severe claustrophobia or implanted medical devices incompatible with MRI. In these patients mammography will need to play a bigger role and may have to be started earlier (e.g. from age 30). Alternatively, at least in the case of BRCA1/2 mutation carriers, risk-reducing surgeries may have to be considered.

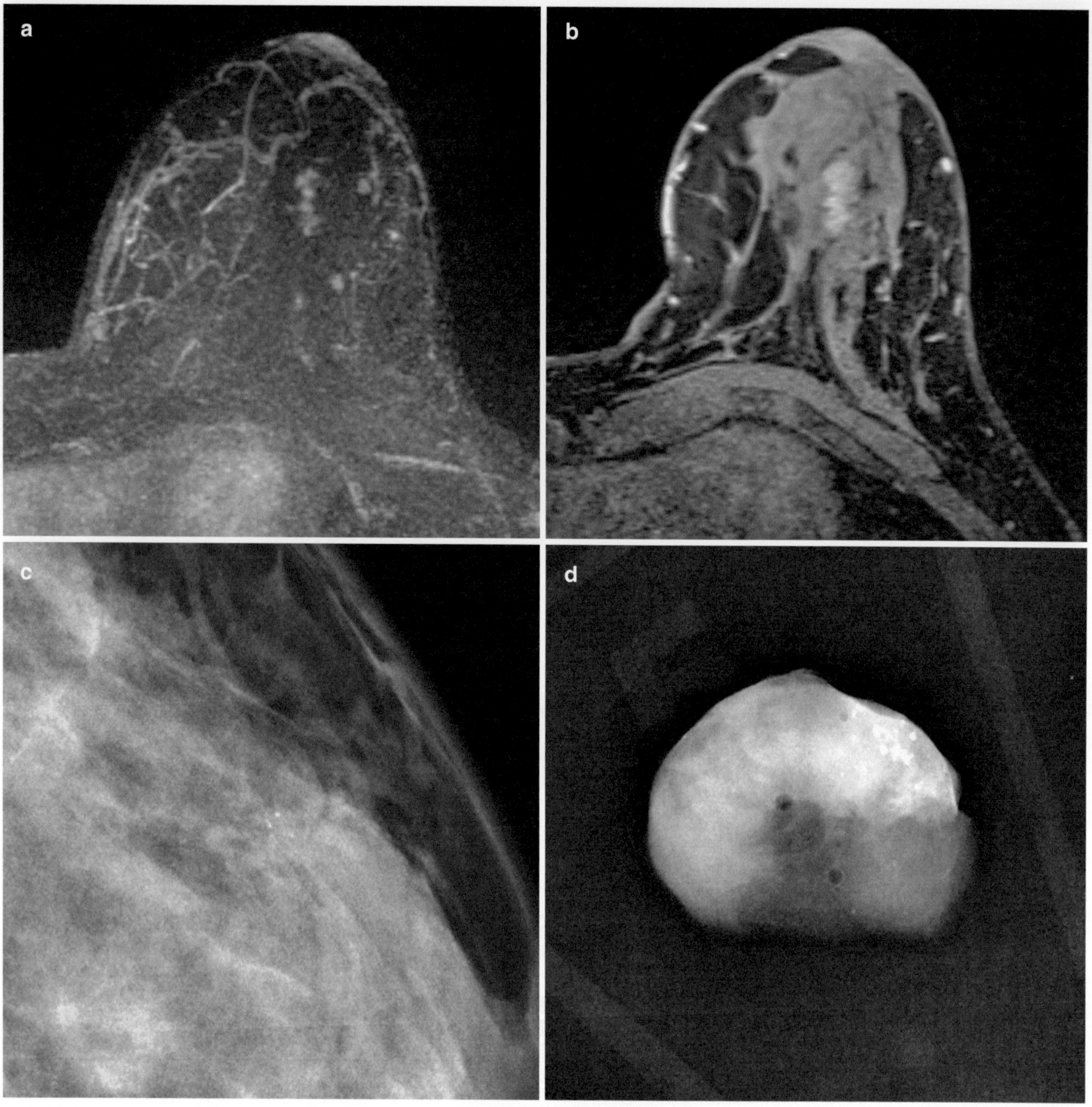

Fig. 2 49-year-old asymptomatic female with a known pathologic BRCA2 mutation attending high-risk multimodal screening. MRI shows a small area of non-mass enhancement with linear distribution in the left breast (**a, b**), which was not present on the prior exam a year ago. In the initial phase after contrast administration the lesion has a "clumped" internal enhancement pattern consisting of several small enhancing foci closely grouped together, best seen on the MIP-projection at 2 min after contrast injection (**a**). The enhancement persists in the delayed phase (**b**) and becomes increasingly confluent over time. On digital mammography (**c**), a corresponding subtle cluster of four or five, predominantly round calcifications is seen, which in itself probably would not have warranted biopsy. Due to the combination of non-mass enhancement on MRI and the presence of corresponding calcifications, a stereotactic vacuum-assisted biopsy (**d**) was performed, which confirmed a 6-mm DCIS intermediate-grade. Because of her BRCA2 carrier status, the patient opted for a bilateral subcutaneous mastectomy, which showed only a small amount of residual DCIS in the left breast in the immediate vicinity of the biopsy cavity

Mammography

The role of mammography in high-risk screening is substantially different from its role in population-based mammography screening, where it represents the primary screening modality. In high-risk multi-modality screening, mammography becomes an adjunct to MRI. Its importance increases in situations, where MRI is more difficult to evaluate, e.g. in cases with very strong background parenchymal enhancement. If a high-quality MRI with little or no background parenchymal enhancement is available, the primary task of mammography is to detect microcalcifications, which cannot be detected on MRI at all, and subtle architectural distortions, which are often better depicted on mammography due to its higher spatial resolution. With this a small amount of additional cancers (usually in-situ or low-grade invasive cancers) can be found in addition to MRI. This effect will be larger in BRCA2 mutation carriers than in BRCA1 mutation carriers, since cancers associated with microcalcifications are less common in BRCA1 mutation carriers [17].

Whenever possible, digital mammography should be used in high-risk screening [5], due to its higher sensitivity in young premenopausal women [18] as well the superior depiction of microcalcifications, the key feature of cancers detected solely by mammography in multimodality high-risk screening.

In younger women, especially in BRCA1 and BRCA2 carriers who may have a higher risk for radiation injury [19], bilateral MLO-views only and/or mammography only every 2 years may be considered. In cases with abnormal findings on MRI, mammography becomes an important second-look tool with additional tailored views as well as the option to perform digital breast tomosynthesis, which due to its cross-sectional nature can more easily be correlated with MRI. In many cases a mammographic correlate for the MRI finding can be found and if necessary biopsy can be performed under stereotactic guidance.

Ultrasound

The likelihood that a breast ultrasound performed after a normal MRI exam will detect additional cancers occult on MRI is very small [5, 20]. One of the main tasks of the ultrasound in high-risk multimodality screening is to further work-up and correlate non-specific findings on MRI. In many cases, ultrasound is able to identify typical small lymph nodes or fibroadenomas as explanation for a small enhancing lesion on MRI, thus increasing the specificity of MRI [21]. Most solid enhancing mass lesions on MRI larger than 5 mm (benign or malignant) will have some correlate on tailored ultrasound imaging and if necessary ultrasound-guided biopsy can easily be performed under ultrasound-guidance. With small lesions biopsied under ultrasound guidance, a marker clip should be placed to allow for correlation with a follow-up MRI in cases with inconclusive correlation between imaging findings and biopsy results.

Due to the virtual absence of side-effects or contraindications, ultrasound is the modality of choice for an additional 6-month interval exam in BRCA1/2 carriers as well as during pregnancy and lactation, as both MRI and mammography are contraindicated during pregnancy and often severely limited during lactation.

Specific Imaging Findings in High-Risk Patients

The underlying genetic abnormalities in high-risk women not only determine the age and frequency, with which breast cancer will occur, but also influence the histological type and imaging presentation of breast cancers [22, 23]. Knowledge of the genetic status of a particular patient is therefore important for choosing the optimal imaging strategy in an individual high-risk patient. Around 69% of all invasive cancers found in BRCA1 mutation carriers are triple-negative, compared to around 16% in BRCA2 mutation carriers [22]. BRCA1-associated triple-negative cancers are particularly fast growing and often lack typical imaging features of sporadic breast cancers, such as irregular margins or spiculation, and microcalcifications are rare in these types of tumors. These tumors are therefore often occult on mammography [24–27] and may be misinterpreted as cysts or fibroadenomas on ultrasound due to the lack of posterior acoustic shadowing and relatively circumscribed margins [28, 29]. On MRI, triple-negative breast cancers are usually easy to recognize despite the relatively benign morphological appearance due to their very strong and fast initial contrast uptake, often combined with rim enhancement in larger lesions [30] (Fig. 3). Imaging findings in BRCA2-associated breast cancers are usually more similar to sporadic breast cancers and microcalcifications-associated in-situ cancers are more common in BRCA2 than in BRCA1 mutation carriers [23].

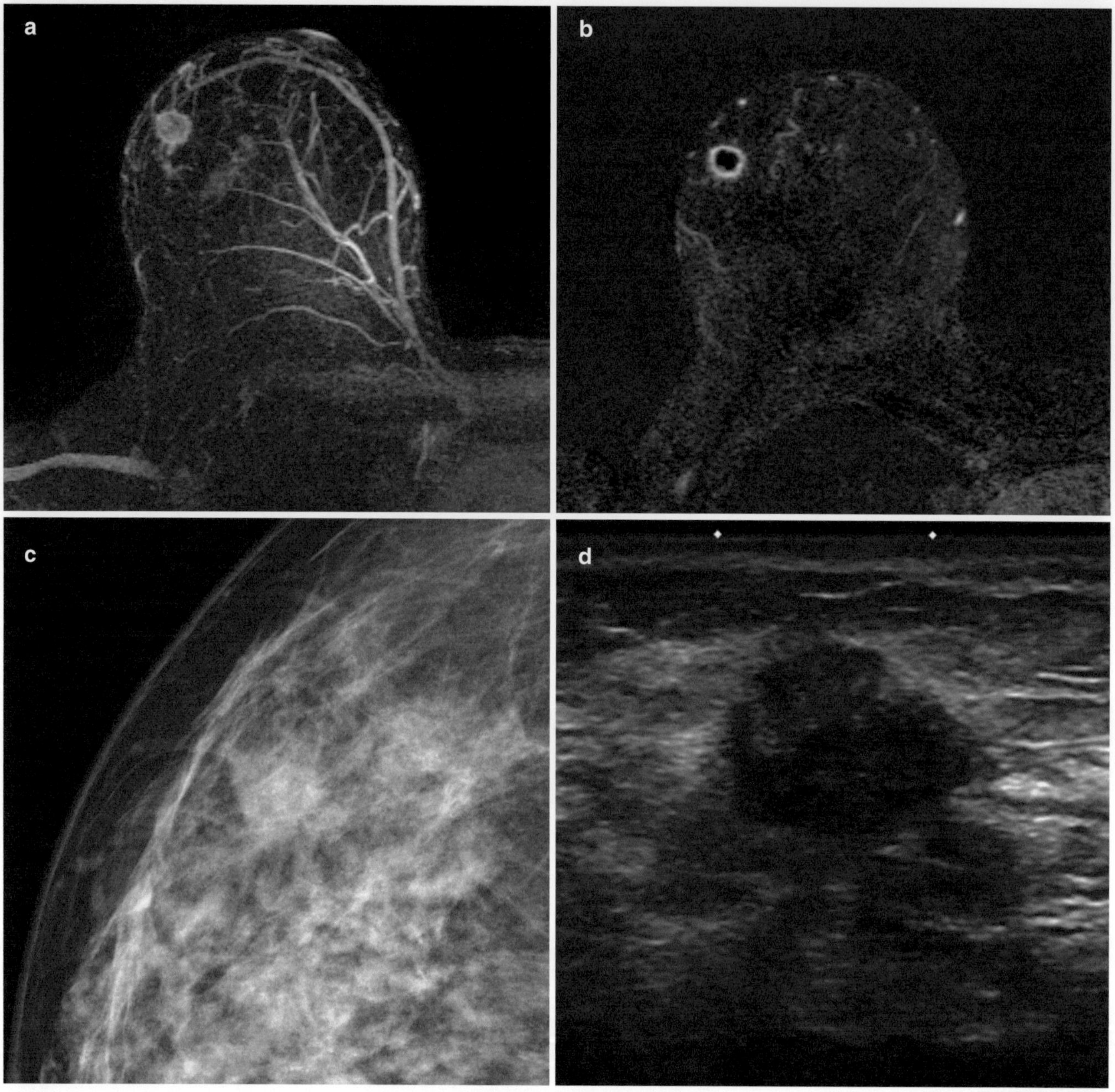

Fig. 3 49-year-old female S/P breast conserving therapy for left breast cancer 9 years ago. The patient has a strong family history of breast cancer, but genetic testing did not show a mutation in one of the known high-risk breast cancer susceptibility genes. At the current scheduled annual high-risk multimodality screening round, the patient reports about a new palpable lump in the right breast, which she had first noticed approximately 4 weeks ago. MRI MIP projection (**a**) and individual slices (**b**) show an 11-mm solid lesion in the right breast with strong, thick and irregular rim enhancement already in the initial phase. Even in retrospect, no corresponding finding could be found at the previous MRI a year ago. On digital mammography (**c**) the lesion corresponds to a very subtle density with just a few associated microcalcifications. On ultrasound (**d**), it is easily seen as a relatively well-defined hypoechoic lesion. Ultrasound-guided core biopsy confirmed an aggressive triple-negative breast cancer with a proliferation rate (MIB-1) of up to 70%

References

1. Mavaddat N, Peock S, Frost D et al (2013) Cancer risks for BRCA1 and BRCA2 mutation carriers: results from prospective analysis of EMBRACE. J Natl Cancer Inst 105:812–822
2. Carney PA, Miglioretti DL, Yankaskas BC et al (2003) Individual and combined effects of age, breast density, and hormone replacement therapy use on the accuracy of screening mammography. Ann Intern Med 138:168–175
3. Bick U (2015) Intensified surveillance for early detection of breast cancer in high-risk patients. Breast Care 10:13–20
4. Sardanelli F, Boetes C, Borisch B et al (2010) Magnetic resonance imaging of the breast: recommendations from the EUSOMA working group. Eur J Cancer 46:1296–1316

5. Chiarelli AM, Prummel MV, Muradali D et al (2014) Effectiveness of screening with annual magnetic resonance imaging and mammography: results of the initial screen from the Ontario high risk breast screening program. J Clin Oncol 32:2224–2230
6. Moller P, Stormorken A, Jonsrud C et al (2013) Survival of patients with BRCA1-associated breast cancer diagnosed in an MRI-based surveillance program. Breast Cancer Res Treat 139:155–161
7. Law J, Faulkner K (2001) Cancers detected and induced, and associated risk and benefit, in a breast screening programme. Br J Radiol 74:1121–1127
8. Nkondjock A, Robidoux A, Paredes Y et al (2006) Diet, lifestyle and BRCA-related breast cancer risk among French-Canadians. Breast Cancer Res Treat 98:285–294
9. Fischer C, Kuchenbacker K, Engel C et al (2013) Evaluating the performance of the breast cancer genetic risk models BOADICEA, IBIS, BRCAPRO and Claus for predicting BRCA1/2 mutation carrier probabilities: a study based on 7352 families from the German hereditary breast and ovarian cancer consortium. J Med Genet 50:360–367
10. Antoniou A, Pharoah PD, Narod S et al (2003) Average risks of breast and ovarian cancer associated with BRCA1 or BRCA2 mutations detected in case series unselected for family history: a combined analysis of 22 studies. Am J Hum Genet 72:1117–1130
11. National Institute for Health and Care Excellence (2013) Familial breast cancer: classification and care of people at risk of familial breast cancer and management of breast cancer and related risks in people with a family history of breast cancer. Update of clinical guideline 14 and 41. (Clinical guideline 164). http://guidance.nice.org.uk/CG164
12. Saadatmand S, Vos JR, Hooning MJ et al (2014) Relevance and efficacy of breast cancer screening in BRCA1 and BRCA2 mutation carriers above 60 years: a national cohort study. Int J Cancer 135:2940–2949
13. Passaperuma K, Warner E, Causer PA et al (2012) Long-term results of screening with magnetic resonance imaging in women with BRCA mutations. Br J Cancer 127:24–30
14. Kuhl CK, Bieling HB, Gieseke J et al (1997) Healthy premenopausal breast parenchyma in dynamic contrast-enhanced MR imaging of the breast: normal contrast medium enhancement and cyclical-phase dependency. Radiology 203:137–144
15. Giess CS, Raza S, Birdwell RL (2013) Patterns of nonmasslike enhancement at screening breast MR imaging of high-risk premenopausal women. Radiographics 33:1343–1360
16. Hao DP, Ai T, Goerner F et al (2012) MRI contrast agents: basic chemistry and safety. J Magn Reson Imaging 36:1060–1071
17. Phi XA, Saadatmand S, De Bock GH et al (2016) Contribution of mammography to MRI screening in BRCA mutation carriers by BRCA status and age: individual patient data meta-analysis. Br J Cancer 114:631–637
18. Pisano ED, Gatsonis C, Hendrick E et al (2005) Diagnostic performance of digital versus film mammography for breast-cancer screening. N Engl J Med 353:1773–1783
19. Speit G, Trenz K (2004) Chromosomal mutagen sensitivity associated with mutations in BRCA genes. Cytogenet Genome Res 104:325–332
20. Berg WA, Mendelson EB (2014) Technologist-performed handheld screening breast US imaging: how is it performed and what are the outcomes to date? Radiology 272:12–27
21. Sim LSJ, Hendriks J, Bult P et al (2005) US correlation for MRI-detected breast lesions in women with familial risk of breast cancer. Clin Radiol 60:801–806
22. Mavaddat N, Barrowdale D, Andrulis IL et al (2012) Pathology of breast and ovarian cancers among BRCA1 and BRCA2 mutation carriers: results from the consortium of investigators of modifiers of BRCA1/2 (CIMBA). Cancer Epidemiol Biomark Prev 21: 134–147
23. Heijnsdijk EAM, Warner E, Gilbert FJ et al (2012) Differences in natural history between breast cancers in BRCA1 and BRCA2 mutation carriers and effects of MRI screening-MRISC, MARIBS, and Canadian studies combined. Cancer Epidemiol Biomark Prev 21:1458–1468
24. Tilanus-Linthorst M, Verhoog L, Obdeijn IM et al (2002) A BRCA1/2 mutation, high breast density and prominent pushing margins of a tumor independently contribute to a frequent false-negative mammography. Int J Cancer 102:91–95
25. Wang YB, Ikeda DM, Narasimhan B et al (2008) Estrogen receptor-negative invasive breast cancer: imaging features of tumors with and without human epidermal growth factor receptor type 2 overexpression. Radiology 246:367–375
26. Kaas R, Kroger R, Hendriks J et al (2004) The significance of circumscribed malignant mammographic masses in the surveillance of BRCA 1/2 gene mutation carriers. Eur Radiol 14: 1647–1653
27. Schrading S, Kuhl CK (2008) Mammographic, US, and MR imaging phenotypes of familial breast cancer. Radiology 246:58–70
28. Mesurolle B, Kadoch L, El-Khoury M et al (2007) Sonographic features of breast carcinoma presenting as masses in BRCA gene mutation carriers. J Ultrasound Med 26:817–824
29. Rhiem K, Flucke U, Schmutzler RK (2006) BRCA1-associated breast carcinomas frequently present with benign sonographic features. AJR 186:E11–E12
30. Uematsu T, Kasami M, Yuen S (2009) Triple-negative breast cancer: correlation between MR imaging and pathologic findings. Radiology 250:638–647

Principles and Management of Imaging Guided Breast Interventions

Christian Weismann

Breast lesions suspicious for malignancy (BI-RADS 4® and BI-RADS 5®) [1] should be preoperatively cleared by needle biopsy. The imaging modality to guide a needle for breast lesion puncture depends on the visibility of the lesion. Whenever a lesion is ultrasound visible ultrasound is the technique of choice to guide the needle to the target. This technique has the advantage to control the needle tip under real time conditions. If a lesion is only perceptible with mammography, e.g., scattered microcalcifications, a stereotactic device is used for guidance. MR lesions without ultrasound or mammography correlate are reserved for MR needle steering.

The **fine needle aspiration biopsy** (FNAB) (needle diameters from 20- to 23-gauge) offers cytology. No differentiation between invasive or in situ cancer can be obtained. Therefore the indication using a fine needle is mostly limited to cyst fluid aspiration and cyst fluid evacuation. To clear suspicious solid or complex solid-cystic lesions a **large core needle** (14-gauge) is widely used. Typically it is combined with a 13-gauge coaxial cannula Fig. 1a, b. The obtained specimen offers histology. In the literature the sensitivity for the 14-gauge core needle has a range from 92 to 99%. The core needle thickness varies from 18-gauge to 12-gauge combined with the fitting coaxial system [2]. A typical 14-gauge large core needle biopsy starts with the infiltration of local anaesthetic using a fine needle (e.g., 20-gauge needle, 7 cm long) under ultrasound-guidance followed by the 2D ultrasound guided positioning of a13-gauge coaxial cannula. The tip of the needle ends in front of the lesion. Via the coaxial cannula the 14-gauge large core needle is inserted and the long axis of the needle has to be parallel to the long axis of the transducer to be in a perfect position with the tip in front of the target (prefire position). After activating the trigger of the biopsy device the needle has to be documented in the postfire position to make clear whether it is a lesion hit or an out of lesion hit [3, 4]. This documentation can be done by two-dimensional ultrasound presenting the postfire long axis needle diameter and the perpendicular needle cross section in relation to the lesion Fig. 1c, d. A perfect lesion hit has to show the needle inside the lesion in both planes. A superior technique to document the correct postfire needle position offers handheld 3D–ultrasound. A three-dimensional dataset is acquired in the postfire needle position. Immediately in all three planes the multiplanar view gives the information whether the needle is in a correct position or the needle has missed the lesion. In the literature this technique is described as 3D–Targeting [5]. After biopsy of breast lesions in particular lesions smaller than 1.5 cm a marker should be inserted.

Vacuum-assisted biopsy devices (VAB) typically use needles from 8-gauge to 11-gauge. They extract with one specimen significant more tissue compared with a 14-gauge core needle. The prior indication for this device is the clearing of suspicious calcifications mostly under stereotactic guidance [3, 6, 7]. For this guidance-technique a + 15 and a − 15 stereotactic image is obtained. In both stereotactic images the target is defined and the depth of the lesion is computer calculated. Pre- and postfire stereotactic images document the needle position (Fig. 2).

The ultrasound guided vacuum-assisted biopsy technique [3, 4] is used to compensate a poor visible ultrasound target, e.g., a diffuse growing lesion with or without palpable tissue stiffening, because of a bigger amount of removed tissue. Performing an ultrasound guided vacuum–assisted biopsy after administration of local anesthesia the biopsy needle is

C. Weismann
Diagnostic and Interventional Breast Unit, Private University Institute of Radiology, PMU, General Hospital Salzburg, Salzburg, Austria
e-mail: christian.weismann@gmx.at

J. Hodler et al. (eds.), *Musculoskeletal Diseases 2017-2020*, DOI 10.1007/978-3-319-54018-4_36

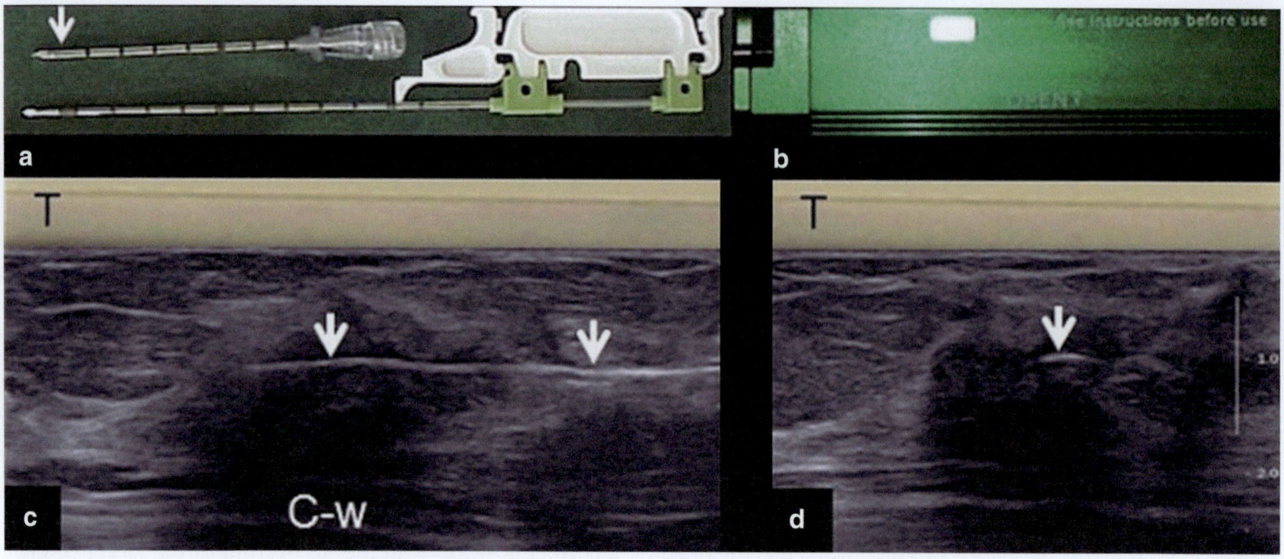

Fig. 1 (**a**) Set of a 13-gauge coaxial cannula (*white arrow*) and a 14-gauge large core needle. (**b**) Typical handheld device for core needle biopsy; the core needle shown in Fig. 1a will be placed into this device. (**c**) 14-gauge large core needle (*white arrows*) within the 13-gauge coaxial cannula in the postfire position; the long axis of the biopsy needle is parallel to the transducer (T), parallel to the chest wall (C-w) and inside the lesion (invasive cancer). (**d**) For full postfire needle documentation: perpendicular cross section of the 14-gauge large core needle (*white arrow*) inside the invasive cancer of Fig. 1c

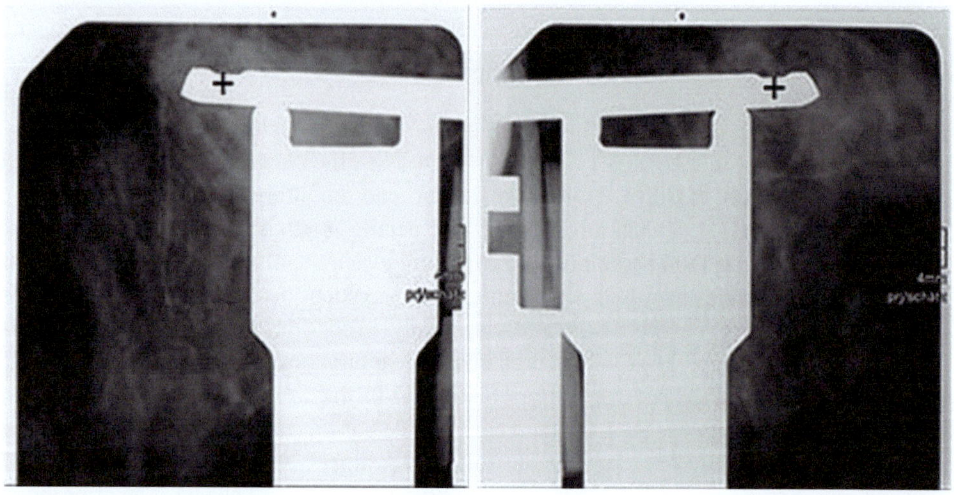

Fig. 2 +15° and −15° stereotactic image of a 9-gauge VAB-needle in the postfire position; the black crosses indicate the calculated target in either +15° and −15° stereotactic image

placed under the lesion not to hide a part of the lesion due to needle artefacts Fig. 3a–c. The option to remove a benign breast lesion of about 2.5 cm long-axis diameter is offered by this ultrasound guided vacuum-assisted biopsy technique Fig. 3d, e [8]. The documentation before biopsy is done in the same way as stated above for the large core needle biopsy in the postfire position. Using 3D–ultrasound a three-dimensional data set is acquired before and after biopsy. After tissue-extraction a marker should be inserted to make clear where the rest of the lesion is or the lesion was located.

Typically the MR-biopsy procedure is performed in prone position using a dedicated breast coil. MR-guided biopsies require MR-compatible vacuum-assisted devices [3, 9, 10]. To guide these needles a grid technology or pillar technology is mainly used. Before performing the MR-guided vacuum-assisted tissue extraction the position of an MR visible indicator has to prove to end in the center of the lesion. Afterwards this indicator is changed by the vacuum-assisted needle device. A MR visible marker has to be inserted after tissue extraction.

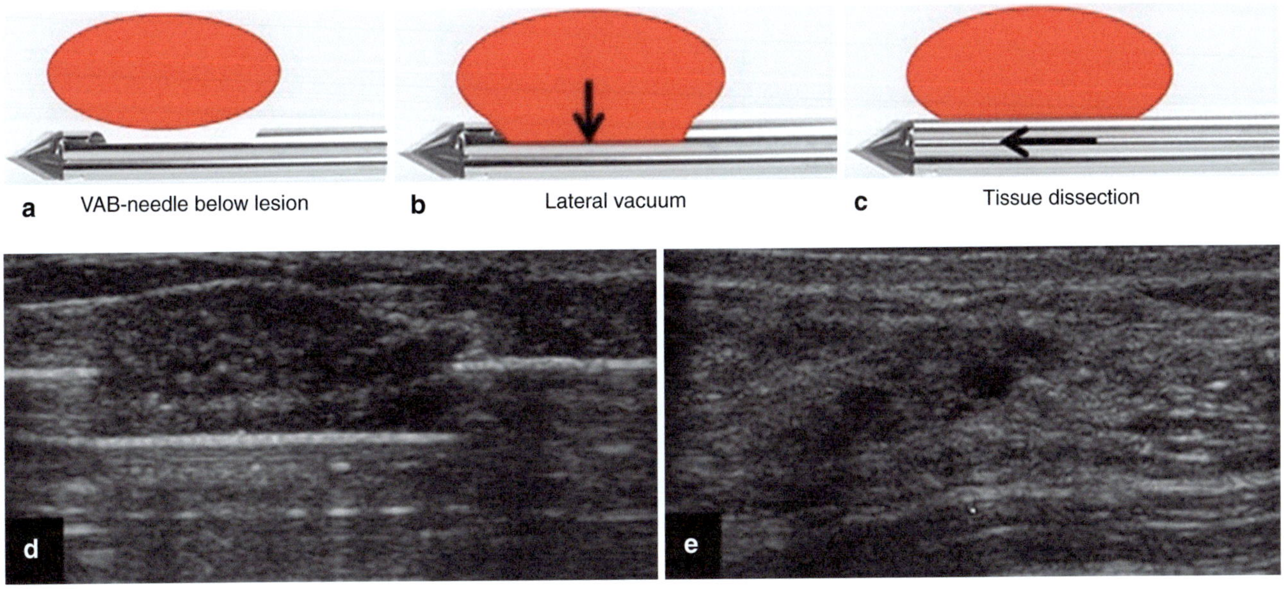

Fig. 3 (**a**) Under US guidance: VAB-needle position below the lesion. (**b**) Lateral vacuum sucks the tissue into the open tissue acquisition chamber (*black arrow*). (**c**) Tissue is dissected by a rotating or oscillating cannula (arrow shows the direction of the movement of the dissecting cannula). (**d**) Before dissecting the tissue the fibroadenotic lesion is partial sucked into the open 8-gauge VAB-acquisition chamber. (**e**) Minimal hematoma in the lesion-bed after VAB-exstirpation of the fibroadenotic lesion seen in Fig. 3d

References

1. Dorsi C, Sickles EA, Mendelson EB, Morris EA (2013) Breast imaging reporting and data system: ACR BI-RADS breast imaging atlas, 5th edn. Reston, VA, American College of Radiology
2. Dershaw DD (2003) Needles and biopsy probes. In: Dershaw DD (ed) Imaging-guided interventional breast techniques. Springer, New York, pp 69–86
3. Mahoney MC, Newell MS (2013) Breast intervention: how I do it. Radiology 268:12–24
4. Youk JH, Kim EK, Kim MJ, Lee JY, Oh KK (2007) Missed breast cancers at US-guided core needle biopsy: how to reduce them. Radiographics 27:79–94
5. Weismann CF, Forstner R, Prokop E, Rettenbacher T (2000) Three-dimensional targeting: a new three-dimensional technique to evaluate needle position during breast biopsy. Ultrasound Obstet Gynecol 16:359–364
6. Berg WA, Arnoldus CL, Teferra E, Bhargavan M (2001) Biopsy of amorphous breast calcifications: pathologic outcome and yield at stereotactic biopsy. Radiology 221:495–503
7. Jackman RJ, Burbank F, Parker SH, Evans WP III, Lechner MC, Richardson TR et al (2001) Stereotactic breast biopsy of nonpalpable lesions: determinants of ductal carcinoma in situ underestimation rates. Radiology 218:497–502
8. March DE, Coughlin BF, Barham RB, Goulart RA, Klein SV, Bur ME, Frank JL, Makari-Judson G (2003) Breast masses: removal of all evidence during biopsy by using handheld vacuum-assisted device—initial experience. Radiology 227:549–555
9. Orel SG, Rosen M, Mies C, Schnall MD (2006) MR imaging-guided 9-gauge vacuum-assisted core needle breast biopsy: initial experience. Radiology 238:54–61
10. Verheyden C, Pages-Bouic E, Balleguier C, Cherel P, Lepori D, Laffargue G et al (2016) Underestimation rate at MR imaging-guided vacuum-assisted breast biopsy: a multi-institutional retrospective study of 1509 breast biopsies. Radiology 281:708–719

MIX
Papier aus verantwortungsvollen Quellen
Paper from responsible sources
FSC® C105338

If you have any concerns about our products,
you can contact us on
ProductSafety@springernature.com

In case Publisher is established outside the EU,
the EU authorized representative is:
Springer Nature Customer Service Center GmbH
Europaplatz 3, 69115 Heidelberg, Germany

Printed by Libri Plureos GmbH
in Hamburg, Germany